Bottom Line's
HEALTH 2020
BREAKTHROUGHS

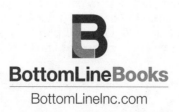

BottomLineBooks

BottomLineInc.com

Bottom Line Books® publishes the advice of expert authorities in many fields.
These opinions may at times conflict as there are often different approaches to solving problems.
The use of this material is no substitute for health, legal, accounting or other professional services.
Consult competent professionals for answers to your specific questions.

Telephone numbers, addresses, prices, offers and websites listed in this book are accurate
at the time of publication, but they are subject to frequent change.

Bottom Line Books® is a registered trademark of Bottom Line Inc.
3 Landmark Square, Suite 201, Stamford, Connecticut 06901

BottomLineInc.com

Bottom Line Books is an imprint of Bottom Line Inc., publisher of print periodicals,
e-letters and books. We are dedicated to bringing you the best information from the most
knowledgeable sources in the world. Our goal is to help you gain greater wealth,
better health, more wisdom, extra time and increased happiness.

Printed in the United States of America

Contents

1 • ALLERGIES AND RESPIRATORY CONDITIONS

Bye-Bye, Allergies! Surprise Treatment for Lifelong Sensitivities 1

You May Depend on Your EpiPen...but Can You Count on It? 2

Clues That Point to an Allergy in Your Dog 4

Get Rid of Those Dust Mites 4

Got Sinusitis That Won't Go Away? 4

Think You've Been Exposed to "Toxic Mold"? Here's What to Do 6

If You Have Asthma, Do This to Protect Yourself from AFib 7

Triple Therapy for COPD: Greater Benefits but Also Greater Risk 8

Lung Disease Linked to Dementia Risk 9

Vitamin D Curbs Lung Attacks 9

"Healthy" Lungs May Have Damage 9

Weak Hands = Weak Lungs 10

Vaping? Your E-Cigarette's Flavor Puts Your Health at Risk 10

Air Pollution Could Ruin Your Vacation 11

Great Travel Destinations with Terrible Air Quality 12

Weird Sleep Apnea Symptom 13

Sleep Apnea Robs Memories 13

Oxygen for Sleep Apnea 13

What Does It Mean When You Drool in Your Sleep? 14

2 • BRAIN HEALTH

The One-Week Plan to a Better Brain 15

New Ways to Make Your Brain Act 20 Years Younger 17

Why Your Brain Needs a Glucose Fix 19

Beware of "Skinny Fat"—a New Dementia Risk 19

Diabetes Medicines Help to Fight Alzheimer's ... 20

Cut Dementia Risk by Lowering Your Blood Pressure 20

Is Dementia Reversible? A Simple Test May Tell 20

Simple Memory Strategy 21

Tip of the Tongue 21

Curcumin Fights Dementia 21

Vitamin D Can Boost Brain Health 22

To Improve Your Memory, Try Pink Noise at Night 23

Contents

To Master a New Skill Follow It Up with
This Workout...23
Probiotics Can Cause Brain Fog 25
Your "Memory Problems" May Actually
Be Due to Hearing Loss 26
When to Start *Levodopa* for Parkinson's
Disease 26
Parkinson's Patients Are Given Drugs That
Work Against Each Other 27
Could You Have Adult Dyslexia? 28
ADHD Breakthrough: A New, Drug-Free
Way to Harness Focus 29
New Help for ALS?...30
Are You Missing the Early Warning Signs
of MS? 30
Surprising Trigger of MS Attacks 31
Better Concussion Treatment 32

3 • CANCER BREAKTHROUGHS

Should I Get Genetic Testing for Cancer?...........33
Cancer Blood Test Advances: From Screening
to Treatment 34
Dinner Time/Bed Time Cancer Risk 35
Are You Missing Out on a Lifesaving
Clinical Trial?..36
Breakthroughs in Lung Cancer 37
Skin Cancer from Your Blood Pressure
Med? Yes, It's Possible 38
Don't Make These Sunscreen Mistakes! 39
Bright Morning Light Helps Insomnia................41
Beware This Colonoscopy Risk 41
Nuts May Improve Colon Cancer Survival 42
Questions to Ask Your Doctor About
Your Colonoscopy 42
Anti-Inflammatory Cancer Fighters 43
A "Game-Changing" Cancer Drug Gets
Fast-Track Approval 43
New Hope for Bladder Cancer 44
A New Approach to Bladder Cancer
Treatment: Watch and Wait 45
Device Fights Brain Tumors...............................46
Brain Cancer Breakthrough 46
Better Liver Cancer Test 46
A New Way to Manage Metastatic Liver
Cancer...47
Are You Putting Your Adult Health at Risk
After Surviving Childhood Cancer?................47
Getting Your Sex Life Back on Track
After Cancer 48

If You've Got Cancer, Stay Out of the ER!...........49
If You Had One HPV Cancer, You're More
Likely to Get Others 51
Is Massage Really Safe for People with Cancer? ...52
Rosey Nasal Spray for Chemo Discomfort 52

4 • CARDIOVASCULAR DISEASE AND STROKE

10 Small Changes for a Healthier Heart 53
6 Heart Disease Prevention Myths: About
Aspirin, Omega-3s, Statins, More.................55
Scuba Diver Heart Danger 56
MINOCA: The Heart Attack You've Never
Heard of 57
The Push-Up Clue to Heart Health....................58
Heart Attack Alert: Daylight Saving Time
Can Be Hazardous to Your Health.................58
Winter Heart Attack Deadlier 60
Turn Up Your Thermostat...................................60
Safe Cooking to Lower Blood Pressure..............60
What's Coffee Doing to Your Blood Pressure?....61
Why Measure Blood Pressure in Both Arms 61
Air Filter for Your Heart 62
Lowering Your LDL Cholesterol: How
Low Should You Go? 62
Triglycerides: The Heart Threat You Should
Not Ignore 63
Eczema Can Kill You in a Surprising Way:
Heart Disease...65
Think You're Having a Heart Attack? How
Chest Pain Is Evaluated in the ER.................65
Is the FDA Approving Dangerous
Heart Devices?...66
Cup of Joe OK with AFib...................................68
You Can Have an MRI Even with an
Older Pacemaker..68
What's Your Stroke Risk If You Have AFib?........68
Diet Drink Stroke Link 70
Stroke Risk Lingers Long After Heart Attack 70
Most People Should Not Take a Daily Aspirin....70
How to Stop a Stroke Before It Happens............71

5 • CONSUMER HEALTH ALERTS

Stop Fibbing to Your Doctor...............................73
Getting to Know Your Pathologist: The
Behind-the-Scenes Doctor 74
New Genetic Test for Chronic Kidney Disease...76
Medicine's Barbaric Little Secret: IVs
Don't Have to Hurt 76

When "Simple" Surgeries Turn Deadly...............77
Older Surgeons Have Lower Patient
    Death Rates 78
Know the Warning Signs of Post-Op Problems ...79
The Best Checkup for Your Kidneys...................80
The Truth About Eyeglass Lens Options.............82
Hidden Toxins: How to Stay Safe 84
Well Water Alert 85
Reduce Your VOC Emissions Footprint:
    Household Products 85
Safer Food and Beverage Containers 87
There's Weed Killer in Your Cereal If You
    Eat These Brands 87
The FDA Banned 6 Artificial Flavors—But
    You're (Probably) Still Eating Them...............88
Not All Bone Broths Are Healthy 89
Radon Testing Concern 89
The Great Sunscreen Debate 89
Drug Recall Alert...90
New Ways to Save Money on Prescription
    Drugs...91
Hospice Warning: What You Need to
    Know to Avoid Poor Care..............................92
Nursing Homes Are Kicking Out Patients..........94

6 • DIABETES BREAKTHROUGHS

The Diabetes Drug Danger Most Doctors Miss....95
This Supplement Fights Diabetes and
    Protects Your Heart 97
The New, Ultimate Diabetes Screening...............97
Hot Baths Can Reduce Diabetes Risk..................98
How Cancer Can Increase Your Diabetes Risk 98
Food to Fight Diabetes......................................99
The High-Fiber Fix for Diabetes.........................99
Intermittent Fasting for Diabetes 101
Medicare Now Covers Diabetes Prevention.......101
The Diabetes Risk Factors That Aren't
    on Your Radar 101
Lower Your Risk for Diabetes with Walking.....103
Blood Sugar–Testing Devices Go High-Tech.....104
Got Diabetes? Here's How to Save Your Feet ...105
Diabetes Meds Linked to Dangerous
    Infection 107
A Dark Side to Certain Diabetes Drugs.............107
Diabetes Fasting Alert 108
Keto Diet: Fighting Type 2 Diabetes with Fat ...108
Easier Eye Screening 110
What Kinds of Rice Are Best for Diabetics?......110
Health Risk for People with Type 2
    Diabetes: Low Iron 112

Insulin Storage Danger.......................................112
8 Ways to Save Money on Insulin 113
Diabetes and Pancreatic Cancer Risk 114

7 • DIGESTIVE DISORDERS

The New Frontier in Healthy Eating.................. 115
Quick and Easy First Aid for Stomach
    Troubles.. 117
Gut Acting Up?... 118
The Brain-Gut Connection 119
Got Stomach Problems? This New Test
    May Pinpoint the Cause................................ 121
GERD Surgery Is Better Than Taking
    More Drugs 122
The Worst Drugs for Gut Health 122
A Sad Way to Fix Heartburn 124
Joint Pain? It's All in Your Gut 125
Gut Health Connected to Heart Disease Risk... 125
The Bad Breath Cause You Didn't Consider..... 126
Diagnosed with Diverticulosis? What to Do...... 127

8 • EMOTIONAL HEALTH

Don't Let Fear About Your Illness Get
    the Best of You 129
Be Kind to Yourself...for Better Health............. 131
Need to See a Psychiatrist? Find the
    Right One 132
Excessive Emotions Could Be Borderline
    Personality Disorder 133
Fast-Acting Antidepressant Receives FDA
    Approval... 134
What to Do If You're Jealous of Your
    Adult Child 135
People with Mild Autism Are All Around
    You: How to Connect.................................... 135
Break the Pain-Isolation-Depression Cycle....... 137
Depression and Seniors: Are You Getting
    the Right Care? 139
Walk Your Way Out of Depression 141
Surprising Way to Deal with a Stressful Task ... 141
You Survived an Opioid Overdose: How
    to Make Sure You Stay Alive 142
Alcoholism Rates Soar in Older Adults 143
Stay Happy All Year 144
If You Have an Eating Disorder Relapse,
    Here's What to Do 146
DIY Anxiety Relief with Acupressure 147
Negative Moods May Signal Poor Health.......... 147

9 • FAMILY HEALTH MATTERS

Surrogate Health-Care Decisions: Are You Sure You Know What Your Loved One Wants? 149

When a Loved One with Dementia Is Hard to Handle… 150

Safer Driving for Elderly Parents 151

Protect a Parent from Caregiver Abuse 152

How to Support Someone with Cancer............. 152

A Way to Give Comfort at the End of Life: Comfort Food..................... 154

After a Suicide Attempt: Keeping Your Loved One Alive 154

8 Ways Pregnancy Has Changed Since You Had a Baby..................... 157

Hold Hands..................... 157

To Prevent Drinking Problems…..................... 159

Keep Your Family Safe in Wildfire Areas......... 159

Obsessed with Feeding Your Kids Healthy? Stop It! 159

Dr. Starbuck's All-Natural Anti-Flu Program for Kids..................... 160

Long-Term Risks of Tonsil and Adenoid Removal..................... 162

Before Giving Your Child a Drug for ADHD: Ask These 7 Questions..................... 162

Better Time-Outs 163

Kids and Toothpaste 164

Pacifier Power! 164

Picture Books Boost Brain Function................. 164

A Dozen Ways to Save Money on Pet Care...... 164

Professor Fido 166

Pot Can Poison Dogs..................... 166

10 • INFECTIOUS DISEASE

Protect Yourself from the Flu..................... 167

Flu Can Be Missed…and Become Deadly 169

Obesity Linked to a New Flu Danger............... 170

How to Survive Sepsis 171

Alternative to Chemical Bug Repellents........... 173

Taking Steroids? Do This to Prevent Deadly Pneumonia 173

What If You Forgot Whether You Got a Vaccination?..................... 174

Can You Have Strep Without a Sore Throat? 175

You're Not Too Old to Get an STD..................... 175

The HPV Test: Why It's Better Than the Pap for Cervical Cancer Screening................. 176

More Grown-Ups Should Get the HPV Vaccination That Used to Be for Kids— Are You One?..................... 178

The "New" and Dangerous Sexually Transmitted Disease HTLV-I..................... 179

Petting Zoo Danger..................... 180

Hand Bit by a Dog? What to Do… 181

6 Germ Hot Spots in Your Doctor's Office 182

The Truth About Fecal Transplants.................. 184

Hepatitis C Treatment Keeps Getting Better..... 185

11 • MEDICAL NEWS ALERTS

Cells Are the New Cure..................... 187

Valuable New Clue in the Fight Against Obesity 189

A New Blood Test May Reveal Your Best Bedtime for the Best Sleep..................... 189

Your Blood Type Offers Clues About Hidden Health Risks..................... 190

What Does Your Blood Type Mean? 192

Marijuana Isn't as Risk-Free as You May Think..................... 192

The Latest in 3-D Medical Printing.................. 193

Lithium: Not Just for Bipolar Disorder.............. 194

Timing Is Everything..................... 196

"Yo-Yo" Cardio Danger..................... 197

Lab-Grown Human Esophagus 198

Ketogenic Diet: More Than a Weight-Loss Fad 198

An Implant That Helps Paralyzed People Move Again 199

"Sniffer" Dogs Hunt Disease..................... 200

12 • MEDICATION SMARTS

Are Your Medications Making Your Life Worse? 201

When Your Medication Makes You Gain Weight 203

Very Common Drugs That Rob Your Body of Nutrients 205

8 Surprising Things Your Pharmacist Can Do for You..................... 206

How to Get Experimental Drugs..................... 207

Does Your Doctor Get Drug Company Perks? ...208

Are You Addicted to Painkillers? 209

Most Powerful Opioid Yet—What You Need to Know..................... 210

Don't Get Addicted to Xanax, Ativan, Ambien or Some Other Sedative..................... 211

How to Tell If You're Hooked on Antibiotics ... 213
The OTC Painkiller Trap 214
The Life-Threatening Drug Reaction You've
    Never Heard of 215
What If You Really Do Need an Opioid? 217
Drugs That Can Damage Tendons 218
Don't Miss a Drug Recall 219
Beware These RX Mistakes 219
Apps for Saving on Prescriptions 220
FDA Approval Doesn't Mean These Drugs
    Will Work Well 220

13 • MEN'S HEALTH

Myths About Male Sexuality 221
Speak Up, Men! Don't Be Embarrassed
    by Incontinence 223
An "ED Gene" 224
Considering a Late Shot at Fatherhood?
    Don't Toss Your Condoms Just Yet! 224
Natural Ways to Reverse Erectile Dysfunction ... 225
Natural Ways to Boost Testosterone 227
Enough Testosterone? 228
To Avoid Prostate Cancer, Eat Soy 229
Men and Melanoma 229
The Right YouTube Videos for Prostate
    Cancer Advice 230
Genetic Testing After Prostate Cancer 231
Testicular Cancer Treatment's Surprising
    Long-Term Side Effects 232
Shorter Prostate Cancer Treatment 233
The Female Hormone That Gives Men
    Migraines 233

14 • NATURAL CURES

20 Cures for 5 Embarrassing Problems 235
Surprising Ways a Top Doctor Uses Nature
    to Stay Healthy 237
A Brand-New Form of Medical Treatment:
    Helps Stroke, Depression, More 239
These 4 "Super Spices" Have Hidden
    Benefits 241
Essential Oils Make Cancer Treatment
    More Bearable 243
Hypnosis for IBS 243
Essential Oils That Relieve the Common
    Cold 245
Natural Cures for a Leaky Bladder 246
This Herb Combo Helps Urinary
    Incontinence 247
Natural Cures for Eczema, Rosacea and
    Dandruff 248
Natural Help for Bipolar Disorder Treatment 249

15 • NUTRITION, DIET AND FITNESS

The Ultra-Healthy Foods You're Probably
    Not Eating 251
7 Surprising Foods That Beat Disease 253
Colorful Cauliflower 254
Better Than Water! How to Stay Properly
    Hydrated 255
Beyond Peanut Butter 256
Give Cheesy "Nooch" a Try 258
Omega-3s for Vegetarians 258
Try Coffee Flour 259
5 Vitamins Nearly Everyone Should Take 259
The Clever Way to Cut Down on Sugar
    (It's Easier, Too) 261
Eating a Variety of Foods Might Make
    You Fat 262
Are You Eating at the Right Time of Day? 262
Easier Than a Diet...and Great for Your
    Health—Intermittent Fasting 264
Want to Lose Weight for Good This Time?
    Don't Go It Alone! 266
8 Surprising Diet Mistakes That Exercisers
    Make 267
Is Your Workout Causing the Wrong Kind
    of Weight Loss? 268
Are You Walking Fast Enough to Live a
    Long Life? 269
Pump Iron for a Healthy Heart and Mind 270
See What's Missing from Your Workout... 270
Smile to Make Exercise Feel Easier 271
Get One Hour of Fitness in 5 Minutes 272

16 • OPTIMUM AGING

How Old Brains Stay Young—and How to
    Make Yours One of Them 273
Look Younger Just by Doing These Face
    Exercises 274
The Secret Anti-Aging Agent You Should
    Be Eating 276
Aging—It's All in the Mind 276
Fight Aging with H2 Therapy 277
Weak or Painful Hands? Try These Helpful
    Kitchen Hacks 279
Gadgets That Make Driving Easier and Safer ... 281
Hearing Assistance at Prices You Can Afford ... 282

Contents

Stay Out of the Hospital....................................284
Fall in Love with Your Hearing Aids................285
Diets Good for the Heart Help Hearing............285
Losing Your Sense of Smell?............................286
See Better Than Ever! New Treatments
    for Cataracts and Glaucoma 288
How Will Glaucoma Affect Cataract Surgery?...290
Glaucoma Usually More Advanced....................290
Muscle Weakness Increases Dementia Risk......291
Surefire Ways to Prevent Muscle Loss: Best
    Foods, Supplements and Exercises...............291

17 • PAIN RELIEF

Headache Sufferers: Are You
    Misdiagnosing Your Pain?.............................293
Safer, Faster Migraine Drug on the Horizon 295
The Confusing Migraine: Aura Without Pain....296
Aimovig Gets FDA Nod as a Migraine
    Preventive Drug 297
Avoid Neck Pain Without Giving Up
    Your iPad...297
How to Really Recover from Whiplash 298
Mysterious Neck, Shoulder, Arm or
    Hand Problems? 298
Is a "Slipping Rib" Causing Your Pain?.............300
Gender Bias with Pain 301
Your Wrist Pain May Not Be Carpal
    Tunnel Syndrome..301
When to Be Concerned About a Bruise............303
Better Movement = Less Pain 304
10 Moves to Prevent Knee, Hip and
    Joint Pain..305
Collagen Supplements for Joint Pain................307
7 Natural Ways to Relieve the Pain of
    Rheumatoid Arthritis 308
The High Risks of Low-Dose Steroids for
    Rheumatoid Arthritis 309
Knee Arthritis Pain Reduced by
    Whole-Body Massage 310
Could You Have Rheumatoid Arthritis and
    Not Know It? 310
How to Exercise Despite Pain 311
How to Talk About Pain with Your Doctor 313

Better Care for Back Pain That Just
    Won't Go Away 313
For Relief from Common Aches and Pains,
    Change the Way You Sleep 314
Relieve Pain Without Drugs..............................314
New Diet for Chronic Pain................................315
Shoe Inserts Do Not Relieve Plantar Fasciitis 315
Could You Use a New Ankle?............................315
Pain-Relieving Stretch for Peripheral
    Artery Disease 316

18 • WOMEN'S HEALTH

What Matters Most When It Comes to
    Breast Cancer Risk..317
Meatless Monday All Week Long......................319
Why Your Screening Mammograms
    Should Be in 3-D 319
Less Side Effects for Breast Cancer
    Treatment 320
Breast Cancer Diagnosis? How to Get
    Needed DNA Testing.....................................320
A Healthy Diet Delays Menopause....................321
Breast Cancer Treatment: Opting Out
    of Chemo..321
Women: Avoid These Heart Attack Traps 322
Red Flags Women Should Watch For.................322
Stroke Risk for Women Is Different...................324
Women: Don't Hesitate to Call an
    Ambulance for Yourself................................324
Ease Endometriosis Pain...Naturally 325
Beware Vaginal Bleeding...................................326
The Endometriosis/Cancer Connection:
    What You Need to Know 326
Minimally Invasive Surgery for Cervical
    Cancer? Not So Fast!.....................................327
Beware: Uterine Cancer Is on the Rise 328
Five Surprising Causes of Post-Menopausal
    Bleeding That Aren't Cancer 328
Licorice Root for Hot Flashes...........................330
Depression During Perimenopause...................330
How Drinking Can Weaken Your Muscles 331
A Woman's Guide to Overcoming Opioid
    Disorder...332

Index...333

CHAPTER 1

Allergies and Respiratory Conditions

Bye-Bye, Allergies! Surprise Treatment for Lifelong Sensitivities

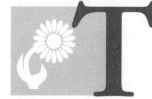**he patient:** "Heather," a woman in her early 60's, who has endured allergic sensitivities as long as she could remember. Her troubling symptoms varied, from skin rashes to intestinal cramping.

Why she came to see me: She initially came to have her diet and allergies evaluated after not having any success with a myriad of other health-care providers over the years. She experienced skin allergies as well as food reactions that came and went without any rhyme or reason. For example, she would react to certain foods at one time and then be tolerant a few weeks later. She developed a skin rash to a wool sweater one season and then the next year tolerated it without a problem. During one of our follow-up visits, I asked her about what other issues she had and she mentioned a persistent cyst on her upper back.

How I evaluated her: The suspicious cyst was located near her shoulder blade adjacent to her spine. It was relatively superficial and the size of a nickel. On palpation, it appeared moderately tender with evidence of some deeper fluid accumulation. At the surface, there was evidence of scar tissue around what seemed to be the opening of a sebaceous gland. (Sebaceous glands are the oil-producing glands that surround hair follicles).

How we addressed her problem: I explained to Heather that even though I had residential training in minor and orificial surgery, the State of Connecticut did not permit naturopathic physicians to perform surgery. I could, however, use a scalpel to remove superficial scar tissue from the area overlying the cyst. This procedure is called "wound debriding," or

Andrew L. Rubman, ND, medical director of Southbury Clinic for Traditional Medicines in Southbury, Connecticut. SouthburyClinic.com removing non-vital tissue, and thus technically not surgery. (*Note:* If it looked either deeply complex, requiring surgical removal, or potentially cancerous, I would have referred Heather to a dermatologist.)

Upon clearing away the overlying scarring blocking the opening to the cyst, I was able to begin to massage out fluid and a small-but-suspicious dark mass the size of a BB. What followed was entirely unexpected. A thin thorn-like spike approximately ⅓" in length emerged and I extracted it with tweezers. It was the remainder of a honey bee poison sack and stinger!

Heather remembered being stung in summer camp when she was eight years old, but never did more than take Benadryl at the time. A few years later she experienced a dramatic reaction to allergy desensitization "therapy" provided by a local allergist who pronounced her "strongly allergic" to bees and gave her an EpiPen after seeing her upper arm weep serum where he had administered her "therapeutic" injections.

I was able to express the remaining contents of the cyst and bandaged the wound.

The patient's progress: What surprised both of us is that in the ensuing months, Heather's chronic allergies began to improve, and a nagging muscular stiffness that she had most of her life in her upper back waned as well. Quite amazing that a foreign body, inserted in one's youth, can cause havoc over one's entire life.

You May Depend on Your EpiPen...but Can You Count on It?

Jay M. Portnoy, MD, professor of pediatrics, Missouri-Kansas City School of Medicine.

If certain foods or a bee sting can put you into sudden anaphylactic shock, you probably carry a self-injecting *epinephrine* device. Most likely that device is an EpiPen. In which case, you really need to read about serious issues with EpiPens that could put your life at risk.

For the 2% of people in the US who have a severe allergic reaction—anaphylaxis—when they are exposed to certain foods or a bee sting or some other allergen, getting epinephrine (adrenaline) immediately is a matter of life and death. Epinephrine is the only drug that can reverse anaphylaxis. Since an anaphylactic reaction can happen too quickly to get to the hospital or even to call 911, people who are known to be at risk for such reactions are advised to carry self-injecting epinephrine devices with them at all times. In the US, an EpiPen is the most common such device. About 3.6 million EpiPens are sold each year, and EpiPen prescriptions have doubled over the past 10 years. For the most part, EpiPens have indeed saved lives. *But there also can be serious problems…*

MALFUNCTIONS

From 2013 to 2014, reports of EpiPen malfunctions increased 400%. This led to an FDA inspection of the Pfizer-owned facility where EpiPens are made…the discovery of epinephrine leaks in some devices and failure to fire when triggered in others…and ultimately the recall of several batches of EpiPens. More recently, the FDA sent the distributor, Mylan Pharmaceutical, a warning letter because the company had failed to investigate 228 reported malfunctions, including several incidents in which patients died.

As of November 2017, Mylan has stated that it is confident that EpiPens currently being manufactured are safe and effective. It also pointed out that people can die from anaphylaxis even when medication is delivered properly…that any medical device in the hands of a nonmedical person has a high risk of being used improperly…and that some people can have a severe adverse reaction to epinephrine itself.

SHORTAGES

Shortages of epinephrine auto-injectors have been an increasing problem not just in the US but also in Canada, where EpiPens are available at pharmacies without a prescription. (While US citizens can buy EpiPens in Canada and use them in Canada, border customs officials might not allow them to be brought into the US.) In 2018 in the US, it was so difficult to fill a prescription—both for the adult version of EpiPen and for EpiPen Jr, the pediatric version—that the FDA extended the usual expiration dates on the devices by a few months. Their reasoning is that a weakened injection of epinephrine is better than none. Nor is EpiPen the only epinephrine device in short supply. Shortages of generic brands marketed by Mylan have been reported, as have shortages of Adrenaclick, an auto-injector made by one of the two EpiPen competitors.

What's causing the current shortage is not known outside of Pfizer and Mylan. It could be a combination of the recall diminishing the supply and an inability of the manufacturer to keep up with increased demand. Food Allergy Research & Education (FARE), a nonprofit advocacy organization, has called on the FDA to declare a national shortage and to demand action from Mylan to explain and address the shortage.

One epinephrine auto-injector is not in short supply—Auvi-Q. The manufacturer, Kaleo, says that it is making sure that commercially insured patients can receive Auvi-Q with no out-of-pocket cost.

Note: Auvi-Q had a voluntary recall in 2015. The new version, which reflects changes made to remedy the problems, is supposed to be reliable. Again, as with EpiPen, there is no way to know for sure.

AFFORDABILITY

When Mylan bought distribution rights to EpiPen in 2007, it raised the price of a two-pack of injectors from $100 to more than $600, making EpiPens too expensive for many people with poor or no insurance. (*Note:* Current recommendations are to carry two injectors at all times. If you are not able to get to emergency medical care within 15 minutes, it is recommended to inject a second dose of epinephrine.)

Mylan's response to complaints about its pricing was to develop its own generic auto-injectors. But at $300 for a two-pack, they are still not very affordable. Patients who can't or don't want to pay the high prices have taken to carrying prefilled syringes of epinephrine…or carrying auto-injectors that have expired. Prefilled syringes are not a good alternative. They are harder to use—a potentially deadly complication for someone going into anaphylactic

shock who is likely to be confused and unable to give himself/herself an intramuscular injection properly.

WHAT YOU CAN DO

To work around the problems of epinephrine auto-injectors' pricing and availability…

•**Ask your doctor for a prescription that doesn't specify a particular brand name.** That way, your pharmacy can dispense to you whatever type is available. Note that other brands do not function mechanically in the same way as EpiPen. If your pharmacist gives you a different brand than you're used to, read the directions very carefully ahead of time…so you'll be able to follow the instructions correctly when you need to use it. Most devices come with a blank "trainer" that can be used for practice. Pharmacists also can show you how to use the device.

•**Plan ahead for refills because it may take several days for your pharmacy to find an auto-injector for you.** EpiPen and Auvi-Q have websites where you can find links for help with availability or financial assistance.

•**In some cases, adult patients have been accepting a pediatric epinephrine auto-injector if an adult one is not available.** The most effective dose of epinephrine needed for an anaphylactic event has not been scientifically established—current doses are more convention than proven by factual data. It is reasonable to carry a pediatric version if that is all that is available. If the dose isn't enough, give a second one.

•**Use the auto-injector if you need it!** You'd think that this advice is unnecessary, but the biggest problem with all auto-injectors is not failure of the device but failure of people to use the device. For example, a recent study found that in more than 2,000 emergency-room visits for an anaphylactic reaction at 34 US hospitals, only about 20% of the patients took or received epinephrine before coming to the ER.

MORE COST/SUPPLY RELIEF?

Relief for at least short supply may be around the corner. The FDA announced in August 2018 its approval of an epinephrine auto-injector made by an Israeli company called Teva. Mylan is suing Teva for patent infringement, but the Teva device is now approved as a generic competitor to EpiPen, although at this writing it is not yet available in US pharmacies. However, currently priced at $300, the Teva auto-injector is not the cost-saver that was hoped for.

Clues That Point to an Allergy in Your Dog

Your Dog.

A common allergy symptom in dogs is scratching, often along with vomiting or diarrhea. If you notice these, see a veterinary dermatologist to find out whether your dog is allergic to something in the air. If so, your pet may need medicated shampoo and possibly medicine. Some people assume that stomach problems and itching are caused by food allergies, but dogs are rarely allergic to specific foods. It is more common for them to react to airborne substances such as pollen, mold or dust mites—and these allergies can cause gastrointestinal disturbance.

Get Rid of Those Dust Mites

HealthLetter.MayoClinic.com

The best ways to reduce dust mites, which can worsen allergies and asthma…

Reduce humidity, which dust mites like—keep home humidity at 30% to 50% by using a dehumidifier or central air-conditioning. Use dust- or allergen-blocking covers on mattresses and pillows. Wash sheets and blankets weekly, in hot water if possible or in cool or warm water with bleach. Vacuum carpets and fabric-covered furniture at least weekly using a vacuum cleaner with a HEPA filter. Clean surfaces with a damp mop or cloth, not dry tools, to avoid stirring up dust. Replace carpets with hard surfaces such

as wood or tile if you are especially sensitive to dust mites—and replace curtains with blinds that can be cleaned.

Got Sinusitis That Won't Go Away?

Richard Firshein, DO, director and founder of Firshein Center for Integrative Medicine in New York City, and author of several books, including *Reversing Asthma, Your Asthma-Free Child, The Nutraceutical Revolution* and *The Vitamin Prescription (for Life)*. FirsheinCenter.com

You've got a stuffy and/or runny nose… swollen and tender sinuses…and fatigue that just won't go away. Sounds like the classic symptoms of a sinus infection (aka sinusitis), so your doctor prescribes an antibiotic. You take a full course of the medication, but you still feel rotten.

Feeling frustrated, you switch to an over-the-counter decongestant, and then you get another prescription…this time for a steroid. When the symptoms drag on for 12 weeks or more, it's official—you've got chronic sinusitis.

Most doctors are quick to blame this condition—the bane of some 34 million Americans each year—on a bacterial infection, nasal polyps or a deviated septum. The problem is, they're all too often wrong.

Eye-opening statistic: In a landmark study published in Mayo Clinic Proceedings, 96% of people with chronic sinusitis were found to have fungus in their mucus—and worse still, the symptoms were exacerbated by mold (a type of fungus) in their environment.

When doctors prescribe antibiotics for acute sinusitis that's not caused by bacteria (a practice that evidence-based medical guidelines do not support), it often leads to chronic sinusitis because these drugs don't eradicate viral or fungal infections or allergic sinusitis—which are the likely root causes.

Here's how to discover whether mold is fueling your chronic sinusitis—and what to do if it is…

THE MOLD MENACE

Most people are scared of mold—but they're not scared enough! Not only is this common environmental toxin (mycotoxin) implicated in a significant number of cases of chronic sinusitis, it also causes or complicates a surprising number of cases seen in clinical practices of allergies and asthma, two conditions that often occur together. *Mold is especially dangerous because it is...*

•**Pervasive.** Outside, it's found in leafy piles, dense vegetation and plant debris. Inside, mold is found in damp areas, such as those near leaky roofs and sinks...behind appliances connected to plumbing (such as the refrigerator, washer and dishwasher)...in basements with high humidity...under carpets...and behind walls. You can even find mold in clothing (such as sweaty gym clothes) that's not washed within a few days of use.

•**Invisible and airborne.** Mold spores can easily find their way into your nasal passages and lungs. Mold can then live in your body as a low-grade, ongoing inflammation/infection. Mold spores are insidious—the toxins from mold may cause serious illness even when the mold itself is hidden from view.

•**Highly allergenic.** Millions of people react to one or more types of mold. This can trigger allergic symptoms (including chronic sinusitis)...or cause or complicate cases of asthma.

DEFEATING MOLD

You can detect and remove environmental mold. And you can strengthen your immune system so that your body is more mold-resistant. *Here's how...*

•**Suspect unhealthy levels of mold** if there's discoloration or black mold on baseboards, wallboards or wallpaper...if there are cracks in shower tile or leaks under the sink...if carpet or padding is in direct contact with a concrete slab...if your air-conditioning or heating has been poorly maintained...if you have a damp basement or crawl space...if there are watermarks or mold spots on walls...or if your dwelling has a musty, moldy odor.

Useful clue: If you have chronic sinusitis, mold may be an issue if you feel worse when you're in a building affected by a recent leak or flood, such as your house, apartment, office or vacation home.

Note: These places may also harbor hidden mold, even in the absence of a known flood or leak.

Another clue: You have been treated repeatedly for acute sinusitis...or have multiple infections that never get better.

Helpful: If you can't see mold but have chronic sinusitis, allergies or asthma, buy a mold-detection kit. These kits are widely available online and at hardware stores.

Don't expect there to be no mold—like bacteria, it can be found everywhere. But high levels (as described on the test kit instructions) are a red alert. If the test detects high levels of mold and you subsequently discover a moldy area that covers less than 10 square feet (about three feet by three feet), you can probably clean it yourself.

What the Centers for Disease Control and Prevention recommends: Scrub with a mixture of one cup of laundry bleach and one gallon of water (never mix bleach and ammonia) to kill mold on surfaces. (For a less toxic cleaner, consider using undiluted white vinegar, which is especially effective on porous surfaces.) Use a fan to dry the area. Wear rubber gloves, goggles and an N95 respirator. Be sure also to wash your clothes carefully afterward.

For larger areas of mold or if a mold test you conducted detected high levels of mold but you can't locate the source, consider hiring an experienced mold-remediation professional. (Mold can hide on the backside of drywall, the topside of ceiling tiles, the underside of carpets, etc.) A mold-remediation specialist can be found online, but be careful to find someone who is certified and/or has years of experience.

In addition to addressing any mold in your surroundings...

•**Try immunotherapy.** If you have chronic sinusitis, see an allergist for a skin or blood test to find out if you're allergic to mold. If you are, ask about immunotherapy—allergy shots or drops that can desensitize you to mold.

•**Ask about antifungal medication.** If you have chronic sinusitis and/or asthma, ask your allergist about getting secretions and/or tissue samples from your sinuses tested to see if you have a fungal infection. If you do, your doctor may want to consider treating you with an oral antifungal medication or steroid.

• **Avoid trigger foods.** Avoid mold- and yeast-containing foods, including bread, beer, wine and certain cheeses (such as Brie, Gorgonzola and Roquefort), as well as fermented foods, such as soy sauce, yogurt and pickles. Reduce or eliminate refined carbohydrates, such as white rice, sweets and pasta—mold feeds on the sugars that are produced when refined carbs break down, leading to the growth of fungi in the body.

• **Consider supplements and other natural treatments.** Nutritional supplements that may help battle chronic sinus infections include prebiotics...probiotics...turmeric or its active ingredient curcumin...and natural antifungals, including caprylic acid and artemisia. Follow the dosage recommendation on the label. Once fungal sinusitis is successfully treated with medication, natural treatments can be used, under your doctor's supervision, to suppress fungal growth.

• **Do nasal irrigation.** Using saline or a neti pot (filled with distilled or sterile water) once or twice daily will help clear your sinuses of fungus.

Think You've Been Exposed to "Toxic Mold"? Here's What to Do

Andrew L. Rubman, ND, naturopathic doctor, founder and medical director, Southbury Clinic for Traditional Medicines, Southbury, Connecticut, and author of the Bottom Line blog "Nature Doc's Patient Diary." SouthburyClinic.com

You've just learned that a building where you spent a lot of time is contaminated by mold—not a surprise, since you've been smelling it and even see it growing on the ceiling and walls. The mold is getting taken care of...but should you do anything else to protect

your health? We posed that question to one of Bottom Line's top health experts.

You may have heard of "sick building syndrome"—illnesses, especially upper-respiratory problems, attributed to airborne contaminants, including "toxic mold." Whether mold really is at the root of the symptoms is controversial and remains unproved. *However, according to the Institute of Medicine (IOM), evidence links indoor mold exposure to...*

• **Upper-respiratory-tract symptoms including coughing and wheezing** in otherwise healthy people.

• **Asthma symptoms** in people with asthma.

• **Hypersensitivity pneumonitis,** a lung disease where lungs of people prone to the condition become inflamed when airborne pollutants, including molds, are inhaled.

Plus, other research suggests that early exposure to indoor mold may be linked to development of asthma in children, especially if they are genetically at risk.

Realistically, you can't completely avoid mold. Scientists estimate that it's been around for 500 million years and forms 25% of Earth's biomass. Nor would you want all mold eliminated—think cheese (especially blue, Roquefort, Gorgonzola), beer, wine, cider, vinegar...and penicillin.

HOW MOLD TAKES HOLD

While many kinds of mold can grow inside buildings, the most common culprit is *Stachybotrys atra,* also called *Stachybotrys chartarum* or black mold. S. atra is greenish black and thrives where there is a continuous supply of moisture (a water leak, condensation, humidity) and nutrients (cellulose-based building materials such as ceiling tiles, wood, wood products...paint, insulation, drywall, carpet, upholstery, etc.). Mold also can grow inside building vents and air-conditioning systems. (*Note:* Legionnaires' pneumonia is caused by the bacterium *Legionella pneumophila*—not mold.)

S. atra is not itself toxic, but it can produce toxins, as can other molds, called mycotoxins. But even when mycotoxins are not present, inhaled spores can cause an allergic reaction...an immune system reaction...or nonallergic irritation of lungs and nasal passages.

People with allergies, asthma or other respiratory conditions such as chronic obstructive pulmonary disease (COPD) are most likely to have a reaction or a worsening of the symptoms of their condition when they inhale mold spores. In otherwise healthy people, typical symptoms include stuffy nose, itchy eyes and wheezing—which usually clear up quickly once the exposure stops.

Mycotoxins, on the other hand, can be nasty. Some mycotoxins are powerful enough to kill bacteria (penicillin, for instance, is a mycotoxin)...and mycotoxins have been weaponized for chemical warfare. Mycotoxins from common indoor molds are not as deadly but still can cause acute and chronic illness.

Acute symptoms from mycotoxin exposure typically include headache, fatigue, disorientation, dizziness and vomiting. Most of the time, these symptoms clear up when exposure is stopped. However, long-term exposure can cause some people to develop more severe symptoms that affect the nervous system, mood, memory and concentration.

"DETOXING" AFTER MOLD EXPOSURE

There are no medications to treat mold toxicity, but you can help your body recover from the effects of exposure to mold by strengthening your immune system.

Obviously, you first need to make sure that you're no longer being exposed to the mold that you suspect is causing your problems. This may be easier to do if the source is your own house than if it's an office building, school, college dorm or some other public building over which you have less say in whether it gets remediated.

But once you've dealt with the source of mold exposure—or while you're waiting for that to happen—take steps to keep your immune system as healthy as possible. Start by making sure you're following basic healthy lifestyle recommendations—stay well-hydrated (drink at least six glasses of water daily)...eat plenty of fresh fruits, including colorful berries, and vegetables...avoid foods that promote inflammation, such as added sugar and fried, refined and processed foods...get enough sleep (ideally, about eight hours a night)...and enough exercise.

Then consider adding the following supplements...

- **Vitamin C.**
- **Vitamin B-12.**
- **Selenium, a trace mineral that increases an important immune system protein called immunoglobulin A (IgA).**

All three are available as supplements and are in most multivitamins, but it's best to consult a naturopathic doctor for appropriate dosages for you. Nasal irrigation with a neti pot and a nasal wash, such as Alkalol, also can help reduce respiratory symptoms.

If you have symptoms that you suspect may be related to mold exposure, besides following these steps you may need a specialized diagnosis and/or treatment. Not all medical doctors (MDs) are familiar with diagnosing and treating illnesses stemming from exposure to indoor mold. You may need to consult a naturopathic physician (ND). Check the site of The American Association of Naturopathic Physicians (Naturopathic.org) to find one near you who can either treat you himself/herself or refer you to a naturopathic environmental medicine specialist.

If You Have Asthma, Do This to Protect Yourself from AFib

Aivaras Cepelis, MSci, researcher at the Norwegian University of Science and Technology in Trondheim, Norway, and lead author of the study titled "Associations of Asthma and Asthma Control with Atrial Fibrillation Risk: Results from the Nord-Trøndelag Health Study (HUNT)," published in *JAMA Cardiology*.

Having asthma puts you at risk for a host of complications, but you may not yet know about a very serious one—atrial fibrillation or AFib. This is a dangerous type of arrhythmia, or irregular heartbeat, and it can lead to a stroke.

Researchers at the Norwegian University of Science and Technology analyzed data from nearly 55,000 adults participating in a long-term health study. About 22% had asthma, but no one had AFib at the start of the study. Researchers found that over a 15-year period, the people with asthma had a greater risk for developing AFib. They were able to quantify the extent of the risk by how well a person's asthma was (or wasn't) controlled. People whose asthma was only partially controlled had a 42% greater risk for AFib than the general population, and those whose asthma was considered uncontrolled (see the signs of this below) had a 74% greater risk. And disturbingly, even those with well-controlled asthma had a 19% greater risk for AFib than people without asthma.

While the average person's risk for AFib increases with age, the researchers didn't find any evidence that age played a role in asthma patients' higher AFib risk. They also didn't find any link between AFib and taking the asthma medications known as beta-2 agonists even though other studies have suggested that these drugs can lead to an increased risk for other types of arrhythmia. However, they concluded that the increased risk for AFib is from a combination of poorly controlled asthma and the frequent need for reliever medication seen in people with more severe asthma.

The bottom line: Following physician advice on asthma management including a good medication plan, not smoking, improving sleeping habits, drinking less alcohol, eating a balanced diet and getting more exercise would improve asthma control and reduce the risk of AFib, said Aivaras Cepelis, MSci, lead author of the study.

REALITY CHECK: SIGNS THAT YOUR ASTHMA IS OUT OF CONTROL

If you have any of the following signs, it's time for a check-in with your asthma specialist to review your asthma care plan…

• **You use quick-relief medications** on more than two days a week.

• **You find yourself coughing, wheezing and experiencing chest tightness** during the day three or more times a week.

• **You have to limit your daily activities** because of your asthma.

Triple Therapy for COPD: Greater Benefits but Also Greater Risk

The study "Triple therapy in the management of chronic obstructive pulmonary disease: systematic review and meta-analysis" by researchers at Guangdong Medical University in China and published in *BMJ*.

Few feelings are as frightening as the inability to breathe, something experienced by most people with COPD, chronic obstructive pulmonary disease. The focus of COPD care is medication-based treatment to avoid breath-robbing flare-ups called "exacerbations," usually using one or two inhaled drugs. But what if that's just not enough? The answer, triple therapy, can help, but it can come at a health cost, as new research shows.

Background: Patients diagnosed with COPD are often started on a single inhaler, usually a long-acting beta 2 adrenoceptor agonist (LABA) or a long-acting muscarinic receptor antagonist (LAMA). If COPD is not well controlled, treatment might step up to either using both of those or one of those plus an inhaled corticosteroid. If exacerbations remain a problem, an aggressive form of treatment is to prescribe all three drugs, which has become a common practice. They can be given with a single inhaler, which is easier on the patient and reduces the risk of dosing errors. But despite widespread use of triple therapy for COPD, questions remain about just how effective—and safe—it is.

Latest research: To answer these questions, researchers analyzed the findings of 21 controlled trials that compared triple therapy to one- or two-drug therapy in patients with COPD.

First the good news: They confirmed that triple therapy reduces exacerbations, improves breathing and improves quality of life compared with either one- or two-drug therapy…and by 25%.

Now the bad news: Triple therapy also increases the risk for pneumonia because of the corticosteroid, a drug known to increase pneumonia risk in anyone with COPD who takes it. The risk for pneumonia is 50% higher than with the two-drug therapy using LABA and LAMA.

Since the risk for pneumonia for anyone with severe COPD is already high due to physical changes that make it harder for the body to fight off infection, a 50% increased risk could be a significant health threat.

Another finding was that triple therapy didn't improve overall survival, so while it's effective, it should be reserved for people with severe COPD who do not respond well to two-drug therapy.

REDUCING YOUR PNEUMONIA RISK

If your COPD is serious enough to warrant triple drug therapy, take all the steps you can to avoid pneumonia. *These are simple enough and bear repeating…*

- **Get your flu, pneumonia and pertussis vaccine shots.**
- **Wash your hands frequently** with soap and water or use a hand sanitizer.
- **Avoid crowds during cold and flu season**.
- **Don't visit sick loved ones,** and yes, even your grandkids.
- **Get plenty of sleep.**
- **Drink plenty of water.**

If you develop symptoms of pneumonia, let your doctor know right away. Some can be similar to an exacerbation, with cough, difficulty breathing and thick or discolored mucus. But with pneumonia, you may also have fever and chills, nausea and vomiting, a rapid heartbeat and/or pain in your chest when you take deep breaths.

Lung Disease Linked to Dementia Risk

Pamela L. Lutsey, PhD, MPH, associate professor, Division of Epidemiology & Community Health, University of Minnesota, Minneapolis.

Compared to those with healthy lungs, people with obstructive lung disease, such as chronic obstructive pulmonary disease (COPD) and asthma, had a 33% higher risk of developing dementia, according to a 23-year study of 14,000 men and women.

Theory: The low blood oxygen levels resulting from these conditions lead to inflammation, stress and damage to the brain's blood vessels.

"Healthy" Lungs May Have Damage

Tillie-Louise Hackett, PhD, associate director, Centre for Heart Lung Innovation, University of British Columbia, Vancouver, Canada.

New finding: A study of lung samples from 34 patients is the first to show that lungs from mild chronic obstructive pulmonary disease (COPD) patients that appear healthy on the surface have already lost more than 40% of their terminal bronchioles (key respiratory passageways).

If you are a smoker, former smoker or have a family history of COPD: Ask your doctor for a spirometry test to assess lung capacity. If you are diagnosed with COPD, even if mild, work with your doctor on a treatment plan.

Vitamin D Curbs Lung Attacks

Background: Flare-ups of chronic obstructive pulmonary disease (COPD), called lung attacks, cause shortness of breath, coughing and increased mucus production. Nearly all COPD deaths are due to lung attacks.

New finding: COPD patients deficient in vitamin D who took supplements had a 45% decrease in the rate of these attacks.

If you have COPD and suffer lung attacks: Get your blood levels of vitamin D tested. If it's below 10 ng/ml, ask your doctor about taking 2,000 IU of vitamin D daily. (For general health, a recommended level is typically 20 ng/ml to 50 ng/ml.)

Adrian R. Martineau, PhD, MRCP, clinical professor of respiratory infection and immunity, The London School of Medicine and Dentistry, Queen Mary University of London, UK.

Weak Hands = Weak Lungs

Study titled "Relationship Between Handgrip Strength and Pulmonary Function in Apparently Healthy Older Women," by researchers at Yonsei University College of Medicine, South Korea, published in *Journal of the American Geriatrics Society*.

Getting older sometimes means needing help with ketchup bottles and pickle jars that used to be easy to open. We might not be happy about it, but it's not surprising. But did you know that the reason you struggle with jar lids can also affect your breathing? Here's why… and what you absolutely should do about it.

Losing muscle strength and mass is a natural process of aging called sarcopenia (see page 291 for more information). How much you lose depends on your health, genetics and lifestyle. Many people think of age-related muscle loss as affecting their arms, legs, torso, etc. But sarcopenia affects all the muscles in the body, including the muscles that control respiration, such as the diaphragm.

Because measuring hand strength is a proven way to infer muscle strength in the rest of the body, researchers at Yonsei University in Korea wondered whether hand strength could predict pulmonary function—how efficiently a person's lungs work. Early detection of impaired lung function can help avert episodic respiratory problems such as bronchitis and pneumonia and help avert cardiovascular disease, chronic obstructive pulmonary disease (COPD), heart failure and early death.

Study: The researchers analyzed data from a health survey of 1,773 healthy women ages 65 to 79. The survey included physical examinations that measured handgrip strength and pulmonary function.

Results: The stronger her hands, the more likely a woman was to have a well-functioning respiratory system—and the weaker her hands, the more likely to have impaired lung function.

Although the study was small and involved only women, and the researchers did comment that research on men is needed, other research has found that grip strength in men is associated with better overall health, including better quality of life and lower risk of dying from heart disease.

While we can't entirely avoid losing muscle as we age, our lifestyle can minimize the loss. Exercise, both aerobic and resistance, and a healthy diet that includes adequate protein are key. There also are things you can do to keep your lungs in top working order, such as breathing exercises, playing a harmonica or even blowing through a straw.

Vaping? Your E-Cigarette's Flavor Puts Your Health at Risk

Study titled "Transcriptomic response of primary human airway epithelial cells to flavoring chemicals in electronic cigarettes," by researchers in the department of environmental health, Harvard T.H. Chan School of Public Health, Boston, published in *Scientific Reports*.

If you vape e-cigarettes (or know someone who does), you'll want to pass on the flavored varieties. Research is finding that the chemicals used to create these flavors damage lung cells…putting vapers at risk for serious respiratory diseases.

Up to 90% of e-cigarettes are flavored, and the variety of flavors keeps growing. Increasingly, the health impact of the chemicals used to create these flavors is coming under scrutiny. For instance, in 2015, Harvard researchers found the chemical diacetyl in 39 e-cigarette flavors they tested. Diacetyl, a synthetic flavor that mimics butter, has been linked to the irreversible lung disease called "popcorn lung," so-named because it was first found among workers who inhaled the chemical while working in factories that produced butter-flavored microwave popcorn.

More recently, Harvard University's T.H. Chan School of Public Health looked at another chemical flavoring in e-cigarettes that is used as a safer alternative to diacetyl—2,3-pentanedione. The researchers cultivated cells from healthy human cilia, the fingerlike projections that line the lungs and bronchial passages and help clear them of mucus, debris and unfriendly microbes. They then exposed the cells to diacetyl or to 2,3-pentanedione and analyzed the results.

Results: Both chemicals significantly affected the cilia cells in ways that demonstrated decreased production and function of cilia. Both chemicals also interfered with a gene that breaks down and removes toxins from lungs and interfered with a gene that has been linked to lung cancer. And impaired ciliary function is closely linked to COPD and asthma—suggesting that 2,3-pentanedione is no safer than diacetyl.

Note: These are only two of approximately 25 chemical flavorings used in e-cigarettes considered high-priority respiratory health concerns. And there are thousands of varieties of flavored e-cigarettes.

Of course, the best way to avoid the health risk of flavored e-cigarettes is to not use e-cigarettes at all. But if you do vape—either to help quit regular cigarettes or because you think it's a "healthier" alternative—stick to kinds that don't list flavoring on the label.

Air Pollution Could Ruin Your Vacation

Claire Westmacott, MPH, public health specialist at the International Association for Medical Assistance to Travellers, a Toronto-based nonprofit organization that strives to make travel healthier. IAMAT.org

Will your next vacation take your breath away—in a bad way? Savvy travelers know the dangers of food poisoning and tropical diseases, but there's one health risk that people often fail to consider until they step off a plane and into the acrid environment of a faraway destination—air pollution. Some of the world's most appealing travel destinations have some of its worst air quality. That pollution could make it challenging to breathe during your visit. It certainly wouldn't be pleasant. And it could even put your health or life at risk, especially if you have a preexisting heart or respira-

tory problem. (See page 12 for the destinations with the worst air quality.)

Here's how to prevent air-quality issues from ruining your travels…

BEFORE YOUR TRIP

Look up the air pollution levels at your destinations. Two excellent online resources for this are BreatheLife (BreatheLife2030.org)—a campaign led by the United Nations and World Health Organization (WHO)—which provides an easy-to-understand gauge of air quality in many cities…and the outdoor-air-quality section of the WHO website (WHO.int/gho/phe), which provides greater detail including air-quality maps for additional areas.

What to look for: A measure of air quality called the mean concentration of fine particulate matter—abbreviated as PM2.5—that is in excess of WHO guidelines. WHO tracks particles of two different sizes in air, and air is unhealthy when particles of either size exceed a certain level.

Example: The mean concentration of "PM2.5" particulate matter in Mumbai, India, is 64 micrograms per cubic meter of air—more than six times WHO guidelines.

• **Pay attention to the season when assessing air pollution levels.** They can be high at any time of the year, but current evidence suggests that winter and summer months can be the most dangerous. Air pollution can be worse in winter because pollutants get trapped by the colder air and more fossil fuels are burned for heating (especially in places that still burn a lot of coal). In the summer months, high temperatures and humidity can increase the concentration of some pollutants. People with preexisting conditions also can be more sensitive to high temperatures and humidity, especially if they're not acclimatized to the hot weather. The best time to travel may depend on which temperatures you fare better with and the seasonal patterns of pollution at your destination.

• **Make a precautionary visit to your doctor.** This is particularly important when traveling to a destination that has air-quality issues if you have a preexisting heart or respiratory problem such as asthma, COPD, chronic bronchitis or emphysema.

Tell your doctor that you intend to visit an area known for its poor air quality, and ask whether it makes sense for you to bring a short-acting bronchodilator metered-dose inhaler (MDI) even if you don't usually use one…corticosteroid tablets…and/or antibiotics—air pollution has been linked to higher rates of respiratory infections. If your health-care provider recommends any of these, make sure that you understand when and how to use them. (Also, confirm that you have sufficient supplies of any medications you already have been prescribed, and refill these prescriptions if necessary.)

If you have a preexisting respiratory or heart condition and/or you are over age 60, also ask your doctor whether you should have a physical exam that includes a stress and lung-capacity test. These tests could help you and your doctor get a more detailed picture of your heart and lung health, which might suggest that additional precautions are needed—or even that the trip is not safe for you at all.

Ideally, any precautionary medical appointments should occur at least six weeks before your trip departure to ensure that there's time to receive any tests or treatments your doctor recommends.

DURING YOUR TRIP

• **Plan indoor afternoons.** Air pollution levels tend to peak in the afternoon, so when visiting places with poor air quality, check off your outdoor to-dos in the mornings and evenings… and save indoor activities such as museum visits for the hours between lunch and dinner. Ideally, these indoor activities should be in buildings that have air-conditioning—the air quality inside an ancient, un–air-conditioned castle or cathedral might be no better than that of the surrounding outdoor air.

Indoor locations where many people smoke cigarettes or where there are woodstoves can be even worse, so avoid these as much as possible.

Safety: Heed any local smog alerts or air-quality warnings that you spot in local news outlets, even if this means spending entire days mainly indoors. The Air Matters app (Air-Matters.com) provides real-time air-quality updates for thousands of locations.

• **Avoid strenuous outdoor physical activity.** Physical exertion makes us breathe more deeply and rapidly, increasing our intake of any pollutants in the air. That means it's a good idea to skip the scenic bike tour during rush hour…and the hike up the mountain during high-smog days.

• **Don't depend on a mask to protect you from air pollution.** You might see people wearing surgical masks outdoors in areas that have air pollution problems. Do not follow their lead—they are not getting the air pollution protection they expect because surgical masks are not designed to filter air. And even with masks that are designed to filter out PM2.5 particles, there is no conclusive evidence to prove that they are effective. If you decide to wear a mask anyway and have a preexisting heart or respiratory problem, ask your doctor whether it is safe for you to wear one or whether the challenges of breathing through a mask will make it even harder for you to get the air you need.

Great Travel Destinations with Terrible Air Quality

Karen Cady-Pereira, senior staff scientist and manager for radiation and climate with Atmospheric and Environmental Research, a Lexington, Massachusetts, weather-and-climate-consulting company. She was lead author of a study of megacity air quality published in *Atmospheric Chemistry and Physics*. AER.com

Some of the most popular travel destinations in the world are also some of the most polluted. Below are five of those, including a key measure of their air quality—the mean concentration of particulate matter that is in excess of World Health Organization (WHO) guidelines. WHO tracks particles of two different sizes, and air that exceeds a certain level in either size is unhealthy.

• **Delhi, India,** is a popular tourist destination because of its history and culture, but its many vehicles, industrial clusters in and around the city, power plants and the use of fires to burn crop residue in surrounding agricultural lands have created some of the worst air quality in the world. The concentration of very fine particulate matter (PM) in the air is 14.3 times WHO guidelines for what is acceptable.

Two more Indian destinations with very poor air quality: Mumbai (PM 6.4 times guidelines) and Kolkata (PM 7.4 times guidelines).

• **Beijing, China,** is among the world's most dynamic cities and most memorable tourist destinations with a rich history dating back thousands of years. But dense traffic, heavy industry in the area and weather patterns that often trap smog over the city contribute to horrible air quality (PM 7.3 times guidelines).

Also: Shanghai, China (PM 4.5 times guidelines)…and elsewhere in Asia, Bangkok, Thailand (PM 2.8 times guidelines).

• **Mexico City** has made strides in improving its air quality in recent decades, but issues remain due in part to a rapidly growing population with an enormous number of cars and trucks and a geographical "bowl" formed by a ring of surrounding mountains (PM 2.2 times guidelines).

• **Paris** is among the world's most popular tourist destinations, but its air quality is among the worst in Europe due in part to heavy industry in northern France and the city's severe traffic congestion (PM 1.4 times guidelines).

• **Los Angeles's** air-quality problems are not as bad as those in the other cities on this list, but it does have the worst air quality of any major travel destination in the US. That's due to terrible traffic congestion, a weather pattern creating a so-called "inversion" layer that acts as a lid and mountains to the north and east (PM 1.2 times guidelines).

Also: Houston doesn't attract as many vacationers as LA, but its air quality is just as bad (PM 1.2 times guidelines).

Weird Sleep Apnea Symptom

Charles Bouchard, MD, professor and chair, department of ophthalmology, Loyola University, Chicago, and corresponding author of a study published in *The Ocular Surface*.

Eyelids that easily flip inside out may indicate sleep apnea. More than half of apnea patients—53%—have floppy eyelids, which means that the upper eyelids are lax, rubbery and easily flip inside out—for example, when you rub your eyes when you are tired. An estimated 34% of men and 17% of women have the condition, but up to 80% of those with apnea have not been diagnosed. Apnea symptoms include loud snoring, excessive daytime sleepiness and fatigue. And sleep apnea is associated with an increased risk for stroke, heart attack, heart disease, diabetes, cancer and death from any cause.

Sleep Apnea Robs Memories

Melinda L. Jackson, PhD, senior lecturer, Monash University, Melbourne, Australia.

Background: Sleep plays a crucial role in consolidating memories.

New finding: More than 50% of people with obstructive sleep apnea (OSA), in which breathing stops intermittently during sleep, had "over-general memories"—those that lack specific detail—versus less than 19% of those without apnea, according to a study of 44 adults.

If you have sleep apnea—or are a heavy snorer, a sign of apnea: See a sleep specialist. Treating OSA may promote better retrieval of memories—and can help alleviate symptoms of depression, which is linked to memory loss and OSA.

Oxygen for Sleep Apnea

Chris D. Turnbull, DPhil, physician, Oxford Centre for Respiratory Medicine, University of Oxford, UK.

Background: Blood pressure often spikes in the morning in people with sleep apnea, increasing risk for heart attack and stroke.

Recent finding: When continuous positive airway pressure (CPAP), the standard treatment for obstructive sleep apnea, was withdrawn, those who got supplemental oxygen didn't experience this spike, compared with the group who received regular air.

What Does It Mean When You Drool in Your Sleep?

Michael Breus, PhD, sleep specialist in Manhattan Beach, California. TheSleepDoctor.com

Many people drool during their slumber. That's because our muscles relax during sleep, and a slackened jaw can allow the mouth to open—especially during the deep stages of sleep. Breathing through an open mouth then dries out the tongue, so the salivary glands produce even more saliva to keep the mouth moist. The extra saliva often drips out of the mouth. This is even more likely to occur if you sleep on your stomach or side. Sleeping on your back may resolve the issue.

That said, drooling also can be a sign of a medical condition. Obvious causes include allergies, a cold or chronic sinusitis, all of which could make it hard to breathe through the nose. Another possibility is a deviated (off-center) nasal septum (the bone and cartilage in the nose that separates the nostrils). This condition can block air flow through the nasal passages and cause mouth breathing. An otolaryngologist can advise you on treatment, which may include a relatively simple surgical procedure. Some drugs can cause excessive saliva production, such as *clonazepam* (Klonopin), a seizure medication also used to treat anxiety, and certain antipsychotics.

Drooling also can be a sign of sleep apnea, a disorder in which breathing briefly stops during sleep. Symptoms include snoring, gasping for breath during the night and excessive daytime sleepiness. If you have any of these symptoms, get evaluated by a sleep specialist. Treatment may include a continuous positive airway pressure (CPAP) device that delivers air via a mask covering the nose during sleep.

If you have a condition that makes it difficult to swallow, such as Parkinson's disease, you may drool during the day and night. The FDA recently approved *incobotulinumtoxinA* (Xeomin) for such patients who drool excessively.

For most people, however, drooling isn't that serious—and can be addressed by treating any underlying condition or switching your sleep position.

CHAPTER 2

Brain Health

The One-Week Plan to a Better Brain

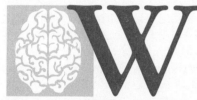

With researchers clamoring to unlock the mystery of what causes memory loss and related cognitive difficulties, it's easy to assume that some elusive discovery will banish these brain problems forever.

The truth is, the key to a better brain—sharper mental focus, improved memory, clearer thinking, balanced emotions and a lower risk for dementia and stroke—is largely within our control now.

Based on the body of research we have analyzed, nine out of 10 cases of Alzheimer's disease could be prevented by changes in lifestyle—what you do day by day, day after day to improve the health of brain cells (neurons) and build more connections between them.

After 15 years of treating thousands of patients with Alzheimer's disease and its frequent precursor known as mild cognitive impairment (MCI), we've devised a simple one-week plan that will help you form habits to protect and enhance your brain in the weeks, months and years to come. *Better-brain lifestyle strategies to adopt…*

***Day #1:* Don't rely on supplements to protect your brain.** There are only two supplements we think are worth taking for brain health—an omega-3 supplement with at least 250 mg daily of *docosahexaenoic acid* (DHA), the most important omega-3 fatty acid for brain health…and 500 micrograms (mcg) daily of vitamin B-12, which is linked to reduced risk for Alzheimer's.*

Our recommendation: Opt for an algae-derived omega-3 supplement over fish oil—it is highly absorbable and toxin- and pollutant-free.

*Before taking any supplement, check with your doctor if you have a medical condition or take medication.

Dean Sherzai, MD, PhD, and Ayesha Sherzai, MD, neurologists and codirectors of the Brain Health and Alzheimer's Prevention Program at Loma Linda University in California. They are authors of the newest book from Bottom Line Inc., *The Alzheimer's Solution* (BottomLine Store.com), and creators of a free brain-health app at BrainXQ.com. TeamSherzai.com

***Day #2:* Add a "superstar" food to your diet.** A whole-food, plant-based diet reduces brain-damaging inflammation and oxidation… protects the small arteries of the brain that are damaged by saturated fats and cholesterol… supplies the brain with the nutrients and phytochemicals it needs for optimal functioning… and minimizes or eliminates refined carbohydrates and other processed foods—all of which weaken neurons and their connections.

Among plant foods, mushrooms are a surprising superstar. In fact, a study published in *Phytotherapy Research* found that older people with MCI had improved cognitive function after 16 weeks of taking dried mushroom powder. Plus, mushrooms deliver umami—the pleasant, savory taste found mainly in cooked meat, making them a great meat substitute.

Our recommendation: Include mushrooms in your meals at least two to three times a week—button mushrooms, portobello, cremini, porcini, maitake, shiitake, you name it.

If you aren't able to follow a strictly plant-based diet, a Mediterranean diet or MIND diet, which focuses on leafy greens, nuts, berries, beans, whole grains, and fish and poultry, is advised.

***Day #3:* Choose the right fats.** More than 60% of the brain is comprised of fat, and the brain constantly uses those fats in the process of rebuilding neurons and their support structures. But for optimal brain health, you need to consume the right kind of fats—not saturated fat, for example, but plant-based fats, such as the mono- and polyunsaturated fats found in nuts, seeds, avocados and olives.

Omega-3 fatty acids—found in nuts, seeds, marine algae and fish—are especially critical for brain health.

Note: We don't recommend fish because it often has high levels of mercury and other toxic chemicals that are bad for the brain. If you must eat fish, stick with small, low-mercury fish such as sardines and anchovies.

Our recommendation: As part of a plant-based diet, get plenty of good fats and limit bad fats. *To do this…*

•**Minimize or eliminate sweets…**processed junk food…sugary cereals…baked packaged goods…chips and other salty snacks…processed white bread products…meats, processed meats and poultry…and canned soups.

•**Maximize fresh and frozen vegetables and fruits…**beans and lentils…100% whole grains…seeds and nuts…brain-healthy oils, such as olive and avocado…low-calorie, plant-based sweeteners, such as date sugar and stevia…non-dairy plant milks…and spices (turmeric is particularly brain protective at a dose of one teaspoon daily—consult your doctor before adding turmeric to your daily diet if you have a chronic condition, such as a gallbladder problem…or take medication, such as a diabetes drug).

***Day #4:* Protect sleep.** During sleep, we "consolidate" memory—turning daily experience into long-term memories. Sleep also detoxifies the brain when "janitor" brain cells (microglia) are activated to remove toxins that accumulate during the day.

Our recommendation: Aim for seven to eight hours of sleep a night.

Avoid foods that are particularly disruptive to sleep, such as sugary foods, high-fat foods, and chocolate and other caffeine-containing foods. Stop eating at least three hours before going to sleep at night…and stop drinking fluids at least two hours before.

***Day #5:* Increase your "klotho" with exercise.** Klotho is a little-known but important antiaging hormone linked in animal studies to protection against cognitive decline. Studies show that klotho levels increase after only 20 minutes of intense aerobic exercise. "Intense" means that you'll have difficulty finishing a sentence.

Our recommendation: Aim for 25 to 30 minutes of intense aerobic exercise, four to five days a week, such as brisk walking, biking or working out on a treadmill, an elliptical, a stairclimber or other type of cardio machine.**

***Day #6:* Get rid of clutter—and clean out your brain.** Stress exhausts the brain. And a surprising source of stress is a cluttered environment—when our homes or offices become disorderly, we experience more stress and anxiety. A clean, orderly space encourages sustained

**Speak to your primary care physician before starting this (or any new) exercise program.

quiet and self-reflection, both of which positively impact cognition.

Our recommendation: As part of a stress-reducing plan, keep your home and office clean and uncluttered.

***Day #7:* Put on your dancing shoes.** Brain-protective cognitive reserve develops from any challenging mental activity, such as learning to play a musical instrument or mastering a new language. But one of the best and most enjoyable ways to build cognitive reserve is dancing. When you dance, it activates various parts of the brain such as your motor cortex…your parietal lobe…your frontal lobe…and your occipital lobe. Plus, dancing is a social activity—and research shows social interaction also builds cognitive reserve.

Our recommendation: Find a dance studio and take dance classes—and then go out dancing. Or buy a DVD and learn to dance at home. Ballroom, jazz, folk—the possibilities are endless!

New Ways to Make Your Brain Act 20 Years Younger

Sandra Bond Chapman, PhD, founder and chief director of the Center for BrainHealth at The University of Texas at Dallas, Dee Wyly Distinguished University Professor at its School of Behavioral and Brain Sciences, lead researcher of the study "Enhancing Innovation and Underlying Neural Mechanisms Via Cognitive Training in Healthy Older Adults" published in *Frontiers in Aging Neuroscience*, and author of *Make Your Brain Smarter: Increase Your Brain's Creativity, Energy, and Focus*, which includes all nine of the strategies used in the study.

If it seems like you've heard conflicting advice in the media about brain games and other ways to make your brain "younger," you're right. A few years ago, pricey brain-game software (and hours at the computer) were thought to accomplish this…and then, soon after, almost completely discredited. In fact, physical exercise, like Ping-Pong and dancing, have held the brain-preservation spotlight recently.

Well, our knowledge about what can really keep your brain humming keeps getting better, and now, according to a recent study from the Center for BrainHealth at The University of Texas at Dallas, simple yet direct brain-training exercises—not games—should be part of any plan to keep your brain young because they can make your brain act 20 years younger. Will this be the last word on brain preservation? Of course not. But when it comes to these latest exercises, they are proved scientifically…they don't take up a lot of time…and it won't cost you anything to try them.

For the 12-week study, 58 cognitively normal people ranging in age from 56 to 75 were randomly divided into three groups—a cognitive-training group, a physical exercise group and a control group.

Members of the cognitive-training group attended weekly 60-minute sessions where they participated in cognitive exercises designed by the researchers that were intended to strengthen "innovative cognition," which is needed for adaptive and flexible thinking—the ability to react to challenging and changing life demands. They also spent two hours a week on homework assignments involving these exercises (we'll share three of them below).

Members of the exercise group did three 60-minute physical workouts per week, alternating between a treadmill and stationary bike. The control group just went on with their lives as usual.

Using MRI scanners, researchers measured how well participants' neurons were working (their "connectivity"), blood flow in the brain and the amount of glucose (energy) their brains used at the beginning, middle and end of the study. Only members of the cognitive-training group showed significant changes—a 30% increase in neuron connectivity on average, an 8% increase in blood flow, the brain's energy supply, and a 17% increase in regional white matter, the fiber bundles that connect different parts of the brain.

Translation? At the end of the study, the cognitive-training group had, on average, improved their brains' fitness so that they worked in many ways like the brains of people 20 years younger. The improved blood flow and regional connectivity were associated with an enhanced ability to think creatively and perform complex reasoning. Thus, greater brain fitness produced higher cognitive performance.

Important: Even though the physical exercise group did not show improved brain function, don't skip fitness workouts. Exercise still conveys benefits ranging from increased fitness and overall physical health to reduced inflammation—and inflammation can be harmful to the brain. So physical exercise does help your brain but in different ways.

BRAIN EXERCISES THAT WORK

Here are three of the study's cognitive exercises that you can use to improve your brain function starting right now…

•**Strategic attention.** Every day, identify two daily tasks that require fairly deep thinking, such as tracking and analyzing your budget, following a complex new recipe, writing meaningful, personal thank-you notes—or pondering the actionable takeaways from an article about the benefits of cognitive exercises.

Then carve out two 30-minute uninterrupted sessions to focus on them. Choose the time of day you usually feel sharpest. But no matter when it is, make sure that the environment is quiet—no cell phones or any other devices to distract you. And don't get up for a snack or a drink or do anything that will take you off your task during these 30-minute blocks. Why? Because it can take up to 20 minutes to get back on track after an interruption.

Benefit: Over time, you'll find that you can accomplish tasks more quickly and with greater focus.

•**Five by five.** Five times a day, intentionally do nothing for five minutes. Stop whatever you're doing—step away from your desk or laptop, for instance—and let your brain rest, empty out and reset. Just as the muscles in your body need a rest after a long run or strenuous workout, your brain needs to rest after working hard. Do not use the time to plan your vacation or the rest of your day in your head or anything of the sort. You can take a walk or sit still, but don't read, play music or listen to an audiobook. Enjoy the silence and lack of stimulation.

Sometimes it will be obvious when you need these breaks, such as when pushing yourself to keep going on a task is netting little result.

Benefit: Taking brain breaks helps you find clarity, collect your thoughts and, often, see things in a new way.

•**Innovative thinking.** Become aware of and increase the moments when your brain innovates—in other words, create more "aha" moments. You say that it's not possible to purposely create innovative thoughts? Oh, yes, it is! The trick is to get yourself out of your familiar ruts—try a new experience, take on a new challenge, seek ways to improve an existing relationship or an ongoing logistical challenge. Brain "aha" moments usually come when you have brain downtime, when you are in the shower, driving without the radio on or in nature with no earbuds. The more you embrace the brain's capacity to improve even routine activities, tasks and conversations, the greater will be your innovative brainpower.

Start by trying to have at least one innovative thought each day, and work your way up from there as you get better at it. But don't just think these thoughts. As soon as you realize that you see a better way to do or say something, write it down and put some aspect of it into practice. Keep an innovation diary, and challenge yourself to see how many times you innovate each day or week. The strongest brain changes come with the implementation of innovative ideas—just thinking them is not enough.

Benefit: By challenging yourself to do and act on innovative thinking, you put your brain in unknown territory and activate the neurotransmitter norepinephrine, the brain's wonder drug that speeds learning and makes it longer lasting. Additionally, innovative problem-solving helps reduce your fear of failure and fear of the unknown—the awe of a new experience actually recharges the brain.

Carving out blocks of time and keeping a tally of your brain breaks and innovation attempts can seem daunting at first. It's OK to start slowly and gradually add to the time you spend on cognitive exercises. Once you start seeing the benefits in your daily life, you'll want to make more time for these exercises, and they will become a habit.

And that's key: For cognitive exercises to work, you need to do them regularly.

Why Your Brain Needs a Glucose Fix

Lisa Mosconi, PhD, associate director of the Alzheimer's Prevention Clinic at Weill Cornell Medical College/NewYork-Presbyterian Hospital in New York City, where she is also associate professor of neuroscience in neurology. She is author of *Brain Food: The Surprising Science of Eating for Cognitive Power.* LisaMosconi.com

For health-conscious people everywhere, "glucose"—a specific type of sugar—has become the enemy. After all, a high-sugar diet has been linked to obesity, diabetes and many more health problems. *But...*

Did you know that while the organs and tissues in your body are mainly fueled by carbohydrates and fats, 99% of the fuel the brain uses comes from glucose? In fact, glucose is essential to keep your brain in top form.

When your brain doesn't get the glucose it needs, memory, focus and reasoning decline. In a worst-case scenario, without sufficient glucose, you could end up with Alzheimer's disease.

THE BEST WAY TO GET GLUCOSE

Getting enough glucose for your brain does not mean eating a diet rich in refined sugar and carbohydrates such as candy, bread, pasta and baked goods. These foods do contain a very small amount of glucose but also a massive amount of other sugars. These other sugars get converted to glucose but, in the process, are hard on the liver and pancreas, increasing insulin levels.

The best foods to provide immediate glucose to the brain are root and other vegetables, fruits and whole grains—key components of the Mediterranean diet.

These foods provide the glucose needed while minimizing the total amount of sugar ingested to avoid high blood sugar and other health problems.

New study: In a three-year study I coauthored and published in *Neurology,* individuals who closely followed a Mediterranean-style diet preserved glucose metabolism in their brains—while those who ate a typical Western diet had decreases in glucose metabolism. Additionally, declining rates of glucose metabolism were associated with increased Alzheimer's plaques.

Glucose-rich foods: 88% of the sugar in scallions is glucose...turnips (76%)...rutabagas (56%)...dried apricots (52%)...kiwifruit (48%)... grapes (40%)...onions (38%)...whole grains (36%)...red beets (31%)...and raw honey (30%).

To put this in perspective—two red beets contain 20% of your brain's daily glucose requirement, which is 62 g of glucose...and one cup of grapes will give your brain 17% of the glucose it needs for a day...but you would need to eat 16 pounds of chocolate chip cookies to achieve your daily goal!

In a study published in *Psychology and Aging,* older adults (ages 65 to 82) were among those given either a drink containing a small amount of glucose or a drink with an artificial sweetener. After consuming these drinks, they were asked to perform difficult mental tasks. The older adults who drank glucose had better memory, a more positive mood and were more engaged with the mental tasks, compared with those given the artificially sweetened drink.

For a quick mental boost: Add one teaspoon of glucose-rich raw honey to a cup of tea. Refined honey, like table sugar, is more likely to give you an energy crash later.

And for a brain-building breakfast or lunch: Try avocado toast with whole-grain bread. It delivers a hearty supply of glucose and brain-healthy monounsaturated fat.

Beware of "Skinny Fat"— a New Dementia Risk

The study "Sarcopenic Obesity and Cognitive Performance" led by researchers at Florida Atlantic University Comprehensive Center for Brain Health in the Charles E. Schmidt College of Medicine in Boca Raton, Florida, published in Clinical Interventions in Aging.

James E. Galvin, MD, MPH, associate dean for clinical research and professor of integrated medical science, Schmidt College of Medicine, Florida Atlantic University, Boca Raton.

In a study of more than 350 people, average age 69, participants who were "skinny fat" (an age-related combination of loss of muscle mass, known as sarcopenia, and high body fat) performed worse on tests of executive function and cognition, including memory, mental flexibility and self-control, than those who were sarcopenic or obese alone. The "skinny" term comes into play because people with sarcopenic obesity tend to look less overweight than those who are simply obese.

If you are "skinny fat": Talk to your doctor about your risk for dementia.

Diabetes Medicines Help to Fight Alzheimer's

Vahram Haroutunian, PhD, professor of psychiatry and neuroscience, Icahn School of Medicine at Mount Sinai, New York City, and leader of a study published in *PLOS One.*

Use of insulin, *metformin* and other medicines routinely prescribed for diabetes treatment is associated with fewer markers of Alzheimer's disease, such as brain abnormalities. Many elderly people with diabetes also have brain changes indicating Alzheimer's disease—and antidiabetes medicines appear to have protective brain effects.

Cut Dementia Risk by Lowering Your Blood Pressure

Heather Snyder, PhD, senior director of medical and scientific operations, Alzheimer's Association, Chicago. Study titled, "Effect of Intensive vs Standard Blood Pressure Control on Probable Dementia," by researchers at the SPRINT Research Group, National Institutes of Health, published in *JAMA.*

Cut dementia risk by lowering blood pressure to a target of 122 (systolic) or below. In a study of 9,361 hypertensive adults, those given medicines to reduce systolic pressure (the upper number) to the target had a statistically significant 19% lower risk for mild cognitive impairment and a 17% lower risk for dementia over the next five years.

Is Dementia Reversible? A Simple Test May Tell

A study, "Gait Analysis in PSP and NPH: Dual-Task Conditions Make the Difference," published in the February 21, 2018, online edition of *Neurology.*

How well can you do two things at once? For people with certain forms of dementia, the answer is quite telling.

Background: A neurological condition known as idiopathic normal pressure hydrocephalus (iNPH) causes symptoms that are often confused with other forms of dementia. When iNPH is misdiagnosed, it's particularly troubling because the symptoms caused by this condition—unlike other forms of dementia—are reversible.

iNPH is caused by excess fluid in the brain, and its symptoms include walking, balance and thinking problems. Because it is so often misdiagnosed, researchers wanted to find a way to help doctors easily identify it. *Here's what they came up with…*

Recent study: Among its symptoms, iNPH causes a distinctive gait disturbance (including difficulty starting to walk and a feeling that the feet are stuck to the ground), so researchers devised a test that involves walking while simultaneously performing a simple task that challenges a person's thinking skills. The speed with which the tasks could be performed was surprisingly accurate in identifying people who had iNPH.

"It is important that people with idiopathic normal pressure hydrocephalus are accurately diagnosed so they can be treated, and their health can improve," explained study author Charlotte Selge, MD, of the Ludwig Maximilian University of Munich in Germany.

Study details: In this study, published in *Neurology,* 27 people with iNPH…38 people with progressive supranuclear palsy (PSP), an incurable condition caused by damaged nerve cells in the brain…and 38 healthy people used as controls walked down a 22-foot-long pressure-sensitive carpet at three different speeds—slow, comfortable and as fast as possible. By assessing the awkwardness of their gaits, researchers were able to accurately identify 82% of the time which participants had iNPH and which had PSP.

The participants were then asked to repeat the walking test while also counting backward...and then while carrying a tray. When the results of the dual-task tests were added to the researchers' original assessments, their diagnostic accuracy jumped to 97%.

Why this matters: When correctly diagnosed, a person with iNPH can receive a surgically implanted shunt that drains excess fluid from the brain to reverse symptoms. More than 80% of people who are properly diagnosed and screened before receiving the surgery will experience rapid improvement of their symptoms—though it may take weeks or months for the full benefits to become apparent, according to the Hydrocephalus Association. People diagnosed early have a higher chance of successful treatment. In future studies, researchers may add more tasks to the test or increase the difficulty of the tasks to boost its diagnostic power even more.

Bottom line: If you or someone you know has symptoms of dementia—including problems with memory, concentration and reasoning—talk to a doctor about the possibility of iNPH. A simple walking test could be an easy, inexpensive way to determine whether the cause of those symptoms is a treatable condition.

Simple Memory Strategy

Want to remember something important? Read it out loud. That was the conclusion of researchers who asked 95 people to use four different strategies to remember material—reading silently...listening to someone else read it...listening to a recording of their own voice reading it...or reading it aloud.

Why reading aloud works: The physical act of voicing the words and then hearing them spoken aloud makes the material more distinctive...and therefore more memorable.

Colin MacLeod, PhD, professor of psychology, and Noah Forrin, PhD, researcher, University of Waterloo, Ontario, Canada.

Tip of the Tongue

Katrien Segaert, PhD, a lecturer in the School of Psychology at England's University of Birmingham.

We've all had moments when we can't quite recall a name or other word that's right on the "tip of our tongue"—and these moments become more frequent as we age.

We might worry that they are harbingers of memory loss, but that's a common misconception. The cause actually is faulty language processing, according to Katrien Segaert, PhD, a lecturer in the School of Psychology at England's University of Birmingham.

When we wish to say a word, the brain must first retrieve the meaning of that word and then figure out which sounds to make. When we have a tip-of-the-tongue moment, our memory recalls the meaning of the word just fine...but the mental process is disrupted before the brain settles on the appropriate sounds.

Encouraging discovery: The more physically fit people are, the fewer of these tip-of-the-tongue moments they have.

Curcumin Fights Dementia

Bill Gottlieb, CHC, a natural health coach in Middletown, California, certified by the American Association of Drugless Practitioners. He is author of 16 health books, including *Speed Healing*. BillGottliebHealth.com

---

Specially formulated supplements of curcumin—the active ingredient in the spice turmeric—improve memory and focus in people who don't have dementia. They also may reduce the risk of developing Alzheimer's disease.

Scientific evidence: Researchers at UCLA Longevity Center recruited 40 healthy middle-aged and elderly people. For 18 months, 21 of them took a curcumin supplement twice daily, while 19 took a placebo. At the beginning and again at the end of the study, their short-term verbal and visual memory abilities—such as recalling memorized words and images—were tested. In addition, their brains were scanned for toxic amyloid plaques and tau tangles, two signs of Alzheimer's.

Key findings: After 18 months, participants taking curcumin had significantly improved results on the memory tests. (*Bonus:* They also had improved mood.) Participants taking the placebo had little or no improvement in memory. What's more, the follow-up brain scans showed that the curcumin group, compared with the placebo group, had lower levels of amyloid and tau deposits.

THE RIGHT KIND OF CURCUMIN SUPPLEMENT

While curcumin in its natural state—in the spice turmeric and in many supplements—is poorly absorbed by the body, there are five formulations that research has shown are well-absorbed. The UCLA researchers used one of them, Theracurmin, at a dose of 90 mg twice daily. (A one-month supply costs about $53.) The other four are Meriva, Curcumin C3 Complex, BCM-95 and CurcuWIN. All are available online.

More research is needed before we know whether curcumin supplements actually prevent Alzheimer's disease. Curcumin supplements have a strong safety record, but they can cause stomach upset in some people. And they act as blood thinners, so doctors generally say that curcumin should not be taken by people using blood-thinning drugs. To determine whether curcumin is safe for you—and what a proper dose might be—it's best to work with a doctor who has studied this supplement.

Vitamin D Can Boost Brain Health

George T. Grossberg, MD, Samuel W. Fordyce Professor of psychiatry and director of geriatric psychiatry at the Saint Louis University School of Medicine and coauthor of the study "The Role of Vitamin D in Cognitive Disorders in Older Adults" published in *Touch Neurology*.

The hardest vitamin to obtain through diet could be one of the most important ones for brain health. You already know vita-min D is a key building block for bones—but it also has a starring role in maintaining normal brain functions and protecting brain cells from damage, a role that grows as the brain ages.

With age, brain cells become more susceptible to damage from calcium-induced stress. Vitamin D may help prevent calcium from entering brain cells by blocking off key channels. It may also prevent braincell loss and increase the ability of nerve cells to communicate with one another, possibly by increasing activity of the neurotransmitter acetylcholine.

Vitamin D helps regulate the brain's immune system and inhibit the inflammatory mediators (cytokines) involved with immunity and inflammation. So when levels of vitamin D are low, the body has less ability to fight inflammation in the brain, inflammation that typically increases with age. This is important because inflammation that destroys brain cells may contribute to the cognitive decline seen in conditions such as Alzheimer's disease and Parkinson's disease. Low levels of vitamin D have also been linked to other forms of dementia, memory loss and depression. A research review in *Touch Neurology* pointed out that 70% to 90% of older adults with cognitive problems are deficient in the vitamin.

MAKING UP THE "D"-IFFERENCE

The National Institutes of Health suggests that people age 50 to 70 get 600 IU of D a day, 800 IU per day for people age 71 or older. It's a challenge to get vitamin D naturally, especially as we age. Vitamin D is made by the skin, but only when the skin is exposed to enough sunlight. Seniors face two problems here. Many people spend more time indoors as they age. And even when you get enough sunlight, "older" skin—skin that has become thinner and more fragile—isn't as efficient at making vitamin D as it used to be. At age 70, your skin makes 50% less vitamin D than it did at age 20.

It also becomes progressively harder to get vitamin D through diet because problems such as gastritis and decreased liver metabolism, common in seniors, limit the body's ability to absorb vitamin D through the digestive system. Some people avoid dairy altogether because of lactose intolerance and/or GERD.

To treat or prevent vitamin-D deficiency, supplements are often the answer. But first it's important to find out your exact level of D with a blood test. In fact, if you're over age 60, you should get your vitamin-D level checked annually, or more often, if needed.

If you are low on D, talk to your doctor about a plan to get up to a brain-healthy level. Studies suggest a daily dose of 1,000 IU. (It's possible to overdose with vitamin-D supplements, but very unlikely as you would need to take the amount associated with toxicity of 10,000 to 40,000 IU per day.) Some people might need a high dose for a short period of time and then a lower maintenance dose. Your doctor can recheck your blood levels after a few months and adjust the dose as needed. The two forms available are D-2 and D-3. Most doctors agree that D-3 is more effective at raising levels.

To Improve Your Memory, Try Pink Noise at Night

Michael Breus, PhD, clinical psychologist, Manhattan Beach, California, and a fellow of The American Academy of Sleep Medicine. He is author of *The Power of When: Discover Your Chronotype—and the Best Time to Eat Lunch, Ask for a Raise, Have Sex, Write a Novel, Take Your Meds, and More.* TheSleepDoctor.com

---

Lots of people use "white noise" machines while they sleep to drown out the sound of snoring bedmates, barking dogs or traffic. But research suggests that "pink noise" is more effective for falling and staying asleep… and sleeping with pink noise might make your memory stronger, too.

White noise sounds like radio static. Pink noise sounds similar, but because it emphasizes lower sound frequencies and deemphasizes the "sizzle" of high frequencies, most people find it calming and restful. Pink noise often is compared with the sound of a steady rainfall.

What about making your memory work better? A study at Northwestern University found that exposure to pink noise while sleeping significantly increased participants' ability to ab-

sorb and then recall information the next day. In the study, the noise wasn't constant all night but was synchronized with the sleepers' brain waves, an effect you can't reproduce at home. But sleeping with pink noise at home might help your memory if for no other reason than it encourages deeper, less interrupted sleep. Anything that does that has a positive effect on your mood and memory.

It's worth trying pink noise if you're struggling to fall asleep or remain asleep, even if there is no significant background noise to block out. Near total silence can keep people awake, too, because the brain becomes more alert to even slight or distant sounds. That's why people who live in cities sometimes have trouble sleeping when they visit the quiet countryside.

If you meditate, pink noise could be beneficial for this as well.

There are numerous free pink-noise apps available, including Sleepo and Pink Noise for Android devices and NoiseZ and White Noise Lite (which includes a pink-noise setting) for Apple devices. Or buy a sound machine capable of generating pink noise (and other sleeping sounds that some people prefer) such as the LectroFan Classic ($49.95, SoundOfSleep.com) or iHome Zenergy iZBT10 ($99.99, iHomeAudio. com), which adds an alarm feature including FM radio and music streaming.

To Master a New Skill Follow It Up with This Workout

Fabien Dal Maso, PhD, assistant professor in the department of kinesiology at University of Montreal and first author with researchers from McGill University in Montreal, Quebec, Canada, of the study titled "Acute Cardiovascular Exercise Promotes Functional Changes in Cortico-Motor Networks During the Early Stages of Motor Memory Consolidation" published in *NeuroImage*.

Want to make a new skill stick? Or make sure you don't forget something you just learned? Follow it up with a bout of high-intensity cardio. That's the finding of the latest study to look at how exercise affects your brain—and you can really use this one to make your brain more powerful.

The study: Researchers had 25 people learn a new motor skill—in this case, using a video game–like joystick to track rectangles on a monitor. Afterward, one half of the participants did some high-intensity cycling on exercise bikes while the other half rested. All participants practiced the skill a few more times that day and then came back and tried it again the next day.

And on that next day, the group that had exercised after the first learning session performed the new skill significantly better that the non-exercisers.

Interestingly, when measuring the exercisers' brain waves while they performed the skill immediately after the high-intensity cycling, the researchers found less activation in the part of the brain that controls hand movement than the nonexercisers, said Fabien Dal Maso, PhD, one of the study authors. And this was a good thing—it showed that the brains of those who had exercised didn't have to work as hard to remember and repeat the task as the brains of those who hadn't exercised. In other words, a single short bout of exercise had led to positive brain changes—improvements in neural connections—that helped "lock in" the skill.

HOW TO IMPROVE YOUR MEMORY SKILLS

Everyone can use exercise to succeed with skill development and learning, said Dr. Dal Maso. His study focused on motor skills, but he said that exercise has also been shown to improve memory skills. Creative tasks, on the other hand, are harder to assess. Creativity can't be evaluated easily in a laboratory the way motor skills and memory skills can. But if you're learning to play the piano, picking up a new sport, perfecting a tennis serve, working on your golf swing, memorizing facts or learning procedures at a new job, exercise can definitely make your brain more of the steel trap you'd like it to be. This finding could also apply to people who need to relearn motor skills after an injury or stroke, as part of a rehab program, Dr. Dal Maso added.

Important: When and how you exercise matters. *To boost retention of new knowledge and skills...*

•**Work out soon after learning.** The participants in the latest study started their exercise 10 minutes after they finished the motor skills task, but other studies have found that there's a window of up to two hours afterward to do a cardio workout, which gives you some flexibility if the learning happens during your workday.

•**Make the exercise vigorous.** Only high-intensity activities have been found to promote higher retention rates among people learning a new motor skill, Dr. Dal Maso said. Those in the study did high-intensity interval training. Their exercise-bike session consisted of three three-minute blocks of pedaling at 90% of their heart rate capacity with two minutes of rest between each block. You can adapt most cardio exercises to high-intensity interval training, or if you want to work out at a vigorous but steady pace for the entire session, choose from fast cycling, running or race walking, swimming laps or even jumping rope, depending on your fitness level, and do it for 15 minutes. How to know whether you're working out at the right intensity? It should be hard to speak more than a few words before you have to stop to take a breath, according to the American Heart Association. (Of course, if it's been a while since you've regularly exercised with intensity, take your relative fitness into account and don't plunge cold turkey into intense exercise.)

•**Don't forget the warm-up and cooldown for safety.** In the study, participants spent two minutes warming up before their intense cycling and then two minutes cooling down afterward. Don't skimp on warm-up and cooldown times, but don't count them as part of your high-intensity minutes.

•**Sleep on it.** Memory retention also is related to getting sufficient sleep.

Dr. Dal Maso's advice: For good learning, exercise afterward...and sleep for a restorative eight hours that night.

Probiotics Can Cause Brain Fog

Satish S.C. Rao, MD, PhD, professor of medicine, director of neurogastroenterology, Medical College of Georgia, Augusta University, and coauthor of study titled "Brain Fogginess, Gas and Bloating: A link between SIBO, Probiotics and Metabolic Acidosis," published in *Clinical and Translational Gastroenterology.*

Andrew L. Rubman, ND, naturopathic physician, medical director of the Southbury Clinic for Traditional Medicines in Southbury, Connecticut, and author of the Bottom Line blog "Nature Doc's Patient Diary."

Taking the healthful bacteria called probiotics can be great for gut health, but new research has uncovered a serious potential side effect—trouble thinking straight, aka brain fogginess.

Why would researchers even look for such a connection? It all started when Satish S.C. Rao, MD, director of neurogastroenterology at the Medical College of Georgia at Augusta University, noticed that a number of his patients with gastrointestinal symptoms had also been experiencing mental symptoms—confusion, impaired judgment, short-term memory problems and difficulty concentrating. The brain fogginess happened intermittently but usually after the patients ate—for four of them, the fogginess was so severe that it was interfering with their careers.

So he conducted a study of 38 patients who had GI complaints of bloating, stomach distention, pain and gas without any obvious cause. Thirty of these patients had not only the GI symptoms but also had complained of brain fogginess.

A variety of tests revealed that the patients with brain fogginess had up to three times the normal level of D-lactic acid, which is made in the gut. Under normal circumstances, D-lactic acid is produced in very small amounts, easily cleared by the kidneys. But when the body produces large amounts of D-lactic acid, the kidneys can't clear it all and it accumulates. The D-lactic acid is then able to enter the brain and cause brain fogginess. (*Note:* This is different from L-lactic acid, which can accumulate in muscle and cause muscle cramps during exercise.)

How did the patients get those high levels of D-lactic acid? The researchers were able to trace it back to their intake of probiotics. They found that in 68% of the patients on probiotics, the probiotics and other bacteria had colonized in the small bowel and produced a condition called SIBO, small intestinal bacterial overgrowth. Every time these bacteria came into contact with sugar—from the carbs in the patients' diets—D-lactic acid production went into overdrive. The result was the brain fogginess along with the GI symptoms. Once they stopped taking probiotics and were treated for bacterial overgrowth with antibiotics, both types of symptoms went away.

PROBIOTICS, THE RIGHT WAY

The problem isn't with probiotics themselves—Dr. Rao does prescribe them to some patients with GI issues. The problem is when people self-prescribe them (only four people in the group of 30 patients with brain fogginess were taking them after consulting with a healthcare provider) and have other aggravating factors that can help set the stage for SIBO and high D-lactic acid levels.

Two known culprits are the heartburn drugs proton pump inhibitors, or PPIs, and opioid pain relievers, says Andrew Rubman, ND, medical director of Southbury Clinic for Traditional Medicines in Southbury, Connecticut.

PPIs make your stomach less acidic, but in doing so they change your gut microbiome and expose the small bowel to bacteria overgrowth. (To ease the occasional acid stomach, Dr. Rubman recommends skipping PPIs in favor of drinking a half-teaspoon of baking soda mixed into a half-cup of water between meals.)

Opioids slow your gut motility and can paralyze the small bowel, making it easier for bacteria to colonize there.

If you'd like to get only the benefits of probiotics, follow these guidelines…

•**Eat probiotic foods.** These include yogurt and kefir, pickled vegetables such as kimchi and sauerkraut, and tempeh and miso.

•**Eat prebiotic foods.** The fiber in these foods basically goes unchanged through the stomach and small bowel and acts as fuel for healthful bacteria in the colon. Prebiotic foods include onions, leeks, garlic, asparagus, Jerusalem artichoke, bananas, whole wheat, yams and sweet potatoes.

•**Get healthful guidance.** Have a medical evaluation to help you determine the right type and amount of supplemental probiotics for you. This is especially important if you have any health conditions, GI or otherwise, in order to avoid an adverse reaction. Don't take a probiotic supplement on your own.

Your "Memory Problems" May Actually Be Due to Hearing Loss

The study "Considering Age-Related Hearing Loss in Neuropsychological Practice: Findings from a Feasibility Study" was conducted by a neuropsychology and cognitive health research team at Baycrest, a geriatric care program affiliated with University of Toronto, and published in *Canadian Journal on Aging.*

Forgetfulness can be frustrating…and frightening, causing you to worry that you have early symptoms of Alzheimer's disease if you can't remember what your spouse told you to pick up at the grocery store, for example, or the name of the restaurant where your friend said to meet.

But don't be too quick to panic.

A Canadian team of researchers recently took a closer look at 20 older adults who were undergoing cognitive evaluations and discovered that "forgetfulness" may have more to do with a person's hearing than an actual memory problem.

When clinical neuropsychologists analyzed the cognitive evaluations of the study participants, along with assessments of their hearing, 56% of those being tested because they were concerned about memory/thinking problems and possible brain disorders had some degree of hearing loss, ranging from mild to severe, with only about 20% of them wearing hearing aids. Interestingly, 25% of the individuals who were worried about potential memory problems had no signs that a brain disorder was causing their forgetfulness.

Because none of us can remember what we never heard, this research suggests that hearing difficulties can masquerade as forgetfulness. Even when a person's brain is otherwise healthy, hearing loss can cause communication problems, social isolation and loneliness—all of which are associated with an increased risk for dementia. Getting treatment for hearing loss can help preserve your physical and mental well-being.

Takeaway: If you're concerned about your memory, ask your primary care doctor to perform a hearing examination in addition to cognitive testing. On the basis of your results, your doctor may give you tips on how to communicate better…suggest an over-the-counter sound amplifier…or recommend that you see an audiologist for a full workup. These hearing professionals can determine the best way to improve your hearing…and if that includes the use of a hearing aid, they can explain how to correctly operate and maintain it. To find an audiologist near you, visit the American Academy of Audiology's website (Audiology.org) for a searchable list.

Important: Today's hearing aids are not the big, ugly, screechy appliances that your grandparents used. They are much more sophisticated now, and some are barely noticeable. They can be expensive, though—typical costs, which aren't covered by insurance, range from $800 to $4,000 per ear—so be sure to work with a professional who can help you find what's right for you.

When to Start *Levodopa* for Parkinson's Disease

Study titled "Randomized Delayed-Start Trial of Levodopa in Parkinson's Disease," led by researchers at University of Amsterdam, the Netherlands, published in *The New England Journal of Medicine.*

Levodopa (Sinemet) is the most effective medicine used to treat Parkinson's disease. In fact, nearly everyone who has the disease will need it eventually. But there has long been a debate over whether it's better to start the drug as soon as symptoms start—or hold out as long as possible to put off dealing with the risks associated with taking levodopa. *New research now has the answer...*

But first, some background...Parkinson's disease (PD) is a progressive brain disease in which nerve cells in the brain that produce the chemical dopamine, a neurotransmitter needed to send signals between cells, gradually die. As the brain cells die, symptoms such as body tremors and slowed movement begin to interfere with daily activities. There is no cure for PD. Instead, symptoms are managed, typically with levodopa, a drug that converts to dopamine in the brain. Some research has found that starting levodopa soon after diagnosis—before symptoms curtail lifestyle—may slow progression of the disease. But other research has found that starting levodopa early actually may speed the loss of dopamine-producing brain cells...that the brain starts to depend more on drug-dopamine than on naturally produced dopamine. The resulting irregular brain levels of dopamine increase risk for dyskinesia, uncontrolled, jerky or writhing movement.

To learn more, researchers from University of Amsterdam in the Netherlands compared early versus delayed start of levodopa in 445 recently diagnosed PD patients whose symptoms were not severe enough to need the drug and who had never received any other treatment for their PD.

Half the patients were randomly assigned to receive a standard dose of levodopa for 80 weeks. The other half received a placebo for 40 weeks...and then levodopa for 40 weeks. Neither patients nor researchers knew which patients were in which group. Patients had their PD rated according to a standard test that measures mental and physical symptoms of the disease, as well as how much activities of daily life are affected. The average score for both groups at the start of the study was between 28 and 29 (out of a possible score of 176, with a higher score meaning more severe disease).

Results: The researchers expected to find that the early starters would have about a four-point advantage in their PD score at the end of the study. But in fact, there was no significant difference between the groups—a one-point improvement for early starters compared with a two-point improvement for late starters.

While it's true that the study didn't find any benefit to starting the drug early, it didn't find any added risk in doing so either—88% of patients in the delayed group and 90% of patients in the early group had no evidence of dyskinesia. These results indicate that it's safe to start the drug whenever a patient (and his/her doctor) feels that it's the right time.

Yet even without dyskinesia, levodopa still has side effects (including drowsiness, nausea, dry mouth, diarrhea, constipation, insomnia among others) that you may want to put off dealing with until the PD symptoms become truly bothersome. But at least now you have more choice.

Parkinson's Patients Are Given Drugs That Work Against Each Other

Allison W. Willis, MD, MS, department of neurology, Perelman School of Medicine, University of Pennsylvania, Philadelphia, lead author of study titled "Patterns of Dementia Treatment and Frank Prescribing Errors in Older Adults With Parkinson Disease," published in *JAMA Neurology.*

People with Parkinson's disease (PD) might be taking "opposing" drugs. About 45% of PD patients taking an acetylcholinesterase inhibitor (such as Aricept) to treat cognitive impairment, which is common in PD, were also prescribed an anticholinergic medication.

Problem: Anticholinergic drugs, which treat overactive bladder, allergies and PD symptoms, decrease cognition.

If you or a loved one is being treated for Parkinson's, review with your doctor and/or pharmacist all medications—prescription and OTC—that are being taken. If it turns out that you're taking both an acetylcholinesterase inhibitor and an anticholinergic, discuss with your doctor whether another medication combination might be better for you.

Could You Have Adult Dyslexia?

Sally E. Shaywitz, MD, Audrey G. Ratner Professor in Learning Development, Yale University School of Medicine. She is coauthor of *Overcoming Dyslexia: A New and Complete Science-Based Program for Reading Problems at Any Level.*

Here's a common scene: A man in his late 50s who has always struggled with reading, hiding the problem from family, friends and coworkers, finally comes in for an evaluation. This person is smart (really smart) and has all the signs of dyslexia. We tell an individual like this that it's not too late to improve his reading skills, be more successful at work and find new tools to make his life much easier. And welcome to the crowd.

While dyslexia can interfere with school and work success, it's also striking how successful some people with the condition have become. Indeed, one clue to the condition is that a person may score higher on an IQ test than you'd expect from his/her reading level.

Examples: Famous performers (Henry Winkler, Whoopi Goldberg, Jay Leno), authors (John Irving, Octavia Butler) and surgeon Toby Cosgrove, MD, CEO of Cleveland Clinic.

It's accompanied by strengths as well as weaknesses. *People with dyslexia often show...*

- **Great ability to learn.**
- **Ability to "see the whole picture"...and think "outside the box."**
- **Resilience and ability to adapt.**

COMMON MISCONCEPTION

Long ago, the most common theory was that dyslexia arose from visual-processing problems. Many people still believe that having this condition means you see letters and words backwards. That's wrong.

People with dyslexia have a brain-based problem processing the distinctive sounds that make up words. The person sees the letter just fine but has trouble naming it, making its sound and blending the sounds of multiple letters into words. The brain systems involved in skilled, automatic reading also do not function efficiently.

HOW TO GET HELP

The first step to getting help is to recognize that you may have the condition (see bulleted questions, on page 29). A thorough evaluation from a professional—such as a psychologist or neuropsychologist who specializes in dyslexia—can help you find out for sure. Costs can vary from several hundred to several thousand dollars and are rarely covered by insurance.

While there is no medical or pharmaceutical treatment for the underlying brain glitch, effective training systems can help you read and process information better. Start with an adult literacy program that can match you to the right instruction. (Check your local library, state department of education or the Davis Dyslexia Association International website, Dyslexia.com.)

One good program is the Wilson Reading System. This program must be done with an instructor and teaches decoding, fluency and vocabulary and helps students read connected text. While not usually covered by insurance, some employers may agree to cover the expense.

"Assistive technologies" also help. Consider "reading pens," such as Voice Dream Reader (about $20), which turn written text into spoken words...and speech-recognition systems for computers, tablets and phones that turn voice into written text.

Note: The Americans with Disabilities Act grants you the right to request "reasonable accommodations" to help you do your job well, although your employer may not be required to pay for certain technologies.

If you learn that you're dyslexic, the good news is that while you may be a slow reader, you can be a fast thinker. Prominent lawyer David Boies—he represented Al Gore before the US Supreme Court in 2000—was diagnosed as a child. He still reads about half as fast as the average person but has developed strategies for getting through large volumes of written material—and says that, in the end, he will have learned a lot and absorbed much more than others.

Finally, if you do discover that you have adult dyslexia, tell your family! There's a good chance that your child, niece or nephew might be struggling with it—and not know it.

GOT DYSLEXIA?

While there's no definitive "test" for dyslexia, there are many signs. *Ask yourself…*

•**When I was a child, did I have difficulty with reading and spelling?**

•**Do I read slowly,** with great effort?

•**Do I ever read for pleasure?** (People with dyslexia rarely do.)

•**Do I struggle with restaurant menus?** (Dyslexic diners fall back on "I'll have what he's having" and "I'll have the special.")

•**Do I feel embarrassment about reading aloud?**

Example: Work presentations, Bible study classes and story time with children or grandchildren.

•**Do I prefer books, reports and articles with lots of figures, charts and graphs—and fewer words?**

•**Do I have problems with spoken language?** People with dyslexia can have problems remembering and pronouncing the names of people and places and retrieving words "on the tip of the tongue."

If you answer "yes" to several of these questions, consider getting a professional evaluation.

ADHD Breakthrough: A New, Drug-Free Way to Harness Focus

Andrew Hill, PhD, the lead neurotherapist at Peak Brain Institute in Los Angeles who has ADHD himself. PeakBrainInstitute.com. Study titled "Effectiveness of neurofeedback versus medication for attention-deficit/hyperactivity disorder" by researchers in Bangkok, Thailand, published in Pediatrics International.

Your brain has five waves—gamma, beta, alpha, theta and delta, each with its own purpose. People with attention-deficit/hyperactivity disorder (ADHD) have a high ratio of the amount of theta to beta waves in the brain's frontal lobe. Theta waves in general are slow and drive daydreaming, creativity, receptive attention, remembering and fantasy. This is a good thing for most people, but not when it happens all the time, as it does in many ADHD brains. When theta is "stuck" at a high level, it's hard for the person to pump the brakes or inhibit the automatic aspects of their attention. When there is too much theta, it overpowers the beta waves, which are more involved in thinking, problem-solving, decision-making and processing information. Addressing ADHD (regardless of how) would result in a better theta-beta ratio. One solution for people with ADHD is to teach the brain how to rein in the high ratio when it's time to focus by reducing theta and increasing beta voluntarily.

The training: Neurofeedback—or biofeedback on the brain—trains the brain to reduce the amount of theta and allow the person to control impulsive, automatic or reactive actions. The biofeedback process starts with capturing a picture of your brain by creating a quantitative electroencephalogram (QEEG) brain map—think of it as the equivalent of an EKG of your heart. An EEG technician will place a cap with electrodes on your head to record resting brain activity. Baseline activity with eyes closed and with eyes open is then compared with a database of age-matched EEGs to determine where your brain is unusual, identify likely bottlenecks and resource limits, and help determine the specifics of your training. Patterns that suggest ADHD are between 80% and 94% accurate, depending on research study, so QEEG serves as a hypothesis generator more than a diagnostic test. Computerized attention testing is usually done alongside the QEEG and helps validate population differences in attention performance.

Training with neurofeedback consists of sessions during which a few electrodes (rather than the QEEG cap) are placed on your scalp to measure your ongoing brain waves as you watch images, play games or listen to sounds. When your brain shifts in the right direction (with a brief reduction in theta and an increase in beta waves, as an example), a reward or an audiovisual feedback based on the brain activity is triggered. The neurofeedback process gently trains the brain to make more or less of different brain waves and attention resources. Moment to moment while playing the game, the brain gets information about the direction it should move in, and it will attempt to learn from this information over the next day or two, much like the time it takes for the effects of a gym workout to show up.

Most people with ADHD need around 40 30-minute sessions, usually done three times a week over a three-month period, with periodic assessments to see how well it's working. Some research using QEEG brain maps has shown that a brain can go from extreme excess theta to typical theta in as little as three months, and the benefits tend to last after training is complete.

While an analysis of a handful of early studies on neurofeedback training showed mixed results, a recent study done in Thailand involving 40 children found it was a promising alternative treatment, and a new analysis review with an international team of researchers is currently under way to further evaluate it. There are many more studies under way or recently completed for ADHD and most show excellent and long-lasting results.

Availability: Neurofeedback training is available in most areas of the country. The key is to make sure that the cognitive-care center you choose has QEEG-mapping technology because this is the most accurate and reliable way to get a training approach tailored to your brain. Insurance may cover some of the costs of the treatment, but it is not generally well-covered, and a course of training to address ADHD can be upward of $5,000.

New Help for ALS?

Pierre Drapeau, PhD, professor, University of Montreal Hospital Research Centre, Canada.

Amyotrophic lateral sclerosis (ALS), also known as Lou Gehrig's disease, is a neurodegenerative disease that affects nerve cells in the brain and spinal cord, causing progressive paralysis of the skeletal mus-

cles. Two drugs are FDA-approved for ALS but are minimally effective. However, a medication called *pimozide* (Orap), which is used to treat psychiatric conditions, including schizophrenia, and has previously been tested successfully in animal ALS models, looks promising. In a preclinical trial of 25 men and women with ALS, those who took the drug maintained control of the thenar muscles, located in the palm of the hand between the thumb and index finger, for six weeks. Loss of control of these muscles is one of the first signs of ALS. It is not known if pimozide could be a cure, or a way to preserve normal neuromuscular function to stabilize the disease. The drug is still experimental, but a larger clinical trial is under way in Canada and recruiting participants.

Are You Missing the Early Warning Signs of MS?

The Position Paper titled "Diagnosis of multiple sclerosis: 2017 revisions of the McDonald criteria" led by an international panel of experts from the Cleveland Clinic, Ohio, and University College London, UK, published in *The Lancet*.

People can get multiple sclerosis (MS) at any age. But it's easy to miss the early warning signs because they can go away as quickly as they showed up. If they do go away, however, that doesn't mean you're out of the woods. If you're in the process of developing MS, it's a sure thing that more is coming.

Missing early clues of MS can delay your getting the right diagnosis and early treatment. And early treatment is your best bet for avoiding not just another MS episode but also the long-term disability that used to be an unavoidable consequence of this disease.

There's something you can do to avoid the above scenario, though—understand, and do, what's explained below.

CHANGES IN HOW MS IS DIAGNOSED

There's no single test to diagnose MS. Instead, doctors use the McDonald Diagnostic Criteria, a combination of symptoms, imaging tests showing damage in multiple locations in the nervous system and some lab tests. It's also typically necessary to rule out other diseases as part of the process.

In late 2017, revisions were made to update the McDonald Criteria. They mostly apply to someone being evaluated for a first attack of MS, called clinically isolated syndrome (CIS). In the past, people with CIS had to wait for a second attack for an MS diagnosis. Now a first attack and a brain MRI showing one or more lesions similar to the kind seen in people known to have MS, possibly along with certain changes in spinal fluid, can be used to make a diagnosis.

These revisions aim to improve the speed and accuracy of diagnosis (and reduce misdiagnoses), but this still typically depends on the patient noticing early signals and bringing them to a doctor's attention so that the process can begin.

To have CIS, you must have one or more key symptoms of MS that last 24 hours or longer…

•**Tingling and numbness in your face, body, arms or legs.** Some people may also experience itching. This can seem like a minor problem, especially if it goes away after a day, but don't minimize it.

•**A sudden change in vision in one eye** that occurs because of inflammation of the optic nerve, called optic neuritis. The change could be blurred vision, changes in perceived color and contrast, or pain when you move your eye.

•**Other symptoms you might experience include dizziness,** clumsiness or trouble walking…muscle spasms, stiffness or weakness… sexual dysfunction…bladder- or bowel-control problems…changes in speech or swallowing… tremor…or hearing loss.

Note: Some of these symptoms can be symptoms of stroke. Stroke is rare in the age range—20 to 40—when MS typically begins. However, stroke can occur at any age, so if you have sudden loss of vision, slurred speech, weakness of one side of your body or drooping on one side of your face, call 911 immediately.

The MS-related "event" that causes CIS is loss of the protective coating around a nerve, which can make nerve signals go a bit haywire, providing you with the above clues that some-

thing's wrong. The fly in the ointment is that a CIS symptom usually gets less severe or even goes away, leaving you wondering whether you simply had a weird bug in your system. But pay attention to what you don't have—CIS is not accompanied by fever or infection.

While you should first contact your regular doctor if you experience an MS warning sign, you have the best chance of getting the right diagnosis if you're then evaluated by a health-care provider who is an expert in MS.

Surprising Trigger of MS Attacks

Tanuja Chitnis, MD, FAAN, professor of neurology, Harvard Medical School, medical director, Partners Multiple Sclerosis Center, Brigham and Women's Hospital, both in Boston.

There is no cure (yet!) for multiple sclerosis, so it is instead managed with drugs to help mitigate the effects of the disease. Lifestyle adjustments, including a healthy diet, can also help. Now research finds that some healthy foods might be a problem for certain people who have MS.

It's already known that certain environmental factors can trigger MS and/or make it worse. But until now, the association between one environmental factor—allergies—and MS has not been clear.

So researchers at Brigham and Women's Hospital and Harvard Medical School had 1,349 adult MS patients fill out questionnaires about their current history of three kinds of allergies—environmental (dust, mold or hay fever), food (eggs, dairy, wheat, soy, fish, shellfish, fruits, nuts or other food) and/or drugs. The patients also had gadolinium-enhanced MRIs of their brains. These scans are taken to show lesions, which confirm that inflammatory cells have crossed into the central nervous system, as happens during an MS attack.

Results: Compared with patients who had no known allergies, patients with food allergies had 27% more MS attacks. The brain scans of these patients also were more than twice as likely to have MS lesions in their brains as patients without food allergies. No association was shown for environmental or drug allergies and either MS attacks or brain lesions.

Note: The study authors point out that they did not distinguish between true food allergy and food sensitivity.

Researchers believe that inflammation may be one reason for the association between food allergy and MS activity and lesions. Since environmental and drug allergies did not have the same effect, the researchers believe that there may be a unique mechanism associated with food allergies and MS relapses. The researchers also suggest that having a food allergy may alter the gut microbiome and produce changes in brain chemicals that affect the central nervous system. This study did not investigate whether active avoidance of the allergen reduced risk. They hope to pursue this important question in future research.

More research is needed to better understand the results of this latest study. But in the meantime, if you or a loved one has MS and a known food allergy (or sensitivity), in light of this research it makes sense to be even more scrupulous about avoiding your allergen. And if you have MS but aren't sure whether you have a food allergy or sensitivity, it's a good idea to discuss with your doctor whether you should be tested. Most adults with food allergies have had them since childhood—but food allergies can also start in adulthood.

Better Concussion Treatment

Sushmita Purkayastha, PhD, assistant professor, department of applied physiology and wellness, Southern Methodist University, Dallas, and leader of a study published in *Journal of Head Trauma*.

Mild problem-solving after a concussion is better for brain function than complete rest. Athletes who were given a simple cognitive test as soon as four days after a concussion were less likely to develop depression and anxiety than ones who followed the usual recommendation of total inactivity. This was true even though the athletes with concussions gave far more incorrect answers on the cognitive test than a control group of athletes without concussions. The accuracy of the answers did not seem to matter—simply engaging in the test produced a positive physiological response.

CHAPTER 3

Cancer Breakthroughs

Should I Get Genetic Testing for Cancer?

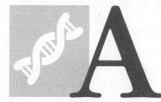**A**dvances in genetic testing for many types of cancer over the past few years have uncovered valuable information for people concerned about their family history of cancer—but also, in some cases, for people with no family history of cancer. *The tests are most likely to be helpful for people with…*

•**A personal history of early-onset cancer…**more than one primary cancer…or a rare cancer.

•**A family history of cancer** where at least two people from one side of the family have had the same or a related kind of cancer.

•**Common cancer patterns in the family** that may suggest an inherited factor—examples include breast, colon, pancreatic, prostate and ovarian cancer.

But even if you do not have a family history of cancer, genetic testing may still be worthwhile. As a genetic counselor, I can see the value even for those who are merely curious—as long as the results are put into the context of personal and family history. And there's always the chance that something unexpected may be uncovered, allowing an opportunity to take steps to avert problems down the road. *Before you have such testing, though, it's important that you get help learning…*

•**What information do I want to know?**

•**Is genetic testing the best way to get that information?**

•**How might the test results change what I do?**

Bear in mind, also, that the current guidelines for reducing risk for cancer are based on data gleaned from families that have a strong history of cancer. It is not known whether the risk

Joy Larsen Haidle, MS, LGC, cancer expert, North Memorial Health, Robbinsdale, Minnesota, and past president of the National Society of Genetic Counselors (NSGC), Chicago.

reduction strategies that have shown benefit for this population would have the same benefit for someone who doesn't have a strong family history of cancer. This is one reason that genetic test results can present difficult choices.

That is where a genetic counselor can help—ideally, starting with deciding whether to get tested. A genetic counselor can help you realistically determine your likelihood of developing a cancer over your lifetime…discuss the various testing options…and explain the results in the context of your personal and family history. You can search for genetic counselors near you at FindAGeneticCounselor.com.

Cancer Blood Test Advances: From Screening to Treatment

Daniel F. Hayes, MD, professor of internal medicine in the division of hematology oncology at University of Michigan School of Medicine, Ann Arbor. The study "Detection and Localization of Surgically Resectable Cancers with a Multi-Analyte Blood Test" was led by researchers from Johns Hopkins University School of Medicine and published in *Science*.

As if a possibly cancerous tumor weren't scary enough, the word biopsy can strike additional fear because of the testing process itself, which often involves using a long needle to remove cells from a tumor or even surgery. Thankfully, advances in cancer research are leading to newer and more informative ways of finding out the nature of a tumor—blood tests. *There are already a few types of such blood tests, and while they all hunt for secrets in patients' DNA, there are differences that you should be aware of…*

LIQUID BIOPSY

The term liquid biopsy was introduced about 10 years ago. It's a way of getting information about a cancer from a blood test (the "liquid") instead of tissue from the tumor itself. When cancers grow or break down, they shed whole cancer cells, proteins, cell fragments or fragments of cancer DNA into the blood. The blood sample taken for a liquid biopsy will have the tumor's cell material and DNA.

A liquid biopsy has many advantages over a tissue biopsy. Different areas of a cancer may have different gene mutations, but a tissue biopsy tells you about only one small area. A liquid biopsy captures genetic information from all areas. Plus, the test is less invasive and less expensive and has a lower risk for pain, bleeding and infection.

Examples of liquid biopsy include the well-known prostate-specific antigen (PSA) test for prostate cancer…the carcinoembryonic antigen (CEA) test for breast, ovarian and colon cancers…the CA 125 for ovarian cancer…and CA 15-3 or CA 27.29 for breast cancer. However, these are all proteins related to cancers that are found in the blood. More recently, scientists have been able to detect and characterize actual tumor DNA by looking at genetic mutations in circulating, cell-free DNA, which is now called circulating tumor DNA, or ctDNA. While you might hear more about its potential, ctDNA testing is still in the early stages, confined mostly to clinical trials.

The main indication for any liquid biopsy has been that when taken over time, serial samples can help determine whether cancer treatment is working. The latest advances in blood testing are starting to guide treatment before it is even started. In 2016, the FDA approved a liquid biopsy test for ctDNA called the cobas EGFR Mutation Test to help guide treatment for the advanced lung cancer called non-small cell lung cancer. This test can be used to direct treatment to a specific type of antineoplastic therapy with a monoclonal antibody directed against EGFR. Other cancers where liquid biopsy may soon be approved to direct treatment are colon, breast and melanoma. It is even hoped that doctors may one day be able to screen for many cancers in a single blood sample.

GERMLINE TESTING

"Germline" mutations are DNA mutations in genes that normally prevent cancer development. Inherited inactivating mutations in these "cancer susceptibility genes" explain why breast, ovarian, colon and prostate cancers run in families. Having a germline mutation (which would appear in every cell of your body, not only in areas susceptible to tumors) makes it harder for your cells to repair errors in DNA, which allows cancer to develop.

Screening blood tests that reveal germline mutations can reliably predict a higher risk for cancer. If one family member tests positive for a germline mutation, other members can be tested to find out whether they're at very high risk for the cancer as well.

One of the best-known examples of a germline mutation is the BRCA genes. Women who have a strong family history of breast cancer and who test positive for BRCA have such a high risk for breast and ovarian cancer that they may elect to have their breasts, and also their ovaries, prophylactically removed before cancer has a chance to develop. Another example is the CDH1 gene mutation, which has a high prediction rate for deadly stomach cancer. Finding that mutation during a screening germline test gives patients the opportunity to consider having their stomach removed prophylactically.

Germline testing can also drive treatment decisions. For instance, colon, prostate and/or ovarian cancers in people with BRCA can be treated with a type of chemotherapy called a PARP inhibitor that works only in patients with BRCA mutations. These drugs have been principally tested in patients with germline BRCA mutations, but there is evidence that in some patients who have not inherited abnormalities in BRCA 1 or 2, the cancer itself may "knock" the gene out. PARP inhibitors may also work in these patients as well. Because of this, there is increasing discussion among experts to test both the germline DNA (which can be done by sequencing DNA from any cell in the body, such as white blood cells or cells lining the inside of the mouth) as well as tumor DNA (such as can be determined in a liquid biopsy).

Newer advances include testing for the cancer gene TP53, which makes it hard to repair radiation damage. Any cancer patient with this gene should avoid radiation treatment.

WHAT'S ON THE HORIZON

Researchers are currently examining how to make ctDNA results more reliable and useful. One problem is that while ctDNA testing may find genetic defects linked to cancer, it may not be able to tell exactly where or what type of cancer the defects came from.

Another hurdle to overcome is that genetic defects can be found in cells that are not cancer. For example, when white blood cells die, they can shed the same genetic defects as some cancer cells, but they will never become cancer.

One advance is taking place at Johns Hopkins where researchers developed CancerSEEK, a ctDNA test to look for proteins associated with the eight types of cancer responsible for 60% of cancer deaths in the US—breast, colorectal, esophageal, liver, lung, pancreatic, stomach and ovarian. By narrowing the focus from all types of cancer to these eight, they were able to limit the number of false-positives. If the results of their 1,005-patient study can be replicated in a larger study currently under way, it's possible that the test could one day be as easy to get at your doctor's office as a blood test for cholesterol.

Note: As amazing as blood biopsies are, it's unlikely that they will completely replace all need for traditional biopsies in the near future, but they are already offering new insights into identifying and treating many cancers.

Dinner Time/Bed Time Cancer Risk

Manolis Kogevinas, MD, PhD, head of the Cancer Research Program at ISGlobal in Barcelona, Spain, and lead author of a study published in *International Journal of Cancer.*

Dining too close to bedtime may increase risk for cancer. Women who ate at least two hours before bedtime had 16% lower risk for breast cancer, compared with women who ate right before going to sleep. For men, the same two hours between dinner and bedtime cut the risk for prostate cancer by 26%. Sleeping soon after eating may affect how food is metabolized, and that may lead to increased cancer risk.

Are You Missing Out on a Lifesaving Clinical Trial?

Elizabeth Anderson, executive administrative director of the cancer clinical trials office at the Stanford Cancer Institute in Palo Alto, California.

If you have a disease that is threatening your life, could you be missing out on a treatment option in a clinical trial? Unless you have a doctor riding shotgun as you plow through all the online medical databases that offer clinical trials, the answer is probably "Yes."

Sorting through treatment options and evaluating whether a particular clinical trial is right for you is complicated. That's why research institutions are taking steps to make information about clinical trials more accessible. For example, the Stanford Cancer Institute in Palo Alto, California, has its own mobile phone app that tells users about every one of its 286 cancer-related trials, notes Elizabeth Anderson, executive administrative director of the institute's cancer clinical trials office. The app gives updates on what the trials' researchers are looking for, notifies specific users when a new trial opens that might be right for them and provides ways to get quick answers to questions about trials.

It's an innovative approach to bringing together potentially good new treatments and the people they can potentially help. But how do you get to even hear about research centers that conduct trials in the first place?

The go-to place for finding clinical trials targeted not only at cancer but at literally thousands of conditions is ClinicalTrials.gov, the government's gargantuan website. In its database at the time of this writing were 48,772 clinical trials recruiting patients.

NIH researchers have tried to update their database with bells and whistles such as live chats, sophisticated graphics, step-by-step directions and other search tips. But the sheer number of listings, the questions they raise about your condition and the choices they offer are mind-boggling. We asked Anderson to suggest approaches to streamline the process and increase the chance that a given patient will find a trial that's a good fit. *She suggested…*

• **Make an appointment with your disease specialist** to understand all the options for treatment, including clinical trials. Chances are that your specialist is aware of at least some relevant trials already and that after a little digging, he/she could explain all of them. Your specialist can assist with reviewing various trials' suitability for your current disease status and inclusion/exclusion information to see whether you meet eligibility requirements before you go any further. Then the two of you can work your way through the possibilities, paying attention to how each trial might advance the knowledge of your condition and how it might help you.

• **Identify any personal constraints** that could affect your ability to participate in a potentially applicable trial. For example, how often would you have to travel to the trial's medical center for monitoring, checkups and tests, and how far away is the center—would you have to fly and/or pay for a hotel? How much time and income would you lose from work, and can you afford this? Your answers will narrow the list of trials you can consider.

• **Look into the researchers conducting the trial.** A research center's description of a trial will identify the doctors and other medical professionals working on it. Check their profiles to see what experience they have with your medical condition. Your own specialist can help you understand and assess the researchers' expertise.

• **Contact the research team to hear firsthand** about the study you're most interested in joining and to see whether you are eligible for the trial. Some of the assessments can be done over the phone, but it is likely you will be asked to come to the research center. One or more of the researchers will go over an "informed consent" document that details the study's purpose…how it is designed, for example, if another treatment or maybe a placebo are part of the study…how long it's expected to last… tests or procedures that will be done…and possible risks and potential benefits. If you decide to participate, you'll need to sign the document before undergoing further evaluations to determine your eligibility for trial participation. Ask how you'll be protected in the event of side effects or unexpected outcomes and, if a treatment helps, whether you can continue it after the trial ends.

•**Circle back with your specialist to discuss everything you've discovered** and get his feedback on how the treatment you'd receive in the trial compares with treatments currently available, how the research treatment could impact your disease and his perspective on the risks versus the benefits. Then use these answers, coupled with the information you've gathered, to help you make your decision about whether or not to join the trial.

Note: Starting a clinical trial may mean that your care will be transferred to the research team for the duration of your trial participation. The researchers would then be working in collaboration with your specialist in providing your care.

Breakthroughs in Lung Cancer

Timothy Burns, MD, PhD, assistant professor of medicine in the department of medicine, Division of Hematology/ Oncology, at UPMC Hillman Cancer Center in Pittsburgh.

Lung cancer kills more Americans—both smokers and nonsmokers—than colon, breast and prostate cancers combined. But the good news is, treatment options are now extending the lives of many people affected by this formidable disease.

Latest development: Recently announced treatment breakthroughs provide new hope for people with non-small cell lung cancer (NSCLC)—the type of malignancy responsible for 85% of all lung cancers.

THE NEW HEAVY HITTERS

•**Immunotherapy.** Some of the newest treatments for NSCLC are immune checkpoint inhibitors—drugs that energize the immune system to kill cancer cells by blocking one of two cancer-promoting proteins, PD-1 and PD-L1. These drugs include *pembrolizumab* (Key-

truda), the immunotherapy treatment credited with saving the life of former President Jimmy Carter when melanoma spread to his brain… *nivolumab* (Opdivo)…*atezolizumab* (Tecentriq) …and *durvalumab* (Imfinzi).

Typically, these drugs are used only as second-line therapies for patients with advanced disease who haven't responded to other types of treatments, such as chemotherapy. But several studies presented at the 2018 annual meeting of the American Association for Cancer Research show that immunotherapy can work as a first-line therapy for people with advanced NSCLC, improving survival.

New scientific findings: A combination of the immunotherapy drug pembrolizumab and chemotherapy worked better than chemo alone as a first-line treatment for patients with metastatic NSCLC—69% were still alive after one year in the combo group, with only 49% alive in the chemo-only group, according to a one-year study published in *The New England Journal of Medicine.*

In a similar one-year study, patients with stage IV lung cancer were given either chemotherapy or two immunotherapy drugs—nivolumab and *ipilimumab* (Yervoy), which blocks CTLA-4, a protein similar to PD-1. Those treated with immunotherapy were 42% less likely to have their disease progress than those who received other treatment.

Meanwhile, research focusing on the use of immunotherapy without chemotherapy as a first-line treatment—reported at a recent meeting of the American Society of Clinical Oncology—also delivered positive results. The stage IV NSCLC patients getting pembrolizumab lived four to eight months longer than those getting chemo. Only 18% of the immunotherapy patients suffered severe side effects, such as inflammation of the lung, liver or colon, versus 41% of those in the chemo group.

Takeaway: With the impressive results of these studies, first-line treatment with an immunotherapy drug with or without chemotherapy is now the standard-of-care for most cases of advanced NSCLC. If a test of your tumor tissue shows that you have a high PD-L1 activity— and one-third of patients with NSCLC do—then single-agent immunotherapy might be the best first treatment for you with or without chemotherapy. Patients whose tumor does not express high levels of this marker still benefit from the combination of immunotherapy with chemotherapy in the majority of cases. Talk to your oncologist.

•**Gene-modulating drugs.** This type of therapy uses drugs to turn off one of several genetic mutations (oncogenes) that can drive lung cancer. An estimated 10% to 20% of NSCLC patients have the epidermal growth factor receptor (EGFR) mutation, which is treated with drugs such as *erlotinib* (Tarceva), *afatinib* (Gilotrif), *gefitinib* (Iressa) and *osimertinib* (Tagrisso). An estimated 5% have the anaplastic lymphoma kinase (ALK) mutation, which is treated with drugs such as *crizotinib* (Xalkori), *ceritinib* (Zykadia), *alectinib* (Alecensa) and *brigatinib* (Alunbrig).

These oral drugs are so powerful that they can, in rare cases, extend life by five years or more. However, the newer and more effective of these drugs—such as alectinib for ALK—has been used as a second-line therapy. Now this treatment paradigm is changing.

New scientific findings: In a study published in 2018, more than 500 NSCLC patients with an EGFR mutation got either osimertinib as a first-line treatment or the previous standard therapy (erlotinib or gefitinib). After 12 months, those taking osimertinib had a 54% lower risk for disease progression or death. In April 2018, the FDA approved osimertinib for first-line treatment of metastatic NSCLC.

In a study of more than 300 metastatic NSCLC patients with the ALK mutation, the disease progressed or death occurred in 41% of those receiving alectinib (a newer more effective drug) compared with 68% receiving crizotinib, an older drug, after about a year and a half. The alectinib group also had fewer side effects. Patients receiving alectinib had control of their tumors for almost three years, on average.

Takeaway: If you are diagnosed with NSCLC, get tested to find out if you have a genetic mutation driving the disease. If you do, talk to your oncologist about the best gene-targeting drug for you—patients with these mutations often do not benefit from immunotherapy.

THE LIQUID BIOPSY OPTION...

The gold standard for biopsies in NSCLC is a tissue biopsy—removing a portion of the tumor and testing it—to identify the specific type of cancer and genetic mutations that inform treatment decisions.

Problem: In many cases, a tissue biopsy isn't possible—for example, the position of the tumor in the lung or other organ may make it too difficult to biopsy, or the patient may have emphysema.

Solution: A liquid (blood-based) biopsy can be used when a tissue biopsy is not an option. The FDA approved liquid biopsy for lung cancer in 2016. A recent study published in *JAMA Oncology* suggests that combining liquid biopsies with tumor biopsies can improve the chance of finding a targetable mutation. Ask your oncologist if this is right for you. FoundationOne and Guardant360 are the two most widely used liquid biopsies.

Skin Cancer from Your Blood Pressure Med? Yes, It's Possible

Anton Pottegård, MScPharm, PhD, clinical pharmacology and pharmacy, department of public health, University of Southern Denmark, Odense, and lead author of study titled "Association of Hydrochlorothiazide Use and Risk of Malignant Melanoma," published in *JAMA Internal Medicine*.

The blood pressure drug you're taking to protect your health could actually be endangering it—by making you more likely to get a deadly form of skin cancer! *Here's the shocking story...*

Hydrochlorothiazide (HCTZ), a diuretic often called a "water pill" because it makes your body excrete more fluid, is one of the most popular blood pressure drugs. It's well known that the drug has a photosensitizing effect, meaning that it makes skin more sensitive to damage from the sun's ultraviolet rays.

Researchers analyzed 10 years of data on about 19,000 people (ages 18 to 90) with melanoma and compared it with data on people who were cancer-free (although some had previously had nonmelanoma skin cancer). Besides checking for HCTZ use, the researchers also checked for use of several other types of blood pressure drugs.

Results: Compared with people who did not have melanoma, people with melanoma were more likely to have taken high cumulative doses of HCTZ. In fact, they were 22% more likely to have taken a cumulative dose of 50,000 mg or more. Of particular concern to the researchers was that people who had taken the highest cumulative doses of HCTZ (100,000 mg or more) were 126% more likely to have nodular melanoma, a form of the disease that isn't clearly tied to high sun exposure. None of the other blood pressure drugs studied were found to be related to melanoma risk at any dose.

If 50,000 mg sounds like a lot, consider that people prescribed blood pressure drugs generally need to take them for the rest of their lives. While a typical starting dose of HCTZ is 12.5 mg/day, doses up to 50 mg/day are prescribed. Taking just the lowest dose of 12.5 mg daily would result in a cumulative dose of 50,000 mg in 10 years—not such a long time in the scheme of things.

Do not stop taking HCTZ (or any other blood pressure medication) without first talking to your doctor. And if you do take HCTZ, in addition to being especially vigilant about sun protection, be sure to get screened regularly for skin cancer. The earlier melanoma is detected and treated, the better the outcome. You can get a free skin cancer screening through the American Academy of Dermatology (AAD.org).

Don't Make These Sunscreen Mistakes!

Barney Kenet, MD, dermatologist and dermatologic surgeon at New York-Presbyterian/Weill Cornell Medical Center and in private practice, both in New York City. He is author of *Saving Your Skin* and *How to Wash Your Face.* KenetMD.com

Remember those days when summer meant baking in the sun after slathering on a baby-oil-and-iodine mixture? Virtually no one makes that mistake any longer! Certainly no one who wants to avoid the dangerous effects of too much sun.

But even with the advent of sunscreen, far too many people are unknowingly increasing their risk for skin cancer.

Sobering facts: Fewer than 15% of men and 30% of women even bother to use sunscreen regularly on their faces and other exposed skin when they are outside for more than an hour, yet the effect can be devastating. In 2019, melanoma, the deadliest type of skin cancer, is expected to be diagnosed in nearly 100,000 Americans. Meanwhile, more than three million Americans are diagnosed each year with other types of skin cancer. *To help protect your precious skin, avoid these mistakes…*

MISTAKE #1: **You neglect this vulnerable spot.** Your eyelids occupy a relatively small part of your body, but thanks to their combination of extremely thin, delicate skin and near-constant ultraviolet (UV) exposure, about 10% of all skin cancers occur there. Scientists may now have an explanation.

In research published in *PLOS ONE*, study participants failed to cover 10% of their faces, on average. And the most frequently neglected area was—you guessed it—the eyelids…and the area located between the inner corners of the eyes and the bridge of the nose.

Not surprisingly, several study participants said that they left those hot spots unprotected out of concern that sunscreen would sting their eyes.

Solution: Choose a gentle sunscreen lotion or cream.

What to try: SkinCeuticals Physical Eye UV Defense, SPF 50 (SkinCeuticals.com)…or "tear-free" Neutrogena Pure & Free Baby Sunscreen, SPF 50 (Neutrogena.com).

Note: Even though these products can be used on the eyelids, keep them out of your eyes.

Don't forget: Sunglasses also help protect the eyelids—and your eyesight. At least 10% of cataract cases can be directly attributed to UV exposure. Look for sunglasses that block 99% or 100% of UV rays.

MISTAKE #2: **You don't wear sun-protective clothing.** Ask a dermatologist for his/her favorite UV-protection tip, and you might be surprised to hear "cover up with clothing" just as often as you hear "wear sunscreen."

Even though you get some protection from regular shirts and pants—think dark-colored synthetic or tightly woven fabrics—"sun-protective clothing" does a far better job. This clothing is rated with a UPF, which stands for Ultraviolet Protection Factor and represents the amount of UVA and UVB rays that can penetrate a particular fabric. A UPF of 50 allows only one-fiftieth of UV radiation to reach the skin.

What to try: Solumbra by Sun Precautions (SunPrecautions.com) has clothing options for men and women.

Don't forget a hat: Golf and baseball caps don't protect the ears from sun exposure. Both men and women should choose a hat with a minimum two- to three-inch-wide brim. Coolibar (Coolibar.com) offers stylish hats with a UPF of 50+ for men and women.

MISTAKE #3: **You skip your "lips and tips."** Lips are prone to developing precancerous lesions called actinic cheilitis—scaly patches that, when untreated, can turn into squamous cell carcinoma, the second most common form of skin cancer.

What to try: Neutrogena Revitalizing Lip Balm, SPF 20 (Neutrogena.com) is a tinted lip balm with moisturizer. Vanicream Lip Protectant, SPF 30 (Vanicream.com) is gluten-free and free of dyes, parabens and other preservatives.

Don't forget your "tips": Tips of the ears, the scalp and tops of hands also are vulnerable to developing skin cancers due to their cumulative sun exposure.

What to try: A stick that allows precise application, such as Kiss My Face Sport Hot Spots Sunscreen, SPF 30 (KissMyFace.com).

MISTAKE #4: **You ignore the label.** Sunscreen ingredients do matter. The FDA has proposed that zinc oxide and titanium dioxide be considered GRASE (generally recognized as safe and effective). On the other hand, para-aminobenzoic acid (PABA) and trolamine salicylate are not GRASE for use in sunscreens due to possible safety concerns. (Trolamine salicylate, for instance, can interfere with healthy blood clotting.)

An additional 12 ingredients, such as the chemical sunscreen ingredients oxybenzone, avobenzone and octinoxate, fall somewhere in between—some experts are concerned about the potential for endocrine disruption, for instance—and more research is needed to determine safety.

New finding: After four thorough applications, the popular chemical sunscreen ingredients avobenzone, oxybenzone, octocrylene and ecamsule were detected in volunteers' blood in concentrations that exceeded the FDA's testing threshold, according to a study published in *JAMA*. For oxybenzone, the threshold level was detected just two hours after the first application and it accumulated at higher rates than the other ingredients. More safety testing will be done.

What to try: Badger's Clear Zinc Sunscreen, SPF 30 (Badgerbalm.com) blends with your skin tone and has 98% certified organic ingredients. Or try Aveeno Baby Continuous Protection Sensitive Skin Zinc Oxide Sunscreen, SPF 50 (Aveeno.com).

Also, pay close attention to terms on the label. *Be sure to choose…*

•**"Broad spectrum."** This means that it protects against UVA rays (which contribute to premature skin aging) and UVB rays (sunburn). Both can lead to skin cancer.

•**"Water-resistant" or "very water-resistant."** This means that it protects wet or sweaty skin for 40 or 80 minutes, respectively.

Also: Throw out sunscreen that is expired… or showing signs of expiration, such as changes in consistency, smell or color. If a product doesn't show an expiration date, use a permanent marker to write the date of purchase on the bottle and use that as a guide.

MISTAKE #5: **You use a combination sunscreen-insect repellent.** Insect repellent ingredients (DEET, in particular) can slash SPF by more than 30%.

What to do: Use a separate sunscreen and insect repellent, and follow the manufacturer's recommendations for each. Apply insect repellent first and wait at least a minute before applying sunscreen. One ounce (two tablespoons) of sunscreen needs to be reapplied every two hours, but insect repellent does not, so be sure you don't apply too much.

Beware This Colonoscopy Risk

Susan Hutfless, PhD, assistant professor of medicine at the Johns Hopkins University School of Medicine and of epidemiology at its Bloomberg School of Public Health, both in Baltimore, and coauthor of the study "Rates of infection after colonoscopy and osophagogastroduodenoscopy in ambulatory surgery centres in the USA" published in *Gut*.

Study titled "Residual moisture and waterborne pathogens inside flexible endoscopes: Evidence from a multisite study of endoscope drying effectiveness" by researchers in St. Paul, Minnesota, published in *American Journal of Infection Control*.

When you're scheduled for a colonoscopy, your thoughts are on getting a clean bill of health at the end of it… not on whether the procedure could give you a dangerous infection. But that is a surprising risk you need to be aware of. It's not that you should forgo this very effective cancer screening…but you should take the simple steps described below to protect yourself.

What we know: Every year, more than 20 million Americans have internal medical tests and treatments done with reusable scopes mounted on the end of tubes that are inserted through either the anus or the mouth and pushed along to various parts of the digestive tract. These tools are marvelous instruments, but they are complex, delicate and very hard to completely disinfect and fully dry between uses.

This can lead to dangerous situations. In a study recently published in the *American Journal of Infection Control*, researchers went to three (unnamed) US hospitals and tested 45 endoscopes that were disinfected after previous uses and ready to be used in additional procedures. They found water-borne germs—germs that bred in water left behind after the scopes were cleaned—on 71% of them. These medical devices were literally breeding grounds for infection.

The danger is not only hypothetical. For example, since 2013, there have been 35 deaths in the US linked to infections stemming from duodenoscopes, scopes often used to diagnose and treat problems with the pancreas.

MORE NEW FINDINGS

To assess the infection risk from reusable scopes, researchers at Johns Hopkins University reviewed records of hospitalizations and emergency department visits in six states over a one-year period to see how many infections developed within seven to 30 days after about two million scope procedures.

The researchers were surprised to find that infections were much more common than previously thought. There were 1.1 infections per 1,000 screening colonoscopies, 1.6 per 1,000 diagnostic colonoscopies and three per 1,000 through the-mouth procedures. *Here's what else they found…*

•**Having been in the hospital and/or having had another type of endoscopic procedure** within the previous 30 days increased a patient's risk for infection.

•**The most common infections were gastrointestinal tract infections and pneumonia.** (The reason for pneumonia, a previously known risk, may be sedation, which can cause patients to aspirate fluids from the respiratory tract and isn't related to contaminated scopes.)

HOW TO REDUCE YOUR RISK

The more of these procedures a center had performed, the lower its infection rate tended to be. So call or e-mail various centers where you might have a procedure and ask how often each center does the procedure and how often patients have gotten infections. Even better, find out whether the center can use (or already is using) one of the disposable scopes recently approved by the FDA.

According to Susan Hutfless, MD, one of the Johns Hopkins researchers, just before your procedure starts, you might also ask your surgeon how confident he or she is that the scope is "clean"—your question might prompt him or her to check this information before using it on you. Even though you might be met with a puzzled expression, the more patients who ask the question, the more likely physicians will be to find out the answers.

If you need a scope procedure for treatment or to diagnose a problem, you may not be able to put it off. But if you've recently been sick or hospitalized or had another endoscopic procedure, consider delaying a screening colonoscopy for a little while to avoid a possible double exposure to infection-causing germs, suggested Dr. Hutfless.

After a scope procedure, be on the lookout for the following infection symptoms…

- **Fever**
- **Chills**
- **Cramps**
- **Nausea**
- **Vomiting**
- **Diarrhea**
- **Cough**
- **Shortness of breath**

Report any and all to your doctor's office right away.

Nuts May Improve Colon Cancer Survival

Charles S. Fuchs, MD, MPH, director of Yale Cancer Center, New Haven, Connecticut, and leader of a study published in *Journal of Clinical Oncology.*

People with stage 3 colon cancer who ate two or more one-ounce servings of tree nuts (such as almonds, walnuts, pecans) weekly had 46% less cancer recurrence and were

53% less likely to die over six-and-a-half years than people who rarely ate nuts. The equivalent of seven almonds a day is enough. Tree nuts have cancer-protective properties that benefit healthy people, too.

Questions to Ask Your Doctor About Your Colonoscopy

National Institutes of Health, NIH.gov…National Cancer Institute, NCI.org…StopColonCancerNow.com…Health CareBlueBook.com…Kaiser Family Foundation, kff.org… Colon Cancer Alliance, CCAlliance.org…American Society for Gastrointestinal Endoscopy, ASGE.org.

No one looks forward to a colonoscopy. But it's one of the few screening tests that can really save your life—if you get it at the right time, the right way and with the right follow-up. *Here are key questions to ask your doctor about your colonoscopy…*

At what age should I start screening for colon cancer? Most people get their first screening test at age 50—but based on your health profile and family history, your doctor might recommend an earlier age.

Which colon screening test should I get? Colonoscopy, which allows a physician to examine your entire colon while you are sedated, is the most widely recommended screen for colon cancer. Other tests such as flexible sigmoidoscopy, which examines only the lower part of the colon, and virtual colonoscopy, which uses a noninvasive CT scan, are available. Your doctor can review the pros and cons of each test—but colonoscopy is the gold standard.

What about a stool test? Stool tests look for blood in the feces, which can be a sign of a digestive problem or colon cancer. The American Cancer Society suggests getting this test every year after age 50. It is not, however, a substitute

*Nongastroenterologists are five times more likely than gastroenterologists, who have specialized training in performing colonoscopies, to miss colorectal cancer during this test. To find a gastroenterologist near you, consult the website of the American College of Gastroenterology at Patients.GI.org.

for colonoscopy. Ask your doctor whether this test should be part of your colon cancer-screening regimen.

Is there any way to make the "bowel prep" less unpleasant? There are a variety of products and tricks to make the bowel-cleansing process more bearable. Your doctor can explain which he/she uses and which might be best for you.

What can I eat and drink prior to my colonoscopy? Not all doctors are still requiring pure clear-liquid diets the day before the test. Check with your doctor for his recommendations.

Should I stop taking my medications and supplements? Anti-platelet drugs, such as *clopidogrel* (Plavix)…anti-coagulants, such as *warfarin* (Coumadin)…and nonsteroidal anti-inflammatory drugs (NSAIDs), such as *ibuprofen* (Motrin), *naproxen* (Aleve) and aspirin, are the medications most commonly stopped a few days prior to a colonoscopy. But there are others. Ask your doctor for advice on stopping any medication or supplements that you take.

Do you offer a choice of sedation type? Most patients are given a "twilight" sedative that leaves them conscious but relaxed—and typically pain-free during the procedure. Other patients receive full anesthesia and are not conscious during the procedure. Ask your doctor what type of sedative you may receive and discuss how deeply you prefer to be sedated.

What is your complication rate for colonoscopy? The main risk of colonoscopy is perforation, a small tear in the colon wall. In research, the incidence of perforation during screening colonoscopy was 0.01%. It's perfectly reasonable to ask your doctor what his complication rate is for the test, and if it is higher than the statistic above, consider working with another colonoscopist whose track record is better.

What is your plan if you find any abnormalities while doing my colonoscopy? If the doctor finds a growth (polyp), it will be removed and sent to a lab to determine whether cancer cells are present. Ask your doctor after the procedure if any polyps were detected, whether they were removed completely and when you'll get the lab results.

Anti-Inflammatory Cancer Fighters

Oncology Letters.

Drugs with anti-inflammatory effects, such as aspirin and *indomethacin* (Indocin), have been shown to help protect against colorectal cancer but often cause side effects.

New finding: Combining the drugs with lecithin, a chemical found in soybeans, may reduce side effects and increase cancer protection.

A "Game-Changing" Cancer Drug Gets Fast-Track Approval

"FDA approves an oncology drug that targets a key genetic driver of cancer, rather than a specific type of tumor," US Food & Drug Administration.

In November 2018, the FDA announced the accelerated approval of a new type of cancer drug, *larotrectinib* (Vitrakvi), the first to target a specific cancer gene rather than a cancer "type," such as breast or colon cancer. This is a monumental shift in cancer treatment because this drug is "tissue agnostic"—it doesn't care where the cancer is, but rather what drives its growth.

Vitrakvi targets the gene mutations known as neurotrophic tyrosine receptor kinase (NTRK) fusions. NTRK genes provide the fuel that helps some solid tumors grow, including infantile fibrosarcoma, soft tissue (muscle) sarcoma and tumors of the salivary gland, thyroid and lung. By targeting NTRK, this drug seeks to stop the growth of these tumors, which often have metastasized to numerous places, can't be removed surgically or have not responded to other treatments. Unlike many cancer drugs that must be given intravenously, Vitrakvi is taken as a pill or oral solution.

FAST-TRACKING CANCER CARE

The accelerated approval of Vitrakvi was based on several early clinical trials with just 55 adults and children with various NTRK positive tumors. These tumors had a 75% response rate to the drug—a complete response for 22% of patients and a partial response for 53%. Before Vitrakvi, many of these cancers were simply untreatable.

In October 2018, an additional year of follow-up data was presented at the European Society for Medical Oncology meeting.

More good news: The overall response rate of the original 55 patients had improved to 80%. There were also 67 new patients who had an overall response rate of 81%. It was also being used to treat NTRK positive tumors in more locations—the colon, gastrointestinal system, breast, bone, pancreas and skin (melanoma).

Patients on Vitrakvi continue to take the drug indefinitely or until it stops working or has to be stopped due to side effects. Common side effects include fatigue, nausea and vomiting, cough, constipation or diarrhea, and dizziness—neurological problems, mostly minor, occurred in about half of patients. But more serious liver damage may occur, so blood tests are needed to check liver function.

New Hope for Bladder Cancer

Brant Allen Inman, MD, MS, a urologist, associate professor of surgery at Duke University School of Medicine and a member of the Duke Cancer Institute, all in Durham, North Carolina. He specializes in diagnostic tests/therapies for bladder cancer and other genitourinary malignancies.

After years without any significant treatment advances or new prevention strategies, bladder cancer is finally getting its due.

Recent developments: The FDA approved five new drugs in 2016–2017 for the treatment of metastatic bladder cancer. It's an important development because these cancers are often deadly, with a five-year survival rate as low as 15% when the cancer is advanced.

Even though the prognosis for people diagnosed with early-stage bladder cancer has been good for quite some time—up to 95% are alive after five years when the cancer is confined to the inner layer of the bladder wall—a late-stage diagnosis now has more treatment options than ever before. In some cases, a new treatment option can double survival time.

What's more, research is uncovering additional steps that can help prevent bladder cancer from recurring after it's been treated—strategies that also will help protect people from developing this malignancy in the first place.

PREVENTION IS BEST

Even though bladder cancer does not get as much public attention as certain other types, it is the sixth most common cancer in the US (and the fourth most common among men), with about 81,000 new cases diagnosed every year.

The good news is that most bladder cancers (about 75%) are non-muscle invasive—that is, they're limited to the lining of the bladder…are usually diagnosed early…and respond well to treatment.

One distinguishing characteristic of bladder cancer is its recurrence rate. More than half of all people treated for this malignancy will have a recurrence. For this reason, it's crucial for anyone with bladder cancer to do everything possible to prevent a recurrence.

Smokers are four to seven times more likely to develop bladder cancer than nonsmokers. The toxins from cigarette smoke are excreted from the body in the urine—and spend many hours concentrated in the bladder, where they can trigger cancer-causing changes. *Other ways to help prevent a bladder cancer diagnosis or recurrence…*

•**Eat more kale.** Cruciferous vegetables (such as kale, broccoli, cauliflower and cabbage) are high in isothiocyanates, chemical compounds that inhibit the ability of cancer cells, including bladder cancer cells, to proliferate. Men who consumed cruciferous vegetables more than five times a week were 51% less likely to develop bladder cancer than those who ate them less than once a week, according to the Health Professionals Follow-Up Study.

•**Stay hydrated.** People who drink more water urinate more frequently, which reduces chemical concentrations and exposure times from cigarette smoke (including secondhand smoke), workplace chemicals (such as polyaromatic hydrocarbons and dyes), air pollution, etc.

Important exception: Research has shown that people who drink water from private wells that may be contaminated with arsenic are at increased risk for bladder cancer. Water that contains high levels of nitrate, a by-product of fertilizers and animal feedlots, has been linked to higher rates of bladder cancer in postmenopausal women.

Take note: If you drink well water, get it checked!

CATCH IT EARLY

After prevention, early detection is, of course, the best way to avoid bladder cancer deaths.

An annual urine test may be worthwhile if you're at high risk—for example, you're already having symptoms (discussed below)…you are exposed to workplace toxins that increase your risk…you're a smoker…and/or you have a personal or family history of bladder cancer.

Important: About 80% to 90% of patients who are diagnosed with bladder cancer will have visible traces of blood in the urine. Blood can appear for many reasons, including urinary tract infections (UTIs) or prostate problems. However, if you see blood in your urine, I advise that you assume it might be cancer and see a physician or possibly a urologist.

Other red flags: Frequent trouble urinating… feeling pain or burning while urinating…and feeling that you need to urinate right away, even when the bladder isn't full. Particularly in women, bladder cancer may be misdiagnosed as a recurrent UTI. A urine culture (not just an in-office urinalysis) is needed to diagnose UTI correctly.

DRUG BREAKTHROUGHS

The recently FDA-approved checkpoint inhibitors target proteins that weaken the immune system. In doing so, the drugs—*pembrolizumab* (Keytruda), *avelumab* (Bavencio), *durvalumab* (Imfinzi), *nivolumab* (Opdivo) and *atezolizumab* (Tecentriq)—intensify immune activity against tumor cells.

An older form of immunotherapy, called intravesical therapy, uses a bacterium (BCG) that's instilled into the bladder. This approach inhibits cancer progression and can reduce the risk for recurrences by about 40%. BCG causes an inflammatory reaction that leads to the recruitment of other immune cells to the bladder, which helps eradicate bladder tumors and helps prevent them from recurring.

Depending on the stage of the cancer, checkpoint inhibitors are an important advancement because they can help patients who didn't do well with BCG or other treatments—or who improved initially but later suffered a cancer recurrence.

The drugs aren't a cure, but they can double the survival time in some cases of metastatic cancer that has not responded to chemotherapy. This means the average survival time of six months is increased to 10 to 12 months.

Another potential benefit: It's hoped that checkpoint inhibitors will control cancer well enough that removal of the bladder, which has been required in those who haven't responded well to other treatments, can be delayed or avoided altogether—but this is still being studied.

Downside: Immunotherapy drugs can increase levels of inflammation throughout the body. Many of these inflammatory reactions are minor and can be managed with topical creams or by stopping the drug temporarily for a couple of weeks. However, in some cases, the reactions can be severe and, in very rare cases, even fatal. When the reaction is more severe, the drug is stopped and the overactive immune system is suppressed by giving steroids and other immunosuppressive drugs.

A New Approach to Bladder Cancer Treatment: Watch and Wait

Study titled "Conservative Management Following Clinical Complete Response to Neoadjuvant Chemotherapy for Muscle-Invasive Bladder Cancer: Contemporary Outcomes of a Multi-Institutional Cohort Study" by researchers at Columbia University Medical Center and Memorial Sloan Kettering Cancer Center and published in *The Journal of Urology.*

The first steps for treating bladder cancer are removing the tumor in a procedure called transurethral resection of bladder tumor or TURBT, followed by chemotherapy. Often these steps eradicate the cancer, yet the standard practice has been for doctors to suggest having the bladder removed in a separate operation, called radical cystectomy, after testing has been completed on the removed tumors and if the cancer was found to have extended into the muscle layer of the organ.

What the researchers wanted to learn was this: If a patient who had muscle-invasive cancer is cancer-free after TURBT and chemo, is it really necessary to then also remove the bladder? What would be the outcome if patients like this were monitored rather than automatically having their bladders removed?

To find out, researchers studied 148 patients who had had muscle-invasive bladder cancer but who had decided on monitoring (also called surveillance) rather than bladder removal after TURBT and chemo. These patients were followed for five years to see how many experienced a cancer recurrence. The average age of the patients was 62, and 80% were men. *Here's what happened over the five years…*

•**The survival rate related to the bladder cancer was 90%.**

•**64%** of the patients were still free of bladder cancer after five years.

•**18%** had a recurrence that ultimately required removing their bladders.

The researchers concluded that the high survival rate supports the option of surveillance for patients with no evidence of cancer after TURBT and chemotherapy.

This is what a surveillance program is likely to involve…

•**Every two to three months,** you will need an overall physical exam, an exam with a bladder scope (cytoscope) and urine testing to look for cancer cells.

•**Every four to six months,** you will need a CT scan or other imaging study of your bladder.

After five years, if there are no signs of recurrence, these tests may be reduced to once a year.

Surveillance does require commitment on your part, but if appropriate, it can be a much easier adjustment than life without a bladder.

Device Fights Brain Tumors

Roger Stupp, MD, chief of neuro-oncology and medical director, Malnati Brain Tumor Institute, Northwestern University Feinberg School of Medicine, Chicago.

A wearable device applied to a patient's shaved scalp slows the growth of glioblastoma (an aggressive brain tumor) by delivering continuous, low-intensity electric currents to brain tissue. The FDA-cleared Optune device is used in addition to chemotherapy. Median survival among patients using the device is about five months longer than for those who do not use the device—and significantly more of the treated group were alive up to two to four years afterward.

Brain Cancer Breakthrough

Michael Vogelbaum, MD, PhD, neurosurgeon and inventor of the CMC, Cleveland Clinic, Ohio, and founder and chief medical officer of Infuseon Therapeutics, Inc.

The blood-brain barrier, a filtering mechanism that protects the brain from toxins, also prevents 98% of chemotherapy drugs from reaching brain tumors.

New option: A device that consists of four ultrathin tubes that are temporarily inserted into the brain, allowing cancer drugs to be delivered directly into the tumor. For details on the first clinical trial of the Cleveland Multiport Catheter (CMC), go to ClinicalTrials.gov.

Better Liver Cancer Test

G. Amit Singal, MD, associate professor of internal medicine and clinical sciences, UT Southwestern Medical Center, Dallas.

When doctors combined a blood test that detects levels of a substance called alpha fetoprotein—a protein that increases in the presence of liver cancer—with abdominal ultrasound (the standard screening method), detection of early-stage liver cancer increased from 45% with ultrasound alone to 63%. Both tests are readily available and should be covered by insurance.

A New Way to Manage Metastatic Liver Cancer

Xiling Shen, PhD, associate professor in the department of biomedical engineering at Duke University in Durham, North Carolina, and study coauthor of "Aldolase B-Mediated Fructose Metabolism Drives Metabolic Reprogramming of Colon Cancer Liver Metastasis," published in *Cell Metabolism*.

Most people who die from cancer don't die from their primary cancer, which can often be surgically removed, but from cancer cells that have metastasized to another part of the body. The liver is one place cancer cells like to go and grow. In fact, metastatic liver cancer is more common than primary liver cancer.

A recent study found that colon cancer cells that migrate to the liver learn to feast on fructose, the sugar that's extremely common in the American diet not so much because it's found naturally in fruit, but because it's added in great quanitities to processed foods.

Why is that so potentially significant for cancer patients? The liver is a major place in the body that stores and breaks down excessive fructose. So the theory is that reducing the amount of fructose eaten could deter the growth of these cancer cells. And if cancer hasn't yet spread to the liver, reducing the amount of fructose eaten might reduce the risk of liver metastasis taking hold.

The enzyme that the liver uses to break down fructose is called ALDOB, and colon cancer cells that find their way to the liver adapt to produce the same enzyme. The metabolized fructose fuels their growth in the liver, which is like a candy store to these cancer cells.

Blocking ALDOB could be a new way to manage liver metastasis, and researchers are working on a drug to do just that. But in the meantime, it makes sense for people with liver metastasis to cut back on fructose consumption.

Here are the foods you unquestionably want to avoid…

•**All types of refined sugar,** such as white, brown and powdered sugars and packaged foods with high amounts of it, such as sweetened breakfast cereals.

•**Corn syrup and high fructose corn syrup**—the primary sweeteners used in candy, sodas, sweetened juices and commercial baked goods.

•**Agave,** honey, molasses, sorghum, maple and pancake syrup.

This study looked at metastasis of colon cancer, but several other cancers also often travel to the liver, including lung, breast, pancreatic and stomach cancers and melanoma. It's reasonable to assume that other cancer cells would also take advantage of any fructose in the liver and grow quickly.

Are You Putting Your Adult Health at Risk After Surviving Childhood Cancer?

Todd Gibson, PhD, assistant member of the faculty at St. Jude's Children's Research Hospital, Memphis, and lead author of the study titled "Perceptions of future health and cancer risk in adult survivors of childhood cancer: A report from the Childhood Cancer Survivor Study," published in *Cancer*.

Jessica Scott, PhD, Memorial Sloan Kettering Cancer Center in New York City, lead author of the study titled "Association of exercise with mortality in adult survivors of childhood cancer," published in *JAMA*.

Surviving childhood cancer is an amazing feat, but if it's left you feeling invincible, you could be putting your adult health in jeopardy.

According to a study done at St. Jude Children's Research Hospital in Memphis, when 15,620 adults who survived childhood cancer were asked how concerned they were about their current health, about one-third said that they were not very concerned or not at all concerned. And nearly 40% weren't concerned about the possibility of facing another bout with cancer.

These responses might indicate that many childhood cancer survivors don't fully understand that they have unique health risks that require a lifetime of vigilance, said Todd M. Gibson, PhD, the study's lead author.

HOW TO FOCUS MORE ON YOUR HEALTH

Cancer treatment, especially radiation and/or chemotherapy, can leave you vulnerable to "late effects," problems that don't show up until many years later, according to the Children's Oncology Group, an international research organization. Late effects can involve nearly every part of the body. They could be chronic health conditions affecting your heart, liver or other key organs, your bones and even your senses, as well as other types of cancers.

There's no cause to live in perpetual anxiety, but it seems that a bit more realism would help. *And for childhood cancer survivors, that means…*

•**Maintain long-term follow-up cancer care.** Keep up with all the screening recommendations for your particular type of cancer as well as for other types (colon, skin, breast if you are a woman, etc.)—ask your doctor.

•**Work with a registered dietitian if you're not at a healthy weight.** Some childhood cancer survivors have trouble gaining weight, while others struggle with being overweight. A nutrition professional can help you develop a plan that includes the foods you like to eat in the correct portion sizes for your weight goals and any unique nutritional needs.

It also helps to pay attention to specific foods linked to cancer risk, according to the National Cancer Institute. For example, while just about everyone knows that cured, smoked and grilled foods are linked with increased cancer risk, few of us really make a point of avoiding them—but you really should.

•**Exercise at a vigorous pace.** A study published in *JAMA Oncology* followed 15,000 childhood cancer survivors for nearly a decade. Researchers found that people who exercised vigorously in their 20s and 30s and increased the amount of exercise they did over an eight-year period had a 40% lower risk of dying compared with those who never or rarely exercised. And exercise can reduce the risks of developing some new cancers later in life, said Jessica Scott, PhD, of the Memorial Sloan Kettering Cancer Center in New York City, lead author of the study. Vigorous activity is aerobic activity that makes you sweat or breathe hard…such as dancing, brisk walking, jogging and playing basketball or tennis, Dr. Scott said.

Note: If childhood cancer left you with physical limitations and that is a reason why you don't exercise vigorously, get some professional help to overcome the barrier—because just about anyone can exercise vigorously with the right tools and training.

Getting Your Sex Life Back on Track After Cancer

Sharon L. Bober, PhD, director of the Sexual Health Program at Dana-Farber Cancer Institute and senior psychologist and assistant professor of psychiatry at Harvard Medical School, both in Boston.

Health-care providers don't bring up the topic of sex while discussing treatment options—partly because they don't want to embarrass their patients, and partly because they're focused on more serious health concerns.

So it's up to you to start the conversation. For instance, you might say, "I'm having a lot of discomfort and things have really changed in my sex life. Can I talk to you about it or can you tell me who I can talk to?"

Here are some common sex challenges that cancer survivors face…

•**You just survived a life-threatening illness**—now you feel guilty for even complaining about something as "trivial" as sex. Sexual health is essential to quality of life and an important contributor to your whole health. And intimacy with a loving partner can help you heal by releasing feel-good hormones, including oxytocin, that ease anxiety.

•**Your genitalia just aren't the same.** Chemo and hormone treatments can dry out the vagina and cause it to atrophy, making sex, masturbation and gynecological exams painful. Radiation, surgery and chemo can cause erectile dysfunction in men, even if their cancer was not directly related to their genital area.

For women: Using a vaginal moisturizer on a regular basis can bring better long-term relief than lubricants.

You may need to apply a moisturizer more often than is recommended on the box for the most effective relief—at least three to five times a week is ideal, applied at bedtime for the best absorption.

Good options: Replens, Hyalo-gyn, Preva-Leaf Oasis…or pure coconut oil. Ask your health-care provider to recommend what would be best for you.

For men: While doctors are quick to solve erection problems with a prescription for a *phosphodiesterase-5* (PDE5) inhibitor such as *sildenafil* (Viagra), there are other options. Penile injections—sometimes called intracavernosal injection therapy—are more effective than taking PDE5 pills. While the idea may seem daunting, men are often glad to hear that there is another option when the "little blue pill" doesn't work. Vacuum erection devices that increase blood flow into the penis to help achieve an erection and penile rings to help maintain one are other options.

For both women and men: A pelvic-floor physical therapist can help restore sexual function with massage, dilators and exercises to build up pelvic-floor muscles, loosen tight muscles and stretch and desensitize scar tissue.

Bonus: These therapies also can reduce urinary and fecal incontinence, a common side effect of cancer therapies.

•**You've tried having sex, but it's just not the same.** Sexual pleasure depends on more than the mechanics of intercourse. Think about ways to achieve intimacy and pleasure without the pressure of reaching an orgasm…or even penile penetration of the vagina. Do what you did when you were dating—hug, cuddle, touch and kiss.

Explore using toys, such as a vibrator, or try new foreplay techniques—experiment with what feels good. Starting slowly, taking your time and expanding your repertoire are all key. A satisfying sex life won't happen overnight. But the journey can be enjoyable, too!

HELPFUL RESOURCES

•**Will2Love.com** is a site founded and run by medical doctors and psychologists that focuses on sexual health for cancer survivors. It's a self-help program that you can do at home and lists psychologists who provide phone counseling.

You also can find providers who specialize in sexual medicine at the International Society for Sexual Medicine, ISSM.info. And there are online forums filled with men and women who are going through the same issues you are at Breast Cancer.org…the American Cancer Society's Cancer Survivors Network, CSN.Cancer.org/forum… and FORCE (Facing Our Risk of Cancer Empowered), FacingOurRisk.org/index.php.

IF IT'S YOUR SPOUSE WHO HAD CANCER…

Framing concerns, fears and wishes using "I" statements instead of "you" can keep the conversation from sounding accusatory.

Example: "I know you feel self-conscious about your body, but you are as beautiful/handsome to me as ever, and I've never stopped wanting you. Can we talk about this?"

Pick a good time and a safe, neutral place to talk, even if you have to schedule it. (For instance, don't launch into this topic when the two of you are getting into bed.) You might be happily surprised at how relieved your partner is to talk!

If You've Got Cancer, Stay Out of the ER!

Nathan Handley, MD, MBA, an oncologist specializing in genitourinary cancers and assistant professor of medical oncology at Thomas Jefferson University in Philadelphia. He is lead author of "Best Practices for Reducing Unplanned Acute Care for Patients with Cancer," published in Journal of Oncology Practice.

Picture this scenario: A 62-year-old widow—let's call her "Mrs. Gand"—has recently been diagnosed with cancer. Two days after her first chemotherapy session, she's at home resting when she is overcome with nausea. It's 9 pm, and she can't get her doctor on the phone. Not knowing what to do, she drives herself to the local hospital ER. After sitting in a cramped waiting room for three hours, the ER doctor admits her to the hospital, where she remains for two days.

What most people don't know: For many cancer patients, a trip to the ER is not only unnecessary, it's time-consuming, costly—and possibly dangerous. For one thing, ER doctors are less familiar with the side effects of cancer treatments—especially newer ones like immunotherapy, which can cause unusual symptoms such as rashes and thyroid abnormalities. A non-cancer specialist may decide that it's safer and easier to admit the patient and wait for more specialized help.

Another important reason to steer clear: After arriving, you'll likely be stuck in a waiting room while more life-threatening cases, such as car accident victims, are seen. Hospitals are notorious sources of hospital-acquired infections. Because cancer patients usually have weaker immune systems due to chemotherapy, they are more susceptible to such infections than people who are healthy.

HOW TO AVOID THE HOSPITAL

Cancer patients have alternatives to the ER… but usually don't know about them. To address this problem, researchers at University of Pennsylvania reviewed the medical literature to identify the best ways for cancer patients to avoid unnecessary visits to the ER and hospitalizations. *The smartest strategies…*

***STRATEGY #1:* Plan ahead.** Many conditions that send cancer patients to the ER can be treated with prescription medications available at the pharmacy. With proper planning, someone like Mrs. Gand would have known that IV antinausea drugs given during chemotherapy usually wear off in 48 hours or less.

She and her oncologist could have then developed a plan to manage potential symptoms, including possibly using a prescription medication, such as *ondansetron* (Zofran) or *prochlorperazine* (Compazine), at home.

Helpful: If a cancer patient can't keep fluids down, IV fluids can sometimes be administered at the clinic where chemo is given so that an ER visit can be avoided.

What to do: Prior to chemo or any cancer treatment, ask your doctor to review any possible side effects—and what to do if any occur.

Important: White blood cell counts drop to their lowest point seven to 14 days after chemo, increasing susceptibility to infection. Knowing this ahead of time allows a cancer patient to take steps, including some of the tactics outlined in this article, to avoid a trip to a germ-laden ER during this crucial window.

Not all infections or fevers warrant hospitalization. If a cancer patient develops symptoms of an infection while at home, such as fever and/or chills, his/her oncologist may be able to see him the same day…or perhaps a colleague can squeeze him in. If you are ever unsure, you should always call your oncologist!

Exceptions: If fever, diarrhea or vomiting is accompanied by shortness of breath, racing heartbeat, stiff neck, new pain or altered mental status, call your doctor—you may have a potentially life-threatening infection known as sepsis. If your doctor is unavailable, head to the ER. When you arrive, say, "I have cancer and am concerned about infection and sepsis" to boost your odds of being seen more quickly.

***STRATEGY #2:* Check out local urgent care.** More oncology practices and hospitals are opening urgent-care clinics specifically for cancer patients, often with same-day appointments and extended hours.

What to do: Before starting treatment, ask your oncologist about alternative places to seek care so you're not scrambling for help should a problem arise. Ask if your oncology clinic offers same-day appointments for symptom management…or if it has an affiliated urgent-care center. Even if the oncology clinic can't accommodate you, some practices are affiliated with specific ERs, allowing for smoother exchange of medical information.

***STRATEGY #3:* Stay connected.** Simply relaying your symptoms to your doctor could keep you out of the ER and the hospital.

New study: Outpatient chemotherapy patients who got weekly e-mails encouraging them to report 12 common symptoms between appointments at Memorial Sloan Kettering Cancer Center in New York City fared better physically, mentally and emotionally than those who didn't get the messages. The patients also lived five months longer, on average.

Why did the e-mails help? They encouraged patients to proactively report side effects, which promotes faster treatment...and relief.

What to do: If your oncologist's office doesn't offer weekly e-mail or text check-ins or other telehealth options, craft a plan with your doctor where you agree to touch base with any unpleasant symptoms, perhaps via a secure online portal. You can also ask if there's a nurse available for such check-ins.

***STRATEGY #4:* Ask about palliative care.** Early palliative care, which focuses on relief from the symptoms and stress of a serious illness, enhances quality and duration of life for patients with chronic or end-stage cancer. Meeting with a palliative care physician early on—soon after diagnosis, ideally—can help ease pain, depression and more.

These specialists are usually covered by insurance and collaborate with you and your oncologist to keep you comfortable and out of the ER. A specialist isn't always necessary, though—most oncologists have some training in palliative care, too.

Important: Palliative care is not hospice. Hospice focuses on a person's final six months, when curative treatment is no longer possible. Palliative care can help nonterminal patients and is used in conjunction with treatment.

If You Had One HPV Cancer, You're More Likely to Get Others

Andrew Sikora, MD, PhD, associate professor of otolaryngology, and codirector of the Head and Neck Cancer Program at Baylor College of Medicine in Houston, Texas, and coauthor of the study titled "Trends in Risks for Second Primary Cancers Associated With Index Human Papillomavirus-Associated Cancers," published in *JAMA Network Open.*

It's scary enough that HPV—the very common human papillomavirus—can cause cervical, vaginal, vulvar, throat, anal and penile cancers. Now a study done at leading cancer centers across the US has found that having one of these HPV-related cancers puts patients at a higher risk for a second one. These are not instances of metastatic cancer (when the original cancer spreads to another area). They are new cancers in a different part of the body.

Why does this happen? The most likely answer is that the virus infects multiple places in the body at once...but it takes different lengths of time for each cancer to develop. Research has also found that some people have variations in their immune genes that make them more susceptible to HPV-associated cancers.

The study, which looked at the records of about 73,000 female and 40,000 male patients with an HPV-related cancer, showed that the risk for getting a second cancer has grown over the past four decades...and that the risk varies depending on where the first cancer was located. The risk of a second HPV-related cancer was greatest in people who initially had HPV-related throat (oropharyngeal) cancer. And if the original cancer was not throat cancer, the most likely second cancer was throat cancer. But risk for any of the HPV-related cancers was elevated.

Here's how you can protect yourself if you've already had one HPV-related cancer...

•**Be vigilant about getting all recommended cancer screenings.** A colonoscopy can find signs of HPV-related rectal or anal cancer. Cervical cancer screenings for women uncover suspicious lesions, often before they have the chance to turn into cancer. Because the area susceptible to this type of throat cancer includes the base of the tongue, tonsils and soft palate, your dentist can visually check for signs of cancer in these areas—ask for this if it's not already part of every visit. And see an otolaryngologist if you experience any of the possible symptoms of throat cancer such as a persistent sore throat, trouble swallowing or a lump in your throat, neck or the back of your mouth.

•**Talk to your doctor about the HPV vaccine.** In October 2018, the FDA extended its approval of Gardasil 9 for people up to age 45. Scientists are also investigating whether it makes sense for people with a history of an HPV-related cancer to be vaccinated against HPV. The prevailing theory has long been that people are exposed to HPV when they are young and then develop cancer later in life. But it could be that later infection as well as infection with a different strain of the virus is occurring more frequently than previously thought and that vaccination could prevent cancer in these situations.

On the horizon: Clinical trials are currently looking at whether HPV vaccination can prevent existing precancerous lesions from developing into cancer and whether certain versions of the vaccine can decrease both the recurrence of an HPV-related cancer and the development of a second one when given as part of cancer treatment.

Is Massage Really Safe for People with Cancer?

Susan G. Salvo, EdD, LMT, licensed massage therapist and instructor at the Louisiana Institute of Massage Therapy. She is author of two massage textbooks, *Massage Therapy: Principles and Practice* and *Mosby's Guide to Pathology for Massage Therapists*. SusanSalvo.com

---

Massage is an enjoyable experience and can play a major role in bringing comfort to someone who is going through the physical and emotional challenges of cancer recovery.

Some people have questioned the safety of massage due to a widely held misconception that massage can cause cancer to spread. But that's not true. In fact, the American Cancer Society and the National Comprehensive Cancer Network, a not-for-profit alliance of leading cancer centers, recommend the use of massage, as long as precautions (described below) are observed. Many cancer centers offer massage to their patients and teach massage to patient caregivers, including spouses and adult children.

Research has shown that massage reduces muscle tension and stiffness, pain and discomfort, anxiety, fatigue and shortness of breath in cancer patients. In addition, studies suggest that massage can decrease neuropathy, reduce nausea and vomiting and lessen lymphedema (swelling in an arm or leg) related to medical procedures such as chemotherapy, radiation therapy and surgery. In the research described above, the frequency of massage varied—study participants may have received a 30-minute massage once daily, biweekly or weekly.

People with cancer should seek out massage practitioners who have credentials beyond licensure such as national board certification and specialty training in oncology massage. To find such a massage therapist nearby check the database of the Society for Oncology Massage (s4om.org).

When a patient goes for a massage, he/she should inform the practitioner of his/her goals for massage therapy and the type of cancer the patient has (as well as any known tumor sites and metastases). The patient should also tell the massage therapist about the cancer treatments received, including surgery, side effects of those treatments and locations of any implanted devices, such as a port that is used to administer chemotherapy, intravenous fluids and blood transfusions. In addition, the patient should be sure to disclose any restrictions placed by the doctor. This may include, for example, lying in a semi-reclining position to promote ease of breathing or avoiding right-shoulder movements because of a recently implanted port on the right upper torso.

Important: Certain types of massage, such as hand and foot massage, are more appropriate for hospital or clinical settings, or for frail and elderly individuals. During subsequent appointments, the patient should notify the massage practitioner of any changes in treatment so that these can be factored into the massage therapy received. If prescribed by a health-care provider, insurance may cover the cost of massage for cancer patients, while some individuals use their health savings accounts to pay for these services.

Rosey Nasal Spray for Chemo Discomfort

Rose geranium spray has been found to relieve nasal vestibulitis, a common (and painful) chemotherapy side effect.

New study: Patients who used the herbal spray daily said that it reduced bleeding, dryness and other symptoms.

BMJ Supportive & Palliative Care.

CHAPTER 4

Cardiovascular Disease and Stroke

10 Small Changes for a Healthier Heart

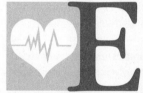

Every year, roughly 610,000 Americans die of heart disease. It is the leading cause of death in the US for both sexes. But there is good news. Research shows that even little shifts in diet and lifestyle can significantly boost your heart health.

Big bonus: Several require little or no effort. *Prominent cardiologist Dr. Joel Kahn suggests 10 surprising lifestyle tweaks that can make a big difference...*

1. Start fidgeting. Yes, you may have been told to sit still as a child, but that was then. Heart disease studies in the UK compared women who habitually sat still with women who regularly fidgeted (e.g., swinging legs, tapping toes, shifting weight) while seated. Over 12 years of follow-up, fidgeters developed heart disease significantly less frequently than women who sat still. Why? Fidgeting is a physical activity, and every bit of movement helps keep blood and oxygen circulating, even if you're glued to a computer all day.

Extra benefit: Little movements burn calories. Fidgeters generally burn around 300 extra calories per day. It's all about movement.

2. See a dentist. You probably already know that periodontal (gum) disease—which half of American adults have—means that you have two to three times greater risk for heart disease than people with healthy gums. But what you may not know is that patients with periodontitis who received treatment—such as special cleanings or, in more advanced cases, surgery—showed an improved cardiovascular risk profile. That's good news! What's the connection? Periodontal disease is a hidden source of inflammation and infection that can age the body, the brain and the heart. There is a growing connection between regular oral health checks and avoiding

Joel K. Kahn, MD, holistic cardiologist and clinical professor of medicine at Wayne State University School of Medicine in Detroit. Dr. Kahn lectures throughout the country on the body's ability to heal itself through proper nutrition. His latest book is *The Plant-Based Solution.* DrJoelKahn.com arterial and heart disease. Simply brushing twice a day and flossing daily, along with limiting sugary beverages and snacks, will reduce your risk significantly. Your dentist can tell you how often you need cleanings, based on your assessed risks for periodontal disease. Insurance usually covers two a year, but if you need more, it's an inexpensive investment in your health.

3. Add ground flaxseed to your food. Just two tablespoons of ground flaxseed a day sprinkled on your cereal, salad, yogurt, smoothie or other foods can make a healthy difference. Ground flaxseed, with its nutty taste, is packed with heart-healthy nutrients, including protein, fiber and omega-3 fatty acids. A meta-analysis of 15 trials published in *Clinical Nutrition* found significant reductions in both systolic blood pressure and diastolic blood pressure after regular supplementation with flaxseed powder or flaxseed oil. Drink lots of water to avoid possible digestive problems.

4. Drink two cups of hibiscus tea daily. The hibiscus plant is a significant source of antioxidants. Hibiscus tea tops the rankings for antioxidant power, even beating matcha (a drink made from powdered green tea leaves), according to NutritionFacts.org. Hibiscus tea also lowers cholesterol and blood pressure, according to a randomized controlled trial reported in *Journal of Human Hypertension*. At the end of the trial, 21% of participants had normalized their blood pressure. This brightly colored tea has a pleasantly tart, fruity taste, hot or cold.

5. Sit in a sauna. Scandinavians and others have sweated it out in the moist heat of saunas for centuries to soothe muscles and relax. But saunas offer other significant benefits as well. Studies from Japan (using dry sauna) and Finland (using wet sauna) demonstrate stronger hearts and longer lives. Why is the sauna experience so powerful? Research published in *Alternative Medicine Review* found that sauna users (with radiant heat or far-infrared units) received multiple health benefits including relief from COPD, chronic fatigue and chronic pain. Try sitting in a sauna at least once a week for 15 to 20 minutes per session.

6. Eat garlic daily. Garlic is a well-known immune system booster and antioxidant. It even can lower blood pressure and cholesterol. In studies at UCLA, aged black garlic extract helped maintain clean arteries in patients with metabolic syndrome by lowering the accumulation of plaque that can cause heart disease. Aged black garlic is available online, but you also can use regular garlic for heart-healthy benefits.

7. Walk barefoot in the grass. Believe it or don't, but growing evidence reveals that direct contact of your body with the earth (called grounding or earthing) helps your heart, eases inflammation and can create a healthier circulatory system. The connection helps reduce blood viscosity—elevated viscosity hinders delivery of oxygen to blood cells. Going barefoot 30 or 40 minutes a day may reduce cardiac events, according to *The Journal of Alternative and Complementary Medicine*. So shake your shoes off, and get your toes on the ground.

8. Give your digestive system a rest. Periodic and intermittent fasting has many benefits, including disease prevention. Studies show that practicing time-restricted eating for at least 12 hours a day (for example, fasting from 8 pm to 8 am) promotes healing and repair of the body. It's an obvious statement, but fasting for certain hours each day means that most people eat less. Fasting and its associated weight loss have been shown to lower blood pressure and reduce the risk for heart disease, diabetes and other diseases.

9. Stand for five minutes every half hour while awake. By now, most people have heard that being sedentary is an independent risk factor for heart disease and stroke. But did you know that this is true even if you exercise regularly? Moderate-to-vigorous physical activity in the morning or evening does not compensate for prolonged sitting, according to an American Heart Disease Scientific Statement. And yet Americans are sedentary for about six to eight hours a day—it's 8.5 to 9.6 hours for those age 60 and over. Move every half hour to help maintain healthy blood sugar and weight. Simply walk away from your desk or stand and stretch for a few minutes.

10. Get busy in bed. A study published in *The BMJ* from Caerphilly, Wales, followed the sex lives of 918 men ages 45 to 59 for 10 years.

The results indicate that frequent (twice a week or more) orgasmic activity can reduce the risk for heart attack by 50%. Research hasn't confirmed whether women would reap the same benefits, but it can't hurt to try.

---

6 Heart Disease Prevention Myths: About Aspirin, Omega-3s, Statins, More

Erin D. Michos, MD, MHS, associate director of preventive cardiology at Ciccarone Center for the Prevention of Heart Disease at The Johns Hopkins University School of Medicine in Baltimore.

Heart disease remains the number-one killer of both men and women in the US today, so prevention is paramount. But conflicting news stories make it tough to figure out what to do. Should you take a baby aspirin…a fish oil supplement…a statin? Since everyone is different, is the risk for some people actually overblown? *Here's what's true about preventing heart disease…what's false…and how to know what you should do…*

MYTH: **A baby aspirin a day keeps heart disease away.** A number of recent studies conducted at major medical research institutions have confirmed that most healthy people without known heart disease shouldn't be taking daily aspirin to prevent heart attacks. The ARRIVE trial looked at more than 12,500 men (age 55 or older) and women (age 60 or older) who were at moderate risk for heart attack, while the ASPREE study included more than 19,000 healthy, low-risk adults over age 65. Both studies were designed to determine whether a daily low-dose aspirin would prevent a first heart attack or stroke. Not only did the low-dose aspirin not reduce that risk in either study—it also increased the risk for major gastrointestinal bleeding. Even more alarming, in ASPREE, the group randomly assigned to take aspirin experienced more deaths from cancer.

Important: Aspirin still is recommended for patients who have had a heart attack already to prevent a second one. But if you're healthy and popping a daily aspirin, my advice is to ask your doctor about stopping your aspirin.

MYTH: **Over-the-counter omega-3 supplements prevent heart disease.** A recent review of major studies found that over-the-counter supplements did not reduce the risk for heart disease or stroke in the general population.

But one type of high-dose omega-3 prescription drug may help certain patients.

New research: The REDUCE-IT trial, conducted at Harvard Medical School, studied Vascepa, a purified form of eicosapentaenoic acid (EPA) given in a high dose (4,000 mg) to patients already treated with statins who were at high risk for cardiovascular disease or diabetes and who had high triglyceride levels. In early results, Vascepa reduced cardiovascular events such as heart attacks and strokes by 25% over five years. While this may turn out to be an effective prescription for certain patients, these results shouldn't prompt healthy people to take over-the-counter fish oil supplements.

MYTH: **The higher your level of HDL "good" cholesterol, the more protected you are from heart disease.** HDL is the so-called "good" cholesterol because it helps remove "bad" LDL cholesterol from your bloodstream. And studies have found that people with high HDL seem to have lower risk for heart disease. But new research casts doubt on whether it's truly protective.

Example: No drug therapies that boost HDL have been shown to reduce heart disease risk.

And too high a level of HDL actually may be harmful. Two recent studies have shown an association between very high levels of HDL (above 80 mg/dL) and increased heart attacks and death from all causes. We don't know why this is, but it may be that very high HDL indicates that your HDL is not functioning properly. Until more is known, focus on the heart disease risks that you can control, such as increasing physical activity, optimizing body weight and keeping triglycerides, LDL cholesterol, blood pressure and blood sugar under control.

MYTH: **If your cholesterol is too high, you need a statin.** Actually, some people with high cholesterol don't benefit from a statin—and some people with low cholesterol actually do. While high cholesterol, especially "bad" LDL cholesterol, is a major risk factor for heart disease, it's not the whole story. Many other factors matter—age, gender, race, blood pressure, family history and whether you smoke, have diabetes or are sedentary. So doctors evaluate your overall risk factors for heart disease to help determine whether to treat you with a statin. They do so by calculating your 10-year risk of having a heart attack or stroke. A score of 7.5% or higher means that a statin is "recommended"—whatever your cholesterol number.

Even if your score is 7.5% or higher, however, you still may not need a statin. Why? The calculator, developed by the American Heart Association and the American College of Cardiology, may overestimate risk, some studies find.

What to do: If your score is high, ask your doctor about a coronary artery calcium (CAC) scan, which detects calcium deposits in arterial plaque. If your CAC score is zero, there's no need for a statin. If it's high (typically 101 or above), that means you have a high risk for heart disease, and a statin generally is recommended. What if it's in the middle, between one and 100? That's a decision to make with your doctor, considering your other risk factors—along with your personal preference about whether you want to start taking a statin.

***MYTH:* Reducing inflammation is a healthy goal, but we don't know whether it will reduce heart disease risk.** Actually, we do. Cardiologists have suspected for some time that chronic inflammation—a state in which your immune system is in overdrive—can fuel the development of clogged arteries (atherosclerosis)…and trigger plaque to rupture and cause a heart attack. But we didn't know until recently whether tamping down inflammation could really help prevent heart attacks and strokes.

Now we know that it can. Last year, the CANTOS study, conducted at Brigham and Women's Hospital in Boston, showed that *canakinumab*, a type of drug called a monoclonal antibody that reduces inflammation, reduces the risk for a new heart attack or stroke by a significant 15% in people who already have had a heart attack.

While the drug still is experimental (and likely will be very expensive if/when it's FDA-approved), the good news is that we already know how to substantially reduce chronic inflammation with healthy habits. These include not smoking…keeping your waist size no more than 40 inches for men and 35 inches for women, regardless of your body weight…eating a Mediterranean-type diet…exercising regularly… getting six to eight hours of sleep every night (the sweet spot for heart health)…and reducing stress (meditation, yoga).

***MYTH:* Unless I have diabetes, my blood sugar levels won't affect heart health.** Blood sugar that's consistently even just a little above normal means that you have prediabetes. As a result, you're not only at greatly increased risk for diabetes but also heart disease. It's a wake-up call to improve your lifestyle, including weight loss (often losing 10 pounds is enough to bring blood sugar back to normal)…increasing dietary fiber… eliminating sugar-sweetened drinks and processed meats…and exercising. Simply by taking a 30-minute daily walk, you can reduce the risk that prediabetes will turn into diabetes by 30%.

Scuba Diver Heart Danger

Peter Buzzacott, PhD, director, injury monitoring and prevention, Divers Alert Network, and adjunct research fellow, School of Human Sciences, University of Western Australia, Crawley. He led a health analysis of nearly 114,000 scuba divers published in *European Journal of Preventive Cardiology*.

Aging scuba divers are at risk for underwater heart attacks. The initial screening for certification to scuba dive lasts for life, so divers, especially those over age 50, should pay special attention to maintaining a healthy cardiovascular system through proper diet, regular exercise, control of blood pressure and cholesterol, and annual physical exams. Recreational diving fatalities are rare, but the number involving cardiac issues is increasing.

MINOCA: The Heart Attack You've Never Heard Of

"Population-level incidence and outcomes of myocardial infarction with non-obstructive coronary arteries (MINOCA): Insights from the Alberta contemporary acute coronary syndrome patients invasive treatment strategies (COAPT) study," by Kevin R. Bainey, MD, assistant professor of medicine in the division of cardiology and colleagues at the University of Alberta in Edmonton, Canada, and published in *International Journal of Cardiology*.

You know the risk stemming from completely blocked arteries—heart attack. But did you know that a minor blockage is enough to cause a heart attack in some people…and that doctors tend to minimize the severity of this type of heart attack? Now, a recent study finds that there is definitely cause for concern, especially among women.

We're talking about MINOCA, the acronym for a myocardial infarction (heart attack) with non-obstructive coronary arteries, somewhat of a mystery compared to more common heart attacks…and under-researched…but dangerous.

Typically, MINOCA has been thought of, and treated, as a less serious type of heart attack. It's not unusual for MINOCA patients to be reassured and sent home from the hospital after experiencing one without the level of care prescribed to other heart attack victims and without a real focus on preventing another heart attack.

But when researchers at the University of Alberta in Canada reviewed the medical records of almost 36,000 patients admitted to hospitals for any type of heart attack, they found startling results…

•**Only 6% of these heart attack patients did not have blocked blood flow to the heart**—meaning their heart attacks were MINOCA. Yet, during the next five years, 11% of these MINOCA patients went on to have second heart attacks or died, showing just how strongly MINOCA can influence future health.

•**Only 25% of heart attack patients with blocked arteries were women,** but 50% of MINOCA patients were women.

•**Only about 40% of MINOCA patients were put on medications to prevent future heart attacks.** And women with MINOCA were likely to be treated with hormone replacement therapy—which does not help to reduce heart attack risk—or antidepressants instead.

•**The average age of MINOCA patients was 59,** about four years younger than for a blockage heart attack.

Although the exact cause of MINOCA remains a mystery, possibilities include a temporarily blocked artery due to a blood clot or a spasm of an artery due to atherosclerosis. In reality, people who get a MINOCA do have diseased coronary arteries. They may have plaques like other heart attack patients and some narrowing of a coronary artery but not enough to cause a complete blockage.

Why women are more affected by MINOCA remains another part of the mystery. Researchers suspect that female hormones may cause a weakening or dysfunction of the inside lining of heart arteries, making them more susceptible to atherosclerosis spasms, but more research needs to be done.

HOW TO PROTECT YOURSELF

Risk factors for MINOCA are similar to risk factors for other heart attacks—high blood pressure, high cholesterol, diabetes, smoking and a family history of heart attack. So, according to the American College of Cardiology, you can reduce your risk of MINOCA with the same heart-healthy lifestyle habits everyone should be following, such as eating healthy, staying active, managing stress and not smoking.

Also, keep in mind that a MINOCA heart attack can feel like any other heart attack with severe chest pain, but it doesn't have to—women, for example, often have milder symptoms such as shortness of breath, nausea, vomiting, dizziness and back or jaw pain. Man or woman, if you have these symptoms, call 911 right away.

The strongest takeaway from this eye-opening study concerns what to do if you do have a MINOCA heart attack: Treat it seriously and do not let your doctors do otherwise. Tell them about this article if that's what it takes. Then, the good news is that you should respond to the same prevention strategies used by people who have had more traditional types of heart attacks, including medications such as statins, beta-blockers and others. But if your doctor persists in telling you that your MINOCA was not that serious, get another opinion.

The Push-Up Clue to Heart Health

Study titled "Association Between Push-up Exercise Capacity and Future Cardiovascular Events Among Active Adult Men," led by researchers at Harvard T.H. Chan School of Public Health, Boston, published in *JAMA Network Open*.

You're not a couch potato. You do exercise regularly. But are you as physically fit as you think you are—enough to protect your heart? How many push-ups you can do might give you an important clue to your heart health.

Because physical activity is one of the best ways to prevent heart disease and prolong life, the American Heart Association urges doctors to check their patients' physical fitness as part of routine physical exams. However, in practice that usually means just asking patients how much they exercise—a predictably unreliable way to measure. Of course, doctors also use treadmill tests to assess cardiovascular fitness. But it's not part of every regular checkup, and it's also time-consuming and expensive. A recent study from Harvard's School of Public Health has found an accurate way to assess physical fitness that's also quick, easy—and free.

For the study, the researchers measured the exercise capacity of 1,000 active, healthy firefighters (average age 40)—who were slightly overweight on average but not obese—when they did push-ups and worked out on treadmills. They were then ranked by how many consecutive push-ups they could do…and for how long they could work out on a treadmill before reaching 85% of their maximum heart rate or were unable to continue (exercise tolerance). The men were followed for 10 years, noting the number of cardiovascular disease (CVD) events (diagnosis of coronary artery disease, heart failure or sudden cardiac death) that occurred.

Results: The more push-ups a man had been able to do at the start of the study, the lower his likelihood of having a CVD event during the following 10 years. Compared with men who had only been able to do 10 or fewer push-ups, those who had been able to do more than 40 had a 96% reduced risk for a CVD event over the 10 years of the study. In fact, of the 37 CVD events that occurred, only one was in a man who could do more than 40 push-ups, versus eight for men who could only do 10 or fewer. (Exercise tolerance on a treadmill also predicted CVD events, but not as directly as the number of push-ups.)

More research is needed to see if these results might apply to women, older men or less physically active adults.

In the meantime, why wait for your next doctor visit? Drop now and do some push-ups. If you struggle to reach even 10, let it be a wake-up call to improve your fitness!

Heart Attack Alert: Daylight Saving Time Can Be Hazardous to Your Health

Michael Terman, PhD, professor of clinical psychology at Columbia University, president of the Center for Environmental Therapeutics, New York City. He is author or coauthor of more than 90 scientific papers in leading medical journals and coauthor of *Reset Your Inner Clock: The Drug-Free Way to Your Best-Ever Sleep, Mood and Energy*.

At 2:00 am on Sunday, March 8, 2020, the US officially switches from Standard Time (ST) to Daylight Saving Time (DST)—you "spring forward" one hour. On November 1, 2020, the US switches from DST to ST—you "fall back" one hour.

Warning: These time changes can be dangerous to your health. *Researchers looked at the rate of heart attacks around the time switches—comparing the seven days right after the switches with the seven days two weeks before and two weeks after the switches…*

In spring there was a 5% to 10% increase in heart attacks during the three days after the switch to DST.

In fall there was a significant spike in heart attacks on the Monday after the switch to ST.

The researchers theorized that sleep disruption from switching the clock may hurt the heart by increasing the activity of the sympathetic nervous system, which speeds heart rate, and by increasing the level of cytokines, immune cells that spark inflammation and damage arteries.

Research also shows that the sleep-disturbing switches can cause other health-related problems, including insomnia, daytime fatigue, a decrease in daytime alertness and negative mood states, such as depression and anxiety.

We asked Michael Terman, PhD, one of the world's leading experts in this field, how to protect your health…

WHO IS MOST VULNERABLE?

Every person has an internal clock that matches wakefulness and sleepiness with the day-night cycle—a phenomenon called circadian rhythm. The science of how circadian rhythm affects health is called chronobiology—and it has shown that each person has a genetically determined chronotype.

"Owls" are chronotypes that usually go to sleep very late and have difficulty waking up in the morning for a normal workday.

"Larks" feel sleepy at a so-called normal hour of the night (such as 10:00 pm) and wake up easily in the morning.

The vast majority of the population is somewhere in between an owl and a lark. But about 10% of the population are owls—and they have far more difficulty adjusting to time switches than larks. Owls are more likely to suffer from switch-caused health problems in the days and even weeks afterward.

If you're not sure whether you're an owl or a lark—or somewhere in between—go to the Center for Environmental Therapeutics (CET.org). On the home page, under the pull down "Assessments," choose "Automated Online Confidential Self-Assessments"…then click on "Your Circadian Rhythm Type," which will open the "Automated-Morningness-Eveningness Questionnaire." The 19 questions take about five to 10 minutes to answer, after which you will receive detailed feedback about your likely chronotype.

PROTECT YOURSELF

If you're an owl, there are many ways to modulate your internal clock so that you're less vulnerable to health problems from the sudden time switches…

•**Gradually set the alarm later.** For the fall switch from DST to ST, your goal is to allow your circadian clock to drift one hour later during the week or so after the switch.

If you typically wake up to an alarm clock at 7:00 am, set the alarm for 6:00 am ST on the Sunday morning of the switch, which is when you'll be inclined to wake up anyway. Over the next six days, set your clock 10 minutes later each day until you arrive at 7:00 am ST.

Reverse this process in the spring, starting six days before the ST to DST switch. Set the alarm 10 minutes earlier each day so that you arrive smoothly at 7:00 am DST on Sunday morning.

•**Exercise daily.** Daily aerobic exercise helps stabilize the circadian system, preventing an owl's tendency to go to sleep later and later. It will help manage both time switches. But avoid aerobic exercise in the hours right before sleep, which can cause insomnia.

To help with the spring transition: As soon as the sun starts to rise after 7:00 am, take a brisk 20-minute walk outside right after you wake up, to jump-start your day. This is the best measure owls can take to prevent health problems caused by the March transition from ST to DST.

•**Eat regular meals.** Owls rarely feel hungry when they first wake up, so they skip breakfast. They then eat a big meal around 1:00 pm and tend to eat again late at night.

Best: Eat breakfast within a half-hour of waking, eat lunch around noon and finish dinner before 8 pm. This helps normalize your circadian rhythm.

•**Take melatonin—the right way.** Melatonin, a hormone produced by the pineal gland in the brain, helps control wakefulness and sleepiness. It's usually not detectable in the blood at midday but begins to rise in the evening, about two to three hours before you feel sleepy.

In the general population, there is a six-hour spread between the average times that melatonin rises. If you're an owl, you tend to have a late onset—in some cases, as late as 1:00 am, so you don't feel sleepy until about 3:00 am. To decrease vulnerability to the time shift, an owl needs to feel sleepy earlier and can do that by taking a melatonin supplement.

Most people who take melatonin mismanage it, taking it like a sleeping pill, 30 to 45 minutes before bedtime. But by that hour, the brain has already started to produce the hormone, and the additional supplement has little effect.

Better: Take a very small amount of melatonin—0.25 milligrams (mg)—five hours before your desired bedtime, starting a week before the springtime switch to DST. Your circadian clock will sense that nighttime has begun and will adjust itself toward earlier sleep onset. Move the melatonin earlier as your sleep adjusts earlier, then stop it when you reach your goal.

After taking melatonin, remain in dim, indoor light because bright, fluorescent light or outdoor light reverses the effect. Also, refrain from intense physical exercise.

•**Use a "dawn simulator."** You can adjust your circadian rhythm using a sophisticated device that plugs into your light fixture and "simulates" the outdoor transition from a starlight level of light to a sunrise level of light. The device allows you to gradually move "dawn" later in the day during the week or so *after* the "fall backward" switch to ST, and later in the day during the week or so *before* the switch to DST.

The subtly intensifying light passes through your eyelids, entraining your internal clock to the time you want to start your day—no matter what is happening outdoors.

Resource: You can order a Smart Lamp Dawn Simulator at CET.org.

Cost: $85.

To read more about daylight saving time versus standard, including a humorous perspective, check out "Sleep and Time Around the World and In Our Own Backyards" on the CET site.

Turn Up Your Thermostat

Stephen Jivraj, PhD, associate professor in quantitative science, epidemiology and public health, University College London, UK.

For every one-degree decrease in indoor temperature reading, there was a 0.48 point rise in systolic (top number) blood pressure readings and a 0.45 point rise in diastolic (bottom number). This study, based on nearly 5,000 people in their homes, may help explain the spike in hypertension rates in the winter.

To help prevent winter increases in blood pressure: Keep the inside of your home at a minimum temperature of 69.8°F, particularly if you have hypertension or a family history of heart disease.

Safe Cooking to Lower Blood Pressure

Gang Liu, PhD, postdoctoral research fellow at Harvard T.H. Chan School of Public Health, Boston.

How meat, poultry and fish are cooked is linked to high blood pressure. People who cook red or white meats more than 15 times per month by grilling, broiling or roasting have a 17% higher chance of developing high blood pressure later on, compared with those who eat meat cooked this way fewer than four times per month. Minimize the amount and frequency of meats cooked by open-flame and high-temperature methods.

What's Coffee Doing to Your Blood Pressure?

Mark C. Houston, MD, associate clinical professor of medicine, Vanderbilt University School of Medicine, and director of the Hypertension Institute at Saint Thomas West Hospital, both in Nashville. He is author of *What Your Doctor May Not Tell You About Hypertension*. Hyper tensionInstitute.com

---

A cup of brewed coffee contains about 100 mg of caffeine, a stimulant that helps us feel more alert in the morning, but it also increases heartbeat and temporarily raises blood pressure. Once the caffeine passes out of your system, which usually takes about five hours or so, your blood pressure should go down.

Some people, however, are more sensitive to the effects of caffeine, whether it be in coffee, energy drinks or certain foods such as chocolate. Caffeine is metabolized in the liver by the CYP1A2 enzyme. *We are genetically programmed to metabolize caffeine in one of two ways…*

•**Rapid metabolizers,** about 45% of the population, can consume up to 400 mg of caffeine (about four cups of brewed coffee) daily with little effect on blood pressure—even in the short term.

•**Slow metabolizers,** about 55% of the population, have very low CYP1A2 activity. Their blood pressure will stay elevated for up to four to five hours. These people also may have tachycardia (fast heart rate) and increased adrenaline levels, which can cause the jitters and wakefulness.

Caffeine sensitivity also tends to increase with age, since the CYP1A2 enzyme works less efficiently as we grow older. Women tend to be more sensitive to the effects of caffeine than men, since estrogen slows CYP1A2 activity.

The only way to know for sure is to have the genetic test CardiaX, which is available from Vibrant America Labs (Vibrant-America.com).

If you think that you're caffeine sensitive, talk to your doctor about the effects of caffeine on your blood pressure, and ask whether it makes sense to cut down on your coffee (and tea—most non-herbal varieties, including green tea and white tea, also contain caffeine!) or switch to decaf.

Why Measure Blood Pressure in Both Arms

Deepak L. Bhatt, MD, MPH, executive director of Interventional Cardiovascular Programs, Brigham and Women's Hospital Heart & Vascular Center, and professor of medicine, Harvard Medical School, both in Boston.

While you might think that a single blood pressure reading is enough for the blood pressure of your whole body, that's not the whole story. Blood pressure readings can differ from arm to arm—and if that difference is significant, it can indicate a likelihood of serious health problems.

Whether you're measuring at home or a health-care professional is taking the readings, it's a good idea to periodically compare the numbers from both arms at least once a year. If there's a significant difference—20 points or more in the systolic (upper) number of your reading—it could mean that you have plaque blocking an artery in your arm.

Plaque buildup in an arm artery is a sign of peripheral artery disease (PAD), a painful and potentially debilitating vascular condition that can lead to claudication, where the narrowed arteries limit blood flow to muscles, especially during exercise.

But that's not all. Plaque buildup in an arm makes it much more likely that you also have plaque in other arteries in your body—including in your heart and brain—putting you at higher risk for heart attack and stroke. In fact, one study found a 38% increased risk for heart attack when the difference in systolic blood pressure between arms was 10 points or more.

If you do find that your blood pressure differs by 10 points or more between arms when you're checking it at home, you should let your doctor know—and continue to monitor it in both arms whenever you check your blood pressure. If, on the other hand, the pressure in both arms is about the same (less than 10 points difference), there's no need to take readings from both arms every time…checking both arms once a year is likely sufficient. And if the periodic check shows that the difference between readings from both arms is climbing, then switch to monitoring both arms—and alert your doctor.

Another good reason to check both arms at least once in a while is to make sure that you get the correct treatment protocol. Treatment decisions, such as whether to start blood pressure medications, should be based on the higher reading. Usually, blood pressure is considered high (and requires medication) if it is at least 140 mmHg systolic/90 mmHg diastolic. But some doctors recommend lifestyle changes for blood pressure greater than 120 mmHg/80 mmHg.

How to take blood pressure at home: The American Heart Association (AHA) recommends using an automatic upper-arm cuff-style monitor. Sit on a chair with your feet flat on the floor. (If your feet don't comfortably reach the floor, use something to raise them, such as a few books.) The arm you're going to use should be supported on a flat surface, such as a table, with the upper arm at heart level. Wait at least five minutes before starting to take your blood pressure. Take two or three readings one minute apart at the same time every day. Write down the results or upload them to a website, such as this online blood pressure tracker from the AHA (Heart.org).

Air Filter for Your Heart

Masako Morishita, PhD, researcher at Michigan State University, East Lansing, and first author of the research published in *JAMA Internal Medicine*.

When study subjects (average age 67) used commercially available, portable HEPA filtration units (costing less than $70 each) at home, they experienced a small but significant decrease in blood pressure—which, if maintained long term, could be enough to decrease cardiovascular events by 16%. HEPA filters remove fine-particulate-matter pollution from the air.

Lowering Your LDL Cholesterol: How Low Should You Go?

Antonio M. Gotto, MD, DPhil, cardiovascular disease specialist. The study "Efficacy and Safety of Further Lowering of Low-Density Lipoprotein Cholesterol in Patients With Very Low Levels: A Meta-analysis" was led by researchers at Brigham and Women's Hospital and Harvard Medical School and published in *JAMA Cardiology*.

Regardless of the drug used, when it comes to LDL cholesterol, the big question is, how low should a given person go? And related—does going lower because of drugs start to present a safety risk at some point?

For example, according to a recent study out of Harvard Medical School and Brigham and Women's Hospital that reviewed four large statin and non-statin drug trials involving people with cardiovascular disease, reducing LDL from 70 mg/dL to 30 mg/dL reduced cardiovascular events by 20%, in essence doubling the benefits found in previous statin-only studies. And this was equally true for statins and statins plus the new type of biologic drug called PCSK9 inhibitors or other nonstatin drugs. This demonstrates that people who can't take or don't benefit from statins can get statinlike benefits from PCSK9 inhibitors. This includes people with very high LDL due to an inherited condition called familial hypercholesterolemia—for many of these people, heart attack risk remains high even with statin therapy.

Not every question has been answered. Most importantly, the "best" low LDL level really hasn't been determined, and yet studies like this one may lead doctors to push for lower and lower levels. Indeed, new guidelines for cholesterol management are being worked on by the American Heart Association and the American College of Cardiology. They could include a drop in what's considered a healthy LDL level to below 70 mg/dL now that it's been shown this can be achieved without incremental side effects—but there are still existing side effects from statins.

Also, consider that the latest study took place over about two years, so any longer-term risks of taking doses that are higher than what's currently being prescribed are as yet unknown—remember that it took 20 years to find out that statins can increase the risk for type 2 diabetes.

For now, talk to your doctor to better understand your personal risk for cardiovascular disease, heart attack and stroke. If a statin is not reducing your LDL to a safe level or if its adverse effects are interfering with your life, a PCSK9 inhibitor could be for you if you have established heart disease or are in a high-risk category. But in terms of going to new lower levels of LDL, regardless of the drug you take to get there, you need to weigh the unknowns as well as the benefits.

There's one more important caution: No drug can fully compensate for not making lifestyle changes to reduce LDL, and they bear repeating…

- **A diet low in saturated and trans fats**
- **Weight management**
- **Physical activity**
- **Stress reduction**
- **Not smoking**

Triglycerides: The Heart Threat You Should Not Ignore

Michael D. Ozner, MD, medical director, Center for Prevention and Wellness, Baptist Health South Florida, Miami, and author of *Heart Attack Proof* and *The Complete Mediterranean Diet*.

When it comes to heart disease risk, most people are aware of the threat high cholesterol poses—in fact, nearly one in three American adults over age 40 takes medication to help control his/her cholesterol… and new guidelines were recently announced to provide better cholesterol management.

What you may not know: According to the latest research, high triglycerides are just as threatening to your heart. But unfortunately, they're frequently downplayed by doctors and their patients.

Background: In prehistoric times, triglycerides (fats, also called lipids, in the blood) were a way for our hunter-gatherer ancestors to store fat—a must when food was sparse and famine common. But the stored fat that saved our ancestors from starvation is killing us now.

Fatty, sugary food is superabundant, and we eat too much of it. As a result, more than 70% of adults in the US are overweight or obese—which means they're storing harmful amounts of triglycerides that increase risk for cardiovascular disease.

Up until now, scientists had not proven that lowering triglycerides also lowers the risk for cardiovascular disease…

Important new finding: In a study published in *The New England Journal of Medicine*, researchers looked at more than 8,000 patients with heart disease, diabetes and other risk factors for heart attack and stroke. All participants were taking a statin, and their low-density lipoprotein (LDL) "bad" cholesterol was at a healthy level (below 100 mg/dL). However, they still had high triglyceride levels.

Adding a triglyceride-lowering drug to their regimen—4 g of *icosapent ethyl* (Vascepa), a highly purified fish oil that delivers the healthful omega-3 fatty acid EPA—lowered triglycerides by 20% compared with a placebo. Over the six-year study, first-time heart attacks were reduced by 31% and strokes by 28%, and there were 20% fewer deaths from cardiovascular disease in patients taking the triglyceride-lowering drug. Additionally, the level of C-reactive protein, a biomarker for artery-damaging inflammation, was reduced by an average of 20%.*

In follow-up research, the results were even better—there was a 30% reduction in the combined rate of first as well as second and subsequent cardiovascular deaths, nonfatal heart attacks or strokes, procedures such as stenting and hospitalization for unstable angina.

*The research was sponsored by Amarin, the manufacturer of Vascepa.

Bottom line: The higher your level of triglycerides, the higher your risk for cardiovascular disease. Based on this new research, lowering high triglycerides will likely become standard practice to curb risk for and treat cardiovascular disease.

GET YOUR LEVELS TESTED

A normal triglyceride level is generally below 150 mg/dL. But research shows that about one-third of Americans have triglycerides in the danger zone—150 mg/dL and above.

To get your levels tested: Your doctor should order a blood test to measure all blood fats that impact the heart, including total cholesterol, LDL cholesterol, HDL cholesterol and triglycerides. Apolipoprotein B levels, which measure the number of potentially harmful particles that carry cholesterol and triglycerides, are often measured as well. The frequency of testing depends on the age and cardiovascular risk of the patient.

While triglyceride levels have previously been measured in standard blood tests, doctors didn't realize their importance in the treatment of cardiovascular disease.

If your triglycerides are high…

Several classes of medications can raise triglyceride levels.

For example: Beta-blockers and diuretics (used for high blood pressure)…estrogen (for menopause)…retinoic acid and retinoids (for psoriasis and other skin problems)…and bile acid sequestrants (used mainly for lowering cholesterol). If you're taking any of these drugs and your triglycerides are high, your doctor may change the dose or prescribe an alternative drug.

Other risk factors for high triglycerides that your doctor should check for include prediabetes and diabetes, kidney disease, thyroid disorder and a family history of very high triglycerides. If an underlying condition is treated, high triglycerides can be resolved.

If the above causes have been ruled out, under the guidance of your doctor and for the amount of time he/she suggests, try the triglyceride-lowering lifestyle plan that follows. This healthy plan is also a good way to help protect against developing high triglycerides.

•**Eat a Mediterranean diet.** The main reason for high triglycerides is a poor diet—namely one that emphasizes processed foods, trans fats (found in baked goods and fried foods), saturated fat (found in meat and dairy products) and sugar and refined starches. Your best strategy is to eliminate or minimize your intake of all these types of foods.

To keep triglycerides under control, I favor the Mediterranean diet, which is rich in vegetables, fruits, whole grains, beans, nuts and seeds, fish and olive oil. In a study published in *Journal of Nutrition*, people who followed a Mediterranean diet for six months had a significant reduction in triglycerides compared with people who ate their usual diet.

•**Exercise regularly.** Regular exercise lowers triglycerides…LDL cholesterol…inflammation…and stress hormones. It also helps control weight, a risk factor for high triglycerides. To start, aim for 20 minutes of moderate exercise (like brisk walking), three to five times a week. Over time, increase to at least 30 minutes, five times weekly. In a recent study published in *Journal of Clinical Lipidology*, daily 30-minute walks lowered triglycerides.

•**Get seven to eight hours of sleep every night.** A new animal study from Japan and published in *American Journal of Physiology-Endocrinology and Metabolism* shows that sleep deprivation increases triglycerides. In a similar study, people with sleep apnea—a disorder in which breathing repeatedly stops during sleep—had higher triglycerides than those without this sleep condition. Sleep apnea is linked to increased cardiovascular disease and is best treated with a continuous positive airway pressure (CPAP) device. See a sleep specialist for advice.

•**Discuss medication.** If the lifestyle measures above don't adequately lower your triglyceride levels, talk to your physician about medication, such as a statin, fibrate and/or the prescription omega-3 fatty acid

•**Vascepa.** It's currently FDA-approved only for patients with triglycerides of 500 mg/dL and above (this level can cause pancreatitis, a potentially life-threatening disease that must be treated). Given the new clinical trial data with Vascepa, it is likely that it will soon be FDA-approved for people at high risk for cardiovascular disease who have well-controlled

LDL cholesterol on statin therapy but continue to have triglyceride levels of 150 mg/dL and above.

Note: Vascepa is pharmaceutical grade and is not the same as the omega-3 fish oil supplements that you can buy in the store.

This study's findings show that eczema must now be considered a risk factor for heart disease. That means people with eczema need to start reducing their risk of heart disease as soon as possible and with more vigorous effort than someone without eczema might.

Eczema Can Kill You in a Surprising Way: Heart Disease

Study titled "Severe and predominantly active atopic eczema in adulthood and long term risk of cardiovascular disease: population based cohort study," led by researchers at London School of Hygiene and Tropical Medicine, published in *BMJ*.

Researchers studied the medical records of more than 387,000 adults with eczema. Compared to an age-matched group of adults without eczema, in general the people with eczema had a 10% to 20% higher risk of developing heart disease over a period of about five years. That's worrisome enough—but the risk rose considerably more for those with very active or severe eczema.

For the study, active eczema meant that symptoms were active 50% or more of the time during the course of the study…and severe eczema meant that a patient had been referred to a specialist or had received treatment with an immune suppressing drug or phototherapy. *Those with active or severe eczema had…*

•**A 20% higher risk for stroke** than people without eczema

•**A 40% to 50% higher risk for angina,** heart attack, atrial fibrillation or death from heart disease

•**A 70% percent higher risk of heart failure.**

WHAT'S THE CONNECTION?

Eczema, sometimes called atopic dermatitis, the most common type, is a disease of inflammation, and the same inflammation that affects your skin can and does affect the rest of your body, including your heart.

Think You're Having a Heart Attack? How Chest Pain Is Evaluated in the ER

Case study titled "Improving Emergency Department Care for Low-Risk Chest Pain" by researchers at Kaiser Permanente Southern California and Oregon Health and Sciences University, published in *New England Journal of Medicine Catalyst*.

Chest pain is the number-two reason people go to the emergency department (stomach pain is number one). While the vast majority of patients are not having a heart attack, the process for ruling out a heart attack can involve extensive testing and a hospital stay. *But there's a better approach now gaining traction in the US—one that was developed more than a decade ago in the Netherlands…*

THE "HEART" OF THE MATTER

For some patients, symptoms along with results from blood tests and an electrocardiogram (EKG) provide indisputable proof that a heart attack has occurred or is occurring. But, for many others, these first tests are inconclusive. It's then up to the ER doctor to make a judgment call about next steps to further investigate what's then termed "low-risk chest pain."

In the US, most patients with low-risk chest pain wind up being admitted to the hospital for observation and further testing, such as a cardiac stress test, to be certain that a heart attack wasn't missed. Yet the "miss rate," or amount of heart attacks that were missed, is just 2.1% of these patients. That means that nearly all of them are having unnecessary and expensive procedures.

As hospitals try to use evidence-based guidelines to improve cost and quality of care, some emergency departments are starting to use the Dutch-developed 10-point scoring system called HEART, an evidence-based, decision-making tool designed to reduce miss rates and unnecessary admissions. (A "miss" is defined as any patient sent home without a diagnosis of heart attack and who went on to have a heart event in the following 30 days.) HEART is an acronym for the five markers that are evaluated—history, EKG, age, risk factors and troponin.

This is how the scoring works…

History: Patients are given 2 points if they have high-risk symptoms such as heavy chest pain, sweating, nausea and vomiting, relief after taking nitroglycerin or pain that gets worse with exertion…1 point if the chest pain is sharp rather than heavy and is not accompanied by other symptoms…and 0 if symptoms are mostly low-risk for heart attack.

EKG: Patients are given 2 points if they have signs of decreased blood flow and other changes…1 point if there are EKG changes that are not specifically indicative of heart disease…and 0 if normal.

Age: Patients are given 2 points if 65 or older …1 point if between 45 to 64…and 0 if under 45.

Risk factors: Patients are given 2 points if they have a history of coronary heart disease, peripheral artery disease, stroke or three or more heart attack risk factors such as obesity, diabetes, high blood pressure, high cholesterol or a family history of heart disease…1 point for one or two of these risk factors…and 0 for no risk factors.

Troponin: Troponin, a protein involved in muscle contraction, is measured with a blood test. It can signal heart muscle damage. Patients are given 2 points for a high troponin level…1 point if it is borderline…and 0 if it is within the normal range.

A score that totals 0 to 3 means there's low risk for heart attack, and patients are likely to be sent home and told to follow up with their primary care provider.

A score of 4 to 6 signals moderate risk, and patients will be admitted for observation and possible cardiac stress testing.

A score of 7 to 10 is high risk, and these patients are admitted to the hospital and referred to a cardiologist for treatment.

THE US GETS HEART SMART

While there have been a few other scoring systems available to doctors, international studies have consistently shown that HEART outperforms them all.

Kaiser Permanente Southern California, a large health-care organization, decided to adopt HEART at 14 of its area hospitals and review the results. An analysis of all 12,000 patients given HEART scoring found that, rather than the expected 2.1% miss rate, it was just 0.18%. Drilling down even further, among the subgroup of patients with low HEART scores who were sent home without a hospital admission, the miss rate was only 0.09%. The results were so positive that Kaiser Permanente plans to adopt the system in other areas of the country that it serves. It may be coming to an ER near you.

Important: If you experience chest pain, always assume it's a medical emergency and call 911. Don't try to diagnose yourself with HEART or any other system, and never drive yourself to the ER.

Is the FDA Approving Dangerous Heart Devices?

Rita F. Redberg, MD, cardiologist, the director of women's cardiovascular services, University of California, San Francisco School of Medicine, and coauthor of the research letter "Assessment of Clinical Trial Evidence for High-Risk Cardiovascular Devices Approved Under the Food and Drug Administration Priority Review Program," published in *JAMA Internal Medicine*.

You've probably heard stories about patients asking the FDA to fast-track new treatments, whether for cancer or diseases such as Parkinson's. But there's a dangerous flip side to quickie approvals, and it's nowhere more evident than with heart devices designed to correct life-threatening conditions.

Overall, 14 of 29 devices approved via a "priority" or fast-track reviewing process between 2007 and 2017 were for high-risk cardiovascular devices, named because of the high-risk nature of the heart conditions they're supposed to treat. But "high risk" could very well apply to some of the devices themselves, according to a research letter from doctors at University of California, San Francisco.

WHEN FASTER ISN'T BETTER

The researchers looked at the clinical trials the FDA used to approve the 14 heart devices, which included stents, heart valves, balloon catheters and implantable defibrillators. *What they found was disturbing…*

•**None of the trials showed whether patients who received the devices did better** than those who received placebo procedures or placebo devices.

•**The number of people in the studies averaged about 500,** and the time they were followed was about 15 months. When it comes to trials in general, these are considered small and short.

•**In most of the trials, the primary objective, or "end point," was something other (read: lesser) than long-term survival** or improved quality of life. For example, an end point might have been merely "non-inferiority," meaning the device was only as good as other devices already available…no better!

•**Two of the 14 devices needed to be re-reviewed** after approval because the FDA realized it needed more information.

•**As of May 2018, six of the 14 devices had safety recalls.** In two of the recalls, the FDA said the devices were likely to cause "serious health consequences or death." In the other recalls, the devices were said to be likely to cause "reversible adverse health consequences."

Important: Recalls do not always result in a device being removed from the market—often there are other versions of the same device that remain on the market.

•**Data from "post-approval studies" for devices,** an important part of the FDA's priority review to make sure a device is safe and effective, is often slow to be collected—if it's collected at all—and not always publicly available. For its part, as of June 2018, the FDA had failed to impose any penalties on any device manufacturers for failing to complete a post-approval study.

These findings are particularly alarming because most of these devices are permanently implanted in patients. Having another operation to remove a problem device exposes patients to risks from surgery itself.

The University of California research letter recommends changes to the FDA priority approval process such as longer clinical trials with more subjects, making primary end points more meaningful to patients, such as improved survival and quality of life, and mandated periodic reviews of these new devices for safety and efficacy.

What should you do if your doctor recommends an implanted device for a high-risk cardiac condition for you or a loved one?

Ask your doctor the following questions: How long has the device been on the market? Are there data to support its approval from at least one randomized clinical trial that measured meaningful outcomes? Were the patients similar to me? (For instance, many device trials enroll mostly younger white men, while women and an ethnically diverse population are not well represented.) If your other treatment options seem inadequate, even a nonoptimal answer to one or more of the above questions might not knock a device out of reasonable consideration. But just exploring these questions helps you make a much more informed decision among all your treatment options.

Also ask whether your doctor has any financial relationship with the device manufacturer—if so, it's a sign that he or she may not be an unbiased source of information.

Cup of Joe OK with AFib

Analysis by researchers at Baker Heart and Diabetes Institute, Melbourne, Australia, of 11 studies on caffeine and arrhythmia, published in *JACC: Clinical Electrophysiology.*

Coffee is safe for heart-rhythm-disorder patients in most cases. Many doctors advise patients with arrhythmia to avoid caffeine, but a recent study shows that regular intake of about 300 milligrams of caffeine—about the amount in three cups of coffee—does not usually trigger arrhythmia. Caffeine also may be safely consumed in tea or other caffeinated beverages. But talk to your doctor, because there are individual differences in reactions to caffeine, and some people may have arrhythmias triggered by it.

You Can Have an MRI Even with an Older Pacemaker

Article titled "Expanding access to magnetic resonance imaging for patients with cardiac rhythm devices," by Collin Culbertson, MD, and Carl Gold, MD, MS, Stanford University, California, published online in *JAMA Neurology.*

If you have one of the newer pacemakers or defibrillators and need an MRI scan, no problem. However, most people who have such devices have the older kind—and are told that an MRI scan is off-limits. So you might be surprised to learn that for years it's been known that you can safely get an MRI scan even if you have an older device—but not everyone who should get this potentially lifesaving imaging is getting it.

The concern about MRI scans with such devices is that the strong magnetic fields used by MRI machines could disrupt the implanted devices' electrical circuits...pull their metal-tipped electrical wires (leads) out of position...and/or overheat the metal and cause damage to surrounding tissue. *Research has shown otherwise, though...*

•**A 2011 study from Johns Hopkins** used a protocol developed at Johns Hopkins and involved 438 people with cardiac implantable electronic devices (CIEDs). They found very low risk of device malfunctioning, moving, heating or causing abnormal heart rhythm.

•**A 2017 study from researchers at Intermountain Medical Center Heart Institute** in Salt Lake City found "not a single problem requiring remediation" in 212 MRIs done on 178 patients with CIEDs.

Furthermore, in 2017, guidelines were published by the Heart Rhythm Society, an international organization of medical and science professionals, with specific protocols that allow MRIs to be safely done with both kinds of CIEDs—newer "conditional" ones and older "nonconditional" or "legacy" ones.

MRI—which stands for magnetic resonance imaging—is the best way to diagnose certain problems in soft tissue areas such as the brain, heart and other internal organs—a diagnosis that can be lifesaving. If you have an older pacemaker or defibrillator, it's smart to find out now—even if you don't have an MRI scheduled—whether your hospital or medical center is set up to give you an MRI. If not, ask what other facility near you could do it.

What's Your Stroke Risk If You Have AFib?

Enrique D. Garcia-Sayan, MD, assistant professor of cardiovascular medicine at the McGovern Medical School at University of Texas and director of echocardiography and associate chief of cardiology at LBJ General Hospital, both in Houston. Study titled "Reassessment of Risk for Stroke During Follow-up of Patients with Atrial Fibrillation" by researchers from National Yang-Ming University in Taipei, Taiwan, and University of Liverpool, UK, published in *Annals of Internal Medicine.*

The main danger of living with atrial fibrillation, or AFib, is that it increases your risk for stroke. With AFib, an irregular (often too-fast) heartbeat causes blood to pool in the left atrial appendage (an upper chamber of the heart), where it can form into a clot that can travel to the brain and cause a stroke.

At the same time, AFib is the number one preventable cause of stroke. Taking a blood-thinning medication called an oral anticoagulant can prevent clots from forming. But there is a downside…anticoagulants can increase your risk for significant bleeding by about 2% to 4% per year. The challenge is to figure out for whom the benefit of taking these drugs outweighs the risk.

To do this, doctors use a scoring system called CHA2DS2-VASc (you can simply say "chad-vasc") that assigns points for various stroke risk factors. *Give yourself one point for each of these characteristics that applies to you…*

- **Congestive heart failure.**
- **Hypertension.**
- **Diabetes.**
- **A history of vascular disease.**
- **Being a woman.**
- **Being between the ages of 65 and 74.**

And two points for the following…

- **Having a history of stroke or transient ischemic attack** (TIA, often called a ministroke).
- **Being age 75 or over.**

People who score zero have no increased yearly stroke risk due to AFib. The yearly risk for a score of one is just under 1%, and the risk increases as your score goes up.

The American Heart Association and other organizations recommend considering aspirin (a medication that prevents blood platelets from clotting) or an anticoagulant (a blood thinner) for anyone with a score of one. Anyone with a score of two or higher is a definite candidate for an oral anticoagulant. *But there are two steps to take to make sure that your CHA2DS2-VASc is as useful as possible…*

- **Recheck your score every year.** Scores change over time, especially as people age. In fact, a study of about 14,600 people newly diagnosed with AFib found that patients initially considered low-risk according to CHA2DS2-VASc and not prescribed an anticoagulant had about a 40% risk of moving into a high-risk range within three years. Within a single year after diagnosis, 16% of the patients in the study had added at least one point to their score.
- **Have your doctor individualize your score.** There are some gray areas in the scoring

system, notably for people with a score of one. For example, if you scored one point only because you're a woman—and you have no other risk factors, taking an anticoagulant might convey more risk than benefit. On the other hand, if you have a score of one and are just one year shy of age 65 or 75, the benefit may outweigh the risk. Similarly, the risk of bleeding is not the same in every patient, and this can be estimated by your doctor by using a different assessment called the HAS-BLED score. These variations are perfect examples of why treatment should be personalized.

If you have AFib, the best decision for you will come from a discussion of drug risks and benefits with your doctor and some shared decision-making.

Important if you take fish oil/omega-3 supplements: Fish oil is not an anticoagulant and should not be used as a substitute for one if you have AFib. That being said, there is much controversy about the perceived increased risk of bleeding in patients taking fish oil for other health reasons. Though high doses of omega-3 fatty acids including fish oil may increase bleeding time, clinically significant bleeding has not been clearly demonstrated in studies of people who were on anticoagulants and took these supplements, nor has evidence been found of increased risk of bleeding or serious adverse events with the addition of fish oil. So, once again, the recommendation is for individualized decision-making and discussion with your physician about whether the benefits of continuing fish oil supplements when starting an anticoagulant outweigh the still-unproved risk of bleeding.

It should be noted, however, that nonsteroidal anti-inflammatory drugs (NSAIDs), such as *ibuprofen* and *naproxen*, should be stopped or minimized while on anticoagulants, as they can increase not only the risk of bleeding but also of stroke. Also, if you were taking aspirin prior to starting a blood thinner, talk to your doctor about whether you should continue to do so because, for many patients, the increased bleeding risk does outweigh the benefits—but don't stop taking aspirin until you have this discussion.

Diet Drink Stroke Link

Yasmin Mossavar-Rahmani, PhD, RD, CDN, associate clinical professor of epidemiology and population health at Albert Einstein College of Medicine, the Bronx, New York, and lead author of a study published in *Stroke*.

A new study found an association between artificially sweetened beverages and a high risk for heart attack, stroke and death among postmenopausal women. Those who drank two diet drinks daily were 29% more likely to have heart disease, 31% more likely to have a clot-caused stroke and 16% more likely to die from any cause than those who drank less than one a week (or not at all).

Stroke Risk Lingers Long After Heart Attack

Study titled "Duration of Heightened Stroke Risk After Myocardial Infarction," led by researchers in the department of neurology at Weill Cornell Medical College, New York City, presented at the annual meeting of the 2018 American Neurological Association.

It's long been known that your risk for a stroke is increased during the month after a heart attack. But after that, it was thought, your stroke risk returns to normal. However, one month is too soon to relax your stroke watch, according to the latest research.

Because a heart attack (myocardial infarction) interrupts normal blood circulation, it's easy for a blood clot to be released into the bloodstream, which then can travel to the brain and cause an ischemic stroke. Studies have found that this risk is highest in the first month after a heart attack. However, those studies were done on small numbers of patients.

To get a more detailed picture of post–heart attack stroke risk, researchers at Weill Cornell Medical College looked at data from 1.7 million people on Medicare over a period of about 4.6 years, including more than 46,000 patients over age 65 who were hospitalized after a heart attack.

Results: As expected, risk for stroke was almost three times higher than normal risk in the first month after a heart attack. However, stroke risk was doubled during the second month… and was still elevated during the third month (about 60% higher). Risk did not return to normal until after the third month.

The researchers surmise that increased stroke risk is partly the result of decreased heart function post–heart attack, during which time the heart is not beating efficiently, and blood tends to pool and form clots. For this reason, heart attack patients typically are prescribed a blood thinner, such as aspirin, after a heart attack. These new findings suggest that patients may need to take a more powerful anticoagulant…and possibly for longer. The researchers suggest that more research is needed to develop guidelines.

Meanwhile, if you or a loved one has recently had a heart attack, alert your doctor that your stroke risk may be higher than previously thought—and discuss strategies to reduce risk.

And stay alert for the "F.A.S.T." warning signs of stroke: Face drooping…Arm weakness…Speech difficulty…and Time to call 911.

Most People Should Not Take a Daily Aspirin

Robert Eckel, MD, professor of medicine at University of Colorado School of Medicine in Aurora, Colorado, and past president of the American Heart Association. UCDenver.edu

Daily low-dose aspirin was long-considered an effective way to reduce the odds of blood clots that could lead to heart attacks and strokes, but recent research suggests that the benefits are outweighed by the risks for dangerous internal bleeding.

Exception: Daily low-dose aspirin is generally beneficial for someone who already has experienced heart attacks or thrombotic strokes.

How to Stop a Stroke Before It Happens

Bruce A. Perler, MD, MBA, a practicing vascular surgeon at Johns Hopkins Medicine and the Julius H. Jacobson II, MD, Endowed Chair in Vascular Surgery at Johns Hopkins University School of Medicine, both in Baltimore.

Feeling perfectly healthy? Chances are, your doctor still orders certain tests—called "screening tests"—that check for conditions such as colon cancer or osteoporosis that might be lurking and could be treated.

So why not a screening test for stroke risk? We know that people living in the US have nearly 800,000 strokes each year and that 80% to 90% of those strokes are caused by blood clots. Many of these strokes originate from clogged carotid arteries—large arteries in the neck that feed blood to your brain. Like the arteries that feed your heart, these can be narrowed by plaque buildup as you age.

This may surprise you: There is a test that can detect such blockages. It's a simple ultrasound of your neck that costs about $70 to $300 (depending on where you live) and sometimes is covered by insurance.

However, no major medical group advises checking the carotid arteries of all adults—due to concerns that many questionable results will turn out to be wrong, leading to needless worry, costly follow-up testing and risky surgeries.

But some medical groups, such as the Society for Vascular Surgery, the American Heart Association and the American Stroke Association, think it makes sense to test certain people who are at increased risk for a stroke from a clogged carotid artery.

The danger: Without testing, too many people, while clinically asymptomatic, will unknowingly suffer one or more symptomless "silent strokes"—small, repeated insults to the brain caused by inadequate blood flow, which over time can lead to decline in cognitive function. Unsuspecting people with blockages also may ignore signs of transient ischemic attacks, or TIAs (also known as "ministrokes")—brief attacks that produce passing stroke symptoms that may last only for a few minutes, such as

weakness of an arm or leg, brief loss of vision or difficulties speaking. Ministrokes can be the precursor to a bigger and permanently damaging stroke. Still other people will get no warning before a stroke that leaves them disabled or dead, further adding rationale for the screening test.

Should you get scanned?

While guidelines from medical groups vary, many doctors—including myself—say that you should consider a potentially lifesaving scan of your carotid arteries if one or more of the following apply to you…

•**A "bruit" in your neck is detected by your doctor.** This abnormal sound, detected by a stethoscope during a routine physical exam, can indicate a narrowed artery—especially when it's accompanied by other stroke risk factors, such as high blood pressure.

Note: Your doctor should listen for a bruit on both sides of your neck. In some cases, patients actually can hear a "whooshing" sound in their ears.

•**You are over age 65 and have multiple stroke risk factors,** such as smoking, elevated cholesterol, high blood pressure and/or diagnosed coronary artery disease.

•**You have been diagnosed with peripheral artery disease (PAD).** This narrowing of the leg arteries can cause leg pain, particularly when walking. If the arteries feeding your limbs are clogged with plaque, the arteries in your neck may be, too.

•**You have worrisome results from an ankle-brachial index test.** With this test, your doctor compares your blood pressure readings at your ankle and upper arm. The test can indicate PAD, so it's recommended for people with suspicious symptoms in their legs, including pain, numbness or weakness, but also is sometimes used as a broader screening tool for artery health.

•**You have had symptoms of a ministroke.** This might include weakness or numbness on one side of your body or slurred speech. Even if the symptoms lasted for just a minute or two, they are serious. People who have a ministroke are at high risk for a bigger stroke, most often in the first few days, but also in the months and years ahead.

If you have possible ministroke symptoms in the future: Treat them as a medical emergency, and call 911 right away.

Important: If you decide, in consultation with your doctor, to get a carotid ultrasound, make sure that you get the gold-standard test, called a carotid duplex ultrasound, from a laboratory accredited by the Intersocietal Accreditation Commission (IAC). The test, which requires no preparation, can take up to 30 to 60 minutes. You will be asked to wear loose-fitting clothing that allows the technician to access your neck. If there is significant plaque in a carotid artery, the lab report should say how extensive the blockage is and describe the characteristics of the plaque in a way that will help your doctor assess your risks.

WHAT'S NEXT?

If your carotid scan shows no significant blockage, continue taking steps to lower your stroke risk—control blood pressure and cholesterol, maintain a healthy body weight and don't smoke.

What if your carotid testing indicates trouble? Here are the rules of thumb...

•**If less than 50% to 60% of your artery is blocked** and you have no symptoms, you will likely be advised to continue or add medications that reduce your stroke risk, such as a statin for high cholesterol, aspirin to reduce clotting and medication to lower your blood pressure. If you smoke, you will have a powerful new reason to quit.

•**If your blockage is 60% or more but you have no symptoms,** surgery (called a carotid endarterectomy) to remove the plaque may be needed, depending on the severity of the narrowing and the character of the plaque... or if there has been increased narrowing over time. If surgery is not indicated, drugs and lifestyle changes are recommended, and scanning should be repeated every six to 12 months to watch for progression.

•**If you have a blockage of 50% to 99% and symptoms, the choices are clearer.** Unless you have a condition, such as severe, noncorrectable coronary artery disease, heart failure or severe chronic obstructive pulmonary disease (COPD), that makes such procedures too risky, endarterectomy or a stent to open your clogged artery likely will be offered. Stenting is considered more appropriate for symptomatic patients who are too high risk for endarterectomy.

Caution: These procedures can reduce your long-term stroke risk, but they both carry risks of causing an immediate stroke or death by dislodging plaque and sending it to your brain.

My advice: If you are considering one of these procedures, look for a highly experienced surgeon and hospital—and ask for their complication rates. With a top-notch team, stroke or death rates following endarterectomy or stenting should be no more than 2% to 3% for asymptomatic patients...and no more than 5% to 6% for symptomatic patients.

CHAPTER 5

Consumer Health Alerts

Stop Fibbing to Your Doctor

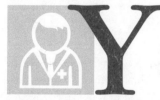

You know the drill. Your doctor asks, "How are you?" and that's your cue to explain that new pain you're wrestling with or that weird rash you've recently noticed. But be honest—do you bare all the facts when talking to your doctor? If you're like most people, probably not.

Shocking research: When more than 4,500 adults were surveyed, 60% to 80% admitted to omissions, distortions and outright lies when talking to their doctors about topics such as how often they exercise, whether they take dietary supplements and how much alcohol they drink, according to research published in *JAMA Network Open.*

Why the cover-up? There are a variety of reasons why patients aren't completely honest with their doctors. *Among the most common…*

•**Shame** (such as not wanting to reveal things they may consider socially unacceptable)…**Embarrassment** (including a reluctance to admit they didn't take their medications because they couldn't afford them)…**A desire to be liked** (wanting to appear to be a "good patient," they may say they've given up smoking, for example, and replaced KFC with kale when that's not true)…and **Fear of bad news** (failing to mention worrisome symptoms because they are afraid the information might point to a serious illness).

A BIGGER PROBLEM

There also can be larger communication issues at play that may interfere with honest dialogue—even if that is the patient's goal—due to today's strained health-care system with shorter doctor visits, electronic record-keeping and overburdened medical personnel.

For one thing, doctors generally dominate the conversation. Even when patients are in-

Danielle Ofri, MD, PhD, associate professor of medicine at NYU Medical Center in New York City and editor in chief of the Bellevue Literary Review. She is author of *What Patients Say, What Doctors Hear.* DanielleOfri.com vited to voice their concerns, research shows that doctors interrupt them within 11 seconds. This isn't simple rudeness—doctors are trained to zero in on diagnosis.

If you start by complaining of a pain in your shoulder, for example, your doctor wants to quickly figure out the source of the pain. But if you wanted to bring something else to your doctor's attention, this may be left unsaid.

Sobering finding: In a recent study published in *Journal of General Internal Medicine*, patients' agendas—what mattered to them—got sufficient attention during only one-third of doctor visits.

Listening also can be a problem in which both doctors and patients fall short. Nervous, rushed and upset by a troubling diagnosis or news about your condition, you may miss much of what you are told. Meanwhile, omissions in your story may occur if your doctor is distracted by the computer on which he/she is entering notes…or is preoccupied with unraveling an earlier symptom.

TRUTH OR CONSEQUENCES

With all these inherent traps in doctor-patient communications, the likely result is overlooked symptoms, misdiagnoses and missed opportunities for the most effective medical intervention.

To avoid such consequences…

•**Make good communication your top priority.** It's the part of your doctor visit that deserves the most time and energy. If this happens, all the other pieces, such as the physical exam, blood tests and X-rays, will fall into place.

•**Bring a list of all your questions and concerns.** But don't expect your doctor to address a dozen symptoms. Instead, show the doctor your list and ask him to pick out what's most important.

Helpful: If there's an item that's especially important to you, let the doctor know by saying, "I want to be sure we get to X."

•**Don't censor yourself.** Don't be ashamed to bring up whatever matters to you—even if you're not sure whether it's medically important.

•**Ask a family member or close friend** to be a second listener and take notes. If you're alone at the appointment and can't take notes,

ask your doctor if it's OK to record the conversation on your smartphone.

•**Be sure the doctor is listening.** If he's not, say, tactfully, "Could you please stop looking at the computer for a minute while I get my story out? I'll be brief."

•**Confirm how to stay in touch.** Whether it's a patient portal, e-mail or number to call, find out how to ask additional questions or request clarifications on anything you don't understand.

•**Don't stick with a doctor with whom you're unable to speak freely.** If you don't feel able to get your story heard, think seriously about changing doctors.

Also: You'll be less likely to lie, fudge or skip over things with a doctor you trust and feel comfortable with.

Getting to Know Your Pathologist: The Behind-the-Scenes Doctor

Michael J. Misialek, MD, associate chair of pathology at Newton-Wellesley Hospital and medical director of the Vernon Cancer Center, both in Newton, Massachusetts, where he directs the Chemistry Laboratory and Point of Care Testing.

Chances are, you have never seen the doctor who is at the front lines of determining virtually all of the key decisions about your health care.

Your pathologist is the behind-the-scenes player who handles laboratory testing that drives nearly 80% of all medical diagnoses and treatments. But this doctor is hardly ever mentioned—much less someone you're likely to meet.

How could that be? On TV shows like CSI, pathologists examine corpses and investigate suspicious deaths. In real life, their work is much more far-reaching. Pathologists are commonly recognized for their role in diagnosing cancer when a biopsy is performed. But these medical doctors also analyze laboratory tests—checking for everything from elevated cholesterol levels and infections to kidney disease and the cause of skin growths.

You can think of it this way—anything that is biopsied, scraped off, drawn from your veins, coughed up or excreted will pass under the microscope of a pathologist, who looks at physical specimens for signs of risk and disease.

INTEGRAL FOR CANCER CARE

If you've been diagnosed with cancer, your initial diagnosis and the subsequent treatment plans always start with a pathologist.

Example: Your doctor might suspect that you have breast cancer—based on a mammogram, physical findings (like a breast lump), symptoms, etc.—but the actual diagnosis will depend on what's discovered from a tissue sample that's examined in a laboratory.

The cancer diagnosis is just the beginning. The pathologist will use microscopic criteria to "grade" tumors according to their severity… identify hormone receptors (such as those for estrogen or progesterone) that predict how tumors are likely to behave…and determine what treatments are most likely to be effective.

Will you do better if you have surgery first, followed by radiation or chemotherapy? Or will your cancer respond more readily to preoperative chemotherapy and/or radiation? The treatments that your doctor ultimately chooses, including the order of treatments, are largely guided by pathology findings.

Recent development: "Liquid biopsy," which is based on a blood draw rather than a tissue sample, is an emerging technology that is transforming not just cancer care but virtually every disease process. To ensure accuracy and precision, pathologists are often involved in the design, validation and oversight of these tests.

Smart idea: If you're diagnosed with cancer or any other serious condition, ask to see the pathologist's report. Pay particular attention to the "diagnosis" section to learn the pathologist's conclusion and the "comments" section, which gives additional information on any subtleties of your case.

TRACKING DISEASE

Many diseases (such as diabetes) and risk factors (including elevated cholesterol) can be diagnosed only by laboratory findings. But about 20% of pathology tests are requested after a diagnosis to determine how well a treatment is working.

An oncologist, for example, might order additional biopsies and/or other tests to track a tumor's response to radiation or chemotherapy…and still more tests to fine-tune the treatments by adding or subtracting drugs, changing doses, etc.

Another example: You'll need laboratory tests to determine if (or how well) medication to treat thyroid disease is working. The same goes for drugs such as insulin, blood thinners and cholesterol-lowering statins.

AN IMPERFECT SCIENCE

Most pathologists will come to the same conclusions when they look at tissue samples—but not always. Doctors are only human.

Example: In a Johns Hopkins study published in *Cancer*, researchers reviewed biopsy slides from more than 6,000 patients and found that 86 patients were given wrong diagnoses that could have led to unnecessary or inappropriate treatments.

Research published in *JAMA*, looking at biopsies for breast cancer, found that 13% of cases of ductal carcinoma in situ (abnormal cells that are found within milk ducts) were not universally agreed upon by pathologists. This doesn't always mean that the pathologists made mistakes—there's disagreement among experts about how to diagnose this condition or interpret laboratory findings. But the study suggests that patients and doctors should view pathology reports with some healthy skepticism.

My advice: Don't hesitate to get a second pathology opinion, particularly if you're dealing with a rare disease…when the treatment for a disease (often the case with cancer) largely depends on pathology findings…or when a pathology report doesn't completely line up with your doctor's best judgment.

Important: A second pathology opinion will not require an additional biopsy—another pathologist is simply asked to review the slides from the first tissue sample.

These second opinions might be covered by insurance, but not always. Also, don't assume that you must use a pathologist who practices in your area for a second opinion. Biopsy slides can be shipped anywhere. Your doctor can often coordinate a second pathology opinion. Just be sure that the pathologist is board-certified and that the work is being performed in a laboratory credentialed by the College of American Pathologists.

MEET FACE-TO-FACE

Most patients never meet the pathologist(s) involved in their medical care, but they should. I urge patients to come forward with questions, particularly when they're dealing with a rare or complicated disease…or when they have questions about the diagnosis that their primary doctor cannot fully answer.

Personal story: I received a call from a breast cancer patient who felt overwhelmed by information. I was familiar with her case because I had made the initial diagnosis. I explained what her diagnosis meant and what the biopsy showed (in terms that a layperson could understand). I was able to give reassurance that her treatment plan was appropriate.

It's not yet routine for patients to consult with pathologists. But where I work, breast cancer patients are always given the chance to meet with a pathologist, just as they meet with oncologists and other members of their care team. While this practice is not widespread, it is gaining acceptance throughout the medical community.

My advice: Ask whether your hospital offers the opportunity to meet the pathologist, how to schedule the meeting and whether there is any cost associated with the visit—most of the time there is not.

New Genetic Test for Chronic Kidney Disease

The New England Journal of Medicine.

A new DNA test can identify a genetic flaw in about 10% of adults with chronic kidney disease…and the test results can help guide better treatment decisions.

Medicine's Barbaric Little Secret: IVs Don't Have to Hurt

David Sherer, MD, an anesthesiologist and coauthor, with Maryann Karinch, of *Dr. David Sherer's Hospital Survival Guide* and *The House of Black and White*, a memoir of growing up in a medical family. DrDavidSherer.com

I recently spoke to an old friend, a fellow physician, about what makes hospitalized patients most uncomfortable. Incredibly, one of the things he told me was that when he is doing rounds in the intensive care unit (ICU), the blood drawings for the daily testing take place around 4:00 AM. I was shocked! How can patients get adequate rest when someone is jabbing a needle in their arms at that ungodly hour?

This led to a discussion about what doctors and nurses do to patients that, in my opinion, border on barbarity. One of them is starting intravenous lines with no local anesthesia on the skin. I consider this one of medical practice's dirty little secrets. *Let me explain…*

When I was an internal medicine intern and medical student, I witnessed the unnecessary infliction of pain on patients who had their IVs started without local anesthesia, often by inexperienced students and interns. This horrible and immoral practice was just considered the norm. It wasn't intentional, it was just the way things were done.

In 1986, as a new anesthesia resident, I was taught how to start an IV and, more importantly, how to do so relatively painlessly—with the use of less than 1 cc of the local anesthetic *lidocaine*. What we were taught is still in practice by many in my specialty today. A small wheal (bubble) of local anesthetic is applied with a tiny (and I mean tiny!) needle just where the IV is to be started in the vein. After five seconds, the practitioner can, with virtually NO pain to the patient, search for and find the proper site for insertion of the IV catheter. I know this to be true because, in my estimation, I've done this an astounding 80,000 times (you read that right) over a nearly 32-year career.

There is absolutely no reason that this should not be standard practice for every patient in need of an IV. The training takes five minutes and the results are dramatic. The amount of lidocaine administered is so minute that it causes no ill effects. And the patients are spared the painful ordeal of IV starts, especially when multiple sticks are involved.

My physician friend and I agreed that another area where this can be employed is when an arterial blood gas is drawn. This procedure is even more painful than an IV start. A needle is inserted into an artery to obtain an arterial blood sample for analysis. Let me tell you, it hurts like hell. Yet health care personnel still inflict it and patients endure it.

It's time for patients to stand up for themselves. Let it be the year that health-care professionals ease the pain from medical practices.

When "Simple" Surgeries Turn Deadly

Frank Overdyk, MD, a patient-safety advocate and anesthesiologist in Charleston, South Carolina. Dr. Overdyk is a member of the board of advisors of the Physician-Patient Alliance for Health & Safety, PPAHS.org. He received the 2018 AAMI (Association for the Advancement of Medical Instrumentation) & Becton Dickinson Patient Safety Award.

Some surgeries and procedures are considered "minor" when compared with lengthy, invasive operations such as heart or brain surgery…or a hip or knee replacement.

The so-called simple procedures—performed about 40 million times each year in the US—often take place in ambulatory surgery centers (ASCs), where you're sent home in a few hours. But what happens when simple surgeries go wrong—or even turn deadly?

NOT SO SIMPLE AFTER ALL

Since their introduction in the US in the 1970s, ASCs have been a valuable resource, helping patients avoid hospital-acquired infections and speeding recovery at home in more comfortable surroundings.

However, the risks are real. Deaths resulting from treatment at ASCs are not officially tracked, but according to a recent investigative report published by *USA Today Network* and Kaiser Health News, more than 260 ASC patients died from surgical complications (such as internal bleeding and cardiac arrest) over the last five years. *Some key risks—and how to protect yourself…*

•**Cosmetic surgery (such as a face-lift).**

What can go wrong: Particularly during any type of cosmetic surgery, in which a surgeon is operating near the mouth, nose, vocal cords or neck, general anesthesia (the use of a drug to make the patient unresponsive and unconscious) or "deep sedation" (similar to general anesthesia but often does not involve a breathing tube) can interfere with a patient's ability to breathe.

To protect yourself: If your surgeon plans to use deep sedation, ask whether a dedicated sedation provider will be involved (by law, general anesthesia requires an anesthesiologist, nurse-anesthetist and/or anesthesiologist assistant). Or ask whether the surgeon can use local anesthesia or a nerve block instead. With a nerve block, local anesthetic is injected near nerves and specific body parts that will be affected by the surgery. Nerve blocks have different risks from general anesthesia and deep sedation but usually don't impede your ability to breathe or your level of consciousness.

•**Tonsillectomy.** Nearly 300,000 tonsil-removal surgeries are performed each year in adults—often prompted by frequent sore throats. But chronically swollen tonsils also contribute to sleep apnea, which raises risks for serious conditions, such as heart attack and stroke.

What can go wrong: Tonsillectomy involves the airway and blood vessels. Persistent bleeding in the airway after tonsillectomy is an infrequent but serious complication that requires immediate attention and can arise hours after the procedure…long after the ASC closes.

To protect yourself: Ask to be the first case of the day. This is the best time to schedule any procedure—but especially this one. Scheduling early in the day gives the most time for any complication to be addressed on-site.

•**Bunionectomy.**

What can go wrong: Recovery from bunion removal can be very painful, and opioid pain relievers often are prescribed for the immediate post-op period and beyond. This can be dangerous, especially for patients with sleep apnea, obesity or advanced age. In addition to depressed breathing, opioids can trigger a variety of side effects, including nausea/vomiting and urinary dysfunction.

To protect yourself: Before your procedure, discuss the plan for post-op pain management. Ask your doctor how you can limit opioid use by instead relying on alternatives, including nonsteroidal anti-inflammatory drugs (NSAIDs) and the COX-2 inhibitor *celecoxib* (Celebrex). These drugs target enzymes responsible for inflammation and pain without such a high risk for side effects.

•**Endoscopy.**

What can go wrong: With endoscopy, which involves the use of deep sedation, both the doctor performing the procedure and the anesthesia provider are working inside your airway. This means that contents from your stomach could get into your lungs (aspiration).

To protect yourself: Make sure you are a suitable candidate and without an acute illness (see below).

ARE YOU AN ASC CANDIDATE?

If you're elderly and/or have chronic health problems that increase your risk for complications during or after your surgery—such as moderate-to-severe sleep apnea, morbid obesity or chronic obstructive pulmonary disease (COPD), discuss with your primary care doctor and the doctor performing the procedure whether you're a suitable candidate for outpatient surgery at an ASC.

Also, if you have a cold, the flu or a fever, call to notify your outpatient facility—you may be asked to reschedule the procedure to a time when you are well. Similarly, if your blood sugar or blood pressure is high or unstable…or you have shortness of breath from asthma or heart failure, notify the doctor performing the procedure and get advice on the best plan of action.

OTHER SAFEGUARDS YOU NEED

Before undergoing treatment at an ASC, also make sure that…

•**The facility only rarely needs to transfer a patient** to a hospital for more advanced care. The hospital also should be relatively close.

•**There will be electronic monitors** and "crash carts" on-site.

•**A dedicated anesthesiologist,** nurse-anesthetist or anesthesiologist assistant will be on hand during the procedure. This is crucial if you will be receiving general anesthesia or deep sedation. Deep sedation carries greater risks than "conscious sedation," during which the patient is able to respond to verbal prompts and commands.

Note: If you are comfortable with taking oral medication for anxiety and prefer not to take the additional risks associated with deep sedation, ask for conscious sedation, and make sure your consent form indicates this.

•**Your oxygen saturation and exhaled carbon dioxide ("capno-graphy")** will be continuously monitored by the dedicated provider mentioned above during all procedures requiring deep sedation or general anesthesia. Oxygen saturation also should be monitored continuously during recovery from deep sedation or general anesthesia. The recovery area should be staffed by a qualified professional trained in basic and advanced cardio life support.

•**The doctor performing the procedure has board certification by a board** that is a member of the American Board of Medical Specialties, ABMS.org. This credential is highly recommended and offers an added layer of safety.

Older Surgeons Have Lower Patient Death Rates

Among 892,187 Medicare patients who had one of 20 types of emergency surgery (such as hysterectomy or a heart valve procedure), those performed by surgeons who were age 50 and older had lower death rates during the four-year study period than procedures done by younger surgeons.

Yusuke Tsugawa, MD, PhD, assistant professor, David Geffen School of Medicine, UCLA, Los Angeles.

Know the Warning Signs of Post-Op Problems

Alana Elise Sigmund, MD, FHM, medical director for arthroplasty at Hospital for Special Surgery, New York City, where she oversees the medical care of postoperative patients.

Now that you're propped up on your familiar sofa and feel an unexpected twinge of post-surgery pain, you realize that you don't really remember all that information about "complications" the nurse warned you about when you were discharged. And that piece of paper with a list of reasons to call the surgeon's office? Suddenly the descriptions all seem very vague.

ARE YOU IN TROUBLE?

It's important to know what's most likely normal and what could be a sign of trouble when you're recovering at home, especially when you're an outpatient and are healing away from the watchful eye of nurses and doctors. Of course, any complications or side effects will depend on the specific type of surgery you had. *Here are some general guidelines…*

Important tip: After an outpatient procedure, you may still feel groggy when you're discharged, so ask the person picking you up to take notes. That way you'll know what your surgeon recommended.

Then use this surgery side effect checklist to quickly recognize a variety of roadblocks on your path to recovery…

***SIDE EFFECT:* Drainage.**

Normal: What's a reasonable amount of drainage—fluid that leaks from the incision after surgery—depends on the type of surgery, and your surgeon should give you a time frame for when yours should slow down and then stop.

Not normal: If you notice drainage increasing, call your doctor. Generally, the fluid should be clear or light pink. If it turns yellow or another color, this could be a sign of infection. If the fluid develops an odor, pick up the phone.

***SIDE EFFECT:* Redness and Swelling.**

Normal: Some redness and swelling around an incision is a normal part of healing. You should see it decrease as you heal.

Not normal: If redness and/or swelling gets darker or starts to spread, you could have cellulitis, an infection in the deep layers of skin and the tissue beneath it, or a surgical site infection that needs to be treated with antibiotics.

Smart tip: If you're concerned or are just unsure, snap a picture of the area with your phone and see if you can send it to the doctor.

***SIDE EFFECT:* Pain.**

Normal: It's almost impossible not to have any pain after surgery and, depending on the type of surgery you had, it could be worse on the second day. But you should start to feel a little better every day after that. If you need pain medication, make sure you take no more than directed.

Not normal: If you feel a sudden and big uptick in pain, that's a red flag, and your doctor needs to know right away. Another reason to give a call is if you just don't feel that your pain is fading over time.

***SIDE EFFECT:* Fever.**

Normal: People often run slight fevers for about two days post-op. If you suspect you have a fever, take your temperature. If it's less than 101.4°F, check again about four hours later to make sure it's going down.

Not normal: If your temperature reaches 101.4°F or higher and occurs two days or more after surgery, there's a greater chance that the fever is due to an infection, especially if you have other symptoms like painful urination or a bad cough. Call your doctor.

***SIDE EFFECT:* Lower Leg Pain.**

Normal: Post-op leg cramps—when the muscle seizes up—are common and often are caused by abnormalities in electrolytes, the various minerals in your body fluids, and you should certainly tell your doctor about leg cramps. You might need nothing more than food and water. If that's not working, reach out to your physician's office.

Not normal: There's another reason you might have leg pain after an operation—and it's a more immediate concern. Pain in your lower leg or calf could be a sign of deep vein thrombosis (DVT), a dangerous type of blood clot that can break free and block an artery in your lung—a potentially fatal condition called a pulmonary embolism (PE). Surgery can raise your risk for DVT. If you have calf pain postoperatively, call your care team. Your doctor may order an imaging test, such as ultrasound, to diagnose a DVT and, if one is found, will then treat you, typically with a blood thinner to dissolve the clot.

ALWAYS CAUSE FOR CONCERN

There's no "normal" for some post-op reactions. *Here are symptoms that definitely require prompt action…*

•**Trouble Breathing.** If you feel short of breath but can still speak in full sentences, alert your care team by phone. The problem may be related to your surgery or another condition you have, like asthma or allergies. But if it's so bad that you can't get out a sentence, call 911. Sudden trouble breathing can be a sign that a DVT has broken free and that you're experiencing a PE.

•**Bleeding.** Normal post-op bleeding can happen after some operations such as sinus surgery. Your doctor should have told you if you're likely to bleed after your procedure and, if so, how much bleeding to expect and when it should stop. If bleeding wasn't mentioned or if it seems different than what was explained to you, contact your doctor. If bleeding is profuse, of course, call 911.

•**Shock.** Shock in medical terms is when the body doesn't have enough blood flowing to its organs. Severe blood loss is a major cause of shock, itself a life-threatening emergency. *Symptoms of shock can include…*

- •Rapid heartbeat and rapid breathing
- •Pale skin and sweating
- •Confusion
- •Weak pulse
- •Unusually cool hands and feet

Call 911 if you think you could be in shock!

•**Chest Pain.** Surgery can stress every system of the body, including the heart. The risk of heart problems after most types of surgery is low for most people, but you're at greater risk if you had major surgery and already have heart disease. In the days after surgery, if you feel pain or any strange sensation in your chest, one or both arms, your jaw or even your stomach that isn't obviously a normal result of the surgery, call 911. You could be having a heart attack.

Special note for women: Women often hurt in other places like the arms, jaw or even the nose.

It's not uncommon for patients to develop an irregular heart beat rhythm called atrial fibrillation (AFib) a day or two after an operation. It's often related to the amount of intravenous fluids you're given to support your blood pressure during surgery, and some people may be especially susceptible to AFib. If you develop AFib, you might notice that your heart is racing or you might feel short of breath. Call your doctor, because AFib raises your risk for stroke. Your doctor will let you know whether it's best to go to the office…or to the ER to determine whether you are experiencing AFib.

The Best Checkup for Your Kidneys

Joseph Vassalotti, MD, chief medical officer of the National Kidney Foundation, Kidney.org, and associate clinical professor of medicine in the division of nephrology at Icahn School of Medicine at Mount Sinai in New York City. His research has been published in peer-reviewed journals such as *American Journal of Nephrology, Kidney International* and *American Journal of Kidney Diseases.*

When you see your doctor for a regular checkup, your kidney health may be getting short shrift. You may think your doctor is staying on top of all the tests you need…but not necessarily.

Screening for chronic kidney disease (CKD)—when it's performed—has traditionally involved a select group of blood and urine tests. But in today's busy doctors' offices, it's common for the urine test to not be ordered. This means that any testing you do receive may be inadequate. Now that's about to change.

Latest development: To simplify testing, the National Kidney Foundation has collaborated with the American Society for Clinical Pathology and other leading laboratory societies and laboratories to identify a combination of specific tests now called the Kidney Profile. When performed together, these tests—a urine sample for albumin-to-creatinine ratio (ACR) and a blood test for estimated glomerular filtration rate (eGFR)—streamline the testing process. These are the two tests recommended by the National Kidney Foundation and the American Diabetes Association to test individuals at risk for kidney disease.

Pairing the results from these tests makes the Kidney Profile more accurate and comprehensive than receiving just one test. The combination not only detects CKD but also identifies the stage of kidney disease and provides a stronger prediction of one's risk for kidney failure, heart disease and other chronic conditions.

If CKD is detected, the test results enable doctors to better determine how a patient's individual case should be managed—typically with medications for those at earlier stages…and with dialysis or even a kidney transplant for people who have later-stage disease.

For example, high blood pressure with high levels of albumin in the urine, or ACR, should be treated with a blood pressure medication that also protects the kidneys—this could be an angiotensin-converting enzyme inhibitor, such as *benazepril* (Lotensin) or an angiotensin receptor blocker, such as *losartan* (Cozaar).

WHO SHOULD GET THE KIDNEY PROFILE?

The people for whom CKD testing is recommended haven't changed—they're the same individuals who should have been getting annual kidney screenings all along. *This includes people in specific high-risk groups for CKD, such as…*

•**Anyone who is age 60 or older.**

•**Adults with diabetes and/or high blood pressure**—chronic conditions that increase risk for CKD.

•**Adults of certain racial or ethnic backgrounds,** including those of African-American, Hispanic, Native American, Asian or Pacific Islander descent.

WHY TESTING MATTERS

If you're wondering whether testing for kidney disease really is that important, the answer is a resounding "Yes!" The condition, which im-

pairs the kidneys' ability to remove wastes and regulate crucial chemical levels in the blood, such as sodium, potassium and calcium, is far more common than most people realize.

Startling statistic: An estimated 30 million Americans have CKD, but only 3.6 million are aware of it, while the others have no inkling that anything is amiss.

Worse yet, more Americans than ever before are now considered to be at risk of developing CKD due to diabetes or high blood pressure. This escalating number stems, in part, from the aging population and the obesity epidemic, both of which drive high blood pressure and type 2 diabetes.

The real danger: Once your kidneys are damaged, the harm that is done usually cannot be reversed. More than 450,000 Americans are now on kidney dialysis. The only other treatment for late-stage kidney failure is a transplant—an option that is limited by the relative lack of available kidneys.

THE KIDNEY PROFILE CAN HELP PREVENT THIS SCARY SCENARIO

When it comes to annual screening for CKD, cost has never been an issue for most people. The Kidney Profile's blood and urine tests cost under $50 and are routinely covered by health insurance. They are easy to get—if your primary care doctor orders both types of tests for the most complete kidney assessment.

Because the Kidney Profile streamlines and simplifies CKD testing for doctors, patients will get the benefit of more complete testing. With leading labs adopting the combination of CKD tests under the heading of "Kidney Profile" on request forms and electronic health records, doctors won't need to search for and order each test separately…and they also can find the results in one place.

Let's face it: When one less click of a computer mouse or check mark on a handwritten form is needed to expedite proper care, your doctor's job gets easier…and the odds of effective care go up.

Important: If you have one of the risk factors (such as diabetes or high blood pressure), be sure to ask your doctor about getting the Kidney Profile. If it's not yet available in your community, ask for the blood (eGFR) and urine (ACR) tests to be ordered individually.

HITTING THE NUMBERS

CKD can be present if one or both tests are abnormal over a period of 90 or more days. *Here are the numbers you should look for in the Kidney Profile (or in the following tests if ordered separately)...*

•ACR urine test.

What's being measured: Albumin is a type of protein that may signal early kidney disease when it appears in the urine. Creatinine, a product of normal muscle metabolism, is filtered by the kidneys as a waste product.

Target numbers: The ACR is a highly sensitive indicator of kidney damage. If you have ever scrambled an egg, you might notice foam on the surface that represents albumin in the egg. Similarly, individuals with high levels of albumin in the urine may notice foamy urine, but the ACR test is more accurate than looking for foam. The ACR test result should be less than 30 mg/g. Higher levels indicate kidney damage, which in turn increases risk for kidney failure and heart disease.

•eGFR blood test.

What's being measured: Creatinine levels are used in a formula that also incorporates your age, weight, race and gender to calculate your eGFR. The number indicates how well your kidneys are filtering blood to remove natural waste products and excess fluid.

Target numbers: You can think of eGFR readings as a percentage of kidney function. A reading of 60 or higher is considered normal, while a reading less than 60 is considered reduced kidney function. The lower the kidney function, the higher the risk for kidney failure and cardiovascular disease. Many people are diagnosed with stage 3 (or moderate) kidney disease when the eGFR result is 30 to 59. A result below 30 is considered severe CKD.

In general, people who have an eGFR of less than 30 should see a nephrologist (kidney specialist). Patients who have an eGFR of less than 15 usually need to be prepared for dialysis or a kidney transplant.

Note: Low kidney function should be considered when prescriptions are being ordered—

some drugs should be avoided, and others need to have the dose adjusted if the drug is eliminated from the body via the kidneys. Approximately half of FDA-approved medications are cleared by the kidneys.

Important: People at risk for kidney disease should be tested at least once every year, but more frequent testing may be advised for more severe kidney disease. Speak to your doctor about the most appropriate testing schedule for you.

For more more information, consult the National Kidney Foundation at Kidney.org/CKD intercept/laboratoryengagement.

The Truth About Eyeglass Lens Options

Jeffrey R. Anshel, OD, an optometrist in private practice in Encinitas, California. Dr. Anshel is founder and past president of the Ocular Nutrition Society and author or coauthor of multiple books, including *Smart Medicine for Your Eyes* and *What You Must Know About Age-Related Macular Degeneration*. EStreetEyes.com

---

Prescription lenses are essentially just two pieces of plastic surrounded by a frame. If you want them to function at maximum capacity and last as long as possible, you probably need to enhance them with some customizations.* *Below, optometrist Jeffrey R. Anshel, OD, tells us what's essential and what's not...*

COATINGS YOU PROBABLY NEED

Most people will want to get both of the following coatings...

•Antireflective coating. With an ultrathin antireflective (AR) coating, your vision will be crisper, with less glare from room lights and fewer distortions, such as halos around headlights at night. This coating will also reduce the reflections others see in your glasses, making your eyes more visible and improving eye contact. For example, if a TV newscaster didn't have AR-coated glasses, bright studio lights would reflect in his/her lenses. In addition, an AR

*Many of these options can be combined and could be included in a lens package for one price. Prices listed here will vary depending on your location in the US. Check with your eye doctor or optician for advice.

coating, which can make computer work more comfortable, will help reduce that "coke bottle" look—reflections in lenses can cause the lenses to appear thicker than they are.

Good to know: AR coatings are constantly improving. Big-box chains often use older technology because it's less expensive, while an eye-care professional in private practice will be more likely to offer the most recent technology. Request at least a one-year warranty. If the coating on your lenses is peeling off…if they seem chronically smudged…or if you notice crazing (cracks), you need a new AR coating. The latest AR treatments are spot-resistant and easily cleaned.

Add-on cost: About $50 to $100.

•**Scratch-resistant coating.** As mentioned earlier, most of today's eyeglass lenses are made of plastic, which is much lighter and softer than glass. Scratch-resistant treatment prevents scuffs and marks that can occur when dropping, storing or even cleaning your glasses.

Tip: For best results, request this treatment on the front and back of the lenses.

Add-on cost: About $50.

WORTH ASKING ABOUT

Ultraviolet (UV) light from the sun or other sources produces radiation that can be harmful to the eyes—it's been linked to cataracts, retinal damage and skin cancer on the eyelids. If you spend any time outdoors without UV-blocking sunglasses or work in an environment in which UV light is prevalent, your glasses should provide protection from UV light. Most prescription lenses (regular lenses or sunglasses) now come with UV protection, but be sure to ask if it's included. If not, the extra cost can be around $20 to $100.

YOU MIGHT WANT TO CONSIDER

•**Transition lenses.** These lenses offer the convenience of not having to switch back and forth from sunglasses to regular glasses. They darken quickly when going out into the sun (it takes about 30 seconds), but take about five minutes to lighten up when going indoors. Transition lenses won't get as dark as traditional sunglasses, especially in a car. These lenses absorb UV light, so they have UV protection built-in.

Add-on cost: About $50 to $150.

•**Polarized lenses.** Outdoor buffs (boaters, skiers, hikers, etc.) and people who drive a lot love polarized sunglasses, which cut the glare from smooth, reflective surfaces like lakes, snow and roads. "Polarized" does not mean "UV light–blocking," so be sure to get both. Because polarized lenses reduce glare, there's no need to add an AR coating to these lenses.

Note: The polarizing film can make it hard to see smartphone and computer screens.

Also: Cataracts can make eyes sensitive to light, and polarized lenses help reduce this sensitivity. Some people use polarized lenses after cataract surgery as well, because the eyes are sensitive to light for a few weeks after the procedure.

Add-on cost: About $100.

FASHION LENSES

•**Tinted lenses.** Tinted glasses (blue, green, pink and, the latest fad, yellow) are a popular fashion trend right now. The deeper the tint, the more it will affect color perception, so you may not be comfortable using tinted glasses for all activities.

Note: Yellow-tinted glasses can block damaging blue light (see below).

Add-on cost: About $35.

•**Mirrored lenses.** The high reflective coating of mirrored lenses lets in less light than other sunglasses—you'll see a gray or brown tint from inside—so they're good for people with sensitive eyes, but they do scratch easily. A mirrored coating can be applied to any lens—prescription or not.

Add-on cost: About $100 to $150.

DO YOU NEED BLUE-BLOCKERS?

High-energy visible (HEV) blue light—emitted by smartphones, tablets, computers, LED television and fluorescent lighting—has been shown to disrupt sleep by preventing the release of melatonin, a hormone in the body that helps regulate sleep. Blue light from electronics and fluorescent lighting has also been linked to eyestrain and headaches. Blue-blocking lenses, with their yellow or amber tint, are thought to reduce the amount of blue light entering your eyes. The lens itself can be tinted or a coating can be applied.

My take: Blue-blocking glasses aren't necessary for most people.

Exceptions: Blue-blockers can help people who have eyestrain, dry eye or headaches from working for long periods on a computer or under fluorescent lights. And if you have age-related macular degeneration (AMD), the leading cause of vision loss, you might want to try them for your regular glasses and sunglasses. Blue light in large doses can damage the retina, which is already deteriorating in AMD.

Sleep disruptions from blue light can be minimized by stopping use of electronic devices about two hours before bedtime.

Blue-blockers do distort color, so they're typically not appropriate for people working on computer graphics. But they now come in lighter tints that distort color less and do reduce glare, so some people like them for driving.

It might cost about $35 to add the blue-blocking tint, but it may be offered as part of a lens package.

If you're buying nonprescription sunglasses: Don't think that a dark tint provides protection from UV light. The label needs to say that they block 100% of UV rays…or look for the term "UV 400."

Hidden Toxins: How to Stay Safe

Joseph Pizzorno, ND, a leading authority on science-based natural and integrative medicine. He founded and served 22 years as president of Bastyr University, the largest fully accredited university of natural medicine in the US.

Asbestos, pesticides, tobacco smoke. We do our best to steer clear of these well-known harmful substances.

But what about the toxins we haven't heard of—the ones that can be found in places we'd never suspect? The truth is, toxins are every-

where—in most rugs and paints…cleaning supplies…cosmetics and perfumes…and the fumes from a gas pump. Even most food cans and the ubiquitous pizza box, designed to hold heat and resist stains, pose risks because of chemicals that, in our bodies, alter our hormones and our immune systems.

Recent development: While most of these hidden toxins are feared for their potential to cause cancer, mounting research shows that these substances also increase risk for serious health problems, such as diabetes and asthma—and more mundane ills like fatigue, poor concentration and memory problems.

Only a few hundred of the more than 80,000 chemicals in use in the US have been adequately tested for safety. But if toxins are everywhere, how can you stay safe? The answer is to limit your "toxic load." *Here's how…*

STEP 1:
EAT ORGANIC

A nutritious diet—lots of fruits, vegetables, whole grains, etc.—can prevent disease. But these foods aren't always as healthful as you would imagine.

Modern agriculture depends on synthetic brews of pesticides, fertilizers and herbicides. Many go-to healthy foods have been flagged by the Environmental Working Group for high pesticide levels.

My advice: I strongly advise patients to buy organic foods—both packaged foods and produce. They contain few (or none) of the most harmful chemicals.

If cost is an issue, be sure that you buy the following 12 foods identified by the Environmental Working Group as the most important to purchase as organic—strawberries, spinach, kale, nectarines, apples, grapes, peaches, cherries, pears, tomatoes, celery and potatoes.

STEP 2:
RID YOUR BODY OF TOXINS

Exposure to toxins increases levels of harmful bacteria in the intestines that overload the detoxifying capacity of the liver…decreases levels of beneficial probiotic organisms…and damages the intestinal lining, which allows harmful substances to pass from the gut into the blood-stream—a condition known as "leaky gut." *My advice...**

• **Take a fiber supplement** (such as Metamu-cil, one to two teaspoons) a half hour before or after meals. Fiber binds to toxins and harmful bacteria to accelerate their excretion.

• **Recolonize the intestine with the probi-otics** *Lactobacillus* and *Bifidobacterium* to help heal the intestinal walls. Many brands contain both organisms. Take one capsule, at least one billion colony-forming units (CFUs), three times daily. I advise taking this supplement indefinitely.

STEP 3:
TAKE A SAFER PAINKILLER

People with arthritis or other painful con-ditions often take daily doses of nonsteroidal anti-inflammatory drugs (NSAIDs), such as *ibu-profen* (Motrin) or *naproxen* (Aleve)...or the pain reliever *acetaminophen* (Tylenol). But all of these drugs can impair the ability of your kidneys to remove toxins from the body.

Safer choices: Take a natural pain reliever, such as the herb butterbur. It reduces inflamma-tion and can relieve pain from headaches and other conditions. Curcumin is another excellent anti-inflammatory. Follow label instructions.

STEP 4:
TEST YOUR TOXIN LEVELS

Your doctor may suggest "target testing" if he/she suspects that you've been exposed to a certain toxin, such as lead in your drinking water. But even if you don't have symptoms (or risk factors), I advise getting a general test for toxins and repeating it every year or two.

One such test is the urinary 8-OHdG, which looks at metabolites that are released when DNA is damaged—a potential sign of elevated toxins. If your results are abnormal, work with your doctor to identify which toxin levels are elevated and their source so you can decrease your exposure as much as possible.

*Before taking any supplement, check with your doctor if you have a chronic medical condition or take medication.

Well Water Alert

Jörg Schullehner, PhD, postdoctoral research fellow, National Center for Register-based Research, Aarhus Uni-versity and Geological Survey of Denmark and Green-land, Aarhus, Denmark.

Most well owners think bacteria and radon are the only risks in well water. But that's not true.

For example, recent research identified unsafe levels of nitrate. When 200,000 water samples were collected from private wells and public water supplies, researchers found an elevated risk for colorectal cancer at less than 1 mg ni-trate per liter...well below the EPA limit of 10 mg/L. (Nitrate accumulation is generally due to fertilizer runoff.) People exposed to more than 2 mg/L over the 35-year study period had a 15% increased risk over those exposed to less than 0.3 mg/L of nitrate in water.

My advice: Get your well water tested for contaminants each year.

Reduce Your VOC Emissions Footprint: Household Products

Jessica Gilman, PhD, an atmospheric chemist at the US National Oceanic and Atmospheric Administration (NOAA) and coauthor of the studies "Diurnal variability and emission pattern of decamethylcyclopentasiloxane (D5) from the application of personal care products in two North American cities" published in *Environmental Science and Technology* and "Volatile chemical products emerging as largest petrochemical source of urban organ-ic emissions" published in *Science,* and Peggy Jenkins, a manager in the research division of the California Air Resources Board.

Can you be creating as much air pollu-tion inside your home as your car does outside? Depending on the products you use, cleaning your bathroom, kitchen or any room in your home could be adding volatile or-ganic compounds, or VOCs, to the air you and your family breathe. Yes, that is the same class of harmful chemicals found in such known haz-ards as turpentine and gasoline.

The combination of emissions from household cleaners, paints, pesticides and personal-care products is now rivaling motor-vehicle emissions as the top source of city air pollution, according to a study conducted by researchers at the National Oceanic and Atmospheric Administration (NOAA) and other institutions across the US.

Here's why you should be concerned: It doesn't take much exposure to some VOCs for health problems to start. You might experience headaches, drowsiness, nausea, eye irritation and other allergic reactions, and respiratory difficulties. And the more you're exposed to VOCs, the greater the health risks—they can harm your lungs, heart, liver, kidneys and central nervous system and could lead to lung cancer.

We're not suggesting that you stop cleaning your home or forgo repainting the family room, but there are steps you can take to reduce your household emissions footprint and therefore protect your health…

•**Become more aware of the range and volume of chemicals you use.** Count all the products under your kitchen sink, in your laundry room and in your garage—you may be surprised at how many you've amassed. Now add items from your home office to the list—from glue sticks to printer ink. If a product smells—good or bad—it's emitting VOCs. *Common household VOC sources include…*

•Air fresheners, deodorizers and scented candles

- •Bathroom and kitchen cleaners
- •Dishwasher and laundry detergents
- •Dryer sheets
- •Furniture and floor polish
- •Glass cleaners
- •Glue
- •Moth balls
- •Paints, stains and related products
- •Printer ink
- •Pesticides
- •Rug and upholstery cleaners

•**Pare down your chemical inventory… and the way you use them.** It's not hard to think of ways you can minimize the number of different products you use—do you really need four or five different cleaners for the surfaces in your bathroom? And by minimizing the number, you can focus on finding a few products that work well and contain a minimum of VOCs. The truth is, a lot less can often clean just as well and exposes you to a lower chemical load in the air. (Using less saves money, too.)

•**Make your own cleaning products.** The only common cleaning solution that doesn't contain VOCs is straight-up water or water mixed with baking soda. The baking soda will create carbon dioxide, a greenhouse gas, when it bubbles, but no VOCs. Just switching to a simpler product, like vinegar, can help. Even though vinegar emits some VOCs, it's a better choice than more noxious and harmful cleansers.

•**Buy VOC-free products when you can.** Keep in mind that so-called low-VOC products are permitted to have up to 50 grams per liter, and "VOC-free" products can have up to 5 grams per liter. So favor "VOC-free" when you can. Check the packaging or look at the manufacturer's website for information on the exact content. The EPA list of hazardous air pollutants is also a good guide when looking to avoid certain chemicals.

•**Ax the air fresheners.** Nearly half of Americans use air fresheners at least once a week, according to Consumer Reports. This means that many of us are literally spraying VOCs into the air to "freshen" it—and actually just adding to indoor air pollution. Surprisingly, the worst culprits are citrus- and pine-scented products. They contain a class of compounds called monoterpenes that are especially reactive in the atmosphere and contribute to the formation of particulates in the air.

•**Bring fresh air in, send pollutants out.** Vow to open your windows and exterior doors more and flip on bathroom or kitchen fans that exhaust outdoors when you're cleaning or cooking. Other options are operating window or attic fans and running a window air conditioner with the vent control open. Ventilation not only helps to reduce levels of air pollutants but also to control humidity, important because many chemicals off-gas at greater rates in higher humidity.

•**Think small quantities.** When it comes to VOC-containing products, buying in bulk is not your best bet even if it saves you money. Instead, buy only what you will use quickly. If you do have leftover product, such as paint or wood stripper, seal the container tightly and consider storing it in a detached shed or at least in the garage. Products can release organic compounds, to some degree, even when they're stored.

Safer Food and Beverage Containers

BPA-free plastic products may be no safer than those containing BPA.

To be safe: Opt for glass and/or metal food and beverage containers, jars and bottles. If you do use plastic, avoid the dishwasher and microwave—heat accelerates chemical release. If plastics show signs of damage such as haziness or cracks, discard them.

Patricia A. Hunt, PhD, Meyer Distinguished Professor in the School of Molecular Biosciences, Washington State University, Pullman, and leader of a study published in *Current Biology*.

There's Weed Killer in Your Cereal If You Eat These Brands

Tasha Stoiber, PhD, senior scientist with the Environmental Working Group in San Francisco.

If oats or oat flour is included in your breakfast cereal or snack of choice, there's a good chance there's also an unwanted herbicide in there.

Two sets of laboratory tests commissioned by the Environmental Working Group (EWG), a consumer-advocacy nonprofit, found glyphosate, the main agent in the weed killer called Roundup, in many popular breakfast cereals and oat-based snacks. While no one wants this in their cereal, the concern is greatest for kids—

most samples were above the EWG benchmark, with a few being 10 times higher.

How does glyphosate wind up in your or your child's breakfast bowl or granola bar? The herbicide is sprayed on wheat, barley, oats and beans. Besides killing weeds, it also acts as a drying agent so the crops can be harvested sooner.

THE RISKIEST AND SAFEST FOODS

Based on the safety threshold set by the California Office of Environmental Health Hazard Assessment, EWG calculated its own health benchmark for glyphosate. But its limit, 160 parts per billion (ppb), is much lower to protect children from glyphosate because they have a higher susceptibility to cancer-causing substances.

Here's where the highest levels of glyphosate were found among samples…

•**Quaker Oatmeal Squares Honey Nut cereal**—2,837 parts per billion

•**Quaker Oatmeal Squares Brown Sugar cereal**—2,746 parts per billion

•**Quaker Overnight Oats Unsweetened with Chia Seeds**—1,799 parts per billion

•**Quaker Old-Fashioned Oats**—1,300 parts per billion

•**Cheerios Oat Crunch Cinnamon cereal**—1,171 parts per billion

While the EWG found glyphosate in some of the samples of organic products, the amounts were well within the group's acceptable limits both for adults and children.

Here are five organic products that had no glyphosate in the samples tested…

•**Nature's Path Organic Honey Almond Granola**—no glyphosate detected

•**Simple Truth Organic Instant Oatmeal**—no glyphosate detected

•**Kashi Heart to Heart Organic Honey Toasted Cereal**—no glyphosate detected

•**Cascadian Farm Organic Harvest Berry Granola Bars**—no glyphosate detected

•**365 Organic Old-Fashioned Rolled Oats**—no glyphosate detected

WHAT'S YOUR LEVEL OF RISK?

The cereal companies maintain that their products are safe and point out that the above levels of glyphosate are within the limit of 30,000 ppb allowed by the EPA. But that limit was set back in 2008 before there was data that linked glyphosate to cancer—and it's 300 times higher than the legal limit that the EPA put on glyphosate about 25 years earlier, before aggressive lobbying by chemical companies. But in any case, the greatest threat is to children.

You can find the complete list of tested foods at EWG.org (search "oat cereals and snacks test").

STEPS TO TAKE NOW

Switching to organic oat–containing products including cereals, granolas, granola bars and flours is the obvious and smart move.

You can also let your voice be heard by contacting the manufacturers of your favorite foods and demanding that they source oats from suppliers that don't use glyphosate.

The FDA Banned 6 Artificial Flavors—But You're (Probably) Still Eating Them

Laura MacCleery, policy director for the Center for Science in the Public Interest in Washington, DC.

The good news: The FDA recently banned six artificial flavors that have been linked to cancer. The final rule initiating the ban was posted in October 2018.

The bad news: You're still eating them, and you might be for a long time.

How could that be? First, as is common with such bans, food manufacturers have two years to actually remove the banned chemicals from their products. Second, because manufacturers are still permitted to label all chemicals used to simulate natural flavors as, generically, "artificial flavors," there's no way to know which products contain these particular offenders. And that's

why, unless you do what we recommend below, you may be chowing down on benzophenone, ethyl acrylate, methyl eugenol, myrcene, pulegone and pyridine for a while to come.

How can this be happening? The ban came in response to a citizen petition from consumer and environmental groups, including the Center for Food Safety, the Center for Science in the Public Interest and the Natural Resources Defense Council, after the six chemicals were linked to cancer in laboratory animals by the National Toxicology Program.

Despite the lab findings, the FDA's position remains that these chemicals don't pose a health risk to consumers and that the animals in the study were exposed to much higher doses than people would ever consume. Fortunately, there is something called the Delaney Clause of the Federal Food, Drug and Cosmetic Act—it stipulates that if a substance is found to cause cancer in humans or animals, it cannot be used in food.

How to protect your health now: Of course, the obvious answer would be to avoid all foods and beverages containing any artificial flavorings. This is easier said than done for many people, however, because sometimes a convenience food is the only food available.

But here's a trick you can use: Many of the banned additives are used to mimic or enhance the flavors of mint, citrus or cinnamon—so just say no to any food or beverage with these flavors and artificial flavoring. And don't forget to check your chewing gum—the banned artificial flavorings are used in gum, too.

In general, knowing which food additives are safe for you and your family is no easy task. The Center for Science in the Public Interest's safety ratings of a wide variety of food additives, Chemical Cuisine (CSPInet.org/eating-healthy/chemical-cuisine), can help you determine what's safe for you and your family to consume and what to avoid.

Not All Bone Broths Are Healthy

Tod Cooperman, MD, president of ConsumerLab.com, an independent group based in White Plains, New York, that tests and reports on the quality of health and nutrition products. ConsumerLab.com

Bone broth's unusual benefits are rooted in the fact that when traditionally prepared, it contains significant amounts of the protein collagen. Studies have found that collagen can reduce joint pain…and somewhat reduce wrinkles, too, for a more youthful appearance.

The trouble is, a laboratory analysis of commercially available bone broths discovered that the amount of collagen these products deliver varies dramatically. Collagen levels often are not listed on product packaging…and the nutritional information that is provided can be wildly inaccurate.

What to do: Purchase a bone broth that delivers lots of collagen at a reasonable price based on independent testing…and that has a reasonably good flavor. *Top picks…*

•**Jarrow Formulas Beyond Bone Broth Spicy Beef Ramen Flavor,** sold as a powder, is the best bone broth value. A 10.8-ounce jar (17 servings) of the powder, which users can add to hot water to make a broth, costs around $21 and provides 11.5 grams of collagen per cup. Jarrow.com

•**Pacific Organic Bone Broth Chicken** is sold as a liquid and is a good choice if you want a bone broth that you can add to soups and recipes without dramatically affecting their flavor. A 32-ounce carton (four servings) often sells for around $6, and one cup provides 4.5 grams of collagen. PacificFoods.com

Radon Testing Concern

Harry Grafton, instructor for the Eastern Regional Radon Training Center at Rutgers University, New Brunswick, New Jersey.

The Environmental Protection Agency (EPA) recommends testing for radon every two years to be sure that levels remain in the acceptable range. (The EPA's acceptable range is under 4 picocuries, or pCi/L, per liter of air, but the World Health Organization recommends a level under 2.7 pCi/L.) You should also retest if you've made structural renovations (such as changing the heating or air-conditioning system).

Why it's important: Radon—a gas formed by the natural breakdown of uranium in soil and rocks—can seep into your house through the foundation and increase your risk for lung cancer. After smoking, radon exposure is the second-leading cause of lung cancer in the US. Retesting is advised even if you already have a radon-mitigation system to be sure that the system is working correctly. Home test kits (under $30) are reliable if you follow the instructions carefully. Or hire a licensed radon specialist.

The Great Sunscreen Debate

Steven Q. Wang, MD, director of dermatologic surgery and dermatology at Memorial-Sloan Kettering Cancer Center in Basking Ridge, New Jersey, and cofounder of Dr. Wang Herbal Skincare.

If you've been using a mineral sunscreen, Consumer Report's 2018 ratings (subscription required for full report) of 73 sunscreens may raise alarm bells. Based on its testing, CR doesn't recommend any mineral sunscreens, which means none were judged to provide "excellent" or "very good" protection from both UVA and UVB radiation—although five got excellent scores for UVA protection. Only sunscreens with chemical ingredients that absorb into the skin have garnered the highest ratings.

You may be thinking, *So are chemical sunscreens the only ones that work?* The answer is no. For one thing, not all mineral sunscreens do poorly in the CR ratings—some were rated as "good." For another, in its 12th Annual Sunscreen Guide, the Environmental Working Group, a nonprofit that examined almost 650 sunscreen products, found that mineral products did well, offering good protection from UVA and UVB radiation without potentially harmful additives.

It's difficult to evaluate the different methodologies that led to these discrepancies in rating mineral sunscreens.

But even if the Consumer Reports methodology is sound (and I have no reason to assume that it's not), I believe that even "good" protection is all you need—but only if you use your sunscreen right. That is my experience with my patients—and in my own testing of sunscreens.

Most of us don't use sunscreen the right way, if we use them at all. And that's a much bigger factor than which kind of sunscreen you choose in determining whether you're protecting yourself from damaging sun radiation that can accelerate skin aging and increase skin cancer risk.

What's more important than which type of sunscreen? Remembering to put it on in the first place, using it correctly—most people don't—and realizing that you can't rely on sunscreen alone to protect your skin.

That last point is the most important one: Your first line of defense should be other forms of protection—hats, clothing, seeking out shade and avoiding the mid-day sun. That advice goes for both adults and children.

MY RULES FOR SUNSCREEN USE

The following simple strategies should help you successfully protect your skin from sun damage…

•**Gear your sunscreen use to where you will be and what you will be doing.** If you drive to an office and work indoors, for example, and then go out briefly for lunch, you need only an SPF 30 sunscreen that you apply once to your face (women should put it on under makeup), neck and exposed areas of your arms. An SPF 30 product is also fine if you're spending more than an hour outdoors. But if you will be outdoors swimming, hiking, playing sports, etc., use an SPF 50 or higher sunscreen that's water resistant, and apply it to all of your exposed skin.

Tip: Don't assume that all mineral sunscreens are water-resistant—some are, others aren't, so check labels.

•**If you're using a chemical sunscreen, apply it 15 to 30 minutes before you go outdoors.** Mineral sunscreens are effective the moment you put them on, but chemical sunscreens need time to be absorbed to take effect.

•**Reapply sunscreen every two hours.** This is true for everyone, but it's especially important if you're sweating or swimming.

•**Don't worry about the exact amount you apply.** Studies show most people don't use enough sunscreen. If guidelines like "one shot glass" or "one teaspoon" are confusing, simply apply sunscreen twice. Like painting a house, you often miss spots (ears, tops of feet, areas of your back) when you apply the first "coat." The second application helps make sure you cover those missed areas and put on enough to really protect yourself.

So choose the sunscreen that you prefer—and then take the steps above to make sure that it's really protecting you.

Drug Recall Alert

Jack E. Fincham, PhD, RPh, professor of pharmacy administration, Presbyterian College School of Pharmacy, Clinton, South Carolina.

If you take prescription medication—especially if it's for high blood pressure or heart problems—listen up!

The FDA recently announced a series of recalls for several lots of blood pressure medications that contain *losartan*, *valsartan* or *irbesartan* after tests found contamination with a suspected cancer-causing chemical.

Not all drug labels include lot numbers (used by pharmaceutical manufacturers to track medications). So anyone taking one of these medications should ask his/her pharmacist if the dispensed generic prescription drug is manufactured by one of the companies cited in the recalls.

Important: Don't stop this—or any—medication without checking with your doctor. The risk of stopping a drug cold turkey could be worse than the risk from any possible impurities it contains. *Also…*

•**Ask your pharmacist about the manufacturer of any drug you're taking.** If there's any question about the manufacturer's track record, ask the pharmacist to get the drug from a different manufacturer.

•**Search for drug recalls.** Go to the FDA website, FDA.gov, and enter a medication name in the search field to see if a drug you're taking has been recalled.

•**Sign up for e-mail alerts at FDA.gov/safety/recalls.** The e-mails provide the latest recall information about drugs and other FDA-regulated products.

New Ways to Save Money on Prescription Drugs

Charles B. Inlander, a consumer advocate and health-care consultant based in Fogelsville, Pennsylvania. He was the founding president of the nonprofit People's Medical Society, a consumer advocacy organization credited with key improvements in the quality of US health care, and is author or coauthor of more than 20 consumer-health books.

If it seems like prescription medication prices have risen nearly as fast as Bitcoin once did, you're not that far off. And it isn't just with exotic drugs.

Examples: In recent years, the price of the heart drug *digoxin*, one of the oldest drugs on the market and historically very cheap, has been raised more than 600%…and the cost of insulin has tripled.

But there are strategies to control your drug costs so that you can afford what you need…

USE DISCOUNT APPS AND SITES

One of the few positive trends in the pharmaceutical business in recent years has been the rise of websites and apps that let you easily search for the lowest prices on prescription medication. None of these services accept insurance, but the prices offered are sometimes even lower than what many people would pay through their insurance plans.

Here are some of the best online drug discount programs (all are free to join)…

•**GoodRx.** Print coupons for discounts or send them to your phone, and then show them at your pharmacy to save up to 80%.

•**RxPharmacyCoupons.com** can save you up to 90% on more than 20,000 name-brand and generic meds at more than 68,000 pharmacies.

•**BlinkHealth.** Buy your prescription at a discount online, then pick it up at your local pharmacy.

Many drug manufacturers also offer discount coupons. Search online for "discount coupons" and the name of the drug you need. These may not be usable along with your prescription drug coverage, so check with your plan.

LET COMPETITION WORK FOR YOU

Prices can vary widely at different pharmacies—even within the same pharmacy chain.

Extra tip: Large-chain drugstores, such as CVS, Rite Aid and Walgreens, and large stores with pharmacies, such as Walmart, Costco and Target, are engaged in a price war over which one can charge the least for some of the most common generic drugs—so call around and take advantage when you have such a prescription to fill. Target, for instance, offers the antibiotic *amoxicillin*, the diabetes drug *chlorpropamide* and the prostate drug *doxazosin* for just $4 a month each (or $10 for a three-month supply). Sam's Club fills some generic prescriptions for free for members.

Keep in mind: Many chains offer drug discount cards, so sign up for them.

NEGOTIATE WITH YOUR PHARMACY

Most people think drug prices at pharmacies are fixed—but often they're not. Simply asking, "Is that your best price?" over the phone or in person is sometimes all it takes to get a discount. A good pharmacist may match a price you find online or search for discount programs or coupons that you can use to reduce the price. It can't hurt to ask—even at big pharmacies.

USE A MAIL-ORDER PHARMACY

If you are taking a medication to control a chronic condition long-term, there's no need to drive to the pharmacy or reorder every month. Mail-order pharmacies—and perhaps even your local one—deliver a 90-day supply to your

91

door and can be set up to auto-refill prescriptions. And it's not merely convenient—it's often cheaper. People who have drug plans with participating mail-order pharmacies typically save as much as one-third compared with using a local pharmacy.

Caution: There are lots of unscrupulous businesses online that present themselves as legitimate pharmacies but that are not. Don't gamble on whether you will receive legitimate medicine. Make sure the site is accredited by the Verified Internet Pharmacy Practice Sites (VIPPS) program from the National Association of Boards of Pharmacy. If you want to see whether an Internet pharmacy is accredited, you can look it up online at NABP.pharmacy/programs/vipps. An example of a good VIPPS-accredited mail-order pharmacy is HealthWarehouse.com. It does not take any insurance, but it's worth comparing prices with those you can get through your insurance plan—you might save money.

GRILL YOUR DOCTOR

When a promising new drug hits the market, doctors are likely to get excited and prescribe it instead of older alternatives. But what if the cost of this new name-brand drug is 10 times that of a time-tested generic or five times that of an older brand-name drug that might be equally effective? Your doctor might not consider the price difference.

Of course, if your condition requires a newer drug for which there's no cheaper equivalent, you should pony up. But whenever your doctor wants to prescribe you a new drug, make sure that you truly need it by grilling him/her about the pros and cons versus older drugs.

THE DANGER OF USING MULTIPLE PHARMACIES

While shopping around can cut your drug costs substantially, there is one potentially large drawback to purchasing your meds in multiple places—dangerous drug interactions. You might have multiple doctors prescribing you different medicines. You should discuss with each of your doctors all the medications you take…but another line of defense against harmful drug interactions can be a pharmacist.

My advice: Make sure that each place that fills a prescription for you enters every med you take into its record on you…even meds that you get elsewhere. Ask a pharmacist to review this complete list every time you add a new prescription. This act of drug due diligence takes only a few extra minutes, and it will help ensure your safety.

Hospice Warning: What You Need to Know to Avoid Poor Care

Linda R. Beck, JD, BCPA, an attorney and board-certified patient advocate who practices at Square One Elder and Health Advocacy LLC, San Luis Obispo, California.

Hospice is designed to ease suffering when a person is expected to live six months or less and has decided not to seek further treatment aimed at curing an illness. Even though most hospice agencies generally do a good job overall—and have the positive caregiver survey data to show for it—some fail to provide crucial services.

Sobering report: While the use of hospice continues to climb in the US, some troubling deficiencies have been revealed in a recent report from the Office of Inspector General (OIG) at the US Department of Health and Human Services.

3 KEY PROBLEM AREAS

Most people who receive hospice care are Medicare beneficiaries.* The OIG, which is charged with ensuring that beneficiaries receive quality care, conducted evaluations and audits of the hospice program from 2006 to 2016. *Key findings…*

•**Care planning often falls short.** Hospices are required to provide a written "plan of care," developed by an interdisciplinary group that includes a physician, registered nurse, social worker and pastoral or other counselor, for each

*Hospice may also be covered by Medicaid and the Veterans Administration. Coverage for hospice under private insurance varies.

hospice patient. The plan also should include a detailed statement of the scope and frequency of services needed. However, the OIG report found that in 85% of general inpatient care stays in 2012, the hospices did not meet these basic care-planning requirements.

Note: Even though most patients receive hospice care in their homes, the plan of care is still required.

•**Important services are sometimes lacking.** The OIG reported that hospices provided fewer services than outlined in the plans of care for 31% of hospice beneficiaries residing in nursing facilities.

Example: A hospice billed for 17 days of general inpatient care for a 70-year-old man but never visited him. Instead, the hospice called his family to inquire how he was doing. Services outlined in plans of care are particularly important to those in general inpatient care because those patients have uncontrolled symptoms— often pain—that cannot be managed in other settings.

•**Many hospices provide only one level of care.** Even though Medicare-certified hospices are required to provide four levels of service when needed, most payments were for only one—"routine care" in the hospice patient's home (whether that's a private residence, nursing home or other facility).

The other levels of care are "general inpatient care" when the patient is admitted to a hospital or other facility to get symptoms under control…"continuous home care" for someone in a crisis…and "respite care" in a hospital or nursing facility when a primary caregiver becomes unavailable or needs a break. When these additional levels of care are not provided, it suggests that the hospice may not be meeting all of the patient's needs.

KNOWING YOUR OPTIONS

When choosing hospice, ask your own (or your loved one's) health-care providers to recommend some high-quality hospice agencies.

Note: Stay in touch with this health-care provider after hospice starts in case you need an advocate at any point. Friends, family members, hospital social workers, nursing-home staffers and clergy members can offer recommendations, too.

Also helpful: Consult Medicare.gov/Hospice Compare, which features consumer survey data showing how each agency compares with national averages on measures such as managing pain and considering patients' values. To dig deeper, check the website for your state public health department, where public complaint information usually appears. If the information is not on the website, call the department and ask how to access it.

TO AVOID POOR CARE

Once you've narrowed your list of possible hospice agencies, here are some key questions to ask…

•**How quickly will the hospice team develop a care plan?** This should happen within two calendar days of the date the patient is admitted to hospice. If you have questions about the plan, talk with the hospice's registered nurse case manager or medical director.

•**How fast is your crisis response time— especially on evenings and weekends?** A crisis could be unmanageable pain, uncontrolled bleeding, vomiting or seizures.

Important: You want to know how quickly a health-care provider will come to the patient's bedside, not just how quickly the hospice answering service will pick up the phone.

•**Will the patient and family see the same nurses, aides and other team members** most of the time? Care is often most consistent when you work with the same individuals.

•**If my loved one is in a nursing home or other long-term facility,** who will be responsible for which aspects of routine care, such as bathing, feeding and monitoring the patient's condition? Facility and hospice staffs may each expect the other to provide these services, which can cause a patient's care to fall through the cracks.

•**Is the hospice accredited by any organization,** such as The Joint Commission or Community Health Accreditation Program (CHAP)? Such accreditations are not required and their absence is not a mark of poor quality, but they do offer some extra reassurance that an agency has been checked out and meets a basic standard of care. All hospices that serve Medicare patients must be certified by Medicare. States have varying licensing requirements, so make sure any agency you pick meets those standards.

You can ask: "What public agency licenses does your hospice have?" For more information, contact the nonprofit Hospice Foundation of America, HospiceFoundation.org.

Nursing Homes Are Kicking Out Patients

Annette Ticoras, MD, physician, patient advocate and owner of Guided Patient Services, Inc., in Westerville, Ohio. GPSColumbus.com

States and the federal government are reporting a rising risk for the 1.3 million Americans now in nursing homes—being improperly evicted. But there are ways to fight back.

In a typical scenario, an elderly person with low income is discharged from the hospital to a nursing home for rehab after a major operation or injury. But after a few weeks—and before the patient is truly able to return home—the nursing home tells the patient that therapy is no longer helping and the bed is going to someone else.

In other words, get out.

What's really going on: The temporary insurance coverage by Medicare is about to run out—typically 20 full-pay days and up to 80 additional partial-pay days. Before lower-paying Medicaid kicks in, the patient is shown the door.

Another scenario: With dementia patients—even some with private pay—the family is told that the patient is a hazard to other residents.

What's really going on: The institution is looking for easier-to-manage patients.

If your loved one is told to start packing, don't panic. Federal regulations require notice, in writing, 30 days before discharge, that specifies a legitimate reason such as patient improvement or endangerment to others.

Important: You have a right to appeal. Do so immediately—your loved one can stay in place for 30 days during the process. Contact your state's long-term-care ombudsman's office. (To find one in your state, go to TheConsumer Voice.org/get_help.)

Another option: Hire a private patient advocate, who can determine if the cause for the resident's status change can be remedied...initiate a plan...get appropriate parties working together...engage new resources...and improve communications. To find one, go to AdvoCon nection.com.

For more information about the rights of nursing home residents, go to TheConsumerVoice. org website and search for "involuntary transfer and discharge." You'll find a wealth of materials that let you know your rights and how to fight for them.

CHAPTER 6

Diabetes Breakthroughs

The Diabetes Drug Danger Most Doctors Miss

Most of the nearly 30 million Americans who have type 2 diabetes are not even aware that cardiovascular problems pose a huge risk for them.

Even more troubling: Your doctor may be facing a knowledge gap, too—for different reasons. A new generation of prescription diabetes medications now is available, and these drugs are particularly effective at helping people with type 2 diabetes control their blood sugar while simultaneously reducing their risk for cardiovascular disease. (One botanical supplement may have similar benefits—see next article.) But the proper use of these medications can be so complicated that your doctor may not be making the right choice for you.

NEW HEART-FRIENDLY DIABETES DRUGS

For many years, there were only three types of drugs—not counting insulin—to help people with type 2 diabetes control their blood glucose levels. *Metformin* typically was prescribed first (and still is)—it's effective, safe and affordable. It has not been shown to increase or decrease cardiovascular risk.

When metformin isn't enough to control blood sugar, sulfonylureas often have been prescribed in addition. They are effective—sometimes too effective, leading to dangerous low-blood-sugar episodes. More disturbing, some studies have found that long-term use of sulfonylureas are associated with an increased risk for heart disease. Similarly, thiazolidinediones, introduced in the 1990s, have been shown to increase the risk for heart failure.

George L. King, MD, chief scientific officer at the Boston-based Joslin Diabetes Center, one of the country's leading diabetes clinical care and research centers. He is a professor of medicine at Harvard Medical School and author, with Royce Flippin, of *Reverse Your Diabetes in 12 Weeks.* Joslin.org

What's new: In the past decade, and especially in just the past few years, a host of new, heart-friendly diabetes drugs have appeared. Most notable are the glucagon-like peptide-1 receptor agonists (GLP-1 agonists, for short) and sodium–glucose cotransporter 2 inhibitors (SGLT2 inhibitors). Both types have been shown in large studies to not just control blood glucose levels but also reduce the risk for heart failure—and reduce mortality in people with type 2 diabetes.

Other new diabetes drugs include dipeptidyl peptidase-4 inhibitors (DPP-4 inhibitors), which don't increase cardiovascular risk, and *colesevelam* and *bromocriptine*, both of which may reduce cardiovascular risk but have significant side effects. Each of these is a different type of drug, and the complexity is leading to some not-so-smart prescriptions and danger for patients.

THE DOCTOR KNOWLEDGE GAP

Metformin remains the "first-line" type 2 diabetes drug. But what should be prescribed when, together with lifestyle changes, it's not enough? Unfortunately, some doctors will not come up with the best answer to that question.

Type 2 diabetes typically is treated by primary care physicians, some of whom are not well-versed in the latest research…or who lack the time to figure out which of the drug options is best-suited to a particular patient. Don't blame your doctor—selecting type 2 diabetes drugs has very quickly become very complicated. Doctors must not only sort through an ever-widening range of drug options with various (and different) side effects, but they also must consider each patient's blood glucose levels, cardiovascular condition, other prescribed medications and, increasingly, financial situation.

Example: New joint guidelines from the American Diabetes Association and the European Association for the Study of Diabetes, presented in October 2018, recommend the use of GLP-1 agonists or SGLT2 inhibitors as the second drug after metformin for patients with type 2 diabetes who have cardiovascular disease. But while metformin and sulfonylureas can cost less than $10 for a 30-day supply, these newer drugs can run $400 or more per month for patients who must pay out of pocket…and might have hefty co-pays. There are many medical caveats, too—such as not using SGLT2 inhibitors in a patient with a certain degree of kidney failure…and how to ramp up the dosage of a GLP-1 agonist to decrease potential side effects.

WHAT DIABETES PATIENTS SHOULD DO

Do not assume that the glucose-control drugs your doctor has prescribed are necessarily the best drugs for you. *In particular…*

•**If you take a drug other than metformin to control blood glucose**—and especially if you take three or more glucose-control drugs—ask your doctor to explain why he/she selected each of these drugs.

•**If you have a history of heart attack or stroke and are taking multiple drugs to control your blood glucose**—but are not taking a GLP-1 agonist or SGLT2 inhibitor—ask your doctor whether one of these might be appropriate for you.

•**If your doctor cannot explain why he chose the drugs** you are taking in a way that you can understand and that sounds reasonable, ask for a referral to an endocrinologist who specializes in the treatment of diabetes.

THE GROWING POWER OF LIFESTYLE

The new diabetes medications give doctors new tools to tailor treatment to an individual's most important risks, including cardiovascular risk. But it's never a good idea to take an additional drug to control your blood sugar if you can do so through lifestyle changes instead, which are more powerful and healthier than any drugs. Fortunately, most of the lifestyle changes that help control blood sugar also protect your heart. Even small changes—such as getting up from your desk and walking around for five minutes every hour—can be very helpful. *My recommendations…*

•**Work up to walking 10,000 steps a day.** You can track this on your phone or with a fitness watch or pedometer.

•**Get 60 minutes of more vigorous exercise every other day**—evenly split between aerobics (such as treadmill jogging) and strength training.

Good news: Those jogging "steps" count toward your 10,000.

•**At mealtime, follow the two-one-one formula**—two portions nonstarchy vegetables (especially dark, leafy greens)…one portion whole grains, legumes or starchy vegetables… and one portion protein-rich food (fish, poultry, lean beef, tofu). For dessert, fruit is best.

•**Get seven or eight hours of sleep a night.**

I know the power of these lifestyle changes from personal experience. About 25 years ago, when my father was age 72, he developed diabetes and was promptly placed on three medications. He took them, but at the same time he began walking an hour a day and eating as I describe above. A year and a half later, while he still technically "had" diabetes, he no longer needed any medication to control it. That's why I have been following this lifestyle myself ever since.

This Supplement Fights Diabetes and Protects Your Heart

Michael Murray, ND, a leading authority on natural medicine. He serves on the Board of Regents of Bastyr University in Seattle and has authored or coauthored more than 30 books featuring natural approaches to health, including *Bottom Line's Encyclopedia of Healing Foods* and *The Encyclopedia of Natural Medicine.* DoctorMurray.com

Expensive drugs are not the only option for people with type 2 diabetes to control blood sugar and protect cardiovascular health. A natural supplement called berberine can provide both of these benefits as well.

The supplement, derived from goldenseal root and other plants, activates an enzyme that makes the body more sensitive to insulin, thus helping to control blood sugar. A 2015 statistical review of 27 clinical trials concluded that berberine can control blood sugar as effectively as the go-to diabetes drug *metformin.*

Bonus: Like the diabetes drugs called GLP-1 agonists and SGLT2 inhibitors, berberine is good for the heart. It reduces high blood pressure, improves the ability of blood vessels to dilate and helps prevent heart failure. Side effects—uncommon and usually mild—can include nausea and stomach upset.

What to do: Before you take any supplement, discuss it with your medical doctor or naturopathic physician to rule out any possible interactions with another medication.

Example: Berberine can interfere with the effectiveness of certain antibiotics and other drugs. A typical dose is 500 mg two to three times daily before meals, but discuss the right dosing for you with your doctor. If berberine works, your doctor might be able to reduce the dose of one or more of your diabetes drugs.

The New, Ultimate Diabetes Screening

Michael Snyder, PhD, researcher, chair of Stanford University's department of genetics and director of the Center for Genomics and Personalized Medicine, Stanford, California, and coauthor of the study titled "Glucotypes Reveal New Patterns of Glucose Dysregulation," published in *PLOS Biology.*

Think you don't have diabetes just because your last blood sugar test said so? Think again! A small but potentially groundbreaking study at Stanford University reveals that annual blood sugar tests—even the vaunted "A1c" test—tell you what's going on in your body only at the moment you had the test.

That can be a problem because, as the study revealed, your blood sugar actually could be spiking to levels throughout the day that would classify you as one of the 30 million adults in the US with undiagnosed, full-blown type 2 diabetes or as one of the additional 84 million adults with prediabetes, diabetes waiting in the wings.

To better understand spikes in blood sugar levels, the researchers recruited 25 men and 32 women, ages 25 to 76, nearly all with no known prior history of diabetes or prediabetes. Interestingly, as part of their screening for participation, two were found to already have diabetes and 14, prediabetes.

Each participant wore a continuous glucose monitor, or CGM, for up to four weeks. (A CGM system includes a tiny sensor that's inserted just under the skin on one side of the abdomen, and it checks blood sugar levels every five minutes around the clock, transmitting data wirelessly to a nearby smartphone or receiver.) Blood sugar levels were recorded as study volunteers worked, slept, ate, hung out with friends or cared for their families...in other words, during all their normal day-to-day activities.

Some of the results were startling. Many participants who did not have diabetes based on initial screening experienced frequent blood sugar surges that put them into the prediabetic or even the diabetic range. The researchers also noted that blood sugar ranges were much higher in some participants than in others in response to specific foods. Other studies have shown that over time, high glucose spikes in people can damage organs including the pancreas, liver and heart.

WHAT WEARING A CGM CAN TELL YOU

While a CGM is traditionally recommended for people with diabetes as an alternative to frequent finger pricks to track blood sugar, for people without diabetes, wearing the device once a year may be a great way to see whether you're in the danger zone for developing the disease, says study coauthor Michael Snyder, PhD. For your first time, you might wear the sensor for three or four weeks, he says, while keeping a journal of everything you eat and noting which foods trigger spikes. By cutting back on these foods, it may be that you can help delay or even prevent the onset of full-blown diabetes. In successive years, wearing a CGM for just one week would enable you to catch any changes and make any needed adjustments, says Dr. Snyder.

To get started, you'll need to ask your doctor for a CGM prescription, instructions on how to use it (it causes only a brief sting as the sensor is inserted) and a follow-up appointment to discuss the readings. You might be met with skepticism at first, but this example of personalized medicine can give you far greater insights into your health than a single test and offer the opportunity to prevent a lifelong condition that comes with serious complications, including heart disease. While insurance won't pay for a CGM for someone without diabetes, Dr. Snyder believes

that these devices will soon become inexpensive and direct-to-consumer, giving people easy access to monitoring their glucose levels.

Hot Baths Can Reduce Diabetes Risk

Christof Leicht, PhD, lecturer in exercise physiology at Loughborough University in the UK and leader of a study of overweight, sedentary men published in *Journal of Applied Physiology*.

Hot baths can reduce blood sugar and chronic inflammation in a similar way that exercise can. Study subjects sat up to their necks for an hour in 102°F water each day for two weeks.

Implication: People unable or unwilling to exercise might be able to reduce the risk for diabetes and other inflammation-related ills. Ask your doctor whether hot baths are safe for you.

How Cancer Can Increase Your Diabetes Risk

Study titled "Incidence of Diabetes After Cancer Development: A Korean National Cohort Study" by researchers at Sungkyunkwan University in Seoul, South Korea, published in *JAMA Oncology*.

What's the one thing that kills cancer survivors more than anything else? Diabetes. That's right—diabetes. And if you're a cancer survivor (or ever become one), new research shows that the importance of taking steps to keep yourself from getting diabetes can hardly be overstated.

THE DANGER IN BOTH DIRECTIONS

Many studies had previously shown that having diabetes increases the risk of getting cancer, but there had been scant information going in the other direction, that cancer may increase the risk for diabetes...until now. Researchers in South Korea recently completed a 10-year study that involved about a half million people, men and women, ages 20 to 70, all free of both diabetes and cancer at the start of the research. *Here's what they found over the course of their work…*

• **Of the 15,130 people diagnosed with cancer, 834, or 5.5%, went on to develop type 2 diabetes.**

• **Those who got cancer had about a 35% higher risk of developing diabetes than those who didn't get cancer,** even after accounting for other diabetes risk factors such as older age, physical inactivity, smoking and obesity.

• **The risk of developing diabetes was highest in the first two years after a cancer diagnosis,** but elevated risk continued through the end of the study.

• **The cancer associated with the highest risk of developing diabetes was pancreatic cancer**—understandable, since the pancreas makes insulin—followed by kidney, liver, gallbladder, lung, blood, breast, stomach and thyroid cancer. The researchers suspect that these cancers may increase risk for diabetes directly because of changes cancer causes in the body… medications used to treat it, such as chemotherapy and/or steroids…and/or the psychological and physical stress of having cancer.

And it's important to know that the risk of developing diabetes after cancer could be even higher for people who have other diabetes risk factors such as being overweight, having a family history of diabetes, having high blood pressure or high cholesterol or not getting enough exercise.

Studies that uncover danger such as this seem like bad news, but they can be good news if they inspire you to make changes that help you avoid the danger. And the especially good news here is that there are many steps you can take to reduce your risk for diabetes after cancer. The National Institutes of Health recommends making sure that you get regular blood tests to screen for diabetes (work with your doctor on how often that should be for you). And don't wait to put an effective lifestyle plan in place to prevent diabetes. Depending on your unique situation, this could involve improving your diet and starting a fitness program.

Food to Fight Diabetes

Magnesium-rich foods could reduce diabetes risk. Scientists tracked roughly 200,000 people for 28 years. Those who reported getting the most magnesium had a 15% lower risk for type 2 diabetes than those who reported getting the least. Good sources of magnesium include whole grains, leafy greens, nuts and beans.

Study by researchers at Harvard T.H. Chan School of Public Health, Boston, published in *Diabetes Care*.

Pecans stave off type 2 diabetes. When people ate a typical American diet—low in fruits and vegetables and high in calorically dense foods—for four weeks, those who consumed 1.5 ounces of pecans daily (a little less than one-half cup) had lower diabetes risk markers than those who did not eat the nuts. Risk markers included insulin levels and insulin resistance.

Study by researchers at Tufts University, Boston, published in *Nutrients*.

The High-Fiber Fix for Diabetes

Liping Zhao, PhD, Eveleigh-Fenton Chair of Applied Microbiology in the department of biochemistry and microbiology at the Rutgers School of Environmental and Biological Sciences, The State University of New Jersey in New Brunswick, and lead author of the study "Gut bacteria selectively promoted by dietary fibers alleviate type 2 diabetes" published in *Science*.

What if you could eat to beat diabetes? You can. New research shows that people who are willing to more than double the fiber in their diets from 16 to 37 grams per day can better control diabetes. It needs to be a high amount of diverse types of fibers, and getting nearly 40 grams may sound like a tall order, but it's actually not that hard—and it could make a radical difference in your blood sugar level.

WHY IT WORKS

Common thinking about why fiber is good for people with type 2 diabetes is that fiber slows down your digestive system. That means less of a sugar spike after eating, important when your body doesn't make enough insulin to handle a high sugar load. Fiber also makes you feel full on less food, and that can help with weight loss, an important goal for many people with diabetes. This means that the benefits are from the physical properties of fiber themselves rather than from improving glycemic control.

But when researchers followed two groups of people with diabetes eating different amounts of fiber, they found that people who ate nearly 40 grams of diverse fibers a day actually regained their own glycemic control back to a higher level than the group that ate only 16 grams—a win-win-win for the 37-gram eaters. The high-fiber-intake group showed a steady increase of insulin secretion and insulin sensitivity, borne out with rigorous medical tests such as the oral glucose tolerance test (OGTT) at the end of each month on the new diet for three consecutive months. This demonstrated that the high-fiber diet actually led to better glycemic control and does not just reduce the sugar load of your diet and make you feel full. Something more fundamental happened.

How that works: By studying the gut bacteria, or gut biome, of the participants, the researchers found that intake of diverse fibers selectively increased a group of bacteria that digest fiber and produce a type of substance called short-chain fatty acids. Higher levels of these acids, acetic and butyric acids, were linked to an increased production of the hormone GLP-1, known to increase insulin secretion.

Interestingly, production of these acids also reduced the pH of the gut, which makes it a less favorable environment for other not-so-good-for-you bacteria, such as producers of indole and hydrogen sulfide, two smelly and toxic compounds that can inhibit GLP-1 production. Endotoxin producers, which can induce inflammation and damage insulin receptors, were also reduced, leading to high insulin sensitivity of all body cells of the patients.

Think of it this way: Picture cultivating a tall tree so that it forms a tight canopy that creates a special environment within the forest. This group of fiber-utilizing gut bacteria are the tall trees of our healthy "gut forest." Eating enough fibers to grow your tall tree gut bacteria may be critical to your health.

In a nutshell, more diverse fibers means more insulin and higher insulin sensitivity, explains lead study author Liping Zhao, PhD, of Rutgers University. Dr. Zhao believes that feeding those short-chain fatty acid-producing bacteria more fibers will not only help people manage type 2 diabetes, it also may help reduce the risk of developing type 2 diabetes, important for people diagnosed with metabolic syndrome or prediabetes.

FIXING YOUR FIBER SHORTFALL

Here's a bit of hominid history you may or may not want to share at your next dinner party. According to Dr. Zhao, studies of fossilized feces from our ancient ancestors shows that they may have eaten 200 to 400 grams of fiber every day! The point being, our modern diets are truly puny in fiber compared with what our bodies might have evolved for. Today, the average American eats only about 16 grams of fiber per day, not nearly enough to get fiber's diabetes-fighting (or many other) benefits.

To get 37 grams of fiber into your diet each day without overeating, you're going to want to choose foods that provide the most grams per serving. When you read nutrition labels, focus on the number of grams rather than the percentage of the recommended daily amount, because that's based on the lower guideline of 25 grams per day. *Here are some of the foods highest in various fibers…*

- **Beans** (15 grams in 1 cup of cooked black beans)
- **Split peas** (16.3 g in 1 cup cooked)
- **Lentils** (15.6 in 1 cup cooked)
- **Fruits,** especially those with edible skins (8 g in 1 cup raspberries, 5.5 g in a medium pear)
- **Vegetables** (10.3 g in 1 medium artichoke, steamed, 8.8 g in 1 cup cooked green peas and 5.1 g in 1 cup cooked broccoli)
- **Whole grains** (5 g in ½ cup rolled oats uncooked, and 6 g in 1 cup cooked pearl barley)
- **Nuts and seeds** (5.2 g in 1.5 ounces almonds, 5.6 g in 2 tablespoons of flaxseed)

Note: If you're wondering if fiber supplements are an easy way out, they're not. You not only need a steady amount of fiber across the day, but you also need the very diverse mix of fibers available through food.

Important: Work with your certified diabetes educator or endocrinologist on the best way to increase your fiber intake as part of your blood sugar management.

The future of fiber and the gut biome may be personalized nutrition. Since everyone's biome is different, tests will measure which bacteria in your gut respond best to which high-fiber foods and in what quantity. With this information, you will be able to get your gut biome into top shape. These tests are already being studied, says Dr. Zhao.

Intermittent Fasting for Diabetes

Peter M. Clifton, MD, PhD, professor of nutrition, School of Pharmacy and Medical Sciences, University of South Australia, Adelaide.

People with type 2 diabetes who ate 500 to 600 calories on two nonconsecutive days each week (and their normal diet on other days) for 12 months had similar blood sugar control as those who ate a calorie-restricted diet (1,200 to 1,500 calories) every day. Intermittent fasting is effective at controlling diabetes, especially for those who do not like restricting calories every day.

Important: Talk to your doctor before starting any new diet if you have diabetes.

Medicare Now Covers Diabetes Prevention

Angela Forfia, senior manager of prevention with the American Association of Diabetes Educators, Chicago. DiabetesEducator.org

Medicare covers the cost of certain diabetes-prevention programs for participants diagnosed with prediabetes. Nearly half of Americans age 65 or older have prediabetes, meaning that they are at significant risk for type 2 diabetes. Unfortunately, most people who have prediabetes do not realize they have it.

Diabetes-prevention programs provide education…personal counseling on lifestyle changes that can prevent or delay type 2 diabetes…and access to support groups with the goals of increasing physical activity, improving eating habits and achieving modest weight loss—weight loss of just 5% to 7% often can dramatically reduce type 2 diabetes risk. According to the Centers for Disease Control and Prevention (CDC), these programs can reduce the odds of developing type 2 diabetes by 71% among people over age 60 who have prediabetes.

Medicare's coverage is provided for free to Medicare enrollees who qualify. (Many private health plans also cover diabetes-prevention programs.)

What to do: Use an online screening tool to determine whether you are at risk for prediabetes.

Example: "Risk Test Hedgehogs (Hedgehogs on Vacation)" is a 60-second prediabetes screening video available on YouTube.

If you could be at risk, ask your health-care provider for a prediabetes blood test. If your doctor tells you that your blood test results meet the criteria for prediabetes, ask whether he/she knows of a Medicare Diabetes Prevention Program (MDPP) in your area. If not, locate diabetes-prevention programs in your area through the CDC's database (NCCD.CDC.gov/ddt_dprp) and contact one to ask whether it is a Medicare program. Even if no program in your area is covered by Medicare, consider paying out of pocket—it is better than getting diabetes.

The Diabetes Risk Factors That Aren't on Your Radar

Aaron Price, LICSW, clinical social worker and lecturer at the Joslin Diabetes Center in Boston, an affiliate of Harvard Medical School. Joslin.org
Study titled "Excess Mortality in Finnish Diabetic Subjects Due to Alcohol, Accidents and Suicide: A Nationwide Study" by researchers at the universities of Helsinki, Eastern Finland and Tampere, published in *European Journal of Endocrinology.*

You know the health consequences of not managing your diabetes. But even when you're doing a good job of it, the lifestyle that diabetes demands—from constantly checking your blood sugar levels to analyzing every bite of food to maintaining a strict exercise schedule—can take a different kind of toll on you. Stress and depression are complications that might not be as openly discussed as getting A1C tests and balancing carbs. Yet left unchecked, they can have devastating emotional consequences such as suicide and alcoholism. Heavy drinking can lead to the fatal liver condition of cirrhosis and accidental deaths from falling or other mishaps while under the influence.

According to a sweeping study done in Finland, deaths from alcoholism—both directly from diseases such as cirrhosis or from accidents related to drinking, such as falling while under the influence—and suicide are higher among people with diabetes than the general public, and even more so for people taking insulin.

The study: Researchers followed more than 200,000 men and women with diabetes over a seven-year period and compared their mortality rates to a similar number of people free from diabetes.

The findings: Men with diabetes taking oral medications and insulin-dependent patients of both sexes, particularly those with type 1 diabetes, had a greater suicide risk than the general population. Alcohol-related and accidental deaths were higher for both sexes. Surprisingly, women with diabetes, including those on only oral medication, had a risk for death related to alcohol use that was 10 times higher than the general population (for men with diabetes, that rate is seven times higher than the general population). In addition to increasing the risk for fatal accidents and suicide—roughly twice the number for men and slightly more than 50% higher for women, excessive drinking impairs self-care and can worsen diabetes itself. It's also linked to severe hypoglycemia (low blood sugar), which can be fatal. Though the researchers can't explain exactly why alcohol has a deadlier impact on women with diabetes than men with diabetes, they suggest that it could be because women in general experience greater levels of depression than men do.

THE OVERLOOKED PART OF DIABETES CARE

Diabetes brings with it a wide range of emotions. Fear over complications can trigger anxiety and depression. You might feel guilty that you're not managing it as carefully as you think you should. Or you're meticulous about managing it and get overwhelmed, developing diabetes burnout as you try to meet the demands of the condition. The CDC estimates that in any 18-month period, 33% to 50% of those with diabetes are suffering from "diabetes distress."

Alcohol isn't the answer, but what is? *These three tweaks to your diabetes management style can help...*

• **Clarify the areas of self-care you need to improve on, and create a clear plan to meet them.** That may sound daunting, but you can make it easier on yourself by breaking down the steps into manageable pieces. Let's say that you should check your blood sugar four times a day, but you can't reach that number on a steady basis. Start with one or two daily checks, and tie them to existing lifestyle habits to make them easier to remember. For example, check your blood sugar every morning before you walk the dog and every evening after you eat dinner. After twice-a-day becomes rote, gradually add in more checks, ideally attached to other existing habits, such as after exercise and after lunch until you reach the best frequency for you.

Important: Working with a diabetes coach can help you establish vital habits.

• **Let your family and friends become your partners in care.** There are many lifestyle changes to make when you develop diabetes, and few of them are easy. Rather than try to tough it out yourself, allow family members and friends to help you stay on track. Maybe one person wants to exercise with you every morning, and another wants to cook meals with you every evening. As a bonus, you'll strengthen your relationships in the process.

• **Get professional support.** If you find that you're feeling down more days than not, are losing interest and pleasure in things, not eating or are overeating, sleeping too much or not enough, and certainly if you're drinking too much (more than one drink per day) or having thoughts of suicide, reach out to your doctor or a licensed mental health professional. A therapist who has been through the Mental Health Provider Diabetes Education Program, a joint program developed by the American Diabetes Association and the American Psychological Association, is specially trained to help people overcome their struggles with diabetes, set reasonable goals and show how to incorporate them into everyday life to avoid much of the anxiety caused by diabetes. You can find a practitioner near you through the search function at the American Diabetes Association website (Diabetes.org).

Lower Your Risk for Diabetes with Walking

Susan Besser, MD, a board-certified family physician, Mercy Personal Physicians, Baltimore.

William Tigbe, MD, University of Warwick, UK, coauthor of a study titled "Time Spent in Sedentary Posture Is Associated with Waist Circumference and Cardiovascular Risk" published in *International Journal of Obesity*.

Study titled "Replacement Effects of Sedentary Time on Metabolic Outcomes: The Maastricht Study" lead by researchers at Maastricht University, the Netherlands, published in *Medicine & Science in Sports & Exercise*.

Have you been warned that you're inching toward diabetes? Just as being too sedentary is a key culprit, being more active can turn the situation around. And with walking, you don't have to jump into a complicated exercise plan. But before you put on comfortable shoes and take off, know the amount of walking that's needed.

Scientists at the University of Warwick in the UK compared the health of postal workers with office jobs to those who walked to deliver mail. The more sitting/less walking, the greater the likelihood of having metabolic syndrome and heart disease risk.

The workers who didn't have risk factors for metabolic syndrome had one thing in common: They walked more than 15,000 steps a day or stood (rather than sat) for more than seven hours a day. Metabolic syndrome has several components—increased blood pressure, high blood sugar, excess body fat around the waist and abnormal cholesterol or triglyceride levels. Each of the study participants who walked fewer than 15,000 steps a day or was upright less than seven hours a day had at least one component of the metabolic syndrome, explained study coauthor William Tigbe, MD. Those who spent most of their time sitting were more likely to have not only metabolic syndrome, but also more belly fat and a significantly higher risk for heart disease.

How long to walk: Gradually build up to 15,000 steps a day. Brisk walkers can log about half that amount in 60 minutes and fill in the rest by taking advantage of "real life" opportunities to walk instead of ride (i.e., in a car, bus, elevator…you get the idea). Use a pedometer, fitness tracker or fitness app on your phone to clock all the steps you take throughout the day in addition to those from dedicated walking. Watching the count increase as the day goes on will motivate you to reach your goal. Yes, 15,000 steps—or about seven miles of walking—can seem intimidating, but don't let that keep you in your chair.

Even some movement helps: Another study, this one done in the Netherlands, found that replacing just 30 minutes of sitting (at work or at home) with 30 minutes of walking can reduce the risk for metabolic syndrome and type 2 diabetes.

How often to walk: Six days a week is ideal. The key is consistency, said Susan Besser, MD, a board-certified family physician with Mercy Personal Physicians in Baltimore, Maryland. Avoid trying to cram in a week's worth of exercise in your weekends. When weekdays are too busy to devote a full 60 minutes to walking, break up daily bouts into four 15-minute walks or six 10-minute walks.

How fast to walk: A brisk walking pace to improve health is four miles per hour. The average person's leisure walk is about 2.5 miles to three miles an hour, so that means making an effort to pick up the pace.

Challenge yourself by adding interval training. Walk faster for one or two blocks (or one or two minutes if you're on a trail) and then return to your normal pace for one or two blocks, repeating the sequence for the entire walking session. As you develop more stamina, change your route to include hills.

Miserable weather? Not an excuse! Use a treadmill or head to a mall and get your steps there.

And how about this: Get a dog. Another UK study found that having a dog—or walking with a friend who had one—helped people with type 2 diabetes stay more active.

Blood Sugar–Testing Devices Go High-Tech

Elena Toschi, MD, insulin pump specialist and type 1 diabetes researcher at Joslin Diabetes Center and instructor in medicine at Harvard Medical School, both in Boston. Joslin.org

Are you ready to make endless finger-sticks and insulin injections things of the past? High-tech devices can help you manage diabetes with less pain and better blood sugar control.

CONTINUOUS GLUCOSE MONITORS (CGM)

Good for: People who need tight glucose control with intensive insulin therapy or don't always know when glucose levels change.

If you rely on 10 or more finger pricks a day or are having a hard time regulating your blood sugar, the newest CGMs can really simplify your life. And you'll have more accurate monitoring, with the equivalent of close to 300 checks per day with minimal finger sticks.

A tiny sensor, inserted under the skin of your belly or upper arm, reads the glucose level in tissue fluid every few minutes and sends it wirelessly to a monitor, smartphone or tablet computer. You can read the results directly on your monitor and use your smartphone or computer to keep track of your glucose levels.

A "stand-alone" CGM can be used with an insulin pump or without—the monitor tells you when your blood sugar is out of range, and then you can do your own insulin injections based on your diabetes management plan. Some models send out an alarm tone to alert you when your glucose level is too low or too high. These benefits make CGMs useful for people with

type 1 diabetes and those with type 2 diabetes who need frequent insulin.

More advantages: You can wear the sensor and transmitter during most everyday activities, including showering and sleeping. A CGM also can relay readings to your doctor's office. *To consider…*

•**Abbott FreeStyle Libre.** This sensor goes on your arm and can stay in place for 10 days. You scan a mobile reader over the sensor to see your glucose reading. A cloud-based software management system allows you to view reports, see trends and change settings. Unlike most CGMs, the FreeStyle Libre does not require finger-stick checks or calibrations. One drawback is that it does not send out alarms.

•**Dexcom G5 Mobile.** This CGM sends glucose results to a receiver and your mobile device. Alarms and alerts warn of high or low glucose limits that you set in advance. This CGM does need to be calibrated with a finger stick every 12 hours. It can be worn for seven days and can be a stand-alone CGM or part of a closed-loop system with the Tandem Diabetes Care t:slim insulin pump (more on this later). You can share your data with your doctor or caregiver. The FDA has recently cleared the Dexcom G6, which is factory-calibrated—no need for finger sticks.

•**Medtronic Guardian Connect.** This CGM is practically a mind reader, with a feature that alerts you an hour before you may hit either your high- or low-glucose limit. The sensor relays readings only to a smartphone app.

Also, you'll need to do twice-daily finger sticks to calibrate it, and when used as a stand-alone and not in concert with a MiniMed system insulin pump (see next page), you'll need to check your glucose level with a finger stick before making a treatment decision.

Cost: There are up-front costs ranging from under $100 for the Abbott reader to $600 or more for the other CGMs listed, plus batteries and sensors. Insurance coverage varies and is changing all the time, so check with your carrier.

Note: Medicare recently started covering some CGMs.

COMBINATION CGM AND INSULIN PUMPS: HYBRID CLOSED-LOOP SYSTEMS

Good for: People who need many insulin injections every day and/or need to adjust insulin dosing based on their blood glucose level, meal type and physical activity.

A computerized insulin pump delivers insulin through a catheter inserted under your skin. The newest pumps and CGMs have been programmed to work together in what's called a hybrid closed-loop system.

The CGM reads sensor glucose levels and sends readings to the pump. Then the pump adjusts the amount of insulin to deliver. You'll still need to monitor your glucose level and perform finger pricks to confirm that the CGM is working correctly, plus make manual adjustments to account for meals and high blood glucose levels. Taking a training program at a clinic or diabetes center will help you become a pro at using it.

Hybrid closed-loop system options typically require a finger stick calibration several times a day, and the glucose-monitoring sensor can be worn for up to seven days at a time. Some are wearable while bathing and even swimming. *To consider...*

•**Tandem Diabetes Care t:slim.** This insulin pump can function as a pump alone or can work with the Dexcom G5 Mobile. You can pick different tones that signal when blood glucose falls below or rises above levels you set.

•**Medtronic MiniMed 670G System.** The latest model of the MiniMed has an AutoMode feature that automatically adjusts basal insulin delivery based on your glucose values and recent insulin delivery. It automatically stops insulin delivery if glucose gets too low.

Cost: The cost of an insulin pump itself is in the thousands, with a monthly cost for supplies. Many insurance companies do cover insulin pumps, but there may be co-pays and deductibles. Medicare may cover it with certain requirements.

INSULIN PENS GET SMARTER

If you don't need the level of insulin management a pump provides but still need insulin injections, the pen format is an advancement over a syringe and vials. You can load a cartridge in a reusable pen or use a single-use throwaway model.

Insulin pens are becoming smarter, too. For example, the reusable Companion InPen with Bluetooth technology and connectivity to Apple Health offers tracking and timing of insulin doses over time and even gives insulin temperature checks—the pen will send a message to your phone to remind you if you miss a dose and if your insulin gets too warm or too cold. An InPen itself lasts for one year, but you'll need to replace its insulin cartridge weekly or monthly.

Got Diabetes? Here's How to Save Your Feet

David G. Armstrong, DPM, MD, PhD, a podiatric surgeon and professor of surgery at Keck School of Medicine of University of Southern California in Los Angeles. He is lead author of "Diabetic Foot Ulcers and Their Recurrence," published in *The New England Journal of Medicine*.

Feet are easy to ignore...unless they hurt. That's one big reason many people with diabetes are at risk for losing their feet—their disease has robbed them, to a large extent, of what doctors call "the gift of pain."

Here's what happens: Diabetes damages nerves, which can lead to a loss of feeling. This means that an ill-fitting shoe or an ingrown toenail can start a silent cascade of injury, leading to a foot ulcer (open sore or wound) and infection.

Many people with diabetes also have poor blood flow, and that can allow an infection to fester—raising the risk that an unnoticed cut or blister could lead to the loss of toes, a foot or even an entire lower leg. Such amputations happen nearly 75,000 times each year in the US.

Even worse danger: Once a person with diabetes has a foot ulcer, his/her chance of dying in the next 10 years doubles. If the foot ulcer leads to amputation, the five-year risk for death is 70%.

But those tragic complications don't have to happen to you. *Here are five simple steps to help prevent foot ulcers and limb loss...*

STEP #1: **Watch your blood sugar—and more.** If you maintain good control of your blood sugar, your heart and kidneys will thank you—and so will your feet. Of course, you need to take your medications, watch your diet, and if your feet are still healthy, use them to stay active—walking is good preventive medicine for your whole body.

Warning: If you already have nerve damage in your feet, talk to your primary care doctor or foot doctor (podiatrist) about the right dose of walking for you. There may be times when you have to stay off your feet to save them.

STEP #2: **Be smart about your shoes and socks.** You need to wear both—whether you're inside or outside your house. (If you've lost sensation in your feet, don't walk around the house barefoot! At least wear house slippers.)

In choosing your socks, start with a clean, lightly padded pair with no irritating seams. Choose well-fitted, supportive shoes with plenty of room for your toes (no pointy-toed shoes!)—and get in the habit of checking inside for foreign objects before slipping them on. Even though high heels aren't recommended, women with diabetes may want to wear moderate heels (no more than two inches) for special occasions.

Buying tip: It's widely known that you should shop for shoes late in the day, when your feet may have swelled a bit, but this is vital for people with diabetes so that they don't buy shoes that are too tight. And stay away from cheap plastic and vinyl shoes—they may be less expensive, but they don't breathe enough, which causes your feet to perspire, increasing the chance for a blister to develop.

If diabetes has already caused changes, such as neuropathy and especially a previous blister or wound on your feet, talk with a podiatrist about the best shoes and inserts for you. These supportive shoes can be pricey (more than $100), but insurers often cover at least one pair per year—though you may want more so that you can allow your shoes to air out for a day between wearings.

Also: See your podiatrist at least once a year to make sure your feet are healthy and you're wearing the right shoes.

STEP #3: **Knock your socks off!** You need to do this every day to get a good look at your feet. Carefully examine the tops, the soles, the heels—and between your toes, where moisture and friction can lead to trouble. Use a mirror (or ask a family member to help if needed).

Goal: Get to know your feet so well that you will notice changes from day to day. Any new redness could signal trouble. Look for swelling, calluses, sores, blisters or ingrown toenails, and let your primary care physician or podiatrist know about these warning signs.

Important: There's one other time to strip off your shoes and socks—each and every time that you see your primary care doctor (not just your podiatrist). Take off your socks as soon as you reach the exam table. That way, both of you will remember to look at and talk about your feet.

STEP #4: **Watch out for hot spots.** If areas of your skin heat up, that can be a sign of inflammation. If you detect that heat early enough, you may be able to head off an ulcer.

Helpful: Consider doing your foot check in the morning before you've been walking on your feet all day. But if that doesn't work for your schedule, just be sure you do your foot check regularly.

Do not be surprised if your doctor asks you to take the temperature of your feet in several spots each day—looking for areas of one foot that are a few degrees warmer than the same areas of the other foot. This can be done with an inexpensive thermometer that can be purchased online, such as Advocate's Non-Contact Infrared Thermometer or Equinox Digital Non-Contact Infrared Thermometer.

Also: If you and your podiatrist are game, you can try out newer heat-sensing socks. These can be paired with your smartphone or other devices to send alerts to you. One such product, Siren's Diabetic Socks, is expected to hit the market soon. You can preorder these socks at Siren.care or 888-459-5470.

STEP #5: **Pamper those puppies.** Dry skin is more easily damaged, so after washing your feet in warm (not hot) water, apply a rich moisturizing cream. Keep toenails trimmed, straight across—and if that becomes difficult for you, ask your health-care providers for nail-trimming help. Make sure to ask your podiatrist before going to a nail salon. *Also, avoid these missteps…*

•**Do not put moisturizer between your toes**—excess moisture there can promote infection. Use talcum powder or cornstarch in those areas.

•**Do not warm your feet with hot-water bottles or heating pads**—you might not feel when it's too hot. Wear warm socks instead.

•**Do not use acids or chemical corn removers,** which could damage the skin and lead to foot ulcers. See a podiatrist for help.

•**Do not attempt "bathroom surgery" on corns, calluses or ingrown toenails.** Consult a podiatrist.

•**Do not smoke.** Quitting is one of the best things you can do to improve blood flow—to your feet and everywhere else. Do not give up trying if you have not quit yet.

Diabetes Meds Linked to Dangerous Infection

Gerald Bernstein, MD, director of the Diabetes Management Program, Friedman Diabetes Institute, Lenox Hill Hospital, New York City.

Common diabetes medications are linked to a dangerous infection called Fournier's gangrene. SGLT2 inhibitors, which include Jardiance and Invokana, reduce blood glucose by stimulating its excretion in the urine. When sugary urine leaks and remains on the skin in the groin area, the tissue can become irritated and infected. Always practice good hygiene, but if you have redness or swelling of the genitals, call your doctor. These symptoms can worsen quickly and lead to serious problems such as blindness, kidney damage and heart disease.

A Dark Side to Certain Diabetes Drugs

Study titled "Sodium glucose cotransporter 2 inhibitors and risk of serious adverse events: nationwide register based cohort study," by researchers in the department of medicine, Karolinska Institute, Stockholm, Sweden, published in *BMJ*.

Three popular diabetes drugs called SGLT-2 inhibitors may have a dark side—they have recently been associated with in-creased risk for having a foot or leg amputated. If your doctor prescribed an SGLT-2 inhibitor for you, should you stop taking it? That depends.

SGLT-2 inhibitors—short for sodium glucose cotransporter 2 inhibitors—work by stimulating the kidneys to remove sugar from the blood. The excess sugar is then eliminated through the urine. *Canagliflozin* (Invokana), *dapagliflozin* (Farxiga) and *empagliflozin* (Jardiance) are the three SGLT-2 inhibitors on the market. While these drugs also have been found to have beneficial effects beyond blood sugar control, such as protecting the heart and kidneys, recent studies and case reports also suggest they carry serious risks.

The FDA has received case reports linking them to kidney infection, blood clots, pancreatitis and ketoacidosis (a serious diabetes complication that causes too much acid to accumulate in blood). In 2016, two large clinical trials found an increased risk for lower limb amputation associated with Invokana, which prompted the FDA to issue a warning for that drug. No such risk was found in the trials for Farxiga or Jardiance.

To get a clearer picture of the risks associated with SGLT-2 inhibitors, researchers from Karolinska Institute in Sweden looked at data from a nationwide registry of type 2 diabetes patients in Sweden and Denmark. The researchers compared about 17,000 patients who were taking an SGLT-2 inhibitor with about 17,000 patients who were taking a GLP-1 agonist, another type of diabetes drug. (GLP-1 agonists include *exenatide*/Byetta, *dulaglutide*/Trulicity and *semaglutide*/Ozempic.) About 1% of the patients taking an SGLT-2 inhibitor were taking Invokana.

Results: Over the three years of the study, patients on SGLT-2 inhibitors were twice as likely as patients taking a GLP-1 agonist to have an amputation or develop ketoacidosis. No increased risk was found for kidney infection, blood clots or pancreatitis.

While a doubled risk sounds scary, the researchers point out that the overall risk for both amputation and ketoacidosis is still very low—in the study, 2.7% for SGLT-2 inhibitors compared with 1.1% for GLP-1 agonists for amputation risk…and 1.3% vs. 0.6% for ketoacidosis risk.

The authors also note that SGLT-2 inhibitors have been associated with important benefits, such as reducing heart disease risk and kidney failure in diabetics, that need to be weighed when deciding what diabetic medication is most appropriate for a patient. They advise doctors to counsel their patients about both risks and benefits of SGLT-2 inhibitors…and to be cautious about prescribing them for patients who are at higher risk for amputation, such as because of a history of peripheral arterial disease, a previous amputation or foot ulcers.

The only warning of amputation risk currently attached to SGLT-2 inhibitors is the FDA's safety alert for Invokana, which they updated in 2017. The European Medicines Agency would like to see that warning extended to all SGLT-2 inhibitors. The FDA is warning that all SGLT-2 inhibitors carry a risk for ketoacidosis.

If you're taking an SGLT-2 inhibitor: Make sure to take good care of your feet. Diabetic foot care includes washing your feet daily…drying them well…checking your feet daily for signs of ulceration or redness…and keeping your feet soft and smooth with lotion to avoid skin cracks. While ketoacidosis is rare, it's smart to know the symptoms.

Diabetes Fasting Alert

Saleh Aldasouqi, MD, professor of medicine and chief of endocrinology, Michigan State University, East Lansing.

Doctors usually ask patients to fast before a blood cholesterol test.

New study: Nearly 20% of 525 people with diabetes experienced fasting-induced hypoglycemia (dangerously low blood-sugar levels) when they stopped eating for the recommended eight to 12 hours before a cholesterol test. The resulting dizziness and confusion are particularly dangerous when patients drive themselves to the clinic.

Also: New research suggests that eating before the test will not affect results. Discuss these findings with your doctor if you have diabetes and are told to fast.

Keto Diet: Fighting Type 2 Diabetes with Fat

James McCarter, MD, PhD, head of research at Virta Health and coauthor of the studies "Effectiveness and Safety of a Novel Care Model for the Management of Type 2 Diabetes at 1 Year: An Open-Label, Non-Randomized, Controlled Study" published in *Diabetes Therapy* and "Cardiovascular Disease Risk Factor Responses to a Type 2 Diabetes Care Model Including Nutritional Ketosis Induced by Sustained Carbohydrate Restriction at 1 Year: An Open-Label, Non-Randomized, Controlled Study," published in *Cardiovascular Diabetology.*

The ketogenic or "keto" diet transforms your body from being a sugar-burning machine to a fat-burning one by flipping the standard American diet on its head. Most Americans eat between 200 grams (g) and 350 g of carbs a day, about half of daily calories. A typical keto diet cuts carbs to between 20 g and 50 g a day, just 5% to 10% of daily calories. Remaining calories come from fat (70% to 80%) and protein (10% to 20%).

Examples of what's emphasized with a ketogenic diet: Eggs, some full-fat dairy, meat and fish, olive oil, nuts and nonstarchy vegetables.

Examples of what's forbidden or strictly limited: Grains, sugar, starchy vegetables and most fruits. Berries, lemons and limes get the green light because they have less sugar than other fruits.

How it works: When your carb intake is this low, your body burns fatty acids and ketones—a form of energy for your body made in the liver when carbohydrates aren't provided. Within about a week on a well-formulated ketogenic diet, your body enters a new metabolic state called nutritional ketosis where this occurs.

Studies show that the diet can improve type 2 diabetes by reducing blood sugar, in turn reducing the need for diabetes medications and triggering significant weight loss.

As your body adjusts to nutritional ketosis, you may feel tired and dizzy and have other flulike symptoms, but these generally go away with adequate salt consumption.

Important: Nutritional ketosis and diabetic ketoacidosis (DKA) are not the same thing. DKA only occurs in diabetes when insulin cannot be produced, mostly with type 1 diabetes. It's an emergency condition in which ketones are produced at a dangerous rate, much higher than what occurs during nutritional ketosis.

KETO DIET + TELEMEDICINE = SUCCESS

For patients with diabetes, following a keto diet should be done only under the watchful eye of a doctor, especially if you take insulin, other diabetes medicine or drugs for high blood pressure. Your blood sugar and weight could drop quickly, so to avoid side effects like low blood sugar (hypoglycemia) or low blood pressure, you'll need to work with your doctor on reducing your medication doses—that's a lot of interaction.

To make monitoring easier and in turn make the diet more available, San Francisco-based Virta Health has developed a way to deliver it through telemedicine and is making a bold claim—the diet plus intensive medical support via the Internet can reverse type 2 diabetes.

Virta patients are paired with a remote health coach and a doctor who formulates a personalized ketogenic diet and provides monitoring. Through a smartphone or computer app, patients upload health data including their weight (through a cellphone-enabled scale), blood sugar, blood ketones, blood pressure (if they have hypertension) and ratings of mood, energy, hunger and cravings. How often this data is uploaded varies from patient to patient. Tracking of biomarkers begins as part of a daily routine and can become less frequent after several months as patients transition from the diabetes reversal phase to long-term success.

With conventional in-person care, a doctor knows about conditions and symptoms only when a patient contacts him/her or when there's an appointment. Virta doctors can see your health data as soon as it's uploaded and are able to reach out as soon as they see trends develop. This means, for example, that medication can be adjusted at intervals as short as one day.

Patients can consult their Virta doctors whenever they want to. But most day-to-day interactions are with the health coach, most of whom are trained as dietitians, nurses or in other allied health professions.

Coaches work with patients to personalize diet recommendations for their specific life circumstances and dietary needs. Planning and support are critical factors in success. Because the system can be personalized, it works for people in diverse situations, from night-shift workers with access to only cafeteria food to long-haul truckers eating at truck stops to stay-at-home parents and grandparents cooking for a large family.

Patients also have access to online resources like keto-friendly recipes and a patient community for more support.

Reaching the goals of reducing blood sugar, weight and blood pressure through nutritional ketosis and reducing doses or completely eliminating medications often happens in the first two months. Virta's founders conducted clinical trials on the keto diet for diabetes before starting the company in 2015, and now more than two dozen studies support various aspects of Virta's nutritional recommendations.

Virta and Indiana University Health are in the process of conducting a five-year controlled trial that compares outcomes of Virta treatment versus that of typical diabetes care. Results from the first year were published in the journals *Diabetes Therapy* and *Cardiovascular Diabetology* in 2018.

Researchers recruited 349 people with long-term type 2 diabetes and obesity. Of those, 262 volunteered to be in the Virta treatment group and 87 chose to stay with their usual diabetes care and saw their regular doctors and diabetes educators.

First year findings: Participants in the Virta group saw some big improvements…

•**On average, A1C** (average blood sugar measured over two to three months) dropped from 7.6% to 6.3%, out of the diabetes and into "prediabetes" range.

•**The group lost 12% of body weight** on average and lessened their need for diabetes medications.

•**94% of those on insulin** were able to reduce or stop its use, and sulfonylurea drugs were eliminated in all patients.

The people in the usual care group saw none of these improvements.

Most heart-health indicators among the Virta group got better, too. For instance, blood pressure and triglycerides went down and HDL ("good") cholesterol went up.

Most of the people in the Virta group stuck with the program, and 83% were still enrolled in the study at the end of the first year.

CAVEATS ABOUT KETO AND VIRTA

A ketogenic diet, whether monitored and managed in person with a doctor and nutritional expert or remotely with a program like Virta's, may reverse diabetes, but it's not a cure. If a patient returns to a typical high-carb diet, blood sugar goes up and, chances are, weight rises again. For many people it's necessary to stay on a ketogenic diet to control diabetes, though some people can tolerate a diet with a slightly higher amount of carbs.

The individualized and varied whole food diet that Virta patients consume provides more than adequate vitamins and fiber for health. Because sodium and fluid retention is also reversed on a ketogenic diet, obtaining adequate dietary salt—often through broth or bouillon—is helpful to avoid side effects of volume depletion. Many patients take a magnesium supplement to counter the magnesium deficiency typical after years of eating the standard American diet.

Virta's specific program of advice and monitoring costs $500 for the starting fee plus $370 per month for the first year and $199/month after the first year. Most insurers including Medicare and Medicaid don't yet pay for it. An employer-sponsored health plan might cover it. Virta offers a payment assistance program that reduces costs for lower income individuals.

What Kinds of Rice Are Best for Diabetics?

Sarah Schenker, RD, PhD (nutrition), registered dietitian and nutritionist based in London. She is a member of the British Dietetic Association, The Nutrition Society, the Association for Nutrition and the Guild of Health Writers and has served on both professional and government committees.

Rice is one of the world's most popular foods. Rice is also a starchy food—bad news for diabetics or others trying to keep their blood sugar at a healthy level. The good news is that not all kinds of rice have the same blood sugar–blitzing effect.

One measure of how fast carbohydrate-containing foods raise blood sugar levels (even for people who are not diabetic) is the glycemic index (GI). Different varieties of rice have different GIs—from as high as 70 or more for short-grain, white sticky rice such as that used in Thai curry or risotto…to about 55 for basmati rice.

There are several reasons that basmati (especially the whole-grain variety) is a particularly good rice choice for diabetics. When cooked, the grain of basmati rice tends to stay intact, keeping it light and fluffy rather than stuck together in clumps. The "light-and-fluffy" property is an indication that the starch hasn't gelatinized, which means that the starch will be released more slowly into the bloodstream, keeping blood-sugar levels more stable—crucial to managing diabetes.

Easier Eye Screening

Vision loss can be prevented by early detection of diabetic retinopathy, a type of damage to the retina caused by high blood sugar.

Problem: About half of people with diabetes don't get annual eye exams.

New: The FDA has cleared a device (IDx-DR) that allows primary care doctors to screen their diabetic patients for retinopathy to determine whether the patient should be referred to an ophthalmologist.

Malvina Eydelman, MD, director, division of ophthalmic and ear, nose and throat devices at the FDA, Silver Spring, Maryland.

Meanwhile, the kind of rice in the high-rice diets that has been linked with worsening diabetes is white, sticky rice, which has the highest GI.

Another reason basmati rice is a good choice for diabetics is its high magnesium content. Magnesium plays a role in insulin regulation, and poor magnesium intake is linked to increased risk for diabetes. Consuming lots of magnesium won't "cure" diabetes, but if you're borderline or prediabetic (still able to produce insulin but not enough of it), an adequate intake of magnesium could help to delay becoming fully diabetic. And the high-fiber content of whole-grain ("brown") basmati rice also improves bowel health, increases satiety and can reduce the risk for type 2 diabetes complications.

But be sure to choose good quality basmati rice—meaning that it is free of broken grains, or at least has very few. Broken grains raise the GI because they develop the stickiness you are trying to avoid. You can't necessarily tell by looking at a container of rice whether it's full of broken grains—especially if it is packaged in a cardboard box. But the price may give you a clue…and a "guaranteed fluffy rice" claim on the container. While in general basmati rice, both white and brown, is better for blood sugar control than white rice, you're better off with any variety of good-quality, long-grain rice that doesn't stick together than with cheap, broken-up basmati that does clump.

BEYOND BASMATI

You don't have to limit yourself to just basmati rice, though. Brown rice of any variety is high in fiber, vitamins and minerals, including magnesium, and generally (depending on quality) has a lower GI than white rice—even white basmati. Unlike white rice, brown rice has not had its bran layer removed (why it's brown), and its fiber and nutrients delay the absorption of starch into the bloodstream, slowing the rise in blood sugar. The fiber makes you feel fuller and for longer, which helps with weight control. And that's important in managing diabetes. Both white basmati and any variety of brown rice are healthful choices for diabetics, so enjoy either according to personal preference or what else you're serving.

Wild rice is also a good choice for diabetics. It is a different genus (Zizania) and not directly related to the more common Asian rice (Oryza sativa). Wild rice has a GI comparable to that of white basmati rice and is high in fiber and many other nutrients that may be helpful in preventing the onset of diabetes.

And in case you were wondering about sushi—which typically is served with short-grain, sticky white rice—you don't have to give it up. Sushi rice has a high GI, but it comes in such small portions that you aren't getting a lot of rice with each piece. And sushi often includes protein—such as fish or egg—which lessens the GI impact.

BLACK, RED, PURPLE RICE

You also may have seen black, red or purple rice—not just in specialty stores but in chain stores such as Walmart and online. What gives these varieties of whole-grain rice their exotic hues are the same health-promoting anthocyanins that give certain fruits and vegetables—grapes, blueberries, strawberries and red cabbage, for instance—their deep colors. Anthocyanins have many healthful properties, including that they are antioxidant and anti-inflammatory, making these kinds of specialty rice another healthy-rice choice for diabetics. Not all of these more exotic rice varieties have been assigned a GI, but they are generally similar in their metabolic effect to brown or basmati rice.

LOWEST GI COOKING METHOD

How rice is cooked also affects its GI. Gentle cooking—most easily and reliably achieved with a purpose-designed rice cooker—keeps the grains intact so they are less starchy. And, since the rice is cooked for the "just right" amount of time and with the exact amount of water, more of the vitamins are preserved.

What you eat along with your rice also matters. Foods with fiber and protein, including vegetables and beans, slow digestion, which helps to reduce the overall GI of your meal. (The protein in meats also slows digestion.)

As you can see, there are many healthy—and delicious—ways to manage your blood sugar and still enjoy rice!

Health Risk for People with Type 2 Diabetes: Low Iron

Milton Fabian Suárez-Ortegón, PhD, Usher Institute of Population Health Sciences and Informatics, University of Edinburgh, Scotland, UK, coauthor of study titled "Decreased iron stores are associated with cardiovascular disease in patients with type 2 diabetes both cross-sectionally and longitudinally," published in *Atherosclerosis*.

When you have diabetes, lowering your heart disease risk by watching your blood pressure and weight is critical. But there's another risk factor that needs to be on your radar, and it's a surprising one—your iron level.

Researchers came to this finding after analyzing data from two different studies on heart disease in people with type 2 diabetes, one done in Spain and the other in Scotland—different populations in many ways, including their diets and levels of alcohol consumption. Yet both groups showed the same pattern of increased risk of heart disease when their iron levels were low. In fact, people with diabetes and low iron were 217% more likely to develop heart disease than those with normal levels of iron.

We don't know whether people with diabetes who increase their iron levels by taking supplements or changing their diets can reduce their risk of heart disease. More research is needed to confirm the link and learn the exact mechanism. But Milton Fabian Suárez-Ortegón, PhD, one of the researchers, said that in the meantime it makes sense for people with diabetes and their doctors to be aware of the finding because, at the very least, an iron deficiency can be a marker of other conditions and can lead to anemia if levels drop extremely low. Remember that simply having diabetes can have as big an impact on your heart and blood vessels as having a heart attack. So, doing everything you can to protect your heart is very important.

PREVENT A DEFICIENCY

All men and postmenopausal women need at least 8 mg of iron a day; all other women need 18 mg. You may be able to get all you need from your diet. Meat, seafood (particularly oysters and mussels), poultry and liver are particularly good sources because they contain both heme and nonheme iron (heme is the easier of the two types for the body to absorb). Plant foods, notably cooked spinach, lentils and beans, quinoa, and nuts including hazelnuts, pistachios and cashews, deliver a good amount of iron but only the nonheme type. (They have plenty of other nutrients, though, so keep eating them!) In fact, eating a food high in vitamin C or one of the iron-rich meats or seafoods along with these plant-based foods will increase the amount of iron your body extracts. Calcium, on the other hand, can interfere with iron absorption—you can lessen this effect when your meal includes a variety of foods.

Yes, you can get iron from a supplement, but it's hard to know how much supplemental iron will be safe and effective without results from blood tests. (Too much iron can cause side effects such as an upset stomach and constipation, and can interfere with absorption of medications.) Your best bet is to check with your health-care provider before supplementing on your own.

Insulin Storage Danger

Katarina Braune, MD, resident physician, department of paediatric endocrinology and diabetes, Charité Universitaetsmedizin, Berlin, Germany.

When sensors were placed near insulin in the refrigerator or a diabetes bag (used for carrying insulin during the day) of 388 patients, 79% of the insulin was stored outside of the recommended temperature range. Insulin stored in the refrigerator was out of the recommended range of 36°F to 46°F two-and-a-half hours a day, on average, during the 49-day monitoring period.

Important: Because temperature deviations are known to affect insulin's blood glucose–lowering effect, always place a thermometer near insulin in the refrigerator—and in a diabetes bag—to ensure its potency.

8 Ways to Save Money on Insulin

Sandra Arévalo, MPH, RDN, CDE, a certified diabetes educator, director of nutrition services at Montefiore Community Programs in New York City and spokesperson for the Academy of Nutrition and Dietetics and the American Association of Diabetes Educators.

If you rely on insulin to manage diabetes, the ouch may be more in your wallet than at your injection site. Even with insurance, you could be laying out hundreds of dollars each month. And no, it's not your imagination. Insulin prices have been steadily rising.

Because of cost, one-third of people on insulin aren't taking it as directed, according to a study in *JAMA Internal Medicine*. This can have disastrous consequences as patients put themselves at short-term risk for dangerously high blood sugar...not to mention the long-term risks for eye, kidney, heart and nerve damage.

1. Review your insulin needs with your doctor. While there's no generic insulin available yet, some brands have been on the market longer and therefore cost less. The long-lasting once-a-day injections are more convenient, but twice-a-day drugs are typically cheaper. Have a frank discussion with your doctor to explore whether a lower-cost insulin regimen will work for you.

2. Know your health insurance plan's drug formularies. This will tell you the price tier for each type of insulin. Formularies are different from one insurance company to another, so if you're on Medicare or are self-insured, be sure to compare the drug prices for different plans during the annual open enrollment period. It may pay to switch plans.

3. Ask about drug programs that help with costs. Your doctor or diabetes educator may have coupons or rebate forms for insulin from the drug companies that manufacture them. However, if they're only for newer drugs, these medications could still be pricier than older ones, even with the discount. Do the math before deciding. All the insulin manufactured in the US comes from just three companies, and they all—Eli Lilly, Novo Nordisk and Sanofi—

offer some level of assistance to people who meet their eligibility requirements.

4. You may be eligible for free or low-cost insulin programs from independent assistance programs such as Needy Meds, Partnership for Prescription Assistance, Rx Assist and Rx Hope. The Charles Ray III Diabetes Association provides meters, strips and other supplies to those who cannot afford them, freeing up some of your budget for insulin.

5. Shop around to compare costs. Prices can vary considerably from pharmacy to pharmacy. Your neighborhood drugstore may charge more (or less) than the chain at the strip mall. Prices can vary even between outlets of the same chain of stores. So take the time to call around and get quotes before you fill your next prescription—and don't forget to include the pharmacy at the discount shopping club you belong to. You also may be able to save money if you use the mail-order pharmacy connected to your insurance plan—buying one 90-day supply is cheaper than three separate monthly refills.

6. Sign up for pharmacy rewards programs. Some national chains offer shopping benefits after you fill a certain number of prescriptions. While the rewards aren't applicable to the cost of medications, you can use them to cut the bill for your other drugstore items. Also look for various discounts offered when you buy online, such as savings when you sign up for auto shipments. These discounts will apply to testing supplies, not the insulin itself. But saving on items such as test strips will reduce your total diabetes medication outlay. There are also independent medication discount plans that offer savings at thousands of pharmacies across the country without any paperwork.

7. Reduce your need for insulin. If you haven't already gotten serious about diet and exercise, doing so now could still have a profound effect on your diabetes. Remember that the more junk food you eat, especially food with refined carbs such as cookies, cake, muffins and sugary beverages, the more insulin you need to control blood sugar. Work with a nutritionist and a fitness trainer to develop a life plan for better blood sugar control.

Note: Never change your medications without consulting your doctor.

8. Consider joining a drug trial. Some research studies include free insulin and supplies for participants. You can find open trials at the National Institute of Diabetes and Digestive and Kidney Diseases (NIDDK.nih.gov). Another, less involved option is to sign up for focus groups where participation is compensated with free supplies. Ask your health-care team members if they know of these in your area.

Stay tuned for more insulin options. That the US supply of insulin is controlled by just three companies helps explain escalating prices for a drug that's nearly 100 years old. (*Note:* There are numerous lawsuits currently being brought against them on the public's behalf.) Biosimilars, which are close but not identical drugs, are coming to the insulin market in March 2020 as part of the FDA's response to sky-high insulin prices. It's unclear how much (or how soon) this new competition will lower prices, but the goal is for it to ultimately make a difference. Talk to your doctor about switching to a biosimilar when one is available.

Diabetes and Pancreatic Cancer Risk

V. Wendy Setiawan, PhD, epidemiologist at Keck School of Medicine, University of Southern California, Los Angeles, and coauthor of a study published in *Journal of the National Cancer Institute*.

Recent-onset diabetes may signal higher risk for pancreatic cancer. The risk is three to four times higher in the first three years after a diabetes diagnosis in people over age 50, compared with those who don't have diabetes. While pancreatic cancer risk is low, if you've been recently diagnosed with diabetes and have pancreatic cancer risk factors, such as family history, ask your doctor about monitoring for early signs of the lethal cancer.

CHAPTER 7

Digestive Disorders

The New Frontier in Healthy Eating

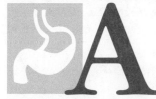**A**t this very moment, trillions of microbes are making themselves at home in your intestines. That's a good thing, because that community of microbes—your microbiome—is key to good health. And the most important factor for a healthy microbiome is what you eat.

Here's how it works: A well-balanced microbiome is chock-full of bacteria that produce certain short-chain fatty acids that positively influence health. These include acetate, propionate and, especially, butyrate—highly biologically active compounds that support gut health, blood sugar regulation, optimal blood fat levels, appetite control and immunity. They also cross the blood-brain barrier and so influence your mood. A healthy microbiome protects against obesity, diabetes, heart disease, certain autoimmune diseases and depression.

Those good-for-you bugs need nourishment, primarily fiber that stays undigested until it reaches the intestines. But the typical Western diet—high in animal protein and fat while low in fiber—effectively starves the microbiome. The solution isn't to just eat more fiber or even more fruits and vegetables—certain foods promote a healthy microbiome in powerful, specific ways. They work in different ways, so eating a bountiful variety is best. *Start by saying "yes" to these foods…*

WALNUTS

People who eat walnuts have more favorable cholesterol levels, as well as less diabetes, than people who rarely eat them. Why?

One key reason: Eating a handful of walnuts each day—about one-third cup, or 16 walnut halves (about 215 calories)—can change the mi-

Laurie Steelsmith, ND, LAc, licensed naturopathic physician and acupuncturist in private practice in Honolulu. She writes Bottom Line's "Natural Healing Secrets for Women" blog and is coauthor of three books—the best-selling *Natural Choices for Women's Health,* the critically acclaimed *Great Sex, Naturally* and her latest, *Growing Younger Every Day.* DrSteelsmith.com crobiome in a good way by increasing the bacteria species that generate butyrate. Other nuts that support a healthy microbiome include almonds, cashews, pistachios, hazelnuts and pecans.

GHEE

Ghee is a type of clarified butter, originally from India, that is simmered and allowed to caramelize before the milk solids are removed. What's left is flavorful and aromatic butter fat without dairy proteins but with high levels of short-chain fatty acids—including butyrate. The flavor is concentrated, so a little goes a long way. One tablespoon a day (about 110 calories) is fine. Ghee is used in cooking and as a condiment.

FOS FOODS

Fructooligosaccharides (FOS) are complex sugars that generally pass undigested through your digestive system until intestinal microbes break them down. FOS are the perfect diet for certain butyrate-producing bacteria. In animal studies, just two weeks on a high-FOS diet significantly increased butyrate production. FOS are found in many everyday foods including bananas, onions, leeks, garlic, asparagus, jicama and Jerusalem artichoke.

Caveat: For some people, FOS-rich foods are hard to digest and can cause gastrointestinal trouble. See "When Gut-Friendly Foods Are Bad for You," next page.

POLYPHENOL-RICH FOOD AND DRINK

The powerful antioxidants called polyphenols found in tea, coffee, berries, grapes, cocoa and certain vegetables (including artichokes, olives and asparagus) are strongly associated with the prevention of diabetes and heart disease. Credit the microbiome, at least in part—90% or more of polyphenols are metabolized by microbes, and they increase levels of the protective bacteria Bifidobacteria and Lactobacillus. *Examples...*

•**Olive oil.** In studies, the microbiomes of animals fed olive oil had higher levels of four bacteria that are known to reduce insulin levels (associated with diabetes prevention) and increase levels of leptin, a hormone that helps control appetite.

•**Cocoa.** Dark chocolate and cocoa powder are rich in flavanols, a type of antioxidant. In a study at University of Reading in the UK, adults who followed a diet rich in cocoa flavanols had an increase in healthful Bifidobacteria and Lactobacilli populations.

My recommendation: Add two or three tablespoons of raw cacao powder to a smoothie a few times a week…or bake with it.

•**Fermented foods.** Yogurt is made when friendly bacteria, usually Lactobacillus bulgaricus and Streptococcus thermophilus, are added to milk. Sauerkraut and kimchi (a salty Korean side dish) are made by allowing beneficial bacteria to digest the natural sugars in cabbage leaves. Other gut-friendly fermented foods include sourdough bread, certain natural cheeses (see below), olives, soy sauce, miso and tempeh. Fermented foods not only contain very high numbers of healthful microbes, but these good-for-you bacteria are particularly likely to survive the passage through the digestive tract—where they can thrive.

Tip: You already know that yogurt has health benefits, but don't neglect cheese. In one study at University of Copenhagen in Denmark, healthy volunteers produced more butyrate when they included cheese in their diets.

Best cheeses for your gut bacteria: Fresh mozzarella, aged Parmigiano, Camembert and raw-milk cheeses.

FOODS TO AVOID

Eating good-for-your-gut foods isn't enough. Certain eating patterns, as well as common additives used by the food industry, can throw a monkey wrench into your microbiome. *Be wary of...*

•**Emulsifiers.** Animal studies show that the microbiomes of mice fed diets with relatively low levels of emulsifiers—chemicals added to stabilize processed foods—were less robust than microbiomes of mice that weren't fed emulsifiers.

Even more concerning: Certain common emulsifiers have been found to chip away at the colon's mucous membrane, which is nature's way of keeping microbes inside the gut so they don't enter the bloodstream where they can do harm.

Avoid: Carboxymethylcellulose (aka cellulose gum, or CMC) and polysorbate-80. You also may want to avoid foods that contain the common emulsifier carrageenan, which can irritate the intestinal wall.

•**Artificial sweeteners.** Sucralose, aspartame and saccharin all have been shown to disrupt the balance and diversity of gut microbiomes.

Example: Mice fed sucralose for six months had higher levels of bacteria that promote inflammation. It's also wise to avoid sugar alcohols such as xylitol, which can cause stomach distress in many people.

Fine to use: Monkfruit sweetener or stevia.

Bottom line: The changes to the microbiome from what you eat may occur quickly, within 24 hours, but they don't last long. Making good diet choices each day is your best strategy to keep your microbiome—and you—healthy.

WHEN GUT-FRIENDLY FOODS ARE BAD FOR YOU

Here's a dilemma—some foods that promote a healthy microbiome can cause gastrointestinal distress for certain people.

Solution: Heal the gut first, then slowly introduce these foods to see if they can be tolerated.

Example: FODMAP is an acronym for "fermentable oligosaccharides, disaccharides, monosaccharides and polyols." Many people have trouble digesting these complex molecules—especially if they have irritable bowel syndrome—and restricting them often leads to symptom relief. But fructooligosaccharides (FOS) in particular help feed a healthy microbiome. Cutting out FODMAPs can reduce Bifidobacterium and other beneficial species.

Solution: If you need a low-FODMAP diet, work with a health professional such as a naturopathic physician on an elimination diet. But as your symptoms improve, gradually reintroduce some foods. Adding them in slowly allows the gut flora to get used to them. You may need to stop eating onions permanently, for example—but bananas might be just fine.

A gluten-free diet poses a similar dilemma. People with celiac disease, as well as those with gluten intolerance, need to avoid wheat and other grains that contain gluten. But skipping wheat often means missing out on fiber that your microbiome needs. People on gluten-free diets have been found to have reduced levels of healthy Bifidobacterium and Lactobacillus and higher levels of unhealthful E. coli and Enterobacteriaceae bacteria.

Solution: If you are avoiding gluten, be sure to eat plenty of high-fiber foods, including whole grains such as oats (be sure they are certified as non-cross-contaminated with gluten), brown rice and millet. You may want to add in psyllium powder to boost your fiber intake, too. As with low-FODMAP diets, people who start out gluten intolerant can sometimes improve their gut health enough that they can reintroduce gluten-containing grains such as whole wheat.

Quick and Easy First Aid for Stomach Troubles

Andrew L. Rubman, ND, founder and medical director, Southbury Clinic for Traditional Medicines, Southbury, Connecticut. He writes the "Nature Doc's Patient Diary" blog at BottomLineInc.com/blogs.

Even if you eat a healthy diet and get plenty of exercise, digestive problems still happen. If they happen a lot, you should check with your doctor to rule out underlying serious health issues. But for once-in-a-while indigestion, constipation and/or diarrhea, there are easy, natural remedies that will soon have your gut feeling better.

FOR OCCASIONAL INDIGESTION

If you ate too much…or too fast…or if something you ate "didn't agree with you," you can try…

•**Baking soda.** Sodium bicarbonate, commonly known as baking soda, neutralizes the acidity in your stomach. Mix about one-half teaspoon of baking soda with four ounces of water, and slowly sip the mixture. Relief should come quickly (and maybe a belch or two).

Important: Wait for at least two hours after eating to drink this remedy—you do not want to partially neutralize the acid that is needed to digest food and absorb nutrients.

FOR OCCASIONAL CONSTIPATION OR DIARRHEA

Both of these conditions can be the result of a poor diet…the wrong mix of organisms in the gut microbiome…and/or certain medications. Not drinking enough water also can cause constipation. *What can help…*

•**Probiotics.** There are many different kinds of beneficial probiotic bacteria that we need to have in our guts for good digestive health. Some of the most well-studied strains with evidence of gut benefit are Lactobacillus casei, Lactobacillus acidophilus and Lactobacillus rhamnosus GG—all particularly good for treating diarrhea but also helpful for treating constipation. Lactobacillus supplements are available over-the-counter in grocery and drugstores.

Align is a good product with a patented strain of another probiotic (Bifidobacterium infantis) that works well with Lactobacillus and that has shown gut benefits in industry-sponsored studies.

Follow the label directions for the correct dose. You should get relief within 12 to 18 hours, although complete healing can take three to five days.

Bonus: Probiotic products containing Lactobacillus have been found to significantly reduce flatulence.

•**Glucomannan.** This water-soluble fiber supplement is made from the root of the konjac plant. It is an effective "bulk-forming" laxative, so it helps with constipation but not diarrhea. As a bonus, glucomannan also helps relieve nausea.

This type of laxative swells in the intestine, softening the stool and making it easier to pass. When using to relieve constipation, take one 575-mg capsule of glucomannan with at least a full eight ounces of water up to three times a day, away from meals.

HOW TO KEEP YOUR DIGESTION WORKING GREAT

While the remedies above are good to have on hand, it's best if you don't have to use them often. *Here are some strategies to keep your digestion functioning smoothly…*

•**Chew thoroughly.** You'll eat more slowly, enjoy your food more—and give your stomach a break. Chewing sufficiently allows enzymes in saliva to start digestion in your mouth, as they're meant to do—and breaking the food into smaller particles lets your intestines better absorb nutrients.

•**Drink water, but not with your meal.** Drinking water or other liquids at mealtime dilutes the hydrochloric acid your stomach needs to digest food, slowing digestion and inhibiting absorption of nutrients.

It's OK to slowly sip just enough liquid at a meal to help you wash down mouthfuls of food if you want—but keep it to no more than four ounces. It's best to not drink close to meals—aim for a half hour before to an hour after. On the other hand, do be sure to drink enough liquids during the rest of the day.

•**Omega-3 fatty acids.** These essential fats not only help fight inflammation, they also promote a healthy gut microbiome. Unless you regularly consume wild-caught cold-water fish, you probably do not get enough from diet alone. One good brand of omega-3 supplements is Nordic Naturals. Whatever brand you use, aim for a daily dose of at least 650 mg of eicosapentaenoic acid and 450 mg of docosahexaenoic acid.

Important: Digestive ailments that are more than just occasional or that are accompanied by other symptoms, such as fever, pain or blood in your bowel movements or vomit, should be checked out by a health-care provider.

Gut Acting Up?

Don't assume that it's something you ate.

New discovery: Some viruses (including the Zika and West Nile viruses) damage nerve cells in the intestine as well as the brain.

Result: Abdominal pain and constipation.

Cell.

The Brain-Gut Connection

Sarah Kinsinger, PhD, a board-certified health psychologist, associate professor of gastroenterology and nutrition and director of Behavioral Medicine for the Digestive Health Program at Loyola University Medical Center in Maywood, Illinois.

Digestive problems—whether it's an upset stomach, diarrhea, constipation or abdominal pain—can make life miserable.

Until recently, doctors have treated these problems by focusing on the gut—approximately 30 feet of tubes and organs through which food is ingested, digested and excreted. Now an increasing body of scientific evidence shows that a new target—the brain—is a missing link in finding relief.

What most people don't realize: Your gut contains more than 100 million nerves, more than what's found in your spinal cord. This "enteric nervous system," connecting the gut and brain, is in constant two-way communication.

For example, signals from the brain play a key role in the day-to-day, moment-to-moment function of digestion. By the same token, feelings like fear, anger and depression are now being increasingly recognized for their effect on digestive functions.

Given the strength of the brain-gut connection, it should be no surprise that top-down treatment with a psychologist (or "brain-gut therapy," as it's come to be called) can help—and in some cases is more effective than conventional medical care, including many medications. *What you need to know...*

THE BRAIN-GUT AXIS IN ACTION

While many details of this "upstairs-downstairs" interaction have yet to be worked out, we know that signals from the brain—via neurotransmitters and nerve signals—control the muscular contractions that move digested food through the digestive tract, regulate secretions such as stomach acid and enzymes that break down food and influence pain sensitivity in the gut.

Because your brain and gut are in such close and constant communication, stress and troubling emotions that alter brain function readily disrupt the smooth workings of your digestive system. These effects are most clearly seen in disorders of brain-gut interaction, where there is no evidence of physiological abnormalities with testing.

Irritable bowel syndrome (IBS), a chronic condition involving abdominal pain accompanied by symptoms like diarrhea, constipation and bloating, is the most common of these. Others include functional dyspepsia (stomach pain, bloating and nausea following meals) and certain cases of heartburn.

But the brain also can contribute to worsening symptoms of organic digestive disorders, such as Crohn's disease or ulcerative colitis, where symptoms are the result of an autoimmune disorder causing inflammation in the gut. In some cases, patients with these disorders continue to experience abdominal pain or diarrhea even when inflammation is well controlled by medication.

The back-and-forth interaction between the brain and gut can create a vicious cycle. When planning to travel, attend a concert or party or simply appear in public, many people with chronic bowel conditions fear that they will pass gas or have an urgent need for a bathroom or sudden, severe pain.

These fears can trigger physiological arousal in the body (the "fight or flight" response) and amplify awareness of sensations that might otherwise be ignored. This stress response can trigger contractions in the intestines and intensify pain sensations. These symptoms and associated anxiety can prevent individuals from enjoying social situations and enjoying life to the fullest.

WHAT BRAIN-GUT THERAPY CAN DO

The brain-gut connection is more than theoretical. There's research showing that when we change how the brain works—the goal of all psychotherapy—it can have profound effects on gastrointestinal symptoms.

Cognitive behavioral therapy (CBT), which changes patterns of thinking and behavior, has the most research support, with at least 20 randomized trials showing its effectiveness in curbing gut-related symptoms. In these studies, typically 60% to 70% of patients are "treatment responders," meaning that they report significant reductions in abdominal pain and improved bowel habits following CBT treatment.

Gut-directed hypnotherapy is the second most researched psychological treatment for IBS and has been validated by several randomized clinical trials. One of the largest observational studies of hypnotherapy for IBS involved 1,000 patients with severe symptoms that had failed to respond to prior medical treatment.

Result: With hypnotherapy, 76% of patients reported clinically significant reductions in IBS symptoms.

While pain reduction is the most prominent benefit, patients also report improvements in bowel habits (more regular bowel movements and improvements in stool consistency) and relief from "non-colonic" symptoms such as fatigue, backaches, headaches and body aches.

Why these treatments confer such benefits is unclear. They may reprogram the brain to tune out or dial down the perception of sensations coming from the gut and help normalize muscular contractions and secretions in digestive organs.

CBT helps patients become aware of the connection between thinking patterns, behaviors and physical sensations in the body and learn to reframe unhelpful thinking patterns.

For example, a patient who gets anxious about travel or parties days before may be encouraged to consider the real probability of an ill-timed episode and the coping strategies he/she might use should one occur. CBT often includes training in relaxation practices, such as mindfulness or diaphragmatic breathing, to reduce physiological stress and empower patients to manage symptoms.

With gut-directed hypnotherapy, patients achieve a deeply relaxed, focused and receptive mental state, where suggestions like a sensation of warmth in the abdominal area can soothe pain and reduce awareness of pain symptoms. Hypnotic suggestions also may modulate nerve function to prevent muscle spasm…or recalibrate the brain's response to signals coming from the gut, easing hypersensitivity to normal sensations.

Both treatments are relatively short-term, typically involving about seven to 12 sessions over the course of three months. But the benefits are often long-lasting. A number of studies show that improvements are maintained for a year or more, and in one trial of hypnotherapy, these benefits were maintained for up to five years. Health insurers often cover these treatments.

IS BRAIN-GUT THERAPY FOR YOU?

Brain-gut therapy has been shown to work for men, women and children with irritable bowel syndrome (IBS). The most important question is, are you open to it and willing to become actively engaged? Both cognitive behavioral therapy (CBT) and hypnotherapy are a kind of brain training, which demands regular practice—that is, homework—to be effective.

Patients most often consider brain-gut therapy after standard medical treatment (such as laxative or antidiarrheal medications) and lifestyle modifications (such as exercise and diet changes) haven't given them the results they want.

People who prefer a drug-free approach may turn to brain-gut therapy earlier. The ideal situation is when a therapist and medical doctor are in regular communication and work together to help the patient. It's best not to wait too long to seek treatment. The more unsuccessful treatment experiences you have, the more stressful the condition becomes.

Your gastroenterologist may know of a mental health provider offering these treatments. Otherwise, look for a provider specializing in CBT or hypnotherapy who is also experienced working with patients with chronic health conditions.

Best resources: The Rome Foundation, a nonprofit organization that researches and educates the public about functional gastrointestinal disorders, has a searchable directory of gastrointestinal mental health providers nationwide, RomeGIPsych.org. The website IBShypnosis.com lists providers who specialize in hypnosis for IBS.

Got Stomach Problems? This New Test May Pinpoint the Cause

Mark Pimentel, MD, executive director of the Medically Associated Science and Technology (MAST) Program at Cedars-Sinai in Los Angeles. *Disclosure:* Dr. Pimentel, who is involved in the clinical trial, is also named on the patent application for the new breath test device.

If you're like most people who suffer from nagging digestive problems, such as bloating, stomach pain and diarrhea or constipation, you've probably been told that you have irritable bowel syndrome (IBS). But that's not the whole story.

Problem: The symptoms of another common intestinal illness, known as small intestinal bacterial overgrowth (SIBO), are similar to those of IBS. As a result, SIBO often gets missed. It's important to recognize SIBO, as this can dictate the type of treatment for this condition.

Good news: Researchers from Cedars-Sinai in Los Angeles recently identified a way to improve the diagnosis and treatment of patients with this IBS-related condition.

Background: SIBO is caused by having too much of certain strains of bacteria in the small intestine. In up to 78% of patients who are diagnosed with IBS, the actual culprit is SIBO.

Even though it's normal (even desirable) for bacteria to live in the digestive tract, the problem with SIBO is that there is too much bacteria—or the wrong type. These bacteria produce excessive amounts of methane gas, one of several types of gas that can lead to flatulence. Methane (along with other gases such as hydrogen) is produced when certain foods (mainly carbohydrates) combine with gas-forming bacteria.

Current test: Even though IBS tends to be the catchall default diagnosis for people with gastrointestinal (GI) problems, a breath test can be used to determine whether SIBO is present.

The test is simple: After a one-day diet that eliminates foods that feed bacteria, you drink a sugar solution and breathe into a device that captures a sample of your breath. A positive breath test for hydrogen or methane gas explains the most common symptoms of SIBO—gas and bloating...flatulence...belching...abdominal pain or cramping...and constipation.

The problem is, methane gas is linked to constipation, but hydrogen has not been linked to the diarrhea that is experienced by many SIBO patients, so doctors knew there was something missing from the routine test for this condition.

Latest development: A large clinical trial has linked the presence of another gas, hydrogen sulfide, to the symptom of diarrhea. That result led to the development of the new breath test device, which is sensitive to four gut gases (carbon dioxide, methane, hydrogen and hydrogen sulfide) that are new hallmarks of SIBO. The new test is slated to become available within the next year or so.

Why this matters: Without an accurate diagnosis, patients with SIBO are unlikely to be prescribed the correct antibiotics (typically a 10- to 14-day course)—the treatment of choice for this condition. The distinction is crucial because IBS is usually treated with self-care approaches, such as diet and stress management...and/or medication, such as dicyclomine, an antispasmodic for bowel spasms—but not antibiotics.

Exception: In IBS patients with high levels of hydrogen sulfide, antibiotics may also provide relief when used in conjunction with IBS medication. *Rifaximin* (Xifaxan), a broad-spectrum antibiotic that is often used to treat SIBO, has been shown to reduce bloating, abdominal pain and loose stools in patients with diarrhea-predominant IBS.

Bottom line: If you struggle with digestive problems, talk to your doctor about both IBS and SIBO. Proper testing will help ensure that you get the best possible treatment.

GERD Surgery Is Better Than Taking More Drugs

Reginald C.W. Bell, MD, founder and director of the Institute of Esophageal and Reflux Surgery in Englewood, Colorado, and lead author of the study "Laparoscopic Magnetic Sphincter Augmentation versus Double-Dose Proton Pump Inhibitors for Management of Moderate-to-Severe Regurgitation in GERD: A Randomized Controlled Trial," published in *Gastrointestinal Endoscopy*. Dr. Bell had the MSA procedure himself three years ago.

Many people don't get enough relief from gastroesophageal reflux disease (GERD) by taking drugs—even the powerful drugs called proton pump inhibitors (PPIs). At the same time, these people rightly worry about the serious side effects of taking even more drugs. The solution may not be more medication, but rather the outpatient surgery called magnetic sphincter augmentation (MSA). That might sound like a drastic solution, but a new study on the six-year-old treatment shows that it has a good safety record—and corrects the problem once and for all.

Heartburn is the most talked about symptom of GERD, but it's by far not the only one. Regurgitation, which feels like a wet, burning burp in your throat or mouth every time it happens, occurs frequently with some patients and can be even worse than heartburn.

Both symptoms are caused by stomach acid creeping up from the stomach into the esophagus due to a weak and leaky lower esophageal sphincter (LES), a valve that's supposed to keep acid in the stomach where it belongs. While PPI drugs can reduce the amount of stomach acid and ease heartburn, they don't fix a leaky LES, and frequently regurgitating even small amounts of acid is still uncomfortable. Worse still, it can over time lead to Barrett's esophagus, precancerous changes in the cells of the esophagus, which can, in turn, lead to esophageal cancer.

Though the MSA procedure was FDA-approved in 2012, most doctors are still treating moderate-to-severe regurgitation by doubling the typical PPI dose, even though that doesn't help most GERD patients.

However, the new study on MSA may have more doctors suggesting it to their patients. An analysis of the procedure from 21 medical centers found that regurgitation stopped in 89% of patients…and so did their heartburn, so they no longer needed to take any PPI medication.

The surgery involves placing a device—basically a bracelet of titanium magnetic beads with the brand name LINX—around the LES. The magnets keep the valve closed when you're not eating or drinking but allow it to open when you are.

Because it's a minimally invasive, laparoscopic procedure—four or five small incisions in the abdomen—most MSA patients can return to normal activities within a few days. The most common side effect is temporary difficulty swallowing (dysphagia), but this can often be avoided by following post-surgery guidelines to eat only one or two spoonfuls of food during every waking hour for the first few weeks. A rare (less than 1%) complication is erosion of the esophagus from the device, which requires removing it.

There are now about 150 surgical centers around the country doing the procedure. Surgeons who are most likely to be experienced in MSA are esophageal surgical specialists. One way to find one near you is to enter your zip code at the website of the company that makes the magnetic device, Torax Medical (ToraxMedical.com).

The Worst Drugs for Gut Health

Anita Gupta, DO, PharmD, MPP, a board-certified anesthesiologist, pharmacist and former FDA adviser. She currently is a physician with Penn Medicine Princeton Health in Princeton, New Jersey, a scholar at Georgetown University's Center for Clinical Bioethics in Washington, DC, and a member of the American Osteopathic Association and American Society of Anesthesiologists.

Antibiotics are known to upset the harmonious balance of the microbiome—the trillions of bacteria in your gastrointestinal (GI) tract that are critically important to maintaining your overall health. As antibiotics eradicate harmful bacteria, they may inadvertently target the good-for-you ones, too, that keep this balance in check.

Shocking new finding: One out of four non-antibiotic drugs also inhibits the growth of at least one strain of healthy gut bacteria, according to a new study in *Nature*.

Among the medications known to disrupt your friendly microbiome flora…

•**Acid-reducing medications.** Proton pump inhibitors (PPIs) such as *omeprazole* (Prilosec OTC) and *esomeprazole* (Nexium) treat heartburn, ulcers and reflux by reducing acid production in the stomach. That ultimately lessens the amount of acid that reaches your gut.

But your gut microbiome wants an acidic environment, which helps healthy bacteria, such as Lactobacillus and Bifidobacterium, thrive and keeps harmful ones at bay. So while changing the gut's pH to a more basic, less acidic level may improve symptoms, it allows dangerous bacteria to proliferate.

Recent finding: A review of studies that included about 300,000 patients found a 65% increase in the incidence of *Clostridium difficile* (C. difficile)–associated diarrhea among PPI patients. C. difficile releases toxins that damage the intestinal wall, causing pain, diarrhea and fever. Unwanted *Streptococcus* and *Staphylococcus* bacteria and *Escherichia coli* (E. coli) also tend to be more prevalent in the gut microbiome of PPI users.

Note: H2 receptor antagonists, known as H2 blockers, such as *ranitidine* (Zantac) or *cimetidine* (Tagamet), exert similar effects on the microbiome, though their impact is less potent than that of PPIs.

Try instead: As many as 70% of PPI patients may be taking them unnecessarily. Ideally, you want to take the smallest dose of these drugs for the shortest duration possible. Talk to your doctor about possibly tapering off by switching to a 20-mg dose of a mild PPI, such as *omeprazole*… then to an H2 blocker for a week or two…then slowly stopping altogether. Lifestyle modifications, including weight loss, smoking cessation and dietary tweaks to curb acid reflux, often are a first line of defense for indigestion.

Algae-based heartburn medicines such as Gaviscon may ease stomach upset by coating the stomach lining and, in turn, have less impact on the microbiome. Most people take two to four tablets after meals and at bedtime, up to four times daily.

Bifidobacterium has been shown to inhibit or prevent C. difficile infections, so consider a Bifidobacterium-containing probiotic, such as MegaFlora for Over 50 ($41.90 for 60 capsules, MegaFood.com) when taking a PPI.

If you use both a PPI and a probiotic, take them separately to avoid canceling out the effects of each one. Most people take the PPI first and wait several hours before taking the probiotic. Talk to your physician to determine the best timing based on the PPI you're taking.

•**Nonsteroidal anti-inflammatory drugs (NSAIDs).** NSAIDs, such as over-the-counter *ibuprofen* (Advil, Motrin) and *naproxen* (Aleve) and prescription *celecoxib* (Celebrex) and *meloxicam* (Mobic), relieve pain by blocking the formation of inflammatory compounds called prostaglandins. But there actually are several types of prostaglandins in the body, including one that protects the lining of the GI tract. Chronic NSAID use can erode this lining, causing leaky gut syndrome. That's when dangerous bacteria "leak" into the bloodstream where they don't belong and can wreak havoc by triggering inflammation, allergies, autoimmune disease and more damage to the microbiome.

Even worse: As the lining erodes, stomach bleeding and ulcers can occur. Patients end up using an acid-blocking medication to get relief, further compromising the microbiome.

Recent findings: NSAIDs also change the composition and diversity of gut microbes. In a study published in *Clinical Microbiology and Infection*, taking celecoxib or ibuprofen was linked with a surplus of *Enterobacteriaceae* bacteria, which can lead to serious infections in older adults.

Other research shows that when NSAIDs alter the microbiome, how the drug itself is broken down is impacted and its effectiveness is diminished. So when you must use an NSAID, take the lowest dose for the shortest duration possible.

Try instead: Yoga and physical therapy may ease pain and help you avoid NSAIDs altogether. Acupuncture stimulates the production of endogenous opioids, your body's own natural pain relievers, and may ease back, neck and shoulder osteoarthritis and headache pain.

A combination of feverfew, an anti-inflammatory plant in the daisy family, and ginger was shown to eliminate or significantly reduce migraine pain in 63% of participants within two hours, according to a study in *Headache*. Run-of-the-mill headaches should respond, too. (*Try:* GelStat Migraine.) Drinking 10.5 ounces of anti-inflammatory tart cherry juice can ease muscle soreness after a workout.

According to a study in *Phytotherapy Research*, rheumatoid arthritis patients who took 500-mg supplements of curcumin, a natural anti-inflammatory compound found in turmeric, experienced more pain relief after eight weeks than those taking an NSAID.

Note: Avoid curcumin if you have ulcers or gallstones or take an anticoagulant.

•**Iron supplements.** Do you take an iron supplement or a multivitamin with iron? Many older adults begin taking these on their own to avoid anemia. If you have colon cancer or a GI disorder such as ulcerative colitis or Crohn's, you may have been prescribed iron pills to counter the iron deficiency that often accompanies these conditions.

The problem: Less than 20% of the iron in most supplements is absorbed, mostly in the small intestine. The rest makes its way to the colon where nasty bacteria, including Salmonella, Shigella and E. coli, depend on it to survive and proliferate. So once that unabsorbed iron reaches the colon, it fuels bad bugs.

Try instead: Most healthy people can get enough iron through diet. In fact, women typically experience an increase in iron stores post-menopause, as they're no longer losing iron through menstruation. A simple blood test can determine whether you need supplements.

If so, try a brand containing ferrous sulfate, which is better absorbed than other forms. (*Try:* Nature Made Iron.) That said, ferrous sulfate is notoriously constipating, so up your daily fiber intake to 30 g, drink plenty of water and get regular exercise to keep things moving.

After a few months, you may be able to switch to less constipating ferrous gluconate (it has less elemental iron by weight than ferrous sulfate, making it a step-down choice).

Tip: Look for the words "Slow Fe" on the bottle. This means the iron is released at a slower rate, which can be less constipating.

A Sad Way to Fix Heartburn

Andrew L. Rubman, ND, founder and medical director, Southbury Clinic for Traditional Medicines, in Southbury, Connecticut. He is a member of Bottom Line's panel of experts and writes the Bottom Line blog "Nature Doc's Patient Diary." SouthburyClinic.com

Easing heartburn shouldn't make you depressed—but it may. Drugs called proton-pump inhibitors (PPIs) such as Nexium and Prilosec treat heartburn by reducing the body's production of stomach acid. But peer-reviewed studies in Italy and Taiwan now find that people who regularly use PPIs are twice as likely to develop depression as people who use them rarely or not at all.

What's the PPI/depression connection? Limiting stomach acid makes it tougher for the healthful bacteria in our guts to thrive because they have adapted to an acidic environment. Changes in the status of gut bacteria have been shown to have profound psychological effects, including depression. The harm done to beneficial bacteria also contributes to other well-known risks of long-term PPI use—heart disease, kidney disease and osteoporosis.

The even sadder part is, none of this is necessary because even people with chronic heartburn often find relief without drugs by changing the way they eat.

Here's how: Signal your body to get ready to digest food so that it produces just the right amount of stomach acid at the right time. Before meals, if you can, spend at least five minutes in the kitchen where you can smell food cooking. During meals, eat slowly and chew each bite thoroughly. And don't dilute those gastric juices—limit beverage consumption during meals.

If heartburn symptoms don't improve, over-the-counter drugs called H2 blockers—such as Tagamet, Pepcid, and Zantac—are somewhat safer than PPIs. But if your symptoms last more than two weeks, see your health-care professional to rule out other conditions.

Joint Pain? It's All in Your Gut

Andrew L. Rubman, ND, founder and medical director, Southbury Clinic for Traditional Medicines, in Southbury, Connecticut. He is a member of Bottom Line's panel of experts and writes the Bottom Line blog "Nature Doc's Patient Diary." SouthburyClinic.com

You can pop an OTC painkiller when your back twinges, your knees ache or your hands cry out in arthritic protest. Or you can skip the drugs and feel much better (maybe permanently!) by getting right to the cause of the pain—your digestion. *Yes! Here's what's going on…*

The connection between digestion and joint pain is inflammation triggered by changes in stomach acid. By the time we reach our 50s, our stomachs produce less hydrochloric acid (HCl), a prime component of stomach fluid. HCl initiates the breakdown of food so that the nutrients can be used by the body and kills potentially harmful bacteria in food. When there isn't enough HCl, the body does not get all the nutrients from the food, because HCl not only starts the digestive process but also triggers enzymes in the small intestine to complete the process. Once the food reaches the large intestine, the incompletely digested particles are often too large and too complex for the bacteria to break them down to create the prebiotics essential to good health—and which benefit the bacteria themselves. Some will putrefy, causing smelly flatulence, constipation…and inflammation.

Chronic stress also suppresses digestive fluids because blood flow gets directed away from the digestive system to other parts of the body, such as the muscles and respiratory system, which are more useful in the fight-or-flight response and digestive enzyme production decreases.

Gut Health Connected to Heart Disease Risk

Improving gut health may lower heart disease risk. Arterial hardening raises cardiovascular risk and is closely related to inflammation, both of which are connected to the balance of gut microbes. In a recent study, nearly 10% of arterial hardening could be explained by gut microbes. Eat a diet rich in omega-3 fatty acids and fiber found in fruits, vegetables and nuts. Supplementation with omega-3s (fish oil) and probiotics also may help.

Ana M. Valdes, PhD, associate professor of musculoskeletal genetics at University of Nottingham School of Medicine, UK, and coauthor of a study published in European Heart Journal.

Note that heartburn most often is not an indication of too much stomach acid, as many think, but of not enough at mealtimes when it's needed. And because HCl signals the sphincter muscle between the stomach and esophagus to close so that food stays in the stomach, low HCl levels also keep the sphincter lax, allowing stomach acid and gas to wash back up the esophagus. Less HCl during a meal means more chance of unwanted organisms setting up shop in the stomach, creating acid-producing inflammation when empty, and voilà, heartburn!

An additional challenge to gut health and contributor to inflammation is the typical American diet, high in foods that are overprocessed and full of sugars.

Result: Inflammatory chemicals, triggered by the hobbled digestive system, circulate throughout the body, including to the joints, where they break down tissue and cartilage and create inflammation—setting the stage for joint problems such as osteoarthritis and rheumatoid arthritis.

WHAT'S GOING ON IN YOUR GUT?

Constipation at least two or three times a month…stools that vary in amount and color… feeling bloated…and passing especially smelly gas are clues that inflammation is likely brewing in your gut. Over time, this intestinal dysfunction can develop into irritable bowel syndrome or leaky gut. Fixing your digestive woes, especially if you've had them for years, may not undo all the damage. And if you frequently have heartburn, it's a good idea to check with your doctor or a gastroenterologist to rule out other health issues. However, you can do a lot to improve your digestion and reduce inflammation—which will dramatically dial down joint pain.

To increase production of HCl…

•**Eat mindfully.** Wolfing down meals doesn't just keep you from enjoying your food. It increases stress levels, reduces production of digestive fluids and doesn't give the enzymes in saliva a chance to start the digestive process. In addition to signaling the production of stomach acid, chewing also signals the lining of the stomach to produce the mucus that protects it from stomach acid. Take time to chew and savor all the flavors, aromas and textures!

•**Avoid drinking during meals.** Drinking beverages while you eat dilutes HCl. A sip or two to help swallow is OK. But if you're chewing thoroughly, you'll produce plenty of saliva and shouldn't need more liquid than that. Have water, wine, coffee and any other beverage either one-half hour before meals or one hour after.

•**Don't cut out salt.** Sodium chloride is an essential component of stomach acid and necessary for good digestion. While sodium does raise blood pressure for people who are sensitive to it, that isn't the case for everyone…and many people do better when they consume more than the recommended daily limit of 2,300 mg (about one teaspoon of salt). But don't go crazy with the salt shaker! A healthy diet, such as the Mediterranean, provides salty foods such as seafood, olives and nuts. And do avoid processed salty foods (pretzels, chips and the like).

•**Take an enzyme supplement with meals.** Consider taking a supplement that contains betaine hydrochloride, a precursor to HCl. I often prescribe DuoZyme, which also contains other digestives enzymes, to my patients. There are many good brands available online and in health-food stores (look for betaine HCl), but it's best to check with a knowledgeable doctor, such as a naturopathic physician, to determine which enzymes would be most effective for you.

To help reduce inflammation…

•**Eat raw foods.** Fruits and vegetables are full of anti-inflammatory phytochemicals. For the most benefit, make raw (or lightly steamed or sautéed) fruits and vegetables half of your diet.

Suggestion: At both lunch and dinner, have a salad that contains a mixture of different-colored fruits and vegetables and a light protein, such as eggs, fish, legumes or chicken. (Beef is fine in moderation.) Add a good brand of olive oil to help your body absorb the nutrients better. You don't have to completely give up sandwiches—or even fast food. Just have them as an occasional treat.

•**Get plenty of omega-3 fatty acids.** Omega-3 fatty acids dampen inflammatory reactions in the body. For example, research has found that omega-3 supplements ease pain for people with rheumatoid arthritis. Foods rich in omega-3s include walnuts, salmon and sardines. You can also take a fish oil supplement. Look for one that contains 650 mg eicosapentaenoic acid and 450 mg docosahexaenoic acid, such as Nordic Naturals.

Follow these steps consistently and within weeks—if not days—you should see your digestion improve. You'll stop degeneration of joint tissue and cartilage, and pain will diminish dramatically. Even if you still need surgery, you'll tolerate it better, recover more quickly and have fewer problems—and less pain—going forward.

The Bad Breath Cause You Didn't Consider

Andrew L. Rubman, ND, founder and medical director, Southbury Clinic for Traditional Medicines, in Southbury, Connecticut. He is a member of Bottom Line's panel of experts and writes the Bottom Line blog "Nature Doc's Patient Diary." SouthburyClinic.com

I t's well-known that certain foods and drinks—think onions, garlic, coffee—can give your breath a foul odor (halitosis). Health conditions, including dental problems and sinus infections, also can lead to bad breath. But there's a common cause of halitosis (and body odor) that often isn't considered—maldigestion. Fortunately, there are simple solutions that can help.

WHAT'S NOT HAPPENING...THAT SHOULD

Maldigestion happens when the normal digestive process doesn't function as it should. This can be caused by several factors, including lactose intolerance or medical conditions such as celiac disease or Crohn's disease. But it grows more common as we age even in people without such conditions.

Foods that are not digested properly create vaporous compounds that can seep out of the stomach or large intestine through the digestive tract's mucous lining instead of passing through and being processed by the digestive tract as they should. If this happens, not only does your body not benefit from absorption and utilization of all the nutrients in the food, but the malodorous compounds that are created are emitted either through the lungs as bad breath...or through our largest organ, the skin, as body odor.

DIGESTION RESCUE

The first step to correcting maldigestion is to chew foods slowly and thoroughly before swallowing. Digestion begins in the mouth as chewing increases food's surface area, allowing it to be more easily processed by acids and enzymes when it reaches the stomach. Chewing also stimulates saliva, which contains digestive enzymes that primarily break down starches.

Step two is to consider what foods you put in your mouth and when you do it.

Reason: Our stomachs are designed to process a healthful mix of complex (unrefined) carbohydrates, fats and proteins, preferably some of each at the same meal.

Simple carbohydrates, on the other hand, are best consumed on their own as a snack because the sweets can be held in the stomach too long if combined with a meal containing heavy proteins and fats and end up fermenting. Consuming sweets at the same time as more complex fats and proteins is asking for digestive trouble.

Step three is to consider stomach acid. A healthy concentration of stomach acid is essential to, among other things, activate enzymes such as pepsin, which breaks down amino acid bonds in protein. Limiting fluids around mealtime helps maintain the correct concentration of acid.

What to do: I recommend that if you want any sort of drink (including water) during meals, sip only enough to help you swallow or clear your palate. If you've chewed your food thoroughly, you shouldn't need lots of liquid to get food to pass comfortably down your esophagus. It's also best to not drink from about a half-hour before meals until an hour or so afterward.

REVIEW YOUR MEDS

Drugs that suppress stomach acid, such as proton pump inhibitors (*omeprazole*/Prilosec, *esomeprazole*/Nexium, *lansoprazole*/Prevacid) and antacids (calcium carbonate/Tums), can have the same bad effect as diluting stomach acid. If you need such medication, for instance to treat heartburn or a stomach ulcer, discuss with your doctor using the medication at the lowest effective dose for the shortest possible length of time and try to take it away from meals rather than around mealtime.

Note: If your bad breath and/or body odor persists even after you've tried these remedies... or if you notice other bothersome signs such as greasy bowel movements or excessive malodorous intestinal gas...check with your doctor to see whether another health issue could be causing your problem.

Diagnosed with Diverticulosis? What to Do...

Anil Minocha, MD, professor of medicine and chief of gastroenterology, Overton Brooks VA Medical Center, Shreveport, Louisiana. Dr. Minocha is author of *Dr. M's Seven-X Plan for Digestive Health*.

Diverticulosis is very common in the US, largely because so many Americans do not eat enough fiber. About half of adults in the US have diverticulosis by age 60—and nearly everyone over 80 has it. Diverticulosis is a condition in which small pouches, called diverticula, form in the inner wall of the colon and bulge outward.

Most diverticula cause no problems and are only found during a colonoscopy, barium enema or other such test for an unrelated condition. Sometimes, though, diverticula can cause mild symptoms such as cramps, bloating and constipation. Increasing the amount of fiber in your diet can help ease symptoms and can help keep new pouches from forming. Doctors used to advise patients with diverticulosis to avoid popcorn, nuts, seeds and certain other foods because they thought that small pieces of these foods might get trapped in the pouches and cause infection. The latest research has found that such foods do not get stuck in diverticula—and are not only safe to eat but are healthy sources of fiber. If bacteria leak through a diverticulum wall, however, the pouch can become infected or inflamed—and when it does, the condition is called diverticulitis.

Let your doctor know if you have symptoms that include abdominal pain (most often, but not always, on the left side), fever, nausea, severe cramping and/or a change in bowel movements. Diverticulitis is usually treated with antibiotics and a liquid diet for a few days to give the colon a rest. You may also need to stick to a low-fiber diet during flare-ups of symptoms because fiber may be too irritating to the inflamed tissue.

That means eating only foods such as chicken and potatoes without skins. Occasionally, a tear of a blood vessel in a diverticular pouch can cause gastrointestinal bleeding—a serious, potentially life-threatening condition. The bleeding may stop by itself or may necessitate diagnosis and treatment of the bleeding blood vessel via colonoscopy and radiological or surgical repair. A perforated pouch can also form an abscess and need to be drained, a hospital procedure.

The best way to keep your diverticulosis from causing problems is to be sure to consume enough fiber. Aim for 25 grams (g) to 30 g daily. Good sources of fiber include beans, whole grains, fruits and vegetables. Discuss with your doctor whether taking fiber supplements is a good idea for you.

Exercising—moderate to brisk walking is a good choice—for at least 30 minutes a day, five days a week helps keep bowel movements regular, which reduces risk for diverticular problems. Keeping your gut healthy with probiotic foods such as yogurt or with a probiotic supplement can help. Look for yogurt that contains live cultures and a supplement that contains at least five billion colony forming units (CFUs) of bifidus and five billion CFUs of acidophilus.

CHAPTER 8

Emotional Health

Don't Let Fear About Your Illness Get the Best of You

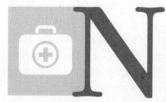

Nothing instills more fear than a diagnosis of cancer or another life-challenging illness. Will your health continue to deteriorate? Will treatments disfigure your body? How will you find the energy to cope with insurance...household responsibilities...and endless rounds of doctor visits and follow-up tests?

Even if the treatments for a serious diagnosis are successful and you (finally!) get a clean bill of health, the fearful feelings won't necessarily stop. You'll always wonder whether you might hear the dreaded words, "Your disease has come back."

Eye-opening research: Among cancer patients—including those who eventually have a full remission—30% to 50% experience some degree of distress, an extreme form of psychological stress. Up to 32% of cancer survivors experience post-traumatic stress disorder (PTSD), compared with just 1% to 4% of the general population.

How do you push through the crushing fear and helpless uncertainty? To learn more, we spoke with Michael E. Ryan, PsyD, a psychologist at Henry Ford Cancer Institute who cares for patients and disease survivors.

What are patients' biggest fears? For those with cancer, the fear of a recurrence is huge. Even those who have been cancer-free for years admit that they often worry the disease will come back and they'll have to go through the same grueling process all over again, or this time they won't be so lucky.

But cancer patients aren't alone in harboring these worries. No one with a chronic or

Michael E. Ryan, PsyD, a psychologist and clinical director of Supportive Oncology Services at Henry Ford Cancer Institute in Detroit. She uses evidence-based methods for assessing patients and intervention techniques to help them cope with the emotional and social challenges that arise from serious illnesses.

life-threatening illness, whether it's heart failure, Alzheimer's disease or Parkinson's disease, feels completely secure. Every exam (especially imaging scans) and follow-up tests can trigger intense "scanxiety," the fear that the other shoe is about to drop. They think about death and mortality—and what will happen to their loved ones should their lives be cut short.

Some people deal with anxiety by avoiding uncomfortable thoughts. Others worry about everything—that every bruise, rash or ache means that the disease has come back. It can be difficult to strike a balance between symptoms that need further medical evaluation and ones that are just part of normal life.

I reassure my patients that their anxiety will tend to lessen over time—but initially it's going to be high.

Isn't it normal to be afraid? It's more important to ask about the degree of anxiety, fear and depression. Everyone deals with stress, but not everyone develops a disorder that requires medication or therapeutic management. Some people have the ability to remain reasonably upbeat and optimistic, regardless of the diagnosis.

Others do need help. Some people experience depression or a traumatic response to a diagnosis and treatment, which can cause symptoms such as anxiety, insomnia, nightmares, memory loss, poor concentration, etc.—long after the initial diagnosis. Up to 58% of cancer patients experience clinical depression, and between 6% and 23% experience anxiety disorders, according to research published in *Seminars in Oncology Nursing.*

How can someone tell the difference between "average" and severe stress? It's normal to feel anxious, worried, down or discouraged when you discover that you have a serious illness. This begins to improve for most people once treatment has started and they know what to expect or as they get further out from remission. They regain a sense of control.

It's reasonable to be concerned, however, when you realize that all you think about is your illness—and that stress/anxiety are interfering with your ability to enjoy a good quality of life. You might lose interest in activities that used to give you pleasure...feel perpetually angry, depressed or morose...or notice that your personal relationships have become strained (or nonexistent).

Are there personal characteristics that predict who will do well/poorly after a frightening diagnosis? We've found that people who perceive that they have good social support—from friends, a spouse, a faith group, etc.—tend to have fewer negative emotions than those who are more isolated or feel they have poor support.

I tell patients that this is a time in their lives when they should reach out to others. You can't always generalize because some people are naturally more solitary and reclusive, but nearly everyone can benefit from some kind of support.

Practically every community has support groups for cancer patients and cancer survivors. Such groups also exist for other serious illnesses, including heart disease and multiple sclerosis.

Does stress increase the risk for a cancer recurrence? We know from laboratory studies that animals that are well cared for respond to treatments better, have slower disease progression and a better response to treatment than animals with high levels of stress.

A study in *Annals of Oncology* that looked at breast cancer patients found that those who took beta-blockers (blood pressure drugs that also block the effects of stress hormones) were more likely to survive their cancer treatments.

Regardless of the medical condition a person is coping with, stress can lead to poor lifestyle behaviors that do affect survival—things like not exercising, smoking, getting poor sleep, eating junk food, etc.

What advice do you give for managing anxiety? It's different for everyone. In general, the most important step is to do anything besides sitting alone and dwelling on your fears. See your friends...take daily walks...join a book club...or take up yoga.

Of course, you should also take advantage of professional resources—psychologists, social workers, hospital programs, etc. In many large hospital systems, these services are often available right where you have other medical appointments for convenience. Behavioral health services often are covered by insurance for a typical co-pay, but check with your insurer.

There are also many free programs available through local medical centers and the community—either in person, over the phone or online. A social worker, if available, can help identify resources and assess the supportive care services that are needed.

I also stress remaining well-informed. Talk to your doctor about your condition and the main treatments. Ask for printed materials or reputable online resources. Independent online searches can provide both good and bad sources of information. Be sure to stick with reliable websites, such as the National Institutes of Health (NIH.gov) and groups that focus on specific chronic illnesses such as the American Heart Association (Heart.org) or American Cancer Society (Cancer.org).

Talk to other patients in a support group. Information is empowering, even when things seem discouraging. However, not everyone thrives on more information, and it can increase sadness and anxiety, which is not helpful. For these individuals, it makes sense to perhaps discuss their illness and treatments only with their doctors.

You don't want to let cancer or any other disease always take center stage. You need to inject joy in your life—whether it's spending time with your grandkids or spending an afternoon in nature. It's important to acknowledge that not every moment will be perfect, but there are often opportunities to find moments of happiness.

Be Kind to Yourself…for Better Health

Study titled "Soothing Your Heart and Feeling Connected: A New Experimental Paradigm to Study the Benefits of Self-Compassion," by researchers at University of Exeter and University of Oxford, both in England, published in *Clinical Psychological Science.*

P ast research has shown that negative thoughts about yourself (and others) are linked to weakened immunity and increased risk for serious health problems ranging from heart disease to dementia.

But could more compassionate thoughts have a positive impact on health?

Researchers divided 135 college students into five groups—each receiving different 11-minute audio recordings that conveyed a range of negative, self-critical messages versus positive, self-compassionate messages.

Not surprisingly, the group that heard instructions to think critically about themselves had increased heart rates and higher sweat responses—both markers for feelings of threat and distress. By comparison, the group that was encouraged to adopt thoughts of "loving kindness," in which they focused kind and soothing thoughts on a loved one and on themselves, had a positive physical response—their heart rates and sweat responses slowed by two or three beats per minute, on average.

"These findings suggest that being kind to oneself switches off the threat response and puts the body in a state of safety and relaxation that is important for regeneration and healing," explains study lead study author Hans Kirschner, PhD, a graduate fellow at the University of Exeter.

This research, published in *Clinical Psychological Science*, gives insight into why people with recurrent depression, for example, seem to benefit from mindfulness-based cognitive therapy that teaches them to become more self-compassionate, according to the study authors.

Caveat: Because the research included only healthy participants, it does not prove that people with depression would benefit from a single self-compassion exercise, as used in the study. However, the researchers believe that a more self-compassionate way of thinking, in general, could be "quite transformative" for many people.

More research is planned to investigate the physiological responses and mood improvement that individuals with recurrent depression may derive from self-compassion practices.

To give self-compassion a try: Notice negative thoughts you have about yourself throughout your day…and replace them with a more positive, self-compassionate message. Even though this may not be easy at first, it will likely become more natural with daily practice.

Need to See a Psychiatrist? Find the Right One

Philip R. Muskin, MD, MA, professor of psychiatry, Columbia University Medical Center, New York City, and current secretary of the American Psychiatric Association.

As long as they have the right credentials, it's helpful—but not critical—that you personally get on with your family doctor, dentist, gynecologist or surgeon. With a psychiatrist, it's a different story. You'll be spending a lot of time together, sharing your most intensely personal thoughts. It can be challenging to find someone who's good...and also makes you feel good about talking to him/her.

Like psychologists, social workers and other kinds of psychotherapists, psychiatrists are trained to provide psychotherapy (talk therapy) to treat mental health disorders. But unlike other kinds of psychotherapists, psychiatrists are medical doctors and also can prescribe psychiatric medication.

Note: Psychiatric nurse practitioners also can prescribe medication and have some training in psychotherapy, but usually psychotherapy is left to other kinds of psychotherapists. Psychiatrists, on the other hand, receive a minimum of four years of education and training in both prescribing medication and several kinds of psychotherapy.

WHO NEEDS A PSYCHIATRIST?

You don't have to be severely depressed or hearing voices to benefit from going to a psychiatrist. Based on your symptoms, your primary care doctor may refer you to a psychiatrist for further evaluation. Or if you're seeing a psychotherapist, he/she may feel medication in addition to psychotherapy might be helpful. *According to the American Psychiatric Association (APA), you may need to consult a psychiatrist if you...*

- **Have a significant change in personality.**
- **Are unable to cope with your daily activities.**
- **Develop strange beliefs,** behaviors or fears.
- **Abuse drugs or alcohol.**
- **Are very depressed or very anxious.**
- **Have extreme emotional highs and lows.**
- **Have thoughts of suicide.**

If you have been treated successfully in the past with medication, or believe strongly that you would benefit from medication, the mental health professional you should contact for the current episode is a psychiatrist.

Besides getting a referral from your primary care doctor, friends or family, you can also...

- **Ask your religious counselor—ministers, priests, rabbis, etc.,** often have experience with local psychiatric providers.
- **Check with your local hospital or university medical center** for a referral to a clinic or provider.
- **Search on the APA website for a provider.**

WHAT TO CHECK

Your insurance may or may not require a "gatekeeper" referral to go to a psychiatrist, so it's a good idea to check what your policy covers before starting treatment. Also, check whether the psychiatrist you're considering is in your plan—many do not participate in insurance at all. Make sure that he is certified by the American Board of Psychiatry and Neurology...and, if appropriate, also certified in a subspecialty, such as child, geriatric or addiction psychiatry. Being affiliated with a medical school or university hospital is another plus—it generally means that he is likely to be up to date on the latest treatments.

While you can search online for patient ratings and/or comments, keep in mind that these are not always reliable. For instance, patients with a gripe might be more motivated to post a rating, while satisfied patients might not bother.

ESTABLISHING A RELATIONSHIP

Depending on the mental health disorder, your treatment options might include different types of psychotherapy (for example, cognitive behavioral, interpersonal or psychodynamic)...lifestyle changes (such as quitting smoking, cutting back on alcohol, maintaining a healthy diet and regular exercise)...and/or medication. You should feel that the doctor takes your preferences into consideration and that you have a choice in decisions that are made.

Example: You might see a psychiatrist for depression and agree that a combination of psychotherapy and medication would be appropriate. However, you're worried about gaining weight from the medication. Does your doctor discuss different medication options and their side effects? Or does he brush off your concerns and push you into the final decision?

You might also ask to have a "trial" period without committing to long-term psychotherapy to see if there is a personality fit between you.

Bottom line: Be patient with the process—but also stay alert for red flags. It might be time to choose a different doctor if, for instance, you feel that you're not improving or are getting worse…your psychiatrist is hard to reach or often unavailable…he seems to ignore medication side effects that bother you…or you become uncomfortable with your treatment plan or your doctor.

Excessive Emotions Could Be Borderline Personality Disorder

Robert O. Friedel, MD, distinguished clinical professor of psychiatry at Virginia Commonwealth University, Richmond. He founded Borderline Personality Clinics at both universities and is author of many scientific articles, book chapters and books, including *Borderline Personality Disorder Demystified*. BPDDemystified.com

D oes your spouse, child or parent sometimes act overly emotional for no obvious reason or behave erratically? Maybe he/she drives recklessly…drinks heavily…acts suspicious of others…becomes inappropriately intense and/or unable to control anger…or even deliberately cuts himself/herself.

Your loved one might have borderline personality disorder (BPD)—a chronic, disabling psychiatric disorder that severely impacts relationships with family, friends and coworkers and is more common than schizophrenia. Unfortunately, the condition is massively under-

diagnosed…and getting the right diagnosis is challenging.

Good news: BPD used to be considered untreatable, but new major advances in treatment allow patients to live full, successful lives.

SYMPTOMS OF BPD

The full spectrum of BPD symptoms typically appears in the teen years or twenties, but sometimes at a later age. It's often not diagnosed until later in adulthood…and sometimes never. BPD is *diagnosed based on having at least five of nine criteria, which fall into four groups of symptoms*…

1. Impaired emotional responses. Periods of intense anguish, anxiety and/or panic attacks…inappropriate, uncontrolled anger…chronic feelings of emptiness.

2. Impulsive, harmful behavior. This includes excessive spending, binge eating, substance abuse, suicidal threats/behavior, cutting oneself or impulsively damaging property.

3. Inaccurate self-perceptions and impaired reasoning. Unstable self-image, often assuming the beliefs, behaviors and speech patterns of companions while having difficulty describing one's own values…high level of suspicion, paranoia, feeling of unreality or that surroundings are unreal…inability to think rationally under socially stressful situations.

4. Unstable relationships. Inclined toward "desperate" efforts in relationships to avoid real or imagined abandonment…having very intense, unstable relationships that vacillate between overidealizing and undervaluing the other person.

Are you or is someone you know at risk? You can take a test that measures risk for BPD on my website. At BPDDemystified.com, click on "Online BPD Test." (You can take the test for someone who refuses to do so by answering the questions based on symptoms you've noticed.)

Note: When the diagnosis of BPD (and the opportunity to treat it) is missed, treatment of a co-occurring condition, such as depression or panic disorder, is less likely to succeed.

Example: A person who abuses alcohol may be able to quit for a while…but unless BPD is also addressed, he is likely to relapse.

THE MOST EFFECTIVE TREATMENT

While treating BPD often includes psychotherapy, I've learned from clinical and research experience that medications also are needed to achieve significant therapeutic results from psychotherapy.

Medications can manage symptoms that don't respond to psychotherapy and can quickly stabilize aggression, excessive suspiciousness, paranoia and other irrational thinking. *Medications that help...*

•**Antipsychotic agents.** This class of medications—which includes *olanzapine* (Zyprexa), *aripiprazole* (Abilify), *risperidone* (Risperdal) and *quetiapine* (Seroquel)—is commonly used to treat other mental illnesses, especially bipolar disorder and schizophrenia. Dosing for BPD is lower than for other mental illnesses.

Prescribed for: Disturbed perceptions such as suspiciousness/paranoia and split ("all-or-nothing") thinking.

Note: I often prescribe the antipsychotic *lurasidone* (Latuda). While its effectiveness against BPD has not been studied, I find that it is equally effective and has fewer side effects (for example, weight gain and high cholesterol) than other drugs in this class.

•**Mood stabilizers.** These include the anticonvulsants *topiramate* (Topamax) and *lamotrigine* (Lamictal), and are often used either with or instead of antipsychotic agents.

Prescribed for: Impulsivity, anger, anxiety and depressed mood.

•**Antianxiety agents and sedatives.** These types of medications, usually benzodiazepines such as *alprazolam* (Xanax) and *diazepam* (Valium), are prescribed with caution (because they are addictive and can make symptoms worse) when the other medications are not effective on their own.

Prescribed for: Co-occurring anxiety or depressive disorder. The nonaddictive antianxiety agent *buspirone* (BuSpar) is also effective and can be a better alternative.

•**Omega-3 fatty acids.** In a study published in *American Journal of Psychiatry*, women with BPD (they were not taking BPD drugs) who took 1,000 mg of an omega-3 fatty acid daily for eight weeks showed a larger reduction in depression and aggression than those who took a placebo. It is thought that omega-3s work in a different way than antipsychotic drugs, so they can be used with BPD drugs—but not in place of them nor at a reduced dosage.

PSYCHOTHERAPY

Typically, someone with BPD sees a therapist once or twice a week for up to two years... and less frequently once symptoms are under control. A therapist will suggest coping mechanisms for dealing effectively with flare-ups of symptoms—such as uncontrollable episodes of anger, suicidal thoughts and intentions, etc.

To find a clinician who treats BPD: Borderline Personality Disorder Resource Center, NYP.org/bpdresourcecenter, 888-694-2273.

To find support for your family: The National Alliance on Mental Illness, NAMI.org, 800-950-6264.

BPD RISK FACTORS

Research suggests that 60% of risk for borderline personality disorder (BPD) is due to genetic abnormalities that affect processing of emotions, impulse control and cognitive activity. These abnormalities can be inherited from someone who has BPD...or bipolar disorder, depression, substance use disorders, ADHD, post-traumatic stress disorder or a related disorder. Emotional, physical or sexual abuse during childhood and other environmental factors further increase the risk and severity of BPD.

Fast-Acting Antidepressant Receives FDA Approval

James Greenblatt, MD, chief medical officer, Walden Behavioral Care, Waltham, Massachusetts, and clinical faculty member, Tufts University School of Medicine, Boston.

Esketamine (Spravato), chemically similar to the anesthetic drug ketamine, has been approved as a nasal spray in combination with an oral antidepressant in people who have not responded adequately to two antidepressant treatments. Found to improve depression more quickly than antidepressants now in use, esketamine's side effects include dizziness, nausea and sedation.

What to Do If You're Jealous of Your Adult Child

Tina Gilbertson, LPC, psychotherapist in Denver and author of Guide for Parents of Estranged Adult Children *and* Constructive Wallowing: How to Beat Bad Feelings by Letting Yourself Have Them. *TinaGilbertson.com*

Parents feeling jealous of their children's success is not unusual. Parents often wrestle with an underlying sense of unfairness. Why should some people reach great success while others never do?

If your life has felt like an uphill battle, it's natural to feel jealous of someone to whom everything seems to come…even if that someone is your child. It's actually quite common between fathers and sons and also between mothers and daughters.

Remember that all emotions are normal—it's who we are as humans—and jealousy about the achievements of your spouse, best friend or even your son or daughter is nothing to feel guilty about. We don't get to decide whether or when we feel jealous!

The trick, though, is to not let the jealousy dictate your actions toward your child.

And ironically, the more room you give the jealousy to run around inside your heart without trying to "fix" it, the less it will influence your relationship with your child. It's when we try to suppress feelings that they start to get out of control and affect how we behave. If you allow yourself to fully experience the jealousy in the privacy of your own heart, you might begin to notice other feelings as well. Maybe there's some pride in there? Perhaps relief that your child is thriving in a world where so many people aren't? But as long as you're battling the jealousy, any positive feelings toward your child will be muted.

Be careful, though—jealousy can make you say things you normally wouldn't say. It also can cause you to keep silent when you should be offering congratulations or praise. Your child will feel you holding back if you allow jealousy to shape your behavior toward him/her.

Bottom line: Don't try to fight your jealousy. Instead, focus on understanding yourself and your emotions. So you wish your life were, or could have been, as great as your adult child's life is shaping up to be? Well, of course you do! Feel the jealousy consciously…don't push it away. That's how you'll process and resolve it—and keep your relationship with your child healthy and strong.

People with Mild Autism Are All Around You: How to Connect

Janet Lintala, DC, an autism mother and author of The Un-Prescription for Autism. *She is a chiropractor in private practice in Beckley, West Virginia. LoveAutism Health.com*

You probably know someone with a mild form of autism. You might not know for sure, and, indeed, that person might not even know. It could be your neighbor, coworker, friend's child or an acquaintance in, say, your book club or bowling league. Maybe it's not readily apparent at first, but over time, you realize that it's tough to make small talk with this person. It is socially awkward, so you stop trying. Maybe you've written him/her off for being rude.

While most attention goes to children, many adults with autism spectrum disorder (ASD) have never been diagnosed with it—partly because we are so much more knowledgeable about it now than we were even 15 years ago. So they have never received help in understanding themselves and communicating in a mostly nonautistic world. And that world often doesn't have a clue how to interact with them.

That's where your understanding comes in. Don't worry—you don't have to know for sure that someone has ASD to improve your approach.

The truth is, it's never a bad idea to reach out to anyone who is struggling in social situations or can't seem to fit in at, say, the office.

DO YOU UNDERSTAND ASD?

Autism is a developmental disability that can affect a person's ability to communicate, socialize and behave appropriately. People on the spectrum can range from those who are not verbal at all to those who have sophisticated vocabulary and strong language skills, yet still struggle with everyday banter.

Common misconception: Many people believe that people with ASD don't need friends—that they're introverts who are happy being alone. This couldn't be further from the truth—most people with autism are socially motivated. They just need your understanding when they reach out. *Here's how…*

YOUR NEW CONVERSATION SKILLS

Although communication skills vary greatly in people with ASD, in general such people have a hard time engaging in what we consider ordinary conversation.

What that looks like: A person with ASD may find it hard to put words together to form longer sentences…to keep up with the rapid-fire exchanges of a spirited conversation…to ask follow-up questions to keep the back-and-forth going…to stay focused on what people are saying. Many with ASD have trouble establishing or maintaining eye contact even during one-on-one conversation. They also may take words literally when the words are not intended literally (which is often)…and misunderstand the meaning of slang phrases. Humor often relies on a play on words, so someone on the spectrum might completely miss a joke. And a nearly universal trait of people with ASD is difficulty picking up nonverbal cues, such as facial expressions, tone of voice or body language.

Result: The conversation never really gets started…peters out quickly…or ends in misunderstanding and maybe even annoyance on the part of the nonautistic person. *Tips for better conversations…*

•**Be patient.** People with ASD frequently have trouble processing spoken words and need time to figure out what you are saying. To help, slow down when you speak…and give them time to come up with a response.

•**Be kind.** Don't assume that someone who doesn't dive into typical conversation is self-centered or aloof. He may have trouble focusing because he's overwhelmed by sensory stimulation—people with ASD find many environments to be too loud, bright and/or smelly. They're not being judgmental—they literally experience these sensory inputs in ways that are different.

•**Be very clear.** Because of their difficulty picking up nonverbal cues, people on the spectrum may have difficulty detecting and understanding sarcasm, irony, innuendo or inside jokes. So be as direct and concrete as you can, and don't take offense when the other person keeps asking questions to clarify what you mean.

•**Be understanding.** People with ASD also can have an anxiety disorder or be nervous around others, often because they were bullied and laughed at when they were younger. That's another reason that they may take longer to answer a question—they're afraid of saying the wrong thing.

MANAGE SOCIAL INTERACTIONS BETTER

Two common behavioral features of autism are intensity and repetitive behavior. A child with autism, for example, may carefully line up his toys again and again—and have meltdowns when he's asked to do something else. Autistic adults, too, may have more trouble than you would expect shifting from the topic or task at hand.

What that looks like: If he's part of a conversation, a person on the spectrum might get very animated chatting about, say, the Beatles—but be utterly unable to chime in when the talk shifts to, say, the Rolling Stones. He may get very anxious when asked to multitask. *How to interact more smoothly…*

•**Manage expectations.** We are used to people looking us in the eye and nodding their heads to show that they are paying attention to our conversation. Your bowling partner with ASD might not look up when you speak, but it doesn't mean that she's not listening.

•**Find creative solutions—and translate them into concrete steps.** Sure, it's irritating when someone in your book club highjacks the discussion about Emma to go on about 19th-century fashion. Instead of banning her from the book club, find a work-around that's good for everyone.

Example: Institute a rule that everyone gets to express her ideas for 10 minutes and then has to relinquish the discussion to the next person.

•**Give everyone a way to contribute.** Your fellow choir member may not be verbally quick enough to share his song suggestions for the upcoming concert when everyone else is brainstorming out loud. So you can propose that members also e-mail their ideas later—or bring them to the next meeting.

Once you're thinking along these lines, you'll get in the habit of solving these little glitches easily.

LIVING AS NEIGHBORS AND FRIENDS

Autism is a spectrum. Some people diagnosed as children may need help with activities of daily living throughout their lives. But many learn to function well in society with a little help.

We often assume that people with disabilities such as ASD can't lead fulfilling lives or fall in love, get married or make lifelong friends. But many can. Many do—and they are all around you. We can help by becoming more knowledgeable about this common disorder and showing empathy as they work on its challenges. We might even find that we've developed new friends.

DEALING WITH AUTISM IN THE OFFICE

Given their challenges in making small talk, understanding typical instructions and deviating from routine, adults with autism spectrum disorder (ASD) often struggle on the job. Many have trouble finding work and keeping it. *Here's what can help make the workplace more kind, inclusive and, yes, more productive…*

•**Promote an atmosphere of understanding.** Share what you have learned about autism with your colleagues. Things will go much smoother around the office if coworkers aren't surprised by someone's ASD-related behavior.

•**Speak concretely whenever possible.** Avoid slang, and use simple, direct language instead.

•**Explain the culture.** There may be unofficial customs that a typical person would simply "pick up," but a person with ASD won't. So tell your coworker if it's the custom that everyone chips in for snacks…and that it's fruitless talking to Jane in accounting before she's had her coffee.

•**Put it in writing.** If you need to give your coworker a set of instructions, e-mail her or write the instructions on paper instead of telling her verbally. Ditto for schedule changes.

•**Be clear about performance expectations.** Let's say that there is an urgent deadline. It might suffice for most people if you hint that this means a little sacrifice, but it's better to say, "For the next three weeks, each of us will need to stay an extra hour each night or work at our desks at lunch to make this happen." Otherwise, your coworker with ASD might take an hour-long lunch—because that's what the employee handbook says.

•**Ask for input.** Many of your coworkers may enjoy grabbing a beer after work occasionally, but the person with ASD may find the tumult of the bar overwhelming. To be more inclusive, offer everyone the opportunity to suggest different venues for out-of-office get-togethers, such as lunch in the park, a potluck at someone's house or drinks at a quiet bar.

Break the Pain-Isolation-Depression Cycle

Shannon Ang, doctoral candidate in the department of sociology and Institute for Social Research, both at University of Michigan, Ann Arbor, and lead author of "Going Online to Stay Connected: Online Social Participation Buffers the Relationship Between Pain and Depression," The Journals of Gerontology Series B. Karen North, PhD, psychologist and clinical professor of communications at the University of Southern California, Annenberg. "Social Media Use in 2018," Pew Research Center.

For most of us, physical or even emotional pain can occasionally hold us back from seeing the people and doing the things we love. But for those suffering from chronic pain, it can be impossible to socialize, isolating people at home, and adding a layer of emotional pain that makes the physical condition even tougher to bear. That combination can be particularly devastating as we get older, when social connections are both less available and even more important for well-being.

Now for some good news: Simple social-media tools provide an unprecedented opportunity to connect socially despite the limitations resulting from physical problems, lack of proximity or problems with scheduling or transportation. Remarkably, social media can be used by all generations to keep isolation from leading to depression.

Researchers at University of Michigan found that connecting with others via social media is an effective substitute for in-person socializing when pain keeps people from engaging in physical activities and face-to-face social events.

The researchers used information from a nationally representative survey of more than 3,400 Medicare patients who answered questions about their depression, pain and social activities online and in person. More than half reported experiencing pain in the previous month and said that it made them less likely to participate in face-to-face social activities. About 17% of all respondents said that they use an online social network. (*Note:* The survey did not ask for other specifics such as what sites people used, what exactly they did when on them and for how long.)

Key finding: Among respondents experiencing chronic pain, just 6% of those who used social media reported symptoms of depression, compared with 15% of those who didn't use social sites. Of course, social media can't completely replace all face-to-face socializing but, according to the study's lead author Shannon Ang, it's a good stop-gap measure until we can find better solutions to remain socially connected when pain and physical limitations stand in the way.

GET CONNECTED WITH SOCIAL MEDIA

While almost 40% of Americans age 65 and older use social media, according to 2018 data from the Pew Research Center, a sizable number of seniors don't take advantage of these tools.

If you're not currently using social media, setting up your accounts on the various social-media platforms can seem a bit daunting. But once you've established the accounts, staying connected isn't hard. The sites/apps are easy to use. Ask a friend or family member already adept at social media to help or consider hiring a local high school or college student—it often takes only a few minutes to set up an account and start using it, and it should only take an hour or two to establish the accounts that interest you and even get a good start at using them.

Choose platforms and groups based on your personal interests and the ones your loved ones like to use—for your friends, that might be Facebook but for your grandchildren, that might be Instagram, said Karen North, PhD, psychologist and clinical professor of communications at University of Southern California.

Facebook: This is the most popular site among seniors, according to Pew. Many people use Facebook to connect with family and friends from different generations, checking out children's and grandchildren's activities and photos and reconnecting with old friends, even friends from childhood. Facebook has fallen out of favor with younger generations and even some older people are posting less, North said, so it might not be as rich of an experience as it once was. Nevertheless, Facebook is set up to let friends and family share pictures, experiences, comments and life events and if your family and friends are using Facebook, then it is a great way to stay up to date and/or to communicate with people in your life.

Instagram: If you're into creative photography, Instagram may be for you. You can scroll through thousands of photos and videos on any subject—from beautiful sunsets and family birthday parties to clips of old movies, and everything in between. It's popular with younger people, too. You can follow your friends' and family's lives through the photos and other images they post—and leave comments for them—and they can see yours. You can save photos to your account and also send private messages. It's also a platform where professionals in many specialties, such as food and fashion, post their news and connect with fans.

Twitter: People use Twitter to be in the know and share what they know in the moment. You can find out what's happening in the world as it unfolds in real time and weigh in with your opinions. Twitter is like a giant information ticker with posted information and images scrolling by in real time. The platform is lightning fast—if you're on Twitter when an earthquake hits, you're likely to read about it before you feel it. The key to Twitter is that people post short messages, just a few short sentences (maximum 280 characters) and often add a label to it called a "hashtag" (abbreviated #) so that you can search for topics that interest you (e.g., "#ArtDeco" will get you pictures of this vintage art form). You can leave and respond to comments and photos both within your circle and with virtually anyone in the world with a Twitter account.

YouTube: There is unlimited content on this widely popular video-sharing platform, including educational and entertainment videos, TV shows and music videos. To keep in touch with family and friends, you can set up a private YouTube channel and share personal videos. You can even make a video to share with your grandchildren or other friends and relatives. For example, you can use your cell phone to make a video of yourself reading a favorite book to your grandchild, showing your face, blowing a kiss and showing pages of the book, even zooming in and pointing with your finger to a favorite picture or a fun detail in the book. Then post it on your family YouTube channel for your grandkids to watch. And your family and friends can share their fun moments by uploading their videos as well. Wouldn't you love watching your daughter do the limbo on her latest cruise or seeing your grandkids build sand castles at the beach?

Note: You can make your account on all these platforms private, meaning only the people who you choose can see or "follow" you. Get more tips from a social media professor about how to stay safe on social media at BottomLineInc.com (search "How a Social-Media Professor Protects His Privacy Online").

Bonus tip: Want to stay connected without any social media platform? The easiest way to connect with friends and loved ones is by using your cell phone's feature that turns your phone call into a video call. On an iPhone, this feature is called FaceTime and on an Android phone it's called Google Duo. Use your phone as the camera and show yourself and the things and people around you. Each person sees the other person live in real time on their phone screens, so it feels like you really are together. This is a great way to "participate" in an event you can't attend in person or simply just read a book to grandchildren. Your grandkids can show off their rooms or their latest art projects or even take you to their class event!

Depression and Seniors: Are You Getting the Right Care?

Marc E. Agronin, MD, geriatric psychiatrist, vice president of behavioral health and clinical research, Miami Jewish Health, and associate professor of psychiatry and neurology, University of Miami Miller School of Medicine, Florida. He is author of six books, most recently *The End of Old Age: Living a Longer More Purposeful Life.* MarcAgronin.com

Depression is not a normal part of aging, but it's often treated that way by primary care doctors and even seniors themselves. The problem can be missed or ignored, and even when it's recognized, you—or a loved one—may not get the appropriate treatment.

IS IT DEPRESSION?

Contrary to the stereotype, depression is actually not more common in healthy seniors compared with younger adults. Unfortunately, many doctors assume that depression is a normal and difficult to treat response to aging, and either miss or neglect the many reversible factors that can be addressed.

Older people are less likely to recognize depression in themselves and, when they do, are more likely to try to tough it out rather than ask for help. There are still many misconceptions about depression—58% of adults over age 65 think depression comes with aging. Even among those who recognize it as a disease, many think it's something they can manage on their own, without professional help.

What does change later in life are some of the risk factors for depression, such as struggling with a debilitating disease like dementia and Parkinson's, heart disease, cancer, arthritis or the after-effects of having a stroke. Losses are another common trigger—losing a spouse or adjusting to retirement can both be stressful. About 17% of seniors who become widowed meet the criteria for depression after one year.

Depression can also be a side effect of a medication you're taking. A study that looked at medication use in more than 26,000 adults found that more than one-third were using a prescription medication that could cause depression. Two of the riskier drug classes are narcotic pain medications and benzodiazepines—these are tranquilizers often taken for anxiety (itself a possible symptom of depression) or sleep.

If you're concerned about depression in yourself or a loved one, know that sadness might not be the only or even the most obvious symptom of depression in later years. Depression does not just affect the mood and the mind. It's a disease of the whole body.

In fact, older people who are depressed are more likely to report physical symptoms than emotional ones, such as...

•**A lack of energy** and/or increase in fatigue.

•**Confusion, memory loss and difficulty making decisions.**

•**Slowed movement or speech.**

•**Either a loss of or increase in appetite** and corresponding weight changes.

•**Sleeping more or less than usual.**

•**Aches and pains,** such as headaches, cramps, an upset stomach or other digestive issues.

•**Acting agitated.**

OVERCOMING TREATMENT CHALLENGES

Complicating the picture, seniors with depression do not respond to treatment as well as younger people. Research that followed over 1,000 patients with depression for two years found that patients age 70 or older were more likely to still have depression after that time, more likely to have frequent symptoms and less likely to show improvement than younger people.

There are specific reasons for this. The longer a patient has depression before getting a diagnosis, the more challenging it is to treat. Seniors may also be less likely than younger people to use psychotherapy (talk therapy), an important part of a comprehensive treatment plan. Antidepressants may not work as well in people who have some cognitive impairment—changes in an aging brain may make brain chemicals that should respond to antidepressants less responsive, making psychotherapy even more essential.

The biggest reason of all is that seniors aren't typically treated by a geriatric psychiatrist, one who specializes in seniors. A primary care doctor or even a psychiatrist without this special training may not be skilled enough for your needs. Indeed, most seniors treated for depression are treated by their primary care doctors—less than 3% of people over age 65 with depression ever see a mental health specialist. If their only treatment is a prescription for an antidepressant, it stands to reason that depression will be worse for them. No antidepressants are better in terms of effectiveness, but their side effect profiles are important to consider. So, while some of the older antidepressants are actually some of the best in terms of effect, their side effects pose too many risks in later life. A geriatric psychiatrist will not only better understand a drug's effect on each individual, but will also be able to tease out symptoms of depression from symptoms of separate medical conditions and help patients overcome resistance to working with a psychotherapist. With this combination of medication and psychotherapy, treatment can be just as effective as for younger people.

Complementary therapies can augment the positive effects of talk therapy and medication. Exercise, such as walking, and a healthy diet can go a long way to improving mood.

Important: Know that unrecognized or undertreated depression in seniors can be extremely dangerous. Suicide is a real risk among the elderly. About 20% of suicides occur in people age 65 and older. Men over age 85 have a six-times higher suicide rate than the average American. Any thoughts or talk of suicide should prompt a loved one to reach out urgently to a mental health specialist or even a suicide hotline.

Still, there's good reason to be positive about managing depression in later life. With age comes better control of emotions, less impulsivity and more resiliency. Combined with the right care, these traits can help conquer depression.

Walk Your Way Out of Depression

Susan Besser, MD, a board-certified family physician with Mercy Personal Physicians in Baltimore.

Study titled "Is There Evidence That Walking Groups Have Health Benefits? A Systematic Review and Meta-Analysis" by researchers at University of East Anglia, UK, published in *British Journal of Sports Medicine*.

On top of feelings of sadness and despair, depression can suck the energy out of you. Getting out of bed is a challenge, let alone getting exercise. But if you can push yourself to go outside and just walk, you can affect real change on your mental condition.

It's almost magical how walking can help with depression, and there's much more at work than the symbolic move from a darkened room to daylight. Yes, exercise releases endorphins, your body's own feel-good chemicals, but it goes deeper than that. It also has a positive direct effect on neuroplasticity—your brain's ability to adapt to changing situations—and that can put the brakes on depression.

Exercise also helps with the physical problems that ride along with depression—including heart disease, often a result of obesity/inactivity, and diabetes, both of which occur at higher rates in people with depression.

Big bonus: If you are able to add a social component to your walking, it turns this simple exercise into an extremely potent depression treatment. That's great news for people who don't want to take medication, want to take less of it, or have taken antidepressants without success. And yet a great many mental health professionals fail to recommend exercise for depression! We've made it easy for you with the following action plan.

How long to walk: According to an analysis of studies on walking for depression, the length of time people walked varied quite a bit and often fell below general guidelines for physical activity. The answer? Aim for walking at least 30 minutes a day at least five days a week, and you'll also meet the fitness recommendations for optimal health, said Susan Besser, MD, a primary care physician with Mercy Personal Physicians in Baltimore. But if that's too difficult at first, do what feels right. Even five minutes can help give you energy when you're feeling exhausted from depression.

How often to walk: Walking most days of the week is ideal, but even three times a week was shown to reduce depression symptoms.

How fast to walk: Walking at any pace is helpful and is better than not walking. But to get aerobic benefits, which have the strongest effect on depression, you'll want to work your way up to four miles per hour—you should be able to have a casual conversation, but not be able to sing or whistle.

A good place: Part of why walking will be so helpful for you if you have depression is that it helps get you out of your own head, Dr. Besser said. Walking in nature—appreciating the beauty of your natural surroundings—can help you achieve this. Walking in an interesting city environment can, too. Whatever your surroundings, the more engaging you find them to be, the better the boost to how you'll feel both during and after your walks. And of course one way to be engaged is to walk with a friend—or two or three.

Surprising Way to Deal with a Stressful Task

Brynne DiMenichi, PhD, Rutgers University, lead author of study "Writing About Past Failures Attenuates Cortisol Responses and Sustained Attention Deficits Following Psychosocial Stress," published in *Frontiers in Behavioral Neuroscience*.

Next time you face a stressful task, think back to a time when you confronted a challenge—and failed. You'll be more likely to succeed. So finds a study published in *Frontiers in Behavioral Neuroscience*. One group of participants wrote about past failures… a second group wrote about unrelated topics.

Both groups then were given the same stressful challenges. They then tried a new task requiring persistent attention.

Results: Participants who had reflected on past failures handled the new task with better physiological responses and less unnecessary rushing, leading to significantly better performance.

It's all about how much stress your brain creates, explains lead study author Brynne Di-Menichi, PhD, of Rutgers University. Stress makes our bodies release the hormone cortisol, triggering the "fight or flight" response. That is great when you need to, say, run away from a tiger but counterproductive when you need to focus.

Why would focusing on a past failure reduce stress? It's the comparison, said Dr. DiMenichi. You might realize that the new challenge seems less daunting than one that laid you low in the past.

To harness the power of past failures before a new challenge, spend perhaps 10 minutes writing or thinking about one of your failures. It should be specific, painful, personal—and, if possible, related to the challenge. For example, before a job interview, you might write about a past job interview that went wrong. Far from undermining your confidence, this could help you keep cool under pressure.

You Survived an Opioid Overdose: How to Make Sure You Stay Alive

Marc R. Larochelle, MD, MPH, researcher at the Grayken Center for Addiction at Boston Medical Center and lead author of the study titled "Medication for Opioid Use Disorder After Nonfatal Opioid Overdose and Association with Mortality," published in *Annals of Internal Medicine*.

You—or a loved one—just survived an opioid overdose. You're relieved and shaken at the same time. You may not realize it, but you're also very vulnerable to repeating the same scenario—the year following an overdose is a very high-risk period for another potentially fatal overdose. And making things worse, there's a good chance that you were sent home without a plan to get the help you need—treatment with a medication to get you or your loved one off the opioid.

A study done at the Grayken Center for Addiction at Boston Medical Center found that only three in 10 survivors of opioid overdoses went on to get what's called *medication for addiction treatment*, or MAT, using one of the three drugs—*methadone, buprenorphine* or *naltrex-*

one—approved by the FDA for this purpose. Yet the researchers also showed how taking one of them saves lives. Deaths from opioids were reduced by 59% among people taking methadone and by 38% among people taking buprenorphine in the year following the overdose, compared with people who didn't take any anti-addiction drugs. (Too few people received naltrexone for the researchers to draw any conclusions about it for this purpose.)

Why aren't more people getting this life-saving treatment? Some aren't told about these medications or aren't told in a strong enough way to inspire them to pursue treatment—they might just be handed a pamphlet or given a casual referral. Other patients, if approached immediately after an overdose, may be too overwhelmed by powerful withdrawal symptoms to process the information about addiction therapy, explained Marc Larochelle, MD, the study's lead researcher. Some simply don't have access to a MAT program.

Tip: You can look for programs in your area on the website of the Substance Abuse and Mental Health Services Administration (SAMHSA.gov).

Misunderstandings about these medications are also a barrier to their use. This is not substituting one addiction for another—these treatments do not produce the highs associated with opioids or heroin. They eliminate withdrawal symptoms and cravings by acting on opioid receptors in the brain.

YOUR OPTIONS FOR ENDING OPIOID ADDICTION

By US law, methadone can be given only through an opioid treatment program certified by SAMHSA. A patient must start treatment by going to the program's clinic every day to get that day's medication—it can't be sent home with a patient from a hospital or picked up at a neighborhood pharmacy. This combination of required clinic visits and medication can be very effective for people who do well with (or need) such a structured program. However, methadone clinics do not exist in many rural areas. On the other hand, if you can make the commitment, once you're doing well on methadone and have not missed any appointments or relapsed, you may be able to start taking the medication at home, depending on your local clinic's policy on home methadone use.

Buprenorphine can be easier to use. It's prescribed by your doctor, and you can get it at any pharmacy. You will see your doctor weekly at first, but these check-ins are spread further apart as time goes on.

While both medications are effective, response is very individualized. Some people feel better with methadone than buprenorphine and vice versa. Trial and error may be necessary.

Both medications are taken over the long term as maintenance therapy. There is no good data on if or when to taper off, so you will need to work with your health-care provider—and understand that while individuals can permanently overcome their addictions, statistically, relapse rates go up when people go off these medications regardless of how long they were taken. In the study, those who used methadone did so for about five months on average, and those who used buprenorphine did so for around four months.

If you are using opioids nonmedically, even if you've never OD'd, don't delay—talk to your doctor or contact an opioid treatment program near you about methadone or buprenorphine therapy. These drugs can help occasional opioid users and those who have only recently become addicted kick the habit, too.

The best way to make a decision on which therapy is best for you is to talk to your primary care doctor about your options and/or visit your state's department of health website to see what resources are readily available in your community.

Alcoholism Rates Soar in Older Adults

Robert L. Doyle, MD, clinical instructor in psychiatry at Harvard Medical School in Boston. He has a private practice in Cambridge, Massachusetts, and is coauthor of *Almost Alcoholic: Is My (or My Loved One's) Drinking a Problem?*

Problem drinking in older adults continues to grow at a frightening rate...but it's not getting the notice it deserves. Shockingly,

72,000 people die in the US each year due to drug overdoses (the majority being opioids), while 88,000 annual deaths are attributed to alcohol.

Why this matters: Heavy drinking is dangerous for anyone—but especially so in older adults, whose vulnerability to alcohol's negative effects increases their risk for everything from diabetes, heart attack and stroke to kidney failure, liver disease, memory problems and osteoporosis.

What you need to know about this troubling trend...

A PROBLEM THAT KEEPS GROWING

Research looking at the extent of excessive drinking among older adults continues to turn up worrisome results.

For example, alcohol use disorder (AUD), a medical diagnosis for what is more commonly known as alcoholism, increased by a whopping 107% among older adults during a recent 10-year study period.

Interestingly, the habit can be insidious, often taking hold only in one's later years. Up to 15% of people don't begin drinking excessively until they are older adults—often during retirement, research has shown.

But the health consequences are severe and mounting among older adults. Alcohol-related visits to hospital emergency departments in the US rose by nearly 50% from 2006 to 2014—especially among females and drinkers who are middle-aged or older, shows a study published in 2018 in *Alcoholism: Clinical and Experimental Research*.

HIDDEN HEALTH DANGERS

Though some studies over the years have linked moderate drinking with a lower risk for heart disease, newer research refutes the notion that alcohol offers any health benefits.

A 2018 global study conducted by researchers at the Institute for Health Metrics and Evaluation at University of Washington found that there's no safe level of drinking if you want to minimize your health risks. Indeed, dying from all causes—and cancer, in particular—rises with increasing levels of alcohol consumption.

Meanwhile, older adults are vulnerable to unique health risks because aging bodies—

even if they are in good shape—can't process alcohol the same as younger bodies can.

Another important factor: Older adults tend to use more medication (prescription and over-the-counter), which raises the risk for dangerous interactions with alcohol. For example, mixing alcohol with blood thinners, such as *warfarin* (Coumadin), can cause gastrointestinal bleeding. Drinking while you're taking heartburn medications, such as *cimetidine* (Tagamet) or *ranitidine* (Zantac), can interfere with alcohol metabolism, causing blood-alcohol levels to spike. When combined with alcohol, cold-and-flu drugs, pain relievers, antidepressants and sleep aids can have intensified medication side effects, such as drowsiness and trouble concentrating.

RED FLAGS TO WATCH FOR

For a person to seek help for alcohol abuse, it requires the drinker to acknowledge that there's a problem. But older adults may be blind to alcohol's negative effects if they're simply drinking the same amount they always have, and alcohol serves as a social lubricant they don't want to give up.

Even if there are signs of problem drinking, they may be mistakenly attributed to "normal" effects of aging rather than the alcohol. So it may be up to others to spot the patterns of problem drinking in family members or friends. *Some red flags...*

•**They're not meeting their obligations** as well as they used to.

•**They're often late** when formerly prompt.

•**They're opting out of social commitments due to illness,** such as colds or the flu, which excessive drinking could be fueling by increasing inflammation levels in the body.

SPOTTING YOUR OWN PROBLEM

If you think alcohol has become a problem for you—even if you've been drinking the same amount for years—try cutting back. Drink half your normal amounts...or try going a month without drinking. If you can't, that may be the biggest sign yet to seek help. Consider counseling combined with medication.

Also helpful: As a psychotherapeutic intervention, Alcoholics Anonymous (AA.org) has a high success rate.

Treatment options: FDA-approved medications for AUD can help you cut cravings and drink less. These medications include *naltrexone* (ReVia, Vivitrol)...*acamprosate* (Campral)... and *disulfiram* (Antabuse). Scientists also are working on genetic tests that can help pinpoint who's most at risk for problem drinking, and which treatments may be most effective.

Stay Happy All Year

Norman E. Rosenthal, MD, clinical professor of psychiatry at Georgetown University School of Medicine, Washington, DC. He is the psychiatrist who first identified seasonal affective disorder and is author of *Winter Blues: Everything You Need to Know to Beat Seasonal Affective Disorder,* now in its fourth edition. NormanRosenthal.com

---

Summer, sadly, doesn't last forever. Soon we'll be wondering where all the light has gone. Then some of us will feel the onset of seasonal affective disorder (SAD), the condition that gives people depressed moods every fall and winter. SAD is no laughing matter—it can make a big chunk of the year a terrible time for sufferers and can hurt their relationships, job performance and overall health.

Not everyone who gets SAD in the fall and/or winter feels sad. Depression is the best-known symptom of SAD, but people who have relatively mild SAD may not become depressed. As a result, they might fail to realize that they have SAD and never seek treatment. But even mild cases can have serious consequences. Mild SAD can produce a decline in energy and productivity and an increase in appetite (especially for carbohydrate-rich foods), easily resulting in unhealthful weight gain.

What to do: If your energy levels are consistently down or your appetite up during times of the year when you do not get much sunlight, you might have SAD—so try a do-it-yourself SAD treatment for a few weeks and see if these symptoms fade. To do this, get outside in sunlight for 30 to 60 minutes each day, even if you must bundle up against cold temperatures to do so…or use a light-therapy lamp for 30 to 60 minutes each day. (More on light-therapy lamps and other SAD treatments below.) Try to get your light (whether from the sun or a light-therapy lamp) in the mornings—that's when research suggests light is most effective at staving off SAD.

Size matters if you buy a light-therapy lamp. You can find light-therapy lamps online and in stores for as little as $30, and almost all of them claim to produce the 10,000-lux light intensity that's recommended and effective for treating SAD. What the lower-end lamp makers tend not to mention is that their lamps might deliver 10,000 lux only if you position your eyes an inch or two from the light, which is impractical and uncomfortable.

What to do: Select a light-therapy lamp that produces 10,000 lux from a lit surface that measures at least 12 inches by 18 inches. Light-therapy lamps this size tend to remain effective over a significantly longer distance.

Examples: Carex Day-Light Classic Bright Light Therapy Lamp, 10,000 lux up to 12 inches away (Carex.com, recently about $115 at Amazon.com)…Sunbox SunRay II, 10,000 lux up to 23 inches away ($359 at Sunbox.com).

Fall/winter SAD treatments need not increase skin cancer risks. It turns out that it isn't the sunlight that reaches our skin that wards off SAD. It's the sunlight that reaches our eyes. When the eyes receive bright light, it triggers the release of mood-regulating neurotransmitters such as serotonin that seem to combat SAD. That means you can apply sunscreen to keep your skin safe when you head outside without increasing your risk for SAD. It also means that you can successfully treat SAD with a light-therapy lamp that filters out potentially dangerous UV rays, as most do. (Though for other health reasons, it's good to let some sun reach your skin—see below.)

Caution: Do wear sunglasses outside on bright days if you are not trying to treat SAD…or when you spend more than an hour in bright sunlight during a day. Excessive amounts of bright light can increase cataract risk.

Exercise and mind-set can help treat winter SAD, too. Light therapy is the best-known treatment for SAD, but if light alone doesn't do the trick, there are other treatments you can try. Exercising causes the body to release SAD-combating neurotransmitters such as serotonin just as bright light does. And a professor at University of Vermont has shown that cognitive behavioral therapy, a form of talk therapy that modifies negative thoughts, can be helpful, too.

What to do: Don't just go outside for 30 to 60 minutes of sunlight in the winter—exercise outside for at least part of this time. If you struggle to drag yourself out of bed in the morning for exercise and sunshine, make plans with a friend or personal trainer to exercise together. Adding another person increases the odds that you will follow through.

When you catch yourself engaging in negative self-talk in the fall/winter, counter with positive responses.

Example: You think, *I'm so lazy.* Immediately question this by reviewing things that you have done that weren't lazy…and then think, *Let's see what I can do today.*

If none of this cures your SAD, ask your doctor about cognitive behavioral therapy with a qualified therapist and about pharmaceutical treatments or supplements—prescription antidepressants can be effective for SAD.

There is a summer version of SAD, but it isn't like its winter cousin. Winter SAD typically brings depressed moods, low energy and an increase in appetite…but there's also a summer version of this condition. Summer SAD, also called reverse SAD, generally produces agitated moods, insomnia, loss of appetite and, in some cases, suicidal ideas. This might explain why there are more suicides in the summer than in the winter in the US, even though winter is the time of year that most people tend to associate with bleak moods. Another difference—while winter SAD is caused by insufficient exposure to sunlight, the cause of summer SAD is less clear-cut. It could be too much sunlight…hot temperatures…or some combination of the two.

What to do: If you regularly experience agitation, insomnia, decreased appetite and/or suicidal thoughts during weeks when you spend lots of time in the summer sun or in hot weather, cut back on time in bright sunlight…take cool showers, baths or swims midday…turn up the air-conditioning…make sure that your bedroom is very dark when you go to bed and until you wake up—add blackout shades/curtains if necessary. If symptoms persist, discuss what you are experiencing with a medical doctor or therapist.

If You Have an Eating Disorder Relapse, Here's What to Do

Laurie Wollman, LCPC, an eating disorders therapist and site director of The Renfrew Center, Baltimore, the nation's first residential eating disorder facility with 19 locations throughout the US.

You've been doing well and maybe even thought that your eating disorder was tucked away, but lately stress has gotten to you and you've started to revert to old habits. Weighing yourself daily…counting every calorie…refusing to eat a single carb…skipping a meal or two. It doesn't take long before you know you're in the danger zone—other people are noticing that you're dropping pounds.

Eating disorder relapses happen, and they can sneak up on you. The highest-risk period for an eating disorder relapse is within about two years of treatment, but they can occur at any point. In fact, the longer you've lived with an eating disorder, the greater the chance of experiencing a relapse.

Here are steps you can take to prevent relapses…and other steps that can stop a relapse in its early stages…

•**Stay connected, or get reconnected, to your original support source.** Whether that's your therapist, medical treatment team or a support group of fellow patients, this support source helped you before—and there's no reason or advantage for you to go it alone now or ever.

•**Review your journal.** Keeping a journal was probably part of your original recovery. If so, periodically go over it alone or with your therapist to preemptively identify triggers that could bring about a relapse and come up with healthy coping strategies. Relapses most often occur during times of stress, such as after a death or a traumatic breakup, because a return to old, familiar habits makes you feel safer and more comfortable and can lead you to think you're in control.

•**Activate your coping mechanisms.** Relapse prevention is an important part of treatment and recovery. If you didn't already develop a strategy to put in place when confronted by a trigger, make a list of action steps that helped you during your recovery and take them, one by one. They might include attending a support group meeting, checking in with your treatment team or confiding in a family member or friend. Also, check to see whether you're really sticking to your meal plan and nutritional guidelines—draw up a meal schedule and eat with other people for accountability. Part of the plan should be to engage in specific activities that bring you joy, such as joining a book club, hiking or taking a painting class.

•**Quickly acknowledge any return to destructive behaviors.** For people recovering from anorexia, warning signs of a relapse might be eliminating specific foods from your diet, being preoccupied with thoughts of food, engaging in food rituals such as eating foods only in a certain order and/or obsessing about weight. For people recovering from binge eating, it might include hiding food (or the food wrappers after eating). For people who are recovering from bulimia, it could be starting to overexercise or reach for a laxative again. As soon as you recognize familiar, destructive thought patterns and behaviors, acknowledge what's happening and restart your former care plan.

•**Let your loved ones into your life, and listen to what they have to say.** Family members and close friends may notice your red flags before you do. Let them be your eyes and ears. Trust that they have your best interests at heart, and listen when they tell you that they see signs that concern them.

•**Ask about additional treatment.** Depression and anxiety often travel with eating disorders and can usher in a relapse. If you are feeling sad, hopeless or overly agitated, talk to your doctor or therapist to make sure you're doing everything that you can to take care of your mental health. This might include taking medication even if only temporarily.

•**Understand that significant weight gain is sometimes fine—even healthful.** There are times in life when significant weight gain occurs naturally, such as during pregnancy or as a side effect of certain medications, and is not a big health threat. Attempting to lose weight can be a slippery slope when you have a history of an eating disorder. Engage a dietitian as well as your therapist to help you lose weight safely when losing weight is truly necessary. It's also important to acknowledge that weight gain isn't a concern unless it brings medical complications with it. Remember that your goal is health at every size.

•**Ditch the scale.** If you're weighing yourself constantly at home, get rid of the scale to stop this behavior. Constantly weighing yourself gives in to the obsession with food and weight and allows you to focus on that instead of healthier coping mechanisms. You can have periodic weigh-ins done at your doctor's or therapist's office instead.

•**Be kind to yourself.** Recovery is a lifelong process, and you want to take it one day at a time. Rather than berate yourself for having a relapse, think about how far you've come in the past. Setbacks happen—the key is to forgive yourself as you take action to prevent it from becoming a full-blown relapse.

DIY Anxiety Relief with Acupressure

Kathleen Lumiere, DAOM, LAc, associate professor and DAOM program director, department of acupuncture and East Asian medicine, Bastyr University, Seattle.

If "anxious" feels like your default emotion you don't have to just accept that. While relaxation techniques such as meditation, counseling and even medication can help, there's another very effective, quick-and-easy way to "get a handle" on your anxiety—literally. We're talking about pressing acupressure points on your body to turn off the angst. *Here's how to do it…*

Acupuncture is commonly used to treat anxiety and the symptoms associated with it. Acupressure works on the same principles and

---

Negative Moods May Signal Poor Health

People who feel sad or angry have higher levels of inflammation—part of the body's response to infections and wounds. Clinical depression and hostility were already known to be associated with inflammatory biomarkers. Now it appears that even lower-level bad moods may increase inflammation—which, if it becomes chronic, can contribute to heart disease, diabetes and some cancers.

Jennifer Graham-Engeland, PhD, associate professor of biobehavioral health, Penn State University, State College, Pennsylvania, and leader of a study published in Brain, Behavior, and Immunity.

---

uses the same pressure points but without the needles. It's also easy to do yourself on your own body, so it's a great remedy that you always have with you.

Like acupuncture, acupressure is based on a theory that energy flows through a system of lines or meridians that crisscross the body. This energy flow can become blocked at pressure points located at the edges of muscles, and anxiety is one of the problems that can result. Stimulating the pressure points opens the flow of energy and relieves the anxiety. Acupressure can relieve not only physical symptoms such as headache, nausea, sweating and heart palpitations…it also can relieve emotional symptoms such as excessive fear, worry, apprehension and irritability.

The seven pressure points below are especially good at relieving anxiety and associated symptoms. When you're working on a particular pressure point, you can either apply steady pressure or gently massage it for a few minutes, whichever works better for you. Repeat as often as you like—acupressure is perfectly safe. You can further enhance the effectiveness by taking slow, deep breaths and/or closing your eyes while you're pressing or massaging. It doesn't matter which points you try, how many of them, in what order or whether you apply pressure to a particular point on one or both sides of the body. Focus on the points (and the side of the body) that work for you. *Seven points to try…*

•**Pericardium 6 (PC 6).** PC 6 is a very well-researched acupressure (and acupuncture) point. In fact, it's the pressure point stimulated by motion sickness wristbands to reduce nausea. (Wearing one of these bands also helps relieve anxiety!) Find it at the center of your inner wrist, about an inch above the crease. PC 6 not only reduces the nausea caused by anxiety, it also can reduce palpitations.

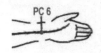

•**Heart 7 (HT 7).** Find HT 7 on the outside of your inner wrist, (the side opposite your thumb), just above the palm of your hand in the crease area. Pressure here may relieve nervousness, fear and palpitations.

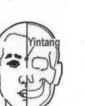

•**Yintang.** Yintang is located right between your eyebrows, an area sometimes called the third eye. It is an especially powerful pressure point for relieving anxiety and calming the whole body. Yintang also is useful for reducing anxiety headaches and insomnia.

•**Jianjing or Gallbladder 21 (GB 21).** This point is located at the top of your shoulder about halfway between your shoulder and neck and in line with your nipple. Since trying to reach your shoulder with the hand on the same side is awkward, you will need to cross your arms to reach each shoulder with the opposite hand (or let someone press this pressure point for you). Pressing GB 21 is wonderful for relieving the neck pain and tension that can accompany anxiety. It also can lower blood pressure.

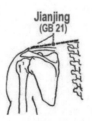

•**Liver 3 (LR 3).** Locate LR 3 by finding the web between your big toe and the next toe (you'll need to take off your shoes and socks), then follow that space up about two inches toward your ankle. Pressure on LR 3 can relieve feelings of tension, irritability and stress.

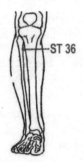

•**Stomach 36 (ST 36).** Find this point about two inches below your knee just on the outside of your shinbone. Pressure here can relieve anxiety-associated nausea and indigestion.

•**Earlobe and Shen Men.** Start by rubbing your earlobe between your fingers, as you would do to wind a watch. You can then run your finger up above the ridge of cartilage that stretches across your upper ear. Right in the center of your upper ear, you will find Shen Men point, which means "calm spirit." Stimulating these ear pressure points may bring you to a calm place and reduce both fear and fatigue.

What else helps: Eating anxiety-reducing foods such as cooked vegetables, leafy greens and mushrooms…avoiding foods that promote anxiety, namely processed, deep-fried and spicy foods as well as sweets (which can relieve anxiety temporarily but then make it worse)… getting regular exercise….and getting enough sleep also help keep anxiety at bay.

Finally, if all these steps don't help or don't help enough, discuss with your doctor what other steps you might need to take. You should also let your doctor know that you have heart palpitations, especially with shortness of breath or dizziness, even if you think they're caused by anxiety, as they could be a sign of a more serious health problem.

CHAPTER 9

Family Health Matters

Surrogate Health-Care Decisions: Are You Sure You Know What Your Loved One Wants?

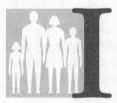

If you've agreed to make serious treatment decisions for a loved one should he/she be unable to, you probably think you know what your loved one would want. So you might be surprised to learn that you very likely don't know your loved one's true wishes. Here's what you need to do—now.

Researchers at Yale University Medical School and VA Connecticut Healthcare System wanted to better understand this gap—and how to close it—so they conducted phone interviews with 349 primary care patients and their surrogates.

Most of the patients in the study were male (68%) and had an average age of about 66. Most of the surrogates were women (78%) and were usually the patient's spouse or partner.

The patients were asked to look at three hypothetical health-care situations that could result from treatment of serious illness…

•**Severe physical disability.** Being confined to bed without the ability to care for themselves.

•**Severe cognitive disability.** Being unable to recognize family members.

•**Severe pain.** Being in severe pain every day.

The surrogates were asked how confident they were that they knew what their loved one's wishes would be for the three situations…and then to rate the situations as "acceptable" or "unacceptable" to their loved one.

Results: While 75% of surrogates rated themselves as extremely confident, when patient ratings were matched with surrogate ratings, only

Study titled "Assessment of Surrogate's Knowledge of Patients' Treatment Goals and Confidence in Their Ability to Make Surrogate Treatment Decisions," by researchers at VA Connecticut Healthcare System and Yale University School of Medicine, published in *JAMA*.

21% of the surrogates correctly matched their loved one's ratings for all three situations.

Overconfidence may be a barrier to having the type of discussion needed to understand a loved one's wishes…and the researchers advise primary-care providers to encourage patients and surrogates to have such discussions. If help is needed initiating such a discussion, they recommend the online Conversation Starter Kit from the Institute for Healthcare Improvement (IHI.org).

This conversation is vital. The researchers also commented that surrogates tend to underestimate the stress, guilt and doubt that they may experience during and after making these decisions. Surrogates frequently experience depression, anxiety and even post-traumatic stress as a result of their decisions.

So if you're a surrogate, it's important to discuss specific wishes with your loved one in detail—and to repeat the conversation from time to time, because wishes may change. Remember, your responsibility is to choose what your loved one wants…not what you want for them.

When a Loved One with Dementia Is Hard to Handle…

Deborah Bier, PhD, a dementia behavior expert in private practice in Lancaster, Massachusetts. She offers in-person coaching and online training and coping tools on her website, FromCrisisToCalm.com. She is also author of *From Crisis to Calm: A Practical Guide to Family Dementia Trouble.*

Caregiving for a dementia patient—whether it's your spouse, parent or some other loved one—is not easy. But the right mind-set will help you defuse and even prevent the troubling behaviors that often occur.

Whether your loved one repeatedly loads and unloads the dishwasher…has conversations with an imaginary friend…or hides the daily mail, you need to respond in a way that will help you change the behavior. You won't get anywhere trying to reason with the person.

You need to dig deep to uncover the hidden meaning of what's going on—in the dementia patient's mind there is always a "reason" for even the strangest behaviors.

What to do: Step back and do a little detective work by reviewing the "Five Ws"— who, what, when, where and why.

For example, let's say a woman with dementia starts screaming in fear whenever she uses the bathroom at night. She insists that an "old woman" is watching her, but her daughter checks and there's no one else in the bathroom or at the window. *Ask yourself…*

•**Who are the people involved in the problem behavior?** Is the behavior triggered by one particular person? Does it only happen when the person is alone? In the example above, the screaming happens only when the mother is alone.

•**What is the exact behavior to be addressed?** Break down large problems into smaller pieces that can be easier to fix. The behavior described above is the woman's fright reaction to seeing or imagining a voyeur.

•**When does the behavior occur?** Look for patterns in terms of time and antecedents. What's going on in the environment just before the behavior? Does it happen only at night, or only when it is time to take medication? The woman above screams only at night when sundowning (also known as late-day confusion) is common.

•**Where does the problematic behavior occur? Is it only in the bedroom, at a doctor's office, outdoors, etc.?** The woman's screaming occurs only in the bathroom, specifically when she is sitting on the toilet.

•**Why is the behavior happening?** This is often the toughest question to answer because it requires delving into the mind of the person with dementia. Is your loved one uncomfortable, frightened, lonely or looking for a purpose? When the daughter of the screaming woman recreated the scene for herself, she realized that the bathroom mirror is directly opposite the toilet. Her mother was seeing her own reflection…but didn't recognize the "old woman" as herself, which is common in the later stages of dementia.

The solution to this problem was not to attempt to convince the mother she was seeing her own reflection. Instead, the daughter simply covered the mirror each night (when the woman's sundowning caused mental confusion).

Important: Medication can often cause or worsen dementia symptoms. Be sure to factor that possibility into any troubling behavior—and consult a doctor for advice.

4 KEY STEPS

When interacting with a person with dementia, try these "rules"...

•**Nurture positive emotions.** Leave your emotional baggage at the door. Let go of anger, guilt or resentment when you are dealing with your loved one with dementia. This is not always easy between family members, but you will be motivated to do this when you see how much it improves dementia behaviors. For example, people with dementia are attuned to body language and tone of voice, so it's very helpful if you are able to remain upbeat and loving.

Also, begin each interaction by "bringing the sweetness." Start with a warm moment—bringing a cup of cocoa in the morning, sitting and holding hands, reading a funny story—before every care task or interaction. It only takes a minute, and it will end up saving you time with the dementia behaviors it prevents or improves.

Work with your loved one's still-present abilities. Rather than dwelling on what your loved one can no longer do, reconnect with what he/she still can do. For example, people with Alzheimer's disease tend to lose fine motor control first—making it difficult to button a shirt, for example—but your loved one can still walk. This means you still can take walks with your loved one and perhaps observe trees, flowers and other elements of nature.

Think when you communicate. Talking to someone with dementia demands attention to details. *You need to...*

•**Remember that body language and emotions often speak louder than words.**

•**Use simple sentences...and slow down.** Allow time for words to be processed. Make sure you have your loved one's attention before you begin speaking by catching and maintaining eye contact.

•**Speak on the same physical level**—sitting or standing—and approach the person from the front, not from the back or side, which can startle your loved one.

Be aware of sensory changes. Dementia changes the way our senses work, which can trigger problems. Understanding these changes will often help you explain the "why" of a particular behavior. *For example...*

•**Vision changes can make it difficult to clearly see and identify objects.** Brighter lights and contrasting colors are needed. Also be sure that your loved one wears all sensory aides, such as eyeglasses and hearing aids.

•**Sounds of favorite music can stimulate memory and keep people with dementia engaged.** But ambient noise—traffic or construction—can be irritating and distracting.

Helpful: Sit down and listen to the music with your loved one so you can share the experience. If he previously played a musical instrument—even years ago—encourage him to pick it up again.

•**Senses of smell and taste can change and are known to become less acute with normal aging**—even more so with dementia. Throwing plates of food or refusing to eat may be due to a changing ability to taste, rather than petulance. Eating with another person may help him mimic the proper actions of eating, and the social interaction of breaking bread together is often an encouragement to eat.

The takeaway: By thoughtfully changing the way you interact with your loved one, you can nudge behaviors in a more peaceful direction, allowing the two of you to reconnect emotionally.

Safer Driving for Elderly Parents

Recommendations from AAA Foundation for Traffic Safety, reported in *USA Today*.

Don't wait until after an accident to talk about safe driving with elderly parents and relatives. About 83% of older drivers never speak to a doctor or family member about their driving ability, so the issue does not come up until there is an accident or other problem.

To make the discussion productive, focus on safety rather than age or ability, and use "I" statements instead of "you" statements—"I am concerned about your safety when you drive," rather than, "You are no longer driving safely." That keeps the talk nonthreatening and prevents it from sounding as if they are about to lose their freedom. Be sure to research, plan for and discuss alternatives to car use so that your relative knows he/she will not be isolated when the time comes to stop driving.

Protect a Parent from Caregiver Abuse

Sandra D. Glazier, Esq., a Bloomfield Hills, Michigan–based partner at Lipson Neilson PC. She specializes in family law, probate and estate planning. LipsonNeilson.com

---

I s the person who takes care of your parent taking advantage of that parent instead? Sometimes there are obvious solutions, such as replacing the caregiver or discussing your concerns with your parent (or the parent's spouse). But what if the caregiver is your sibling…or the parent trusts the caregiver?

Here's what to do if a caregiver might be robbing your parent of his/her freedom or assets…

•**Confirm your suspicions.** Is it suddenly difficult to contact your parent? When you do reach him, is the caregiver always nearby monitoring the conversation? As a start, ask the parent's other relatives and friends whether their observations match yours.

Next: Visit your parent in his home. Controlling caregivers often isolate their victims to deepen their dependence—so observe whether your parent has time outside the caregiver's presence (ideally with friends) and whether he is housebound despite being mobile. Also check whether valuables are missing…and whether the parent has access to all of his own mail. (And scan that mail to make sure that he still is

receiving his bank, credit card and investment statements—abusive caregivers often change addresses on file so that mail is sent to them.)

•**Focus outside eyes on your parent's situation.** To do this, offer to pay for visits from a professional care manager. This person will coordinate your parent's care—and watch for signs of elder abuse. The local Area Agency on Aging or the Aging Life Care Association likely can help you find a care manager. Expect to pay $100 to $200 per hour.

Also ask your parent whether he stays in touch with a financial adviser. If not, suggest that he do so. You can alert a financial adviser (or estate planner) to watch for suspicious transactions.

•**Consider corrective steps.** *If you determine that a caregiver is exerting undue control and your family cannot remedy the situation on its own…*

•Report your concerns to the Adult Protective Services department in your parent's state. This agency can assess the situation and might take steps to protect your parent.

•Hire an attorney to petition for your guardianship or conservatorship (depending on the state) of your parent. This is an option if the parent is no longer capable of looking after his own affairs. The bar association in your parent's home state may direct you to appropriate attorneys. This can be a lengthy and expensive process and usually is a last resort, but it's needed in some cases to stop an abusive caregiver.

How to Support Someone with Cancer

Alan Wolfelt, PhD, founder and director of Center for Loss & Life Transition and author of Healing a Friend or Loved One's Grieving Heart After a Cancer Diagnosis. CenterForLoss.com

---

Y ou'd never consciously abandon a friend who has cancer, and yet that's the message many people inadvertently send… either by not reaching out at all or by changing the topic to something less threatening whenever the friend brings up his/her illness.

Of course, you want to be supportive—it's just that you feel helpless or unsure of what to say. Some people blurt out platitudes ("This is all part of God's plan") or share their own cancer stories (or those of people they know), none of which is helpful.

If you find yourself in this situation— and most of us will someday—the most compassionate thing to say first is actually simple and straightforward: "I'm so sorry to learn this. I want you to know that, if you want to talk, I am here for you."

Then take these steps to be part of the support network that's so vital to everyone facing cancer...

• **Acknowledge your helplessness.** It's OK to be at a loss for words after your initial expression of sorrow. What's important is to take your cues from your friend, and that starts with listening to find out what he needs.

• **Reach out repeatedly.** Maybe your friend didn't respond to your initial e-mail or phone call because he was feeling overwhelmed. Don't give up! Let him know you're thinking of him with a text, an e-mail, a card or a phone call every other week. Is he your best friend? Then reach out more often—at least once a week. One of the trickiest parts of being a cancer companion is knowing when to reach out and when to stay away. While you do need to respect boundaries and overt requests to be left alone, remember this mantra—when in doubt, reach out. People who are struggling often need time and space to go into exile. Grief and coming to terms with mortality invite interior struggles and demand this alone time. But remember—if you do end up "bothering" him, chances are your efforts to be present will far outweigh any inconvenience you may cause.

• **Lend a hand.** When you do call, be straight-forward and ask, "What do you most need help with right now?" Then follow through, whether it's cleaning his house, doing laundry, shopping for groceries, buying birthday gifts for a loved one or transportation to doctor appointments. And keep offering every so often, even if your friend turns down your request the first time, realizing it can be hard for him to admit needing such help at first. It may help to be specif-

ic—for instance, if you know she has children who need to be shuttled to soccer practice, offer to drive them. It's easier for your friend to say, "Yes, thank you," than to try to figure out what to ask for.

• **Squelch your inner cheerleader.** It's important to frequently ask "Is there anything you'd like to talk about?"—and then let your friend guide the conversation. If he's feeling pessimistic, don't try to "talk him out of it" by telling him that he's got a great doctor or that the odds are in his favor. The last thing he needs is a cheerleader. That's because you need to match his emotional tone or he'll feel disconnected from you. If he needs to befriend sadness, let him be sad. If you project that you can only accept happy emotions, he cannot be authentic with you and will often not want to be in your presence. Instead, simply allow him to express his fears, grief and any other emotions he's going through. Your empathetic reaction can make him feel hopeful again.

When words seem inadequate, simply remind yourself of a great way to support your friend: Mouth closed, ears open, presence available. Empathy is being in tune with what someone feels, not trying to change it.

• **Get comfortable with long pauses.** It's easy to feel uneasy when conversation tapers off. But if your friend doesn't want to talk—or is too distressed to speak or simply isn't really a talker—stay silent until he's ready to open up. Remember that just your being there is meaningful for your friend. Often, it means listening and overcoming the need to say something in return. How do you "listen" to silent types? By simply spending time with them. You might play cards, watch a movie or fold laundry together...and find that communication—verbal or nonverbal—happens naturally.

One thing that may help your friend communicate more easily is the EmPat Project—special "cancer" emojis created by artist Nina Beaty when she was undergoing treatment for lung cancer. Available through a free, downloadable app that you can add to text messages, these emojis rely on cute, funny drawings to telegraph a person's thoughts and moods. They're excellent shortcuts for saying "I'm overwhelmed" or

"I'm having a good day" without having to over-explain.

The bottom line: It's not always necessary to talk, but always keep your ears open, and be available and present. Your friend will quickly realize that he can count on you to be part of his support system.

A Way to Give Comfort at the End of Life: Comfort Food

Margaret L. Campbell, PhD, RN, professor, adult palliative care specialist, Wayne State University College of Nursing, Detroit.

When a loved one is dying, you naturally want to do anything that might ease his/her last days, if at all possible. Pleasure feeding is one way to give comfort—and even joy—at this stage. It can also help ease your own distress. Here's how to do it.

Someone who is dying no longer needs food or water, which can be hard for families to understand and accept. At some point, even the healthiest foods won't help your loved one live longer, and actually can make him more uncomfortable by causing bloating or nausea.

Pleasure feeding, on the other hand, is a way to allow a dying person to still experience the taste and feel of a favorite food or drink…in very small amounts. It's something that can be done for anyone who is conscious, even someone whose swallowing is impaired. In fact, one patient with a feeding tube was still able to swallow soda and melted orange sherbet. Not only did it make the patient happier, his family also was delighted at his pleasure.

HOW TO PLEASURE FEED

Use these guidelines when providing pleasure feeding to your loved one…

•**Let your loved one choose.** Pleasure feeding should be done only on request, and the patient should choose the food and amount.

•**Honor the choice even if it is not "healthy."** When a dying person isn't eating much, concerns about high cholesterol, heart disease, diabetes, etc., are immaterial. Coffee, cookies, ice cream—even beer—are appropriate for pleasure feeding.

•**Raise the head of the bed.** The safest way to offer pleasure feeding is when your loved one is upright to reduce the risk of choking.

•**Stick with small bites and sips.** Small amounts given slowly are sufficiently satisfying and, again, reduce the risk of choking.

•**Don't force.** Even with a food that was always enjoyed, don't try to force your loved one to eat. It's natural for people who are dying to eat and drink much less.

Important: Don't try to offer food and/or liquids to someone who is unable to swallow or who is unconscious.

OTHER WAYS TO COMFORT

If your loved one can't or doesn't want food, offering ice chips or small sips of cold water helps relieve a dry mouth—and that, too, is comforting. *Here are other ways to ease a dying loved one…*

•**Moisten his mouth with a damp cloth or swab.**

•**Apply lip balm.**

•**Gently rub lotion on dry skin.**

•**Play his favorite music.**

•**Read a book.**

•**Pray.**

•**Talk about favorite memories.**

After a Suicide Attempt: Keeping Your Loved One Alive

Heidi Bryan serves on the National Suicide Prevention Lifeline Consumer Survivor Subcommittee, is a trained facilitator for suicide bereavement support groups and the coauthor of *Now What Do I Do?* a guide for suicide-attempt survivors. HeidiBryan.com

Most people who attempt suicide are not likely to die…at least not the first time. But they are likely to try again. The biggest risk comes within the first three months of a suicide attempt, but risk remains elevated throughout their depression recovery, which can be years long.

It's common for people close to someone who attempted suicide to say that they didn't see it coming. Loved ones tend to put blinders on, says Heidi Bryan, a member of the National Suicide Prevention Lifeline Consumer Survivor Committee. But once a suicide attempt has occurred, what you do and don't do, and what you say and don't say, matter—a lot—she says.

Bryan speaks from the heart and from experience. She has battled depression most of her life. Not only is she a suicide-attempt survivor, she also lost her brother to suicide in 1995.

A suicide attempt is traumatic for everyone involved, the depressed person and everyone who loves him or her. But you don't have to stand by and feel helpless, says Bryan.

Know that some people will be resistant to your intervening and that there's only so much you'll be able to do to persuade them to get help or cooperate, said Bryan. But it also has been her experience that when you show empathy—recognize the severe emotional pain that he is in, know that he didn't really want to die but wanted to end his pain—and approach him with compassion, the majority of suicide-attempt survivors will be cooperative. When feeling understood and having a sense of collaboration, they also have ownership of their life and aren't just being told what they need to do. This goes a very long way for someone who just attempted suicide.

•**First, make your home safer.** Remove all guns. Just locking them up isn't enough. If you don't want to permanently get rid of them, see whether a friend or family member who lives elsewhere can safeguard them for you. At the very least, store ammunition separately from any gun, and keep both under lock and key. Only you should know where the key is kept.

•**Some people attempt to overdose with drugs.** That's why you don't want the attempt survivor to be in charge of his/her medications. Hide or lock up over-the-counter medicines, too, especially Tylenol, Bryan says.

Though people often think of Tylenol as safe, teens tend to use it to try to commit suicide, and overdosing with it can cause severe liver damage. It's in a lot of households and often overlooked as being potentially dangerous.

Do the same with liquor, pesticides and other poisons, razors, knives and rope. It can be difficult for you to live this way, but think of it as a small sacrifice to make sure that your home is a safe zone, Bryan says.

If the suicide-attempt survivor doesn't live with you, to make his environment safe, go with him to his home and remove as many access to means—items that could be used to attempt suicide—as possible.

If someone was hospitalized after a suicide attempt, it's recommended that he not go home to an empty house for the first few weeks. Have him stay with you or stay (or have someone stay) with him temporarily. If being with him around-the-clock isn't possible, maybe during the day is doable, supplemented with one or two check-in calls in the evening until his suicidality subsides. See if you can form a safety network of friends and relatives to support the person during the initial period of crisis.

•**Try to keep your emotions in check.** It's understandable if the suicide attempt left you angry or upset. But lashing out with statements such as, "What were you thinking?" or "How could you do this to me?" aren't helpful and could be very harmful, Bryan says, causing your loved one to withdraw rather than share what made him want to end his life.

•**Say thoughtful and kind things.** How would you treat someone who had just had a heart attack? Reach out to your loved one with the same type of concern, Bryan says. Help him focus on reasons for living and making life more positive and meaningful. Unsure of how to take the first step?

Bryan suggests saying this to your loved one: "You may not feel loved, but you have to know that you are. Trust me to know that I'm right about this. So let's work together to get you feeling better. And always remember, you are not alone. I am here for you."

•**Educate yourself.** Learn the warning signs of suicidal thoughts so that you can tell whether you need to step in before your loved one tries again. Sleeping too much or too little and losing interest in favorite pastimes are well-known signs of depression, but talking about being a burden to others or saying that life has no purpose are the kind of statements that often lead to suicide. For more signs, go to SuicidePreventionLifeline.org.

• **It can be painful and frightening for you to acknowledge that your loved one could be on the verge of another suicide attempt, but don't ignore any signs.** Face them head-on.

Try this: Sit down with your loved one, and through loving conversation, identify three to five negative emotions that he's wrestling with. These might include, for example, anger, feeling overwhelmed or trapped. Determine a scale he can use to describe their severity—for instance, one is mild and five is bubbling over. Then have a daily check-in—ask whether the levels of these emotions are rising, and if they're nearing the top of the scale, agree that it's time for intervention, such as more intensive mental health therapy.

• **Walk the line between concern and smothering.** Yes, you want to keep a watchful eye on your loved one and be in a position to take action to prevent another suicide attempt if needed, but you don't want to be constantly hovering—that will make him feel trapped and aggravate the situation, Bryan says. You and your loved one need to determine how much space feels right. It may take some trial and error, but don't give up.

While the majority of suicide-attempt survivors, when approached with empathy, compassion, and collaboration, will respond positively to working together, that's not the case for everyone. If your efforts are met with a response such as, "Leave me alone," there isn't much you can do but leave him alone for a period of time. You might express concern about doing that and then wait for an opportunity to talk with him, Bryan said. He will need to process what happened. You can only do your best—the rest is up to the attempt survivor.

• **Fill out a "safety plan" together.** This is a written plan that details a series of progressive steps he can take to address suicidal thoughts. First, list his specific warning signs that suicidal

thoughts are starting to grow, such as the emotions listed above. Experiencing these are the signal to take action.

The next section of the plan lists at least three self-soothing steps that he can do himself to distract his mind from these thoughts. These can be as simple as meditating, journaling, cleaning out a drawer, holding ice cubes in his hand and letting them melt, or petting a dog. There should also be a list of external resources—a change in scenery, so to speak—such as going for a walk, to a movie or to a coffee shop to distract himself and stop the thoughts if the initial distractions don't work. You might also suggest that he try an app with a mood journal, distraction techniques and other resources, says Bryan, who recommends the free app Mood-Tools-Depression Aid for iOS devices.

The safety plan next lists at least three people he can call to talk to about his feelings—family or close friends—when self-soothing doesn't work.

It must include numbers for a crisis center such as the Suicide Prevention Lifeline at 1-800-273-TALK (8255), for a text such as Crisis Text Line at 741741 (patients can text with a trained crisis counselor), and for his doctor to contact for help.

The plan should also detail at least one thing that's important to him and makes life worth living so that he can look at this on his safety plan and be reminded of it when life looks bleak, Bryan added.

• **Deal with your feelings, too.** It may not be an easy conversation to have, but you and other family members should openly discuss what happened and everyone's feelings about it. You might all benefit from therapy, not just the person who attempted suicide, because you all need support, says Bryan. Make sure that the professional you choose is a good fit for everyone, is knowledgeable about specific treatments and practices that can help prevent suicide attempts and has an approach to care that feels like a good fit for you and your loved one.

You can find even more resources at…

• **ReportingOnSuicide.org**

• **PleaseLive.org/after-attempt/**

• **SpeakingOfSuicide.com/**

And the online booklet, *A Journey Toward Health and Hope* from the Substance Abuse and Mental Health Services Administration (https://store.samhsa.gov).

---

8 Ways Pregnancy Has Changed Since You Had a Baby

Kathy Hartke, MD, an obstetrician/gynecologist in Brookfield, Wisconsin. She is past chair of the Wisconsin Section of the American College of Obstetricians and Gynecologists as well as its current legislative cochair. She also serves on the board of the WI Association of Perinatal Care. She has seven grandchildren.

If your daughter, granddaughter or daughter-in-law (or niece!) is expecting, you may be tempted to give all sorts of "helpful" advice. *Here's a tip:* Most of it will be dead wrong.

What medical science now knows about pregnancy and labor has changed enormously since you had a baby. *Here are the latest evidence-based "best practices" for having a baby—so that you can be a truly helpful advice giver…*

You may think: Bed rest prevents preterm labor.

But the truth is: Bed rest does most pregnant women no good—and even may be harmful. Doctors used to order women who were at risk of delivering prematurely to take to bed day and night. The goal was to prolong the pregnancy. But then studies showed that bed rest didn't actually accomplish that or, indeed, improve outcomes in any way. Plus it comes with dangerous side effects, including an increased risk for blood clots. Today doctors recommend bed rest only in rare medical circumstances—and often in a modified form that allows for walking around.

You may think: Epidurals slow down labor and lead to C-sections.

But the truth is: Epidurals are safe. Epidurals—regional anesthesia or "nerve blocks" used to dull pain during labor—have been around for decades. But they fell out of favor in the 1980s and early 1990s because they often reduced a woman's ability to push or feel anything below the waist, thereby increasing her chances of needing a cesarean section.

Update: New epidural drugs are more effective, easy to calibrate and safe for both baby and mother. They don't slow labor and don't lead to more C-sections. A woman can safely get an epidural during the earliest stages of labor so that she can experience less pain right away.

You may think: Once a C-section, always a C-section.

But the truth is: Doctors now encourage most women to try for vaginal birth after cesarean (VBAC), especially if they want to have more kids later. Doctors used to be reluctant to have a woman give birth vaginally after she had delivered a child via cesarean—they believed that the risk for a rupture at the site of the uterine incision, leading to excessive bleeding and possible brain damage to the baby, was too high. That's no longer the case. Successful VBAC, which occurs between 60% and 80% of the time, means less risk for hemorrhage, infection and blood clots, shorter recovery and a reduced chance of complications in future pregnancies. But a failed VBAC can lead to complications, so it needs to be done in a facility capable of emergency delivery via C-section.

You may think: A woman who exercises during pregnancy should take it slow and stop exercising if her heart rate gets high.

But the truth is: Pregnant women should work out! If you exercised during your own pregnancy, you were probably told to not let

Hold Hands

Holding a spouse's hand reduces stress in challenging situations. A recent experiment presented 80 married people with an intentionally stressful task and then monitored pupil dilation, a measure of physiological stress. Participants who held a spouse's hand experienced much less stress during the task than those who faced it alone—even though their spouses didn't do or say anything.

Tyler Graff, PhD candidate in the department of psychology at Brigham Young University, Provo, Utah, and lead author of a study published in *PLOS ONE*.

your heart rate go too high—and to bring it down if it did. Now doctors are encouraging moms-to-be to swim laps, lift weights, take fitness classes—even compete in 5K runs. Being sedentary is as harmful for expectant women as it is for anyone else, and it's not good for the fetus either, so moms-to-be should exercise at a moderately intense pace for at least 20 to 30 minutes, four to five times a week. But while they don't have to watch their heart rates, they should stay away from activities where there could be trauma to the abdomen such as skydiving, horseback riding and martial arts. Scuba diving also is off limits because the fetus may be harmed during decompression.

You may think: Just eat! It's OK to gain 25 pounds or more.

But the truth is: It depends on how much the pregnant woman weighed before. Weight-gain guidelines are tailored now to a woman's prepregnancy weight. While 25 pounds still is the guideline for women who were normal weight before they got pregnant, those who were overweight or obese should gain less.

Example: A woman with a body mass index (BMI) of 30—that's 180 pounds for a five-foot, five-inch-tall woman, which is considered obese—will be advised to keep her weight gain to between 11 and 20 pounds.

You may think: Never eat sushi when you're pregnant.

But the truth is: It's no more likely to be unsafe than many other foods if you know your restaurant. For years, sushi was off the menu for expectant women because of the chance of parasites from undercooked or raw fish. But in the US (as in most developed countries), the fish common in sushi, such as salmon, flounder and tuna, almost never have parasites, according to *Obstetrics and Gynecology*. Pregnant women are encouraged to avoid raw and undercooked fish in general, but sushi that is prepared in a clean, reputable establishment is unlikely to pose a risk. Pregnant women should eat two or three servings of fish a week, but avoid fish high in mercury such as swordfish, shark and marlin. Canned light tuna is OK.

Bonus advice: Caffeine is safe for most pregnant women up to 300 milligrams a day, about the amount in two or three cups of coffee.

You may think: If a woman's labor isn't progressing rapidly, it's time for medical intervention.

But the truth is: Most of the time, it's best to let labor progress at its own rate. Physicians have come to view childbirth the way midwives always have—if they're patient, it usually will progress naturally, and every woman progresses at her own rate. During the latent (early) phase of labor, if the fetal heart tracing is normal, mothers may be sent home until contractions get stronger. Hydrotherapy, massage, self-hypnosis training, walking and changing positions may provide pain relief for mild contractions. Active labor officially begins when a woman has dilated to six centimeters, but new research shows that this can take from just a few hours to eight, 10 or more—and that's fine. Today if an expectant mom dilates to four centimeters—and stays that way for two hours—doctors will give her more time rather than rush to do a C-section. Labor and delivery tend to be patient-led these days. If her pregnancy is considered low-risk, she doesn't need to be hooked up constantly to fetal monitors or IVs…told to push as soon as she's fully dilated (in most cases, she can wait until she feels the need to push)…or have her water broken artificially. Most women will go into labor within 12 hours of water breaking, but there still are some circumstances in which it makes medical sense to induce labor.

You may think: Babies deserve a cozy place to sleep.

But the truth is: Bare cribs are best. Before you splurge on a gift of crib décor, be advised that bumper pads, pillows, quilts, sheepskins and stuffed animals for the crib are considered unsafe. To reduce the risk for sudden infant death syndrome (SIDS), babies must sleep on a firm mattress covered with a tight-fitting sheet—and nothing else. It's still OK to swaddle a newborn or put him/her in a sleep sack (on his back, of course), but there shouldn't be anything soft or loose in the crib. After one year, these precautions aren't necessary.

Now that you know the facts, you can be a source of wisdom as the mom-to-be in your family prepares for the big event. To stay up to date, visit the website of the American College of Obstetricians and Gynecologists (ACOG.org) and click on the "For Patients" section.

To Prevent Drinking Problems...

Craig R. Colder, PhD, professor of psychology at University at Buffalo, New York, and leader of a study published in *Addictive Behaviors*.

Letting children sip alcohol may lead to drinking problems later. Children under age 13 who were allowed to taste alcohol under parental supervision were more likely to have alcohol-related problems in late adolescence compared with those who weren't.

What adults can do: Do not give alcohol to children, and when they become teenagers, talk together about alcohol use so that they don't feel alone when facing drinking decisions.

Keep Your Family Safe in Wildfire Areas

Shirleen Loloyan Kohn, MD, pulmonologist, Children's Hospital, Los Angeles.

Stay indoors as much as possible. Use an air purifier with a HEPA filter if you have one. Leave the air-conditioning turned off unless you can set the air conditioner to recirculate the air inside rather than taking in air from outside. Wear an N95-rated face mask if you must go outdoors—and be sure it fits properly. If anyone in the family has breathing issues, such as asthma, get out of town to an area with better air quality. Anyone with asthma should also have extra rescue inhalers on hand.

Obsessed with Feeding Your Kids Healthy? Stop It!

Joanne Labiner, LCSW, psychotherapist and eating disorders specialist in practice for 36 years in New York City.

To set your kids up for a lifetime of good health, you're on a mission to feed your family only healthy choices—but doing this can backfire, especially when your idea of healthy is at an extreme. When concepts of "good" and "bad" are linked to food and eating in children's minds, negative emotions such as stress and anxiety (and worse) can result—and that can set the stage for an unhealthy relationship with food as they grow up.

How could that happen? Your kids don't live in a bubble, and inevitably they will be outside your presence and be offered foods that are forbidden in your household, whether that's soda or anything less than a tofu burger on a whole grain bun. For example, kids don't want to be different from their friends, so they're naturally going to want to eat pizza, a hot dog, cake and treats at play dates and birthday parties. The problem is that when they eat something you would never allow, they may feel guilty... ashamed...anxious—as if they've done something very wrong.

You might be thinking, *Yes, I hope that would be their response*, much the same way you hope that would be their response to other forbidden things like cigarettes and alcohol. But forbidding foods can engender negative feelings at a much younger age and worsen throughout childhood. With food, as with everything else in parenting, it's important to embrace moderation and to pick one's battles. Assuming that there are no serious food allergies, eating white bread, for example, is not dangerous to one's mental or physical health in the way that cigarettes or alcohol are.

Additionally, figuring out what, when and how much to eat are fundamental ways that children learn about themselves. If they're allowed a reasonable amount of autonomy in this area, they will develop healthy self-esteem. If too much control is exerted, it will interfere with their developing sense of self, which can undermine healthy self-esteem.

When kids start believing that they're "bad" people, that belief is hard to shake and can follow them into adulthood. Some people develop what's called the "imposter syndrome"—to the world, they present a very successful façade, but inside they're constantly worried that people will find out that they are really "no good."

Another risk when parents are too controlling about diet is that kids will feel compelled to sneak forbidden foods. For example, they may use allowance money to secretly binge on cookies or another treat and then feel ashamed afterward. This could put them at risk for an eating disorder, for which secrecy and shame are hallmarks.

KIDS AND FOOD: CREATE A HEALTHY RELATIONSHIP

Consider these tips to foster a positive relationship between your kids and food…

•**Resist making every meal a teachable moment.** You might be tempted to talk about all the reasons your family should gobble up the healthy foods on their dinner plates, but don't. That turns every meal into an unpleasant, stress-filled experience. Use mealtime to reconnect with your family about other aspects of their lives.

•**Don't make hunger a flaw or a crime.** For example, if your child is hungry at 5 pm but dinner isn't until 6, don't deny him/her a snack, and don't make him feel bad for wanting one. Children should learn to pay attention to what their bodies tell them. Ignoring hunger can confuse children and make them hate their needs and then, possibly, themselves.

•**Resign from the clean-plate club.** Your kids will eat what they naturally need to, so don't hound them to clean their plates or take just "one more bite" of broccoli. Hounding your children will "load" eating and food with a lot of negative emotion, which actually creates emotional eating, the basis of all eating disorders.

•**Include all food groups.** Keep in mind that your kids need a variety of foods to grow properly. So unless there's a confirmed allergy or condition such as celiac disease, don't rule out entire categories of food. Talk to your pediatrician about what a healthy diet means for your children at different stages. For instance, young children need a significant amount of fat in their diets for their brains and nervous systems to develop properly. If you want to deviate from the doctor's advice, ask yourself, *Why am I doing this?* It's possible that you have some emotional issues with food that need working through, maybe with the help of a professional therapist.

•**Don't demonize treats.** Yes, they're in a category by themselves—after all, no one needs cookies, candy, soda or chips. Have a conversation with your kids about this kind of food. Explain that it doesn't help their bodies grow healthier. But then give them some wiggle room—while fruit, vegetables and nuts might be your go-to, everyday snacks, acknowledge that chips and cookies taste good and can be "sometimes" treats rather than making them completely off limits.

Dr. Starbuck's All-Natural Anti-Flu Program for Kids

Jamison Starbuck, ND, a naturopathic physician in family practice and writer and producer of Dr. Starbuck's Health Tips for Kids, a weekly program on Montana Public Radio, MTPR.org, both in Missoula. DrJamisonStarbuck.com

Whether or not your child gets vaccinated for the flu is a personal choice that only you as a parent should make. But regardless of your decision, it's essential to take other steps to support your child's immune system to reduce his/her risk of catching the flu…and to increase the child's ability to recover quickly if illness does occur. And the good news is, you don't need harsh drugs to do this! *My advice…**

•**Sleep.** No medicine is a substitute for adequate and quality sleep. Make sure your child gets eight to 10 hours a night. (Kids younger

*Consult your child's doctor before giving him/her these or any other supplements or homeopathic remedies.

than 14 need even more.) If falling asleep is difficult, I often prescribe L-tryptophan, an amino acid that's found in turkey but may be needed in supplement form to get adequate amounts. It's generally safe for children age 10 and older who weigh at least 75 pounds but should be avoided if the child is taking an antidepressant and/or sleep medication. Check with your child's doctor for dosing instructions.

•**Fish oil.** Though it does not directly act as an antiviral, a fish oil supplement strengthens the body, which promotes a robust immune system. Fish oil is generally safe for children ages four and older. Check with your child's doctor for dosing instructions.

•**Elderberry and Echinacea root.** These immune-supporting herbs are safe to take on a daily basis for several months. Research shows that people who take both of these plant medicines throughout flu season have a lower risk for viral illnesses, including colds. Kids who take these herbs also get better more quickly if they do get sick. These herbs are available in varying strengths in tinctures and syrups. Follow the manufacturer's label for dosing.

My advice to my patients: Take daily October through March.

•**Muco coccinum.** I prescribe this homeopathic flu medicine as an alternative to the flu shot. It contains infinitesimal amounts of flu virus—much less than is present in a flu vaccine—and helps the body defend against the flu.

My advice to my patients: Take once a month from October to March. One tablet should be dissolved in the mouth, 30 minutes before or after eating food.

Note: Even though you may be more familiar with the homeopathic flu remedy Influenzinum, I tend to prescribe that formula for acute illness and find Muco coccinum to be a more effective preventive.

TREATING FLU

If your child gets the flu, your best bet is to see your doctor. You'll get an accurate diagnosis and rule out any complications or related concerns, such as a concurrent bacterial infection on top of the flu or bronchitis—especially if your child has a high fever and/or pain in the ears or chest.

I suggest seeing a naturopathic doctor—we are well-trained in treating the flu and viral illnesses in general. Herbal and homeopathic medicines, teas and baths can hasten a child's recovery and be safely combined with any other medicine you may use—whether it's an over-the-counter decongestant or pain medication or a prescription flu medication such as *oseltamivir* (Tamiflu). To find a naturopathic doctor near you, consult the American Association of Naturopathic Physicians (Naturopathic.org).

When patients see me with obvious flu symptoms, the first step is prescribing Influenzinum 9 C—a general homeopathic flu remedy—two pellets twice daily for three days.

I also often recommend one of the following four homeopathic remedies to relieve flu symptoms…

•**Gelsemium.** If the child appears dull, droopy and drowsy.

•**Bryonia.** If the child's mucous membranes are dry…and/or he/she is irritable, thirsty and feels worse with any movement.

•**Arsenicum.** If the child is fearful, anxious, restless and complains of burning pains in the chest and limbs.

•**Pulsatilla.** If the child is weepy and clinging and/or has lots of thick mucus from the nose.

Typical dose that I prescribe to my patients: I choose the homeopathic remedy that seems closest to the child's symptoms. A 30 C potency remedy is given, and the parent is instructed to place two pellets under the child's tongue 30 minutes before or after eating food twice daily for one to three days.

•**Throat Coat tea (by Traditional Medicinals) contains slippery elm and licorice root.** It helps when a child has symptoms that may accompany the flu, such as a sore throat or cough, and can even help with an upset stomach. I often recommend that parents have this on hand.

•**Epsom salt baths are great for kids.** A 20-minute soak is relaxing, warming and helps with achy muscles. Kids are often able to sleep shortly after an Epsom salt soak. Increase the medicinal effectiveness of the bath by having your child drink a cup of either ginger or peppermint tea while in the bath. Both herbs have a mild antiviral action and can reduce fever. This is another common adjunct to my care.

Long-Term Risks of Tonsil and Adenoid Removal

Sean Byars, PhD, research fellow, school of biosciences, University of Melbourne, Australia, and coleader of an analysis of a database on more than 1,180,000 Danish children, published in *JAMA Otolaryngology Head and Neck Surgery*.

Tonsillectomy to treat chronic tonsillitis and adenoidectomy to treat recurrent middle-ear infections both increase the risk for respiratory, allergic and infectious diseases in later life. The risk for diseases of the upper-respiratory tract almost triples when children have had tonsillectomies. For children whose adenoids have been removed, the risk for chronic obstructive pulmonary disease more than doubles—and the risk for upper-respiratory-tract diseases and conjunctivitis nearly doubles.

Before Giving Your Child a Drug for ADHD: Ask These 7 Questions

Andrew Hill, PhD, founder of Peak Brain Institute in Costa Mesa, California, and a lecturer in psychology, neuroscience and gerontology at the University of California, Los Angeles. Diagnosed with ADHD as an adult, he has successfully addressed his own ADHD, as well as that of hundreds of others with attention difficulty, using nondrug therapies.

The Centers for Disease Control and Prevention (CDC) estimates that 11% of children between the ages of four and 17 have attention deficit/hyperactivity disorder (ADHD)—leaving many parents with the difficult decision of whether to treat their child with powerful (and potentially risky) drugs.

The decision is particularly fraught because ADHD has a low threshold for diagnosis—that is, there aren't any definitive physical tests to identify the condition. It's usually diagnosed by a primary-care physician (probably a pediatrician), who runs through a checklist of possible behavioral—and subjective—symptoms, such as inattention, excessive talking, not paying attention, etc. If a child is found to have a certain number of these symptoms, he/she could be diagnosed with ADHD.

Problem: Many other conditions, including anxiety, sleep problems and learning disabilities (such as difficulty with language processing or dyslexia), can cause similar symptoms. But despite this inherent uncertainty, children in the US are about 14 times more likely to be given a prescription for ADHD medication than children in the UK.

My take: Children who display such behaviors often need emotional support more than a prescription drug. *To find out, ask these questions of any health-care provider who believes your child has ADHD…*

How can you be sure it's ADHD and not a behavioral problem? A doctor will evaluate your child by running down a list of 18 possible symptoms. These include "does not seem to listen"…"often fidgets"…and/or "talks excessively." The problem is that every child has some degree of these behaviors. Maybe your child drops things just to hear the noise…fidgets in his seat…or always forgets to take out the trash. Most children will outgrow the behaviors—or learn to control them—as they get older.

Important: ADHD rarely develops after the age of 12. If your child didn't exhibit problems in elementary school but is starting to struggle with issues in eighth grade, he probably doesn't have ADHD. (In adults who have ADHD, the condition would have been present in childhood regardless of whether it was diagnosed at that time.)

To help diagnose ADHD, the FDA has approved a device that uses an electroencephalogram (EEG), a test that detects abnormalities in brain waves, to measure theta and beta brain waves. Children with ADHD tend to have a higher theta-to-beta ratio between the waves than children without ADHD. The test isn't conclusive, but it can help doctors feel more confident that an ADHD diagnosis is correct.

Why are you suggesting drug therapy? Even if your doctor is unsure about the diagnosis, he/she might say something such as, "Let's try medications and see if they help."

But for the majority of children, the nondrug treatments discussed below can be equally effective—and safer. For example, neurofeedback (see below) is recognized as being as effective as medication for ADHD.

That said, drugs can be a smart choice in some cases. Drugs can quickly change behavior (and make life easier for parents) and may be essential for children with extreme impulsivity.

Example: A child who keeps reaching toward the flames on a gas stove, despite getting burned in the past. This type of risky behavior is a clear indication for drug therapy.

What's the difference between methylphenidate (Ritalin) and amphetamine/dextroamphetamine (Adderall)? And which one would work best for my child? They're the two most widely used prescription drug treatments for ADHD. Both are stimulants that increase levels of dopamine and norepinephrine, neurotransmitters that speed up brain activity and increase attention and reduce impulsivity.

Better Time-Outs

Time-outs must be carefully managed to be an effective discipline. *Some tips…*

•**They are only for children ages two to six**—older kids should have privileges revoked instead.

•**Time-outs should occur only in cases of specific behaviors** that parents and children discuss and agree upon in advance—for example, hitting and disobeying direct requests.

•**Less serious toddler behavior,** such as whining or begging, should be handled through compromise or by giving a simple explanation of why a particular behavior is not acceptable.

Ennio Cipani, PhD, clinical psychologist, Visalia, California, and author of the free e-book *Punishment on Trial,* quoted at LiveScience.com.

Both drugs have about a 70% success rate, but there are some important differences. Ritalin targets the parts of the brain that control focus and attention—but not the parts that control arousal. So it is less likely than Adderall to be misused or cause addiction. Serious side effects (Adderall sometimes causes an increase in blood pressure and heart rate, while Ritalin can cause numbness/tingling in the fingers, hands and face, etc.) are rare, but I worry that children who depend on drugs won't develop the skills to deal with normal variations in their personality and temperament.

Are there any better drug treatments? Ritalin and Adderall are the most common treatments because they work almost immediately and are unlikely to cause serious or long-lasting side effects. But your child's doctor might recommend starting treatment with the antidepressant *bupropion* (Wellbutrin), for example, *atomoxetine* (Strattera), which affects norepinephrine levels, or other nonstimulant drugs.

They're less likely to dampen the motivational part of the brain (a possible side effect of Ritalin/Adderall) but can take weeks or months to fully kick in.

What are the best nondrug drug treatments?

•**Neurofeedback.** The American Academy of Pediatrics ranks it a "Level 1 Best Support" treatment for ADHD. During regular sessions, a child will wear an electrode-studded cap that maps brain activity while he plays a computer or video game. The game stops when brain activity shows that the child is losing focus and resumes when he uses the focus-centered part of the brain.

A meta-analysis of research published in *Clinical EEG and Neuroscience* found that neurofeedback caused large-scale improvements in inattention and impulsivity, along with more modest improvements in hyperactivity. One drawback is that a series of brief sessions (about 30 minutes each) can cost more than $2,000 and is probably not covered by your insurance.

•**Mindfulness meditation.** Children attend weekly classes in which they learn to focus their attention on objects or activities (such as their breathing rhythms)…acknowledge the presence of distracting thoughts…and learn to prevent distractions from interfering with their thoughts. A study published in the *Journal of Attention Disorders* found that 78% of participants in a mediation program had an average reduction in ADHD symptoms of 30%.

•**Nutritional supplements.** They're not effective for everyone, but there's some evidence that omega-3 fatty acids and other supplements (see below) can help in some cases.

Examples: Children given fish-oil supplements (high in omega-3s) for three months showed improvements in behavior as well as reading and spelling, according to a study in *Pediatrics*. (A typical dose might be 2.5 g daily). Meanwhile, research published in *The British Journal of Psychiatry* found that patients given a mix of vitamin B-12, vitamin D, folate and other nutrients had more improvements in inattention and hyperactivity/impulsivity than those who were taking placebos.

Can drugs/behavioral approaches be combined? They're often used together. A study published in *Journal of Clinical Child & Adolescent Psychology* found that a combined approach allowed children to take much lower doses of medication.

Are there any groups that offer support to kids with ADHD? Children and Adults with Attention-Deficit/Hyperactivity Disorder (CHADD.org) has a nationwide network of affiliates and provides evidence-based information on the condition.

Kids and Toothpaste

Recommendations by Centers for Disease Control and Prevention and American Dental Association.

Using too much toothpaste can damage kids' teeth, causing pitting and discoloration of developing teeth. Children ages two to three should use only a rice-grain-size smear of toothpaste on their brushes. Kids ages three to six should use a pea-size amount. Parents should supervise children's brushing for two to three minutes at a time, twice a day.

Pacifier Power!

American College of Allergy, Asthma and Immunology.

Parents do their infants a favor if they clean pacifiers by popping them into their own mouths. "Parental pacifier sucking" lowers infant levels of IgE, an antibody linked to allergies and asthma.

Picture Books Boost Brain Function

Study by researchers at Cincinnati Children's Hospital, presented at a meeting of the Pediatric Academic Societies.

The sight of illustrations that stay still and allow children time to explore them visually engages the deep cognitive functions of developing brains.

Recent study: Simply listening to a story being read did not cause the brains of four-year-olds to become fully involved. Neither did stories told using moving visuals, as on a TV screen or tablet—there was too much happening too quickly. Young children were pulled most strongly into picture books that provided a story with illustrations that they could spend time looking at and absorbing.

A Dozen Ways to Save Money on Pet Care

Lauren Greutman, dog owner and author of *The Recovering Spender: How to Live a Happy, Fulfilled, Debt-Free Life*. She writes and speaks about frugal living and household finance on her website and on TV shows such as *Today* and *Good Morning America*. LaurenGreutman.com

Our furry friends (plus feathered friends and other pets, too) can be costly companions.

Example: Add up the bills for pet food, veterinarian visits, kennels and other expenses, and the typical dog will cost its owner around $15,000 over the course of its lifetime, according to the ASPCA—much more if the animal experiences major medical problems. The average cat costs nearly as much, and even smaller pets such as guinea pigs, rabbits and birds can cost thousands of dollars to keep.

It's worth it, but wouldn't it be nice to spend less? *Here are several ways to reduce the cost of pet ownership...*

VETERINARY CARE AND DRUGS

•**Buy pet medicines online or in affordable pharmacy chains.** Many veterinary practices add large markups to medicines. In nonemergency situations, check for lower prices on 1800PetMeds.com and PetCareRX.com —you might save as much as 50%. (For nonprescription pet medicines, also try Amazon.com, which recently purchased Wag.com.) Most Costco, Kroger and Walmart pharmacies sell veterinary medications at low prices, too, though they tend to stock only a modest selection of pet meds.

•**Buy pills meant for larger pets and cut them to size.** Because dogs vary greatly in size, dog medicines tend to be available in dramatically different dosages for large, medium and small animals. But while a pill meant for a 100-pound dog likely contains four times as much medicine as one meant for a 25-pound dog, it often costs only a little extra. With many drugs, it's safe to buy pills meant for a larger animal and use a pill splitter to divide them into the appropriate dosage for a smaller animal. Never do this, though, unless you have confirmed with your vet that it is safe to do with the specific medication.

•**Use the vet in a nearby small town.** Veterinarians in upscale cities and suburban areas often charge significantly more than those in more rural or economically modest areas. Call veterinary offices within a half-hour drive of your home, particularly those in areas with lower real estate prices, and ask their rates for basic checkups as a quick gauge of their overall prices. You might save $20 to $100 or more per visit.

Alternative: If there's an accredited veterinary college in your area, it likely offers veterinary services at low rates. These services usually are provided by veterinary students, but those students are overseen by highly experienced veterinarians.

•**Ask local humane societies and SPCA chapters** about affordable pet-vaccination programs in your area. Some pet-oriented nonprofits offer vaccinations on certain days of the year for less than a vet's office is likely to charge—often just $10 to $15 per vaccination, compared with $15 to $30 for the same vaccinations from the typical veterinary practice.

TRAINING AND BOARDING

•**Find affordable dog boarding, walking and sitting services on Rover.com.** This is the Uber of dog care—people make a few extra bucks by offering animal-care services through the website. In many areas, you can find people willing to walk a dog for as little as $15...or take a dog or cat into their homes (or dog/cat sit in your home) for as little as $20 or $30 per night, though rates vary. Sitters must pass background checks and the site includes ratings and reviews of care providers from other pet owners.

Alternative: Make a deal with another animal lover in your area to take in each other's pets when you travel.

•**Ask pet stores whether they offer special deals for owners of recently obtained pets.** If you get a new pet, there's a good chance that you can get some great deals from nearby pet-supply stores. Many stores, in particular chain stores, offer valuable coupon books to new pet owners in hopes of earning their ongoing business.

Example: PetSmart's "Adoption Kit" includes a free private-training session...a free day of doggie day care...a free overnight boarding stay...a free bag of food...and a half-price grooming session.

•**Take training classes on YouTube.** Before you pay hundreds of dollars for pet-training classes or one-on-one sessions, try the free training videos on YouTube. Just type in the species of animal, the word "training" and the specific skill you are trying to teach or troubling behavior you are trying to stop.

Professor Fido

The presence of a friendly dog improves the speed and accuracy with which young children handle mental and physical tasks, including reading. Dogs seem to reduce anxiety while building motivation, confidence and feelings of support—helping children who have difficulty with reading.

Sophie Hall, PhD, research fellow, School of Life Sciences, University of Lincoln, UK, and leader of a study published in PLOS ONE.

PET FOOD AND TREATS

•**Choose pet food based on price per serving, not price per pound.** Inexpensive pet food is not a money saver if it's so full of "fillers" such as rice and corn that you have to give your pet larger-than-normal servings so that the pet gets the nourishment it needs. Dog- and cat-food packaging usually includes a "Recommended Daily Feeding Chart" that lists serving amounts for different-sized pets by weight. These guidelines report the amount of the food that an animal of a particular size is likely to need to obtain a balanced diet, according to the guidelines of the Association of American Feed Control Officials. Compare brands by comparing how many servings your pet would get for each dollar spent.

•**Price pet food online and in chains that beat grocery store prices.** Websites such as Amazon.com, Chewy.com and Walmart.com often undercut grocery store and pet-supply store prices on pet food by 10% to 20% and frequently offer free or low-cost shipping. (As a bonus, the potentially heavy bags of pet food will be delivered right to your door.) If you prefer to shop in brick-and-mortar stores, Walmart and Tractor Supply Co., a chain with 1,700 stores across the country, often charge less for pet food than do supermarkets and pet-supply stores. Some pet-supply stores will match other retailers' lower prices.

•**Use a food dehydrator to make pet treats.** Most dogs and cats love dried meat treats, but these can be pricey in stores. With a food dehydrator, you can buy meat when it's on sale at your market and then make inexpensive dried meat treats at home. Enter the terms "dehydrator," "treats" and "dog" or "cat" into a search engine to find recipes.

PET TOYS AND ENCLOSURES

•**Purchase pet toys that were not meant to be pet toys.** If your dog plays with tennis balls, they're usually significantly cheaper in the sporting-goods section of a store than in the pet-supply section. If your pet likes to play with stuffed animals, you often can find these used at thrift stores for just 25 or 50 cents apiece. (Wash them before giving them to your pet.) Most cats would just as soon chase a piece of string tied to the end of a stick or the dot of light from a laser pointer as they would play with something that's marketed as a cat toy. Enter "cat toys" and "homemade" or "DIY" into a search engine to find many more options.

•**Buy fish tanks and animal cages at thrift stores...or look for postings on Craigslist.com.** Just be sure to thoroughly clean any secondhand cage (or tank) before using it for your pet.

Pot Can Poison Dogs

Your Dog.

Marijuana can poison dogs—and this is happening more frequently as cannabis use becomes more widespread.

Dogs may eat a discarded joint or food containing cannabis. *Symptoms:* Urinary incontinence, disorientation, respiratory difficulty, tremors, unconsciousness. Mild effects usually wear off in a few days. But to be safe, take your dog to the vet.

Self-defense: Keep cannabis away from anywhere that dogs can reach—and do not let dogs into any room where cannabis is being smoked or has recently been smoked, since they will react to the residue in the air.

CHAPTER 10

Infectious Disease

Protect Yourself from the Flu

The 2017–2018 flu season was the worst in the US since the 1970s —49 million people got sick…960,000 were hospitalized…and nearly 80,000 died. It was a perfect storm—a particularly nasty influenza virus…a vaccine that was less effective than usual…and a growing population of older people, who are most susceptible to the flu and related complications. About 70% of flu hospitalizations and 90% of deaths were among people age 65 and older.

It's hard to tell how bad a flu season will be, so it makes sense to protect yourself no matter what the predictions. We interviewed an infectious-diseases expert and an integrative physician to bring you a powerful toolkit to help you avoid the flu—and if you do get sick, to help you get better fast.

FLU SHOTS, BOOZE AND SHUT-EYE

Infectious-diseases specialist William Schaffner, MD, advises everyone to…

•**Get an annual flu shot even if you're skeptical.** Fewer and fewer Americans are doing so. Recent research from the Centers for Disease Control and Prevention (CDC) shows that skipping the shot was a significant contributor to the record-high hospitalizations and deaths during that dangerous 2017–2018 span. According to the CDC, only 37% of US adults got vaccinated—down significantly from more than 43% the year before. If you're skeptical about the flu shot based on what happened during a rampant flu season—the vaccine was less effective than usual—keep in mind that things would have been even worse without it. If you are vacci-

William Schaffner, MD, professor of preventive medicine in the department of health policy and professor of medicine in the division of infectious diseases at Vanderbilt University School of Medicine, Nashville.

Fred Pescatore, MD, a practitioner of natural and integrative medicine in New York City, author of several books including *The A-List Diet* and former associate medical director of the Atkins Center for Complementary Medicine.

nated and still get the flu, you're likely to have a milder infection. It also will be shorter in duration, and you'll be less likely to get pneumonia, to be hospitalized—or to die.

If you're age 65 or older, make sure that you get one of the vaccines licensed for use in older adults. There are two—the high-dose flu vaccine and the adjuvanted flu vaccine. Either one is fine and will give you a bigger immune response than the standard shot. I don't recommend the nasal vaccine for older people.

•**Get extra protection if you think you've been exposed to the flu.** If flu is rampant in your community or a family member brought it home, your doctor can prescribe an antiviral medication (see next page). These not only help reduce flu symptoms, especially if taken within 48 hours of the start of symptoms but, according to the FDA, also may help prevent flu if you are exposed. It's still important to get a flu shot, of course, but an antiviral medication can provide additional protection if needed.

Tip: If you're planning a trip between early fall and spring, ask your doctor about prescribing an antiviral for you to have on hand in case you find yourself surrounded by people with the flu. Cruise ships, in particular, are hotbeds for the flu.

•**Cut back on or avoid alcohol during flu season.** Alcohol negatively affects the body's immune response and can increase the likelihood of getting an infection as well as the severity of an infection. Do stay hydrated, though—that helps your immune system function at its best.

•**Stay active.** Regular exercise boosts immunity, so keep up your fitness routine throughout the winter even when you feel like hibernating.

•**Keep a solid sleep schedule.** Healthy men and women who average less than seven hours of sleep per night are three times more likely to catch a cold, compared with those who get eight hours or more of sleep, and good sleep likely helps ward off the flu, too.

•**Be smarter about hygiene.** Besides frequently washing your hands and using an alcohol-based hand sanitizer, regularly sanitize shared surfaces such as those in bathrooms and kitchens…and doorknobs throughout the

house. Don't get too close to sick people if you can help it—viruses can be spread not only by sneezes but also by simply breathing. And stay home if you're sick so that you don't become a dreaded spreader of germs.

NATURAL WAYS TO PREVENT FLU

Integrative medicine practitioner Fred Pescatore, MD, often prescribes dietary supplements for the fall and winter to help his patients prevent colds and flu. *It's fine to take one, two or all three of the following…*

•**N-acetyl cysteine (NAC).** This antioxidant can help prevent the flu, and clinical studies have found that it helps ward off flu symptoms even in people who already are infected with the virus.

Typical dose: 500 milligrams (mg) per day.

•**Olive leaf extract.** This supplement contains a bitter compound called oleuropein that has strong antiviral properties.

Typical dose: 500 mg per day.

•**Monolaurin.** This antiviral is derived from lauric acid, one of the main fats in coconuts. It destroys viruses by breaking down their outer membranes.

Typical dose: 300 mg per day.

OTHER NATURAL PREVENTIVES

Sunlight helps your body produce vitamin D, a potent immune booster. Some scientists think that the lack of sunlight and reduced vitamin-D production in the darker months help explain why flu is so common then. For extra protection, give yourself some full-spectrum light inside your home, too. Light therapy has been shown to enhance the immune system in the winter, and a full-spectrum light box is well worth the investment for this purpose.

IF YOU DO GET THE FLU— FROM DR. SCHAFFNER…

Antiviral drugs can make your illness milder… shorten the duration of the time you are sick… and may prevent serious flu-related complications that can lead to hospitalization. It's best to take an antiviral within 48 hours of symptom onset, so call your doctor the minute you start to feel sick. Classic flu symptoms include sudden onset of fever, aches, chills and tiredness.

Even if you've had the flu for more than a few days, an antiviral drug still may lessen symptoms. That's especially important for people at high risk for flu-related complications, which includes people who are age 65 or older and people with medical conditions such as heart disease, diabetes or asthma.

Oseltamivir (Tamiflu) is the standby, and it's still effective, but now there's a new option—*baloxavir marboxil* (Xofluza), which was approved by the FDA in October 2018. Unlike Tamiflu, which is taken over the course of five days, it's a single dose. It also dramatically cuts "viral shedding," so you're less infectious (Tamiflu hasn't been shown to do this). Overall, Xofluza and Tamiflu are about equally effective, and their costs are very similar.

FROM DR. PESCATORE...

The following remedies can help reduce the severity and duration of the flu. *It's fine to use one or any combination of these remedies...*

•**Oregano oil gargle.** Put two drops of oregano oil in one-quarter cup of water, gargle and spit. It is fine to gargle up to four times a day. Keep in mind—it has an intense flavor, and you'll smell like pizza!

•**Active hexose correlated compound (AHCC).** This mushroom extract has been shown to shorten the duration of flu and ease symptoms. It also improved the immune response in people who took it right after getting a flu shot.

Typical dose: 500 mg three times a day.

•**Elderberry tea** is an antiviral that's effective for treating flu symptoms and shortening the duration of the illness. Drink one cup a day. You also can take it as an extract or a syrup.

•**Robuvit,** an antioxidant supplement derived from French oak wood, helps people recover more fully after flu symptoms have passed. In a study, people who took the supplement daily for three weeks after their flu symptoms subsided had better post-flu strength, sleep quality and attention span, compared with people who didn't take it.

Typical dose: 200 mg three times a day.

Flu Can Be Missed...and Become Deadly

Leslie Kernisan, MD, MPH, a geriatrician and founder of the aging health podcast and website, BetterHealth WhileAging.net. Study titled "Underdiagnosis of Influenza Virus Infection in Hospitalized Older Adults," by researchers at Vanderbilt University School of Medicine in Nashville, Tennessee, published in *Journal of the American Geriatrics Society*.

Did you know that you can have the flu without having flu symptoms? It's particularly true for people over age 65—and it can be really dangerous.

A recent study found that older people going to hospitals with respiratory illnesses—during flu season—were less likely than younger people to be tested for the flu! *Here's what the study found—and how to protect yourself...*

UNDERCOVER OPERATION

Researchers analyzed how often flu tests were ordered for 1,422 patients who were admitted to four Tennessee hospitals during several of the past flu seasons. Many, but not all, had symptoms that can signal the flu, including cough or fever. The researchers looked at the rates of testing for the flu according to doctors' orders. They also independently—and surreptitiously—tested each patient for the flu themselves.

Results: Doctors flu-tested only 28% of patients, and were only about half as likely to order flu testing for patients 65 or older than they were for patients who were younger.

Important finding: More than one-quarter of the older people with confirmed influenza infection in this study did not have classic influenza-like signs such as cough and fever.

Here's why: Older people often don't develop the cardinal signs of infection from the flu—their immune systems do not respond as vigorously as younger people's. For example, they're less likely to develop a fever, which is one of nature's defenses against many viruses and bacteria. Plus, older people may have lower normal temperatures, so the typical definition of fever (above 100.4°F) may not be the right guide.

As a result, in older people with the flu, it might initially seem like a worsening of symptoms of chronic conditions they already have, such as asthma, congestive heart failure or chronic obstructive pulmonary disease (COPD). Or they might just feel fatigued and under the weather. But doctors should know better—especially during flu season—because these patients are actually in grave danger.

WHY PROMPT DIAGNOSIS MATTERS

Knowing that you have the flu is critically important. Even though early symptoms of the flu may appear less worrisome in older people than in younger people, the flu can—and often does—ultimately come roaring forth in these older people and turn very serious very quickly. Research suggests that in people who are "high-risk"—and everyone age 65 or older is considered high-risk—early use of antiviral medications can significantly reduce the risk for serious complications of the flu, including bronchitis, pneumonia and death.

Important: The 15-minute rapid-flu test often used in doctors' offices and hospitals frequently results in "false negatives," meaning you may have the flu but the test doesn't detect it. So if your rapid test is negative, ask your doctor to also give you a follow-up test, which can take a few hours.

If you get the flu shot and you feel ill during flu season, ask to be tested for the flu anyway. It is quite possible to get the flu even though you've been vaccinated.

INSIST ON GETTING TESTED

If you are over 65 and you don't feel well, get tested for the flu even if you do not have a fever or cough. Don't wait to see what happens or until you get much sicker—anti-influenza medication works best the sooner you start it and can help you avoid hospitalization. It's possible that doctors and hospitals may be more attuned to flu testing during a bad-flu year, but if it is not offered, ask to have the test.

More ways to protect yourself…

•**Be sure to get a flu vaccination.**

•**Ask your doctor about getting vaccinated** against pneumococcal disease to protect you against pneumonia and other illnesses that can make the flu particularly deadly. The one-time-only vaccination series (usually two shots

administered one year apart) is recommended for all people age 65 and older.

Obesity Linked to a New Flu Danger

The study "Obesity Increases the Duration of Influenza A Virus Shedding in Adults," led by researchers at University of Michigan and published in *The Journal of Infectious Diseases.*

Obesity has long been known to increase a person's risk for diabetes, heart disease, stroke—and complications from the flu, such as bronchitis, pneumonia and even death.

Now: Researchers from University of Michigan have recently discovered that obesity—defined as a body mass index (BMI) of 30 or above—may play an important role in how the flu spreads from person to person.

Study results: After monitoring nearly 1,800 people in 320 households for three flu seasons (2015 to 2017), the research team found that flu sufferers who were obese shed the influenza A flu virus 42% to 104% longer than people who weren't obese. (Viral shedding is considered the time when a person may be contagious.) Interestingly, obese individuals with lab-confirmed flu who were only mildly ill or had no symptoms were the most likely to shed the virus, while the effect was less pronounced in those with two or more flu symptoms.

Note: The nose and throat swabs used in the study detected flu virus RNA but did not indicate whether the virus was actually infectious.

What this finding means: Researchers aren't sure why obesity may extend viral shedding in people with the flu. They theorize, however, that chronic inflammation triggered by obesity may be at least partially to blame. If further research confirms that the virus shed for longer periods is, in fact, infectious, efforts to reduce the number of people who are obese may also help minimize the spread of viral diseases.

Bottom line: Because the flu is a life-threatening condition that claims the lives of tens of thousands of Americans each year, it's crucial to do everything possible to protect yourself and your family from this serious illness.

The CDC recommends annual flu vaccination (with rare exceptions) for everyone age six months and older. Even though the effectiveness of the vaccine varies from year to year, it generally decreases the duration of the flu if you do get sick and also decreases your risk for complications.

Also: Wash your hands frequently with soap and water for at least 20 seconds and try to avoid contact with sick people. If you must be around people who could have the flu, consider wearing an inexpensive over-the-counter surgical mask. If you feel the symptoms of the flu coming on (fever, chills, body aches, cough, sore throat, runny or stuffy nose, headache and fatigue), ask your doctor about an antiviral medication, which can lessen symptoms, shorten the time you are sick by about one day and reduce risk for complications if taken within two days of becoming ill with flu symptoms.

Meanwhile, further studies will be needed to confirm whether flu transmission risk increases along with obesity prevalence. Stay tuned as researchers discover more about this intriguing question.

How to Survive Sepsis

Steven Q. Simpson, MD, professor of medicine at University of Kansas, Kansas City, and chief medical officer of the Sepsis Alliance, Sepsis.org. He was among the authors of the *2016 International Guidelines for Management of Sepsis and Septic Shock.*

When it comes to medical emergencies, we all know that heart attack, stroke and asthma attacks are among the most serious. But there's a medical emergency that most people don't know about even though it kills 270,000 people in the US each year. That's one death every two minutes…and more deaths than those caused by prostate cancer, breast cancer and AIDS combined.

This runaway killer is known as sepsis. It is a life-threatening condition that occurs when the body goes into overdrive to fight an infection, such as pneumonia, the flu or even a urinary tract infection.

Sepsis causes a deadly cascade of events when the chemicals that the immune system releases into the blood to fight infection trigger inflammation throughout the body that leads to tissue damage, organ failure and death. If not recognized and treated promptly, sepsis can worsen—and kill—within a matter of days…or even hours.

Latest development: New efforts are under way to help people identify sepsis more quickly and get the right treatment promptly so they can survive this devastating illness.

What you need to know to protect yourself and your family…

THE DANGER SIGNS

While anyone who is battling a bacterial, viral or fungal infection can develop sepsis, the old and very young are at particular risk. So are people with chronic diseases such as diabetes, cancer, chronic obstructive pulmonary disease (COPD) and kidney disease.

Sepsis is commonly misdiagnosed because its symptoms—including fast breathing (greater than 20 breaths per minute—the normal rate is 12 to 20)…a racing pulse (above 90 beats per minute)…the chills…pale, clammy skin…and extreme fatigue—can be mistaken for any number of health problems such as heart attack, stroke, pulmonary embolism, exacerbations of chronic lung disease or heart failure.

Misdiagnosis also can occur because there is no definitive test for sepsis—it is diagnosed based on a checklist of signs and symptoms.

To help people identify the red flags of sepsis, the Sepsis Alliance has created the TIME acronym…

Temperature: It can be either above normal (such as 100.4°F or higher) or below normal (such as 96.8°F or lower). Severe chills or burning fever are common.

Infection: It may be obvious, such as the flu or an abscess, or there could be less obvious signs and symptoms, including intense pain in some part of one's body, profound weakness or loss of appetite for both food and water.

Mental decline: People with sepsis are often confused or disoriented. They may be very sleepy and hard to rouse.

Extremely ill: Sufferers often experience intense, sharp pain in the chest, belly or elsewhere. They may be short of breath. Many survivors recall, "I felt like I was going to die."

If you think you may have sepsis, seek immediate medical attention. If your doctor isn't available, call 911 or get to an emergency room.

Important: Whether you're seeing your own physician or an ER doctor, make sure he/she knows your concerns.

Ask straight out: "Could this be sepsis?" Don't be shy about pushing for tests for impaired organ function such as creatinine for kidney function, lactate (lactic acid) level, platelet count, bilirubin and liver enzyme studies.

Keep in mind that the diagnosis of sepsis is missed completely about half of the time—and a delay in treatment can be fatal. Untreated sepsis can rapidly turn into shock, in which blood pressure plummets and tissues are starved for oxygen and nutrients. For every hour that treatment is delayed, the likelihood of septic shock increases.

NEWEST TREATMENT OPTIONS

The latest sepsis practice guidelines, jointly issued by American and European critical care medicine societies, more strongly emphasize the urgency of sepsis diagnosis and treatment.

Under these guidelines, a main goal is to eradicate infection with antibiotics that cover a wide variety of bacteria. Equally important is raising blood pressure to restore delivery of oxygen and nutrients to the organs and normalize their ability to function. This means intravenous fluids and, if needed, vasopressor drugs, such as *norepinephrine*, that stimulate the heart and tighten blood vessels to improve function.

Drugs to reduce immune system activity, once a mainstay of treatment, are no longer standard, reflecting a better understanding of the complex biology involved. Instead, researchers are exploring the use of anti-inflammatory drugs early in the condition's course and immune-stimulating drugs later.

Another change involves medical centers' adoption of highly organized procedures to bring optimal treatment to their patients in the shortest time.

For example, in New York State, which mandates this approach, patients who were diagnosed and treated for sepsis after three hours (and up to 12 hours) of an exam were 14% more likely to die in the hospital than those treated within three hours, according to a study published in *The New England Journal of Medicine*.

To be alert for possible sepsis: If you have a loved one in the ICU, ask the doctors every day if there are signs of infection, especially if the person is on a mechanical ventilator.

LINGERING AILMENTS

Scientists are discovering increasing evidence that the effects of sepsis can linger. Up to half of survivors suffer "post-sepsis syndrome" (PSS). Physical aspects of PSS reflect damage to vital organs and other tissues. There can be impaired breathing and liver and kidney function, which are often irreversible. Gangrene due to tissue death caused by infecting organisms can necessitate amputation. Fatigue and muscle and joint pain are sometimes disabling.

Recent discovery: The long-term mental impact has only recently been recognized. This may include insomnia, hallucinations, panic attacks, poor concentration, impaired memory and even post-traumatic stress disorder (PTSD).

While the reasons for such mental effects are not yet known, it's believed that sepsis may disrupt the protective blood-brain barrier, leaving the brain vulnerable to damaging inflammation.

Medications used in the ICU—especially sedative agents, including benzodiazepines such as *midazolam* (Versed)—also may have negative effects on mental functioning, sometimes lasting for years.

Much remains to be learned about PSS, but it seems likely that quick action early in the course of sepsis could cut the risk.

AVOIDING SEPSIS

The key to preventing sepsis is to prevent infection. *To do this…*

• **Get recommended vaccinations,** including yearly flu shots and vaccination against pneumonia.

Also: Sepsis can occur with shingles if the skin becomes infected with bacteria. This is an additional reason to consider getting the shingles vaccine.

• **Practice good hygiene.** Wash your hands frequently and thoroughly (for at least 20 seconds).

• **Clean any cut, scrape or burn quickly and apply antiseptic or antimicrobial cream.** If a wound shows signs of a worsening infection—redness, swelling, red streaks radiating up the arm or leg—seek immediate medical attention.

Note: Sepsis is not generally contagious, but some infections that cause sepsis are, such as plague or meningococcal meningitis.

Alternative to Chemical Bug Repellents

Joseph M. Conlon, MSc, technical advisor, American Mosquito Control Association, Mount Laurel, New Jersey.

Since mosquitoes spread diseases, it's important to steer clear of them. Fortunately, there are several nontoxic ways to do that.

Use a small electric fan to create a gentle breeze…pleasant for you, but like a wind tunnel for tiny mosquitoes! Besides making it difficult for them to fly, it disperses the carbon dioxide and human scents that attract them. You can also light your patio with a yellow "bug light" bulb. It won't attract the little bloodsuckers the way that white lights will. It helps to dress in light-colored, loose-fitting clothing, too, since mosquitoes are attracted to darker colors, and it's easier for them to bite through tightly fitted clothing. In addition, eliminate all sources of standing water since mosquitoes need standing water to lay their eggs. Keep the grass cut short and the bushes trimmed so they're less hospitable to mosquitoes.

Taking Steroids? Do This to Prevent Deadly Pneumonia

Study titled "Prophylactic effect of trimethoprim-sulfamethoxazole for pneumocystis pneumonia in patients with rheumatic diseases exposed to prolonged high-dose glucocorticoids" by researchers at the Seoul National University College of Medicine, Republic of Korea, and the University of Alabama at Birmingham, published in the *Annals of Rheumatic Diseases.*

People with autoimmune diseases, such as lupus or rheumatoid arthritis, can be more susceptible to infections because their immune systems don't tend to work as they should. At the same time, autoimmune diseases often involve flare-ups of damaging inflammation. A high dose of a steroid—often prescribed by doctors in these situations—can provide relief by reducing inflammation…but here's the catch. The steroids also further weaken the immune system, leaving autoimmune patients even more vulnerable to infection.

And one kind of infection is particularly opportunistic and nasty—the lung infection called pneumocystis pneumonia (PCP). It's not caused by anything exotic. In fact, the culprit is a common fungus. The fungus is rarely a problem if you have a healthy immune system—your body clears it easily. But for someone whose immune system is already compromised, taking 30 or more milligrams of steroids a day for four weeks or more increases not only the risk of acquiring PCP but also the risk of dying from it.

The study: Researchers analyzed the records of 1,092 people with autoimmune diseases who were on just such a course of steroids. They followed the patients for a year from the day that treatment started…that's the time span in which the infection tends to develop. In addition to the steroids, about one-quarter of the study subjects also took the antibiotic combination *trimethoprim/sulfamethoxazole*—you probably know this treatment by the brand names Septra and Bactrim. They started the antibiotic on the same day that they started the steroid and stopped when the daily steroid dose was tapered off.

This antibiotic has been used against PCP in other kinds of patients, such as organ transplant recipients and people with HIV, but it had never been rigorously tested for autoimmune diseases such as lupus or rheumatoid arthritis. The goal of the study was to learn whether it could prevent participants from getting pneumocystis pneumonia, how well it did this job and how safe it was.

The findings: Just one person developed the pneumonia among people given the antibiotics, and that person had to discontinue the antibiotic because of side effects. In comparison, there were 29 cases of pneumonia among the participants who weren't given the antibiotics (and 11 of them died).

The researchers concluded that the benefits of giving this specific antibiotic treatment, along with long-term, high-dose steroids, far outweigh any risks.

In the know: You should still be aware of the signs of PCP. Any time you're on high-dose, long-term steroids, tell your doctor right away if you have…

- **High fever or chills**
- **Cough or trouble breathing**
- **Chest pain**
- **Extreme tiredness**

What If You Forgot Whether You Got a Vaccination?

William Schaffner, MD, professor of medicine, division of infectious diseases, Vanderbilt University School of Medicine, Nashville.

When it comes to keeping track of immunizations, many people consider it a no brainer for children but tend to let it slip as adults. Even doctors' offices can miss recording it. Many assume that somewhere, somehow, someone else has been keeping track of what you got.

No one is doing that. And while each state does have its own vaccine registry, they are pri-marily used to record childhood vaccinations. So the responsibility for keeping adult vaccination records lies with the patient. Ideally, everyone should have an up-to-date record detailing all vaccinations from childhood on, and their dates, stored in some safe place.

A good way to start is by printing out the Vaccine Administration Record for Adults from the Centers for Disease Control and Prevention. The form lists the 13 most commonly immunized-against illnesses and gives spaces to enter the type of vaccine received…the date it was given…the route (e.g., injection in left arm)…plus other details. Fill in any information that you can remember.

Next, try to track down what's missing. To do that, contact previous doctors and ask whether they kept records of your immunizations. You can also try asking any pharmacies where you got a vaccination…and contact the state registry for any state where you ever lived, just in case something got recorded. *Here are some important vaccinations adults should get…*

- **Flu (yearly).**
- **Pneumonia twice**—one vaccine when you turn 65 and then a second vaccine a year later.
- **Shingles,** starting at age 50 if you are not immune-compromised. The CDC recommends the Shingrix vaccine over an older one called Zostavax. If you've had the older shingles vaccine, or if you've had shingles, you should still get the newer vaccine. There are no recommendations yet for people with compromised immunity.

Once you've got your form as filled out as much as possible, take it with you whenever you get a vaccination—including any immunizations that you get for travel—so your doctor or pharmacist can fill in the new information and sign and date it.

If memory and detective work fail and you still can't determine whether you've had a pneumonia vaccination—or another of the adult vaccinations listed above—there is no danger in getting a repeat shot (or a repeat two shots in the case of the pneumonia vaccination). You may get more redness, swelling and soreness at the site of the injections than you would if it were your first immunization, but it would not harm your health. Just remember to record it this time, and store the record in a safe place!

Can You Have Strep Without a Sore Throat?

Chris Van Beneden, MD, MPH, senior epidemiologist, National Center for Immunization and Respiratory Diseases, Centers for Disease Control and Prevention, Atlanta.

To be diagnosed with strep throat (known medically as group A strep pharyngitis), there are two requirements—a sore throat (pharyngitis) and laboratory confirmation of an infection caused by bacteria known as group A Streptococcus.

You can be a carrier for the bacteria that causes strep throat but not actually have strep pharyngitis.

Here's what can happen: People can have the group A strep bacteria in the back of their throats without being sick. We call this being a carrier. In general, group A strep carriers do not need antibiotics, since they are unlikely to spread the bacteria to other people or become ill themselves.

Even though strep throat most often affects children from ages five to 15, the illness can occur at any age. Symptoms include a sudden onset of sore throat that causes pain when swallowing…fever (typically 101 degrees Fahrenheit or higher)…red, swollen tonsils (with or without white patches)…and tender lymph nodes in the front part of the neck. However, children are more likely than adults to also have a headache, stomach pain, nausea and/or vomiting. In adults, throat symptoms caused by strep are often mild. A person with a sore throat due to strep may also have a bright red rash—when accompanied by a high fever, this illness is called "scarlet fever." The rash looks like a sunburn and feels like sandpaper.

A doctor cannot diagnose strep throat just by looking at a person's throat. Testing for group A strep includes a rapid test (a throat swab is performed in a doctor's office, and results are available in 10 to 20 minutes) or culture (a throat swab specimen is sent to a lab for analysis, and results come 24 to 48 hours later). Even though strep throat is more common in children, adults should ask their health-care provider about getting tested if they have the symptoms described above.

An important distinction: When a person has a cough, runny nose (rhinorrhea), hoarseness and oral ulcers (small, painful lesions that can develop in your mouth or at the base of your gums) along with a sore throat, it's more likely that a virus is to blame rather than a strep infection. In fact, most cases of a sore throat are due to a viral infection, which does not require antibiotics. A viral infection will typically improve on its own within a few days. Giving a test for strep to people who have these symptoms is not recommended.

If an adult or child has a sore throat, you can…

• **Soothe the sore throat with ice chips,** sore throat spray, popsicles or lozenges (do not give lozenges to young children).

• **Gargle with salt water.**

• **Drink warm beverages.**

• **Use a clean humidifier or cool-mist vaporizer.**

• **Take *acetaminophen, ibuprofen* or *naproxen*** to relieve pain or fever.

You're Not Too Old to Get an STD

Edward Hook, III, MD, professor in the division of infectious diseases at the University of Alabama at Birmingham School of Medicine, codirector of the UAB Center for Social Medicine and STDs and director of the STD Control Program for the Jefferson County (Alabama) Department of Health.

You might think that sexually transmitted diseases, or STDs, are health issues that mostly teens and young adults have to worry about. But anyone of any age who's not in a totally (and we mean totally) monogamous relationship where both partners have been tested for STDs is at risk.

Right now, there's a dramatic surge in cases of chlamydia, gonorrhea and syphilis in the

US, with all three hitting record numbers in 2016 and again in 2017. The number of people over age 45 getting these diseases more than doubled between 2012 and 2016, according to the latest record-keeping from the CDC. Better news is that HIV is on the decline—but it's still a concern along with HPV, the human papillomavirus, which causes cervical cancer in women (and can cause other cancers in women and men), and trichomoniasis, a sexually transmitted parasite that can increase your risk of getting an STD including HIV.

What in the world is going on? Put simply, Americans have become lax about practicing safe sex because of advances in the treatment of HIV—the fear of getting AIDs from HIV is not as strong as it used to be. We have, as a country, gone backwards in protecting ourselves.

But here's what hasn't changed: STDs can still be dangerous or even deadly…you can never fully rid yourself of some of them once you have them…and most STDs don't produce early symptoms, so you can't "spot" warning signs in a potential partner any more than you can in yourself, leaving you open to infections.

If you're at a time in your life when you don't want to be in a serious relationship yet want to enjoy an active sex life, here's how to keep yourself from becoming another STD statistic…

•**Keep practicing safer sex.** Use a condom every time, especially if you don't know for sure that your partner has been screened and is negative for all STDs. This also keeps your partner safe should you have an infection you're unaware of. Condoms alone don't do it, though—that's why the term is "safer"—it's not possible to protect yourself 100%.

Condom use is even lower among people engaging in oral sex than in purely genital contact. Since more and more STDs appear to be transmitted through oral contact, infections could be prevented with use of condoms and oral barriers or dams (placed over the vulva during oral sex).

•**Get regular sexual-health checkups.** This includes a physical exam and screening tests. Advancing age might not make it feel any less awkward to talk to your doctor—primary, ob-gyn or urologist—about your private life, but

he/she needs to know if you have new partners because this helps determine whether and when you should have STD tests.

This talk about your sex life need not be complex.

Just two facts will tell your doctor whether additional history is needed: How many sexual partners you have had in the past six months…and whether you think that any of your partners currently has or might have had other partners in the past six months.

•**STD screening isn't painful or complex.** Women are tested for chlamydia, gonorrhea, trichomoniasis and HPV with a vaginal swab or a urine sample. Men are tested for gonorrhea and chlamydia with a urine sample…trichomoniasis is harder to detect in men, but a urine sample or swab can be used if there's a discharge. Both men and women are tested for syphilis and HIV with a blood sample.

If you and your partner decide to be exclusive—and avoid condoms and/or engage in oral sex in the process—you should both have a sexual-health checkup first. Remember that monogamy doesn't confer protection from an STD that came from a former partner.

The HPV Test: Why It's Better Than the Pap for Cervical Cancer Screening

Diane Harper, MD, MPH, MS, professor in the departments of family medicine and obstetrics and gynecology at University of Michigan, physician director for Community Outreach, Engagement and Health Disparities at University of Michigan Rogel Cancer Center and one of the country's leading experts on HPV.

Guidelines for how to screen and when to screen for cervical cancer had been a moving target until late 2018, when the US Preventive Services Task Force clarified very simply what techniques work and how often screening needs to happen. But those guidelines are different depending on age. *Here's what you need to know…*

FOR WOMEN AGES 30 TO 65

The guidelines state that you can choose between…

•**Having the HPV (human papillomavirus) test every five years.**

•**Having the Pap test every three years.**

•**Co-testing with the Pap and HPV tests every five years.**

Why all the choices? Although research has shown that for women 30 years and older the HPV test picks up more suspect lesions sooner than the Pap test does and with fewer false positives, it will take time for the medical community to adopt such a landmark change (some doctors are still doing annual Pap tests even though the move to every three years is already over a decade old—know that since insurance reimbursement follows the current guidelines, patients may then be billed for screening too frequently). So, for the time being, the Pap is still one of the stand-alone options. It is also used after a stand-alone HPV test if that test comes back positive. The most expensive way to use the Pap test is to do it at the same time as the HPV test (co-testing)—it may provide a convenience but at a cost.

Discuss all three options with your doctor to find the most appropriate one for you. Your unique personal or family health history might lead your primary care physician to recommend one over another.

HOW HPV TESTING WORKS

Many experts believe that, ultimately, the HPV test will be the one standard. It looks for 14 high-risk strains of HPV including HPV-16 and HPV-18, the two responsible for 70% of all cervical cancers.

If you choose to have the HPV test and…

•**The test is negative,** you won't need any cervical cancer screening for five years.

•**The test is positive,** it does not mean you have cancer, but does mean you'll need to follow it up with a Pap test to give your doctor more information—whether the virus has caused any changes in your cervix or is just sitting there.

Your doctor may just be able to use the liquid from your HPV test to do the Pap test and not need to call you back for an exam.

What typically happens next…

•**If that Pap test is normal or shows that any changes are minor,** in a year you'll repeat the HPV test to see if the virus cleared on its own and if not, have a repeat Pap to check for any further changes to the cervix.

•**If the changes on your Pap are more severe,** then you'll likely have a colposcopy with biopsy. A colposcopy uses a lighted instrument to look for precancerous changes or lesions in the tissue of your cervix—a lesion is an indicator that there is usually more disease than is showing. Biopsies, or tissue samples, will be taken from both the outside and the inside of your cervix and examined.

•**If all the results are negative,** you'll need to have two normal tests (a negative HPV and a normal Pap) six months after the biopsy and again six months later before you can return to every five-year screening.

•**If the biopsies show severe changes,** then you'll have another procedure called LEEP, which uses electrical current to remove the abnormal cells from the cervix.

Note about the HPV test methods: Both the Pap and HPV tests can be done during a gynecological exam. However, you can also collect your own HPV sample at home with a swab and send it to a lab for testing.

Two recent studies looked at the effectiveness of self-collected HPV tests and found that the results were comparable to those done in a doctor's office. These kits are already available online—examples include Selfcollect.com and Mylabbox.com and can be a good option for women without easy access to screening clinics.

FOR WOMEN AGES 21 TO 29

The guideline for this age group is for only the Pap test to be done every three years.

Why is there a difference based solely on age? Most sexually active young women have been exposed to at least one strain of HPV. The body will usually be able to rid itself of the virus on its own in two or three years. During that time, women will automatically test positive for HPV even though it's unlikely that there's any cancer. For those under 30, the Pap test is the more sensitive way to screen for cervical cancer.

FOR WOMEN OVER AGE 65

Although the guidelines don't recommend screening for women in this age group who had adequate prior screening and are not at high risk, if you're very sexually active—or your partners could be, talk to your doctor about continuing HPV screening.

FOR WOMEN WITH CERTAIN HEALTH CONDITIONS

All the above guidelines are for women at average risk of cervical cancer. They don't address women who have a high risk for cervical cancer because of HIV-1, having had an organ transplant or their mothers took the drug DES to prevent miscarriage. If you're in any of these situations, talk to your doctor about how often you should be screened and what tests are most appropriate.

Note: The BRCA gene is not associated with cervical cancer, so cervical cancer screening recommendations are independent of BRCA status.

TESTING FOR OTHER HPV-ASSOCIATED CANCERS

HPV is also associated with head and neck and anal cancers…and for women, vaginal and vulvar, and for men, penile cancers. There are no guidelines for routine screening for these cancers, but there are tests that can look for them. For instance, there's an anal version of the Pap test that can look for precancerous changes…if you have itching or bleeding from your anus, talk to your doctor about this right away. The main warning sign for head and neck cancer is laryngitis that doesn't seem to go away.

And to help keep your immune system strong and able to clear the virus, practice these essentials: Eat a healthy diet…exercise regularly…drink alcohol in moderation…get appropriate screenings…and if you smoke, quit. Smoking makes your immune system less effective and speeds up the transition from healthy cells to cancerous ones.

More Grown-Ups Should Get the HPV Vaccination That Used to Be for Kids—Are You One?

Anna Wald, MD, MPH, head of the allergy and infectious diseases division, professor of medicine, laboratory medicine and epidemiology, University of Washington, Seattle.

You may have heard that the age limit for getting the HPV vaccine was increased to 45, but what does that really mean if you're over the previous ceiling of age 26? After all, when the vaccine was first introduced, the idea was to offer protection against key strains of the virus before people became sexually active. The answer is simple—it can still be a lifesaver. And the reason is that the vaccine can prevent reinfection as well as new infections.

The CDC estimates that 80 million Americans carry one or more strains of HPV (human papilloma virus), a dangerous family of viruses that can cause not only genital warts but also cervical, vaginal and vulvar cancers in women…penile cancer in men…and throat cancer in both sexes. Research shows that, unlike with most other viruses, contracting one strain of HPV may not confer immunity—not only can a person still be infected by other HPV strains (there are more than 100 in all), but also reinfected by the same initial strain.

While it's ideal to be vaccinated during the preteen years, people up to age 45 still will benefit from the vaccine's primary goal—protection against the most dangerous strains of the HPV responsible for the cancers mentioned above.

HOW THE AGE CHANGE CAME ABOUT

The FDA extended its approval of the Gardasil 9 vaccine up to age 45 for both sexes after a groundbreaking study of more than 3,000 women, ages 27 to 47, for whom Gardasil was found to be 88% effective in preventing HPV infection, genital warts, vulvar and vaginal precancers, cervical precancers and cervical cancers related to the virus. Because men have been shown to have the same immune response as women, experts anticipate that the vaccine will also offer men in this age group protections against genital warts and cancer. This is especially important considering the recent steep rise in HPV-related cancers in men.

Why this should matter to you: HPV is the most prevalent sexually transmitted disease in the US—the CDC states that nearly all men and women will get at least one type of HPV at some point within their sexually active lifetimes. If you have new sexual partners or if there's any chance that you and your current partner aren't completely monogamous, you're at risk of being infected with one or more HPV strains and should consider getting vaccinated. Note that teens age 15 and older and adults need a total of three shots unlike younger teens, who need only two.

About the vaccine: There are no serious or long-lasting side effects of the vaccine. As with any shot, you might have soreness, swelling and/or redness at the injection site. Some people have reported getting a headache soon afterward.

Also, there is more to learn about the vaccine, including how long its protection lasts.

Important: Even if vaccinated, women still need regular tests to identify cervical cell changes. The vaccine does not replace these screening measures.

The "New" and Dangerous Sexually Transmitted Disease HTLV-I

Robert C. Gallo, MD, professor of medicine and of microbiology-immunology and cofounder and director of the Institute of Human Virology at the University of Maryland School of Medicine, and cofounder and international scientific director of the Global Virus Network, and Yutaka Tagaya, MD, PhD, assistant professor at the Institute of Human Virology at the University of Maryland School of Medicine, both in Baltimore.

A very old viral infection in humans is becoming a substantial threat. It is devastating people in central Australia, among other locations. Could it be the second coming of HIV…and headed for the US and everywhere else, too? For answers, we turned to Robert C. Gallo, MD, the scientist who with his colleagues reported the discovery of this virus, HTLV-1, in 1980, but whose attention turned to HIV/AIDS when that virus swept across the globe.

A DEADLY "NEW" DISEASE THAT ISN'T NEW

Most people have never heard of HTLV-1, and it was even off the radar of many health professionals until quite recently. But researchers renewed the alarm about HTLV-1—that stands for "human T-cell leukemia virus Type 1"—at the 2017 international meeting of Dr. Gallo's Global Virus Network in Melbourne, Australia. HTLV-1 had already been identified as the first human virus known to directly cause a human cancer, specifically an adult T-cell leukemia and lymphoma, and the first human retrovirus ever shown to cause disease at all. Later a French group showed that it also causes a severe paralytic neurological disease. But now, it's also been found to cause a deadly lung infection, called bronchiectasis, and it is killing one particular group of people in far less time than the decades it takes for those cancers to develop, Dr. Gallo said.

HTLV-1 is a retrovirus. It's not as immediately infectious as most other viruses, such as the flu virus, but rather it takes some time to find a way into the DNA of people exposed to it. An astonishing 45% of the indigenous people in Alice Springs, Australia, are infected with HTLV-1. And that's not the only place. Other pockets of rampant HTLV-1 infection around the world are in New Guinea, Japan, Haiti, Jamaica, Peru, Chile, Brazil, Colombia, West Africa and Florida, primarily involving immigrants from the Caribbean region. There is an important difference between the outbreaks in Australia and elsewhere, according to Yutaka Tagaya, MD, PhD, a colleague of Dr. Gallo's. The virus currently affecting Alice Springs is a different subtype than the one seen in the other hot spots and may be more infectious—the lung infection is killing more people and doing so much faster than any other illness caused by HTLV-1. But the how and why of the rampant lung infection are still mysteries.

Important note: According to a study on HTLV-1–infected patients in Florida published in *Blood Advances*, the leukemia/lymphoma caused by the disease is very aggressive and ultimately fatal. There are currently trials of antiviral drugs under way and anti-CCR4 antibody therapy is approved in Japan to combat the disease.

DO YOU NEED TO BE WORRIED?

Other than a few news headlines that followed the Global Virus Network meeting, we haven't heard much about HTLV-1 in the US because it is still relatively rare here—less than 0.1% of Americans overall are infected. But it is disproportionately hitting certain groups—while very few Americans of European descent have been infected, 1% to 2% of African Americans have been infected, a comparatively huge number.

Being infected does not mean a particular person will necessarily develop cancer or another illness—some people are just carriers. But because HTLV-1 is similar in important ways to its cousin HIV, it's important to be aware of it. Like HIV, HTLV-1 is a sexually transmitted disease and can be spread through exposure to infected blood and from mother to child through breastfeeding.

The US, Australia, Japan, Peru, Brazil and most European countries test their blood banks for the virus, but not all countries do. Medical centers in the US used to, but no longer do, test transplant organs for HTLV-1, the government's rationale being that there are too few cases of HTLV-1 to justify the cost, especially in view of a high rate of false positives from the test. Dr. Gallo points out that the risk may need to be reevaluated in light of recent studies in Japan in which the HTLV-1 infection associated with organ transplants was shown to substantially increase the chances of developing aggressive neurological disease.

As one of the scientists who first connected the dots between HIV and AIDS, Dr. Gallo is advocating for HTLV-1 to be added to the list of sexually transmitted diseases maintained by the World Health Organization, which recognizes it but has not given it the importance of other diseases. Greater recognition by the WHO would almost certainly speed up efforts around the world for development of treatments and a vaccine and for additional countries to test their blood supplies and transplant organs. Dr. Gallo believes that if all focus hadn't completely shifted to HIV when it was discovered, science could have prevented what's happening now to the indigenous people of central Australia.

Until this all happens, he suggests the following to protect yourself from being infected by HTLV-1, particularly if you're a world traveler…

•**Practice safe sex,** get tested and ask any partners to be tested for the virus, as many people do for the HIV virus.

•**Be aware of the blood-testing practices** of the country you're in, and if there's any way to avoid it, don't get a blood transfusion in a country that does not test its blood supply for HTLV-1.

•**If you need an organ transplant,** ask that the organ be tested for HTLV-1.

Note: If you're pregnant, get tested for HTLV-1 and, if you test positive, don't breastfeed.

Could HTLV-1 take us by surprise and become a ubiquitous killer the way HIV did in the 1980s? Both Dr. Gallo and Dr. Tagaya think that type of global epidemic is unlikely because HTLV-1 is not nearly as easily transmitted as HIV. It's an older virus, and mankind has already somewhat adapted to it biologically. But more and more people are being exposed to

Petting Zoo Danger

Petting zoos can spread antibiotic-resistant germs. A recent Israeli study of 228 petting zoo animals found that 12% carried strains of bacteria that are resistant to antibiotics and capable of infecting humans. Children who cannot yet be trusted to keep their hands out of their mouths should not directly touch the animals or go to petting zoos. Everyone else should wash their hands vigorously and repeatedly after touching these animals.

Howard Smith, MD, a pediatric ear, nose and throat physician and former radio talk show host, broadcasts the weekly podcast "Dr. Howard Smith OnCall." DrHoward Smith.com it. For instance, HTLV-1 hotspots in Japan used to be only in the southwest and northern parts of the country, but now there is one in Tokyo as well. Both Drs. Gallo and Tagaya said that we're probably seeing the early stages of what will become a global problem, but not with the speed or prevalence of HIV.

Hand Bit by a Dog?
What to Do…

William Schaffner, MD, professor of preventive medicine in the department of health policy and professor of medicine in the division of infectious diseases at Vanderbilt University School of Medicine in Nashville.

Even if you know that the dog is up to date on rabies shots, a dog bite to the hand requires immediate medical attention.

Not only should you see a doctor—you should go to the ER!

Why? As a general rule, dog bites on the hand need specific care unless they are very minor and superficial—and seeing just any health-care provider won't be enough.

There's a tendency to want to minimize a bite, especially when it's your own dog, but that's a mistake.

The reasons: Even when there isn't a lot of pain, a dog bite can result in serious injury to soft tissues and tendons. It can cause nerve damage as well as infection and leave you with limited motion in your hand if not properly—and quickly—treated, and it doesn't matter whether it's your dog, a neighbor's or a stranger's.

Dog bites are not just puncture injuries but also "crush injuries," and either way, they can be more serious than they look. The amount of force from a dog's jaw can be substantial, so a bite can mash tissue well beyond any broken skin. If the dog grabbed you and then moved its head side to side while holding on—an instinctive attack behavior—it can worsen the injury.

What about germs? Dogs' mouths tend to be somewhat cleaner than people's mouths, but they are still teeming with bacteria. A dog's bite is therefore also an injection of bacteria. If those germs are injected deeply enough, they can easily cause not only a local infection but also a dangerous systemic infection. People with weakened immune systems or diabetes are even more susceptible, but no one is immune.

Here are the steps that should be taken if a dog bites your hand: Wash your wound with soap and water immediately, wrap it with some gauze or, in a pinch, a clean towel and head to the ER.

Why the ER? Your primary care provider and even a typical "urgent care" facility aren't equipped to handle the protocols for a dog bite.

Tip: Don't go alone—getting bitten by a dog is a traumatic experience (especially if you own the dog), and you'll likely be shaken up, so if possible, let someone else drive even if you think you can drive yourself. Don't waste time rummaging around for your dog's rabies certificate—if you're sure that it has been vaccinated, you don't need it.

At the ER, your care may include X-rays to make sure there are no broken bones, an exam to determine the depth of the injury, cleaning and debriding the wound (removing any damaged tissue to promote healing) and any needed surgery. (If you were bitten on the face, the emergency department can also bring in a plastic surgeon.) The doctor will also make sure that the injury didn't involve a compartment—the various tendons in the hand that enable the muscles to make your fingers move are separated into compartments. If you get an infection in a compartment, it can injure the corresponding tendon.

Since it's impossible to isolate the type of bacteria that got from the dog's mouth into the wound, a weeklong course of broad-spectrum antibiotics is the standard treatment. If you don't remember when you had your last tetanus shot, you'll likely be given a booster, possibly the Tdap vaccine, which protects against tetanus, diphtheria and pertussis (whopping cough) and is commonly the one used.

You may need a follow-up visit with a specialist if you had surgery or rehab after your hand heals. If the emergency department you go to isn't part of your health-care provider's electronic network, you'll likely be told to let your doctor know about the incident and the care you received…and to give his or her office a call if you see signs that your wound is getting worse—swelling, pain, redness (especially if it's extending beyond the area of the bite), discharge and/or a low-grade fever.

If it was your own dog that attacked, consider whether you need to call your vet to discuss the situation. Ask yourself if this was a provoked bite—were you playing roughly with your dog, did he get startled or was a stranger involved? In these cases, it was likely an isolated incident. But do be more concerned if your dog became aggressive spontaneously and talk to your vet about steps to take.

6 Germ Hot Spots in Your Doctor's Office

Miryam Z. Wahrman, PhD, professor of biology at William Paterson University in Wayne, New Jersey, where she specializes in microbiology, hand hygiene and the interactions between bacteria and environmental surfaces. She is author of *The Hand Book: Surviving in a Germ-Filled World.*

There's a secret that doctors know but don't always talk about—one of the most germ-laden places to visit may be a medical office.

While doctors, nurses and medical assistants have gotten more conscientious about washing their hands, millions of Americans still develop health-care related infections every year. As you'd expect, hospitals are among the most germ-laden places, but even routine doctor visits can present risks.

Troubling development: Bacteria that can lead to life-threatening Clostridium difficile infection (commonly referred to as "C. diff"), a diarrhea-related illness that once was found almost exclusively in hospitals and nursing homes, has been linked to visits to doctors' and dentists' offices, according to a 2015 study published in *The New England Journal of Medicine.*

If you know where the germs are most likely to hide out in medical offices, there are simple steps you can take—beyond handwashing—to reduce your risk of picking up microorganisms that spread colds, flu and other diseases.

IN THE WAITING ROOM

Even though it's impossible to find a germ-free doctor's office (or really any place that people frequent), you shouldn't let that stop you from seeing your physician if you're sick or need a checkup. *When you go, just be sure to follow these steps to avoid germs that lurk in these common hot spots…*

•**Dirty pens.** Patients are accustomed to the pen-and-clipboard check-in ritual, but have you ever wondered what lives on the clipboard pen? It's been touched by hundreds of germy hands, including those of people who are seriously ill. If your check-in involves an electronic tablet, many fingers have touched that as well.

Test swabs taken from doctors' offices show that the average writing implement harbors vast quantities of pathogens—far more than door handles, the armrests of the waiting-room chairs or the doctor's computer keyboard. Because people grip pens with unwashed hands… put them behind their ears…or even in their mouths, pens are also germier than the clipboard you get at check-in.

My advice: Carry your own pen for filling out forms in your doctor's office, signing receipts and to use anywhere you might need to give your signature—at the supermarket, department stores, etc.

•**Germy magazines.** The well-thumbed magazines on a waiting-room table can carry whatever germs were on the previous reader's hands…or were sprayed like an aerosol from a sneeze or cough.

My advice: Bring your own reading material to the doctor's waiting room. Our research, conducted at William Paterson University, found that germs can survive for weeks or even months on paper.

•**Other patients.** Pediatrician offices often have "sick" and "well" areas in the waiting rooms. This hasn't become common practice for doctors who treat adults—perhaps because adults tend to be more careful about hygiene than young children, covering sneezes and coughs and using tissues—and few doctors have waiting rooms big enough to accommodate separate areas.

My advice: Don't sit near patients who are coughing or sneezing, wiping their noses or are otherwise visibly ill. If possible, schedule routine visits so that you're not in the office during flu season. And definitely keep up with vaccines, including those for flu and pneumonia.

Helpful: Consider wearing a face mask in the doctor's office, particularly during flu season. Experts used to think that the flu virus was mainly transmitted through coughing and sneezing and by touching contaminated surfaces. But we now know that these infectious aerosols, airborne droplets produced by coughs or sneezes, can hover in the air for hours. New research shows that these aerosols are also transmitted simply during normal breathing.

You can buy surgical-style face masks in pharmacies…or ask for one at the front desk if your doctor's office provides them for patients who could be contagious. They don't provide a perfect barrier, but a snug-fitting mask will help protect you from other patients—and protect them from you. Even though you may feel self-conscious wearing one, the other patients will appreciate it if they think you're the one who is sick.

THE DOCTOR

•**Handheld devices.** Doctors routinely carry cell phones, tablets or other electronic devices when they make their rounds or see patients in the office. They use them to take notes, check your medical history and look up drug information—and unwittingly to pass germs, in some cases, from one patient to the next.

Shocking research: In a study published in *Online Journal of Health and Allied Sciences,* 75% of the cell phones carried by health professionals were contaminated with disease-causing germs, including methicillin-resistant Staphylococcus aureus (MRSA) and other dangerous pathogens. Equally concerning was that more than half of the health-care workers said that they never cleaned their phones…and 87% admitted that they didn't wash their hands after using them.

Even if your doctor is conscientious about handwashing, the device will reinfect his/her fingertips every time it's touched.

My advice: Ask your doctor to wash his hands after touching the device—and before touching

you. Gloves can help, but only if they're new. You can say to your doctor, "I see that you just touched your tablet. Would you mind putting on a new pair of gloves?"

•**Contaminated stethoscopes.** The stethoscope is the classic emblem of medical care. It's also one of the most contaminated.

Scientific evidence: When researchers measured bacterial concentrations both on stethoscopes and on the hands of doctors who used them, in 71 out of 83 cases, the stethoscopes carried more germs than any part of the doctors' hands except for the fingertips, according to a study in *Mayo Clinic Proceedings.*

Unless a stethoscope is wiped down with alcohol after every use, assume that you're being exposed to bacteria or viruses from the patients who came before you.

My advice: Doctors have gotten better about cleaning their stethoscopes with alcohol wipes, but they may forget…so remind them!

•**White coats.** Most doctors wear a white coat and keep it on all day. It's not as clean as it may look.

Research published in *American Journal of Infection Control* found that 23% of physician white coats carried disease-causing microorganisms, including, in some cases, antibiotic-resistant MRSA.

My advice: Whether or not the doctor is wearing a white coat, be aware of what the doctor touches before he touches you. He should don his gloves right before examining you. If the doctor adjusts his necktie (another germ hot spot) or gets something from a pocket, he should put on a clean pair of gloves. Politely ask your doctor to use an alcohol pad to swab skin areas that have been accidentally brushed with a necktie or jacket sleeve.

When the appointment is over, feel free to give your doctor a fist bump instead of a handshake…or, better yet, just a friendly smile. He will respect your nod to the latest trend in hand-hygiene practices!

After your appointment: Don't forget to wash your hands before leaving the doctor's office—ideally, with soap and water for 20 seconds, but with an alcohol-based hand sanitizer if a sink is not readily available. Research has shown that hand jewelry—and particularly rings, which are rarely removed—is a common cause of bacterial contamination (and transmission), so scrub well, including on and around rings.

Grab a clean paper towel on your way out of the restroom and use that as a barrier when you open doors and push elevator buttons. Then throw it in the trash on your way out of the building.

The Truth About Fecal Transplants

Henning Gerke, MD, gastroenterologist, University of Iowa Health Care, and clinical professor of internal medicine, gastroenterology and hepatology, University of Iowa, Carver College of Medicine, Iowa City.

Admittedly, a fecal transplant—putting someone else's poop into your body—sounds unpleasant. However, it may be the only way to cure some very serious gastrointestinal conditions that resist conventional treatment. And the procedure is not really as gross as what you're probably imagining.

The medical name for the procedure is fecal microbiota transplantation (or FMT)—and the serious condition it most commonly treats is C. difficile (C. diff), a bacterial infection that sickens half a million Americans and kills up to 30,000 each year. In fact, both the Infectious Diseases Society of America and The Society for Healthcare Epidemiology of America have recently added FMT to their official guidelines for treating C. diff.

AN ANCIENT THERAPY MADE MODERN

The concept of curing illness with donor fecal matter dates back to 4th-century China, when a cruder version of the procedure (which truly was gross—it involved making a soup!) was used to treat severe food poisoning and diarrhea. Today's procedure administers FMT via colonoscopy, enema or a tube run through the nose and into the stomach. (An oral capsule is being tested in clinical trials.) The procedure is simple and usually performed outpatient. In most cases, the patient leaves the hospital the same day and C. diff symptoms ease within days.

The fecal matter used in FMT comes from either a local donor (someone you know or the hospital's donor program) or from a national nonprofit stool bank called OpenBiome. In all cases, donors are screened first for illnesses, the same as for blood donors. With a local donor, medical staff mixes the stool with saline (often in a basic kitchen blender) to prepare for a transplant. OpenBiome stool donations are filtered and homogenized, then sealed and kept frozen.

The risk for side effects is low—for instance, abdominal discomfort or a mild fever. FMT has become so accepted as a treatment for C. diff that 97% of Americans live within two hours of a facility that performs the procedure, according to OpenBiome.

HOW FMT WORKS

The main culprit behind C. diff and many other gastrointestinal upsets is a disruption of the gut microbiome. This can be caused by medical conditions, such as a compromised immune system, diabetes or obesity…or from taking certain drugs, such as antibiotics. FMT transplants gut organisms from a healthy donor into a sick patient's gut, repopulating the disrupted gut and helping to restore the natural balance. Numerous studies show FMT to be about 70% to 90%—or more—effective for treating recurrent C. diff infections. (If you're wondering why probiotics don't help, they contain only a few strains of microorganisms, not the wide, diverse spectrum contained in the stool of a healthy donor.)

C. diff bacteria actually are present in a normal, healthy gut in small numbers. But when antibiotics—even a single course—kill off healthy gut bacteria while they're killing the pathogens that made you sick, C. diff can take over, triggering severe diarrhea. Ironically, the standard first line of treatment for C. diff is more antibiotics, which explains why recurrent C. diff is a common problem. Especially vulnerable are children, people over age 65 and those who have a compromised immune system.

THE FMT FRONTIER

While the effectiveness of FMT has only been established for treating C. diff—which is the only FDA-approved use outside of research—the procedure shows promise for other conditions. Because your gut microbiome is critical to your whole immune system and your general health, scientists are studying how FMT might also treat irritable bowel syndrome (IBS), Crohn's disease, diabetes, obesity, peanut allergies and melanoma.

The National Institutes of Health is currently funding a large study that is being conducted by the Fecal Microbiota Transplantation National Registry under the guidance of the American Gastroenterological Association's Center for Gut Microbiome Research and Education.

The study plans to track about 4,000 FMT patients for a decade after their transplants. The researchers will be gathering data on FMT's effectiveness for C. diff and other illnesses, including information on the short- and long-term effects. Currently, more than 20 hospitals, medical centers and medical schools across the country are participating—a number that's expected to grow to 75.

Meanwhile, you can search for a doctor who performs FMT by going to OpenBiome.org.

Hepatitis C Treatment Keeps Getting Better

Eric Lawitz, MD, a professor of medicine at University of Texas Health San Antonio and vice president of scientific and research development for the Texas Liver Institute, also in San Antonio. TXLiver.com

Sometimes progress seems to happen very slowly…and then all at once. Such is the case with treatments for the potentially lethal hepatitis C virus.

For years, Americans with hepatitis C suffered through grueling therapies requiring as many as 18 pills a day, as well as injections of the medication interferon, known for dreadful side effects such as extreme fatigue, rashes, muscle aches, anemia, anxiety and depression.

During this time, hepatitis C killed more Americans than any other infectious disease.

A new era: The dismal track record for hepatitis C therapies began reversing five or so years ago with a variety of much more effective antiviral medications…but with a catch. The first-generation antivirals were genotype specific, which means different treatment regimens were required depending on the specific genotype of the patient's infection. Hepatitis C genotypes are strains that represent the genetic variation of the virus. People can be infected with one of six major genotypes of hepatitis C, which include multiple subtypes of each genotype.

Now: Second-generation antivirals have come on the scene, curing the vast majority of patients with all genotypes of the disease…regardless of their previous interferon therapy…and despite the presence or absence of severe scarring of the liver (cirrhosis), a serious complication that can develop within 20 years of contracting the infection.*

THE GAME-CHANGERS

The first round of game-changing drugs treated genotypes 1 to 6. The first pill to treat all six genotypes of hepatitis C was FDA-approved in 2016. *Sofosbuvir/velpatasvir* (Epclusa) is a 12-week regimen for patients with or without cirrhosis.

The latest breakthrough drug is *glecaprevir/pibrentasvir* (Mavyret), which was approved by the FDA in 2017 as an eight-week regimen effective for all hepatitis C genotypes in people without cirrhosis. (Patients with cirrhosis require 12 weeks of treatment with the drug…those with genotype 3 who have been treated with interferon take the drug for 16 weeks regardless of the presence or absence of cirrhosis.)

The cure rate for the latest two drugs is about 98% in many populations. For the 2% who fail the first round of therapy, there is a three-medication antiviral combination of *sofosbuvir/velpatasvir/voxilaprevir* (Vosevi), and this cures 96% of the remaining 2% who failed the first-line therapy. All told, this leaves only one in 1,000 hepatitis C patients uncured.

*Impressive cure rates can be achieved only if the treatment course is completed.

NEW THINKING ON TESTING

Along with the new medications, there's no longer a need for needle biopsy. Doctors have traditionally relied on a liver biopsy, which involves extracting a small piece of tissue with a needle, to determine the extent of a hepatitis C patient's liver damage. Now the FibroScan, a painless, noninvasive test that measures the amount of liver scarring, is the preferred way to determine the presence or absence of cirrhosis. If your doctor does not advise FibroScan testing, ask for it! Insurance typically covers the cost.

THE FOLLOW-UP

Hepatitis C patients who have liver cirrhosis before successful treatment are at higher risk of developing liver cancer, as cirrhosis is a risk factor for cancer. If you have cirrhosis, you should receive twice-yearly screening via a blood test and ultrasound. The extra caution is well worth it, since small liver tumors can be removed surgically, treated locally or with a liver transplant, while large cancers tend to be life-threatening.

IMPORTANT NOTE ABOUT TESTING

Hepatitis C is often present for decades before symptoms (such as fatigue, nausea and/or jaundice) or complications occur, suggesting a weakening liver or development of liver cancer. Speak to your doctor about testing for hepatitis C.

CHAPTER 11

Medical News Alerts

Cells Are the New Cure

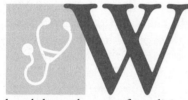

While stem cell therapies have been on the radar for decades, the recent successes in this breakthrough area of medicine are remarkable. Twenty years ago, these accomplishments would have sounded fantastic and otherworldly. But now they're a reality.

NOTEWORTHY SUCCESSES

The science is moving very quickly. It seems like every day doctors are announcing yet another advance in stem cell therapies. These successes will revolutionize the way that medicine is practiced.

Stem cells have now been used to…

•**Build a new bladder.** It's now possible to grow a new bladder in a laboratory—stem cells are removed from the patient's injured organ and "seeded" in a bladder-shaped mold. In one patient, a made-to-order bladder continues to function more than 15 years after it was implanted.

•**Create insulin-producing cells.** Type 1 diabetes is an autoimmune disease in which the body's immune system destroys insulin-producing beta cells in the pancreas. Patients can survive only with daily injections of insulin, a treatment that's expensive and time-consuming—and not optimally effective.

There are a variety of ways to produce beta cells that can be implanted in a patient—existing beta cells can be induced to multiply using medications…non-insulin-producing cells can be manipulated to convert into beta cells…and stem cells from the patient, or more often a donor, can be induced into beta cells. The cells do not necessarily have to be injected into the

Max Gomez, PhD, a CBS News medical correspondent who has spent more than three decades producing health and science segments for network stations in New York City and Philadelphia. He has earned nine Emmy Awards and was named "Man of the Year" by the American Health Foundation. He is coauthor, with Robin Smith, MD, of *Cells Are the New Cure: The Cutting-Edge Medical Breakthroughs That Are Transforming Our Health*.

pancreas, but they do need to be protected from destruction by the autoimmune system.

•Aid in heart failure recovery. In the largest study of this type, the University of Utah found that heart failure patients whose hearts were injected with stem cells had a 37% lower rate of death/hospitalization than those given a placebo. The stem cells, extracted from the heart patient's bone marrow, helped existing heart cells work more efficiently.

•Repair an esophagus. In an experimental procedure, a patient who had a damaged section of esophagus was given metal stents that were then populated with stem cells from the patient's muscle and donated skin. Four years later, the cell therapy had caused all five layers of the esophageal wall to regenerate. The patient could swallow normally, and the stents were removed.

•Speed stroke recovery. Even when patients survive a stroke, they often suffer from permanent neurological damage. A study conducted by researchers at Stanford University and University of Pittsburgh found that stroke patients who were injected with modified stem cells had significant improvements.

Details: Stem cells were genetically manipulated to secrete chemical factors that have been shown to support and protect damaged cells. Patients were given a onetime injection of these stem cells into an area of the brain damaged by stroke. Patients saw improvements in mobility—for example, weakened legs began to work better and some patients in wheelchairs reported the ability to walk again. It's possible that the stem cells (which began to die off a month after the treatment) secreted chemicals that improved neural circuits and reactivated impaired sections of the brain.

Outlook for the future: Right now, there are thousands of ongoing clinical trials involving stem cells.

IMPORTANT CAVEATS

Hundreds of private clinics throughout the US are getting ahead of science and offering stem cell treatments that have not been FDA-approved for conditions as varied as Parkinson's disease, spinal cord injuries and multiple sclerosis.

Some of the treatments might be helpful, but many others won't pan out…and may draw a patient away from standard treatment that could be helpful. In some cases, stem cell treatment at private clinics can be dangerous, since the source and purity of cells aren't known—for example, cells that have been multiplied in unknown labs may have been transformed into cancer cells. Also, without FDA approval, the treatments are not likely to be covered by insurance…and the cost can be enormous.

My advice: Avoid private clinics. If your doctor determines that you have a condition that might be improved with stem cell therapy, ask him/her to help you enroll in a clinical trial in your area. ClinicalTrials.gov is a good place to review ongoing stem cell clinical trials. In many cases, the sponsors of the study will pick up some or all of the costs.

HOW STEM CELL THERAPIES WORK

Most serious diseases—heart disease, diabetes, cancer and arthritis, among many others—are caused by damaged (or aging) cells in the body's tissues. The theory behind stem cell therapies is that these diseases can be cured by replacing defective cells with pristine, disease-free cells. With this groundbreaking approach, stem cells can be extracted, isolated, purified and multiplied in a lab and then implanted in the body, where they continue to divide and differentiate to regenerate healthy adult tissues. Stem cells also can act as natural healers, rather than actually replacing aging cells.

Early in your body's development, embryonic stem cells are undifferentiated. Each has the potential to eventually become any of the different types of cells that your body needs—for example, skin cells, brain cells, heart cells, etc. For medical research, embryos have either been created in the lab or obtained from in vitro fertilization clinics. But this practice is controversial—to obtain the cells, an embryo has to be destroyed.

For practical as well as moral and ethical reasons, most researchers now work with adult stem cells—stem cells that persist after birth and are found in virtually every tissue of the body. Adult stem cells have probably lost some of the potential to become any type of cell, but they can be manipulated.

Example: Adult stem cells taken from fat tissue can be coaxed to become cartilage, bone or even heart cells.

Another source of stem cells: Induced pluripotent stem cells (iPSCs). These are fully differentiated adult cells that can be transformed into embryonic-like cells via genetic manipulation in a lab.

Valuable New Clue in the Fight Against Obesity

Study titled "The Inhibitory Innate Immune Sensor NLRP12 Maintains a Threshold against Obesity by Regulating Gut Microbiota Homeostasis," by researchers at University of North Carolina and published in *Cell Host & Microbe*.

While 40% of Americans are obese, some of them actually eat less—and exercise more—than their thinner peers. So what's at work here? Could obese people really have a "fat gene" that prevents them from losing weight? In fact, recent research indicates that it's the lack of particular gene activity that might cause the trouble…

•**Previous recent studies have linked inflammation to obesity and diabetes.** But scientists have now found that a specific anti-inflammatory gene—called NLRP12—protects mice against obesity and insulin resistance when they eat a high-fat diet. It appears that NLRP12 promotes the growth of a beneficial gut bacteria that wards off inflammation and weight gain. So an NLRP12 gene that isn't firing on all cylinders may contribute to obesity.

Breakthrough implication: This finding may ultimately lead doctors to an effective new way to fight weight gain…and thereby lower the risk for obesity-related diseases such as cancer, heart disease, stroke and diabetes.

Study details: Investigators at University of North Carolina genetically altered mice to eliminate the NLRP12 gene. They then fed these mice and a group of ordinary mice a high-fat diet for several months. The mice without the gene did not eat or drink any more than their peers, but they gained significantly more fat, became heavier and had signs of inflammation in the gut.

When researchers later fed the beneficial bacteria Lachnospiraceae to the mice who lacked NLRP12, the harmful inflammation was reversed and the mice were protected from further weight gain. Researchers explained that Lachnospiraceae contain enzymes that convert carbohydrates and fiber into short-chain fatty acids, such as butyrate and propionate, that have anti-inflammatory properties.

Can this work for humans? A follow-up investigation indicates that it might. Scientists in the Netherlands studied fat cells from obese humans and found that the higher a subject's body mass index, the lower his/her NLRP12 gene activity (as explained earlier, NLRP12 promotes good bacteria that curb inflammation). This finding supports recent research that human obesity is also influenced by inflammation, not just by eating and exercise habits.

What's next? Further studies are needed to determine if supplementing with beneficial bacteria or short-chain fatty acids could be a relatively inexpensive way to promote weight loss and lower the risks for diabetes and other obesity-related diseases.

A New Blood Test May Reveal Your Best Bedtime for the Best Sleep

Rosemary Braun, PhD, MPH, assistant professor of biostatistics and researcher at Northwestern University Feinberg School of Medicine, Evanston, Illinois, and lead author of "Universal Method for Robust Detection of Circadian State from Gene Expression" published in *PNAS*.

Is insomnia keeping you from the sleep you need or do you just want to feel more refreshed when you wake up in the morning? A revolutionary new blood test may one day be able to unlock your ability to get a good night's sleep, enabling you to wake energized and ready to start the day.

First, forget the notion that your sleep/wake cycle is run by the rising and setting of the sun. It's actually determined by the body's circadian clock, the internal system that runs 24 hours a day—give or take a few minutes—and by 10 circadian clock genes, each of which leads to the production of certain proteins. Whether we're alert and ready for action or ready to fall asleep on our feet depends on how slowly or quickly those proteins break down over a 24-hour period.

If you're someone who falls asleep before the sun sets, that suggests that your genetic clock is likely to be a bit slower than the 24-hour cycle of the clock on your wall. If you're someone who's still fired up in the late evening, it's likely your genetic clock runs a bit faster.

The inability to get a good night's sleep is often due to a faulty circadian clock. And when a person's circadian clock is far off from the way it's supposed to work, it can influence not only nighttime sleep and daytime energy levels but also the time of day when side effects from medications are more likely to occur and when certain drug treatments are most likely to be effective. This has enormous implications for people with chronic conditions such as diabetes, heart disease or high blood pressure, with cancer, or with mental health issues such as depression or anxiety.

So how do you know whether your circadian clock is working normally? The current gold standard is a test that profiles melatonin, a hormone in your blood. It involves spending several hours in a sleep lab and having a blood sample drawn every hour so that scientists can track melatonin levels—a degree of testing most people are not willing to do.

That's about to change in the near future, thanks to the development of "TimeSignature," a blood test that looks at your circadian clock genes. It requires just two blood draws, between eight to 12 hours apart, and uses a mathematical formula to determine when and which circadian clock genes are on the job, taking a rest or slacking off. With more research, TimeSignature may one day be able help in the diagnosis of circadian problems such as delayed sleep-phase

syndrome, advanced sleep-wake phase disorder, irregular sleep-wake rhythm, non-24-hour sleep-wake rhythm (often caused by a shift-work disorder or even just by jet lag). This will be invaluable information not only for getting a good night's sleep but also for effectively treating many health conditions. For instance, armed with this information, a doctor should be able to target the time of day when some kind of intervention will get your sleep cycle back on track and/or help optimize treatment for conditions other than sleep disorders, such as when to take blood pressure medication or even administer chemotherapy for cancer patients.

TimeSignature is currently going through the regulatory process required for any new test to come to market, but in the interim the researchers have made the formula available to other scientists who can use it to investigate more precisely the mechanisms by which circadian alignment impacts health.

Your Blood Type Offers Clues About Hidden Health Risks

Mary Cushman, MD, a hematologist and professor of medicine and pathology at Larner College of Medicine at University of Vermont in Burlington, where she is also a board director of the university's Cardiovascular Research Institute. Dr. Cushman's research interest is the study of causative factors for diseases of aging. She completed a term as board director for the American Heart Association National Center in 2017 and is editor in chief of *Research and Practice in Thrombosis and Haemostasis.*

Your blood type is as fundamental as your eye color, determined by genes and equally unchangeable. But while you may have learned long ago which of the four principal blood types you possess—A, B, AB or O—mounting evidence suggests that your specific type may actually influence your health risks.

THE RISKIEST TYPES

Scientists first began theorizing about the links between blood type and disease risks decades ago, but now the research is stacking up. An increasing body of evidence shows that people with certain blood types do, in fact, have higher odds of developing an array of common medical conditions, including heart attack, stroke and other serious health problems.

To be clear, no specific blood type causes a health problem to develop—researchers have uncovered an association, meaning that some medical conditions are more likely to occur in people with certain blood types.

When it comes to health risks, type O appears to be the least hazardous. Non-O blood types—that is, A, B or AB—are linked to higher risks for certain health problems.

So what is it about these blood types that leads to greater health risks? It's not the blood type itself that's the problem…it's the enzymes associated with non-O blood types that affect other substances in the body known as clotting factors. Type AB, in particular, appears to have the highest clotting potential, meaning it sometimes clots when it shouldn't.

Non-O blood also tends to have higher levels of proteins called cellular adhesion molecules that can serve as a "glue" between cells in the inner lining of blood vessels, effectively trapping white blood cells as they stream by.

When white blood cells burrow under the inner lining of blood vessels, they promote the kind of inflammation that's considered a hallmark of atherosclerosis (narrowed arteries that can wreak havoc in the brain, heart or other key areas) or even form a dangerous blood clot.

KEY SCIENTIFIC EVIDENCE

Here are common conditions for which your blood type may play a role…

•**Blood clots.** People with non-O blood types experience, on average, 60% to 80% higher risks for clotting problems such as deep vein thrombosis (DVT) and pulmonary embolism (PE), according to a sweeping 2016 review published in *WIREs Systems Biology and Medicine*. With DVT and PE, blood clots form in the legs and can break off and travel to the lungs in a devastating fashion. Together, these conditions kill up to 100,000 Americans yearly.

•**Heart attack and stroke.** In an analysis of more than 1.3 million people presented at the professional meeting Heart Failure 2017 and the 4th World Congress on Acute Heart Failure, researchers found that those with non-O blood types had, on average, a 9% higher risk of experiencing a heart attack or stroke. Dutch scientists uncovered the association after reviewing 11 different populations from nine individual studies. People with type A, in particular, tend to have higher cholesterol than other blood types, a significant risk factor for coronary events.

•**Memory problems.** People with blood type AB were 82% more likely than those with other blood types to develop precursors to dementia such as thinking and memory impairments, according to 2014 University of Vermont research examining more than 30,000 people and published in *Neurology*.

While AB is the least common blood type, found in only about 4% of Americans, those with this blood type comprised 6% of the group who developed cognitive issues, compared with 4% of study participants with other blood types.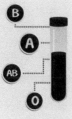

•**Cancer.** When it comes to cancer risk, for unknown reasons, type A individuals are 20% more likely to develop a stomach malignancy than those with type O blood, according to research published in *American Journal of Epidemiology*. On the flip side, people with type O blood are significantly more likely to be hospitalized with peptic ulcers than those with other blood types.

•**Traveler's diarrhea.** A type of E. coli infection commonly known as "traveler's diarrhea" strikes people with type A or AB blood more severely than those with other blood types, a 2018 study published in *The Journal of Clinical Investigation* has found. E. coli, which leads to millions of cases of diarrhea and kills several hundred thousand people worldwide every year, comes in various strains.

Using data from 106 people, scientists found that those with type A or AB blood were far more likely to get sicker—and sooner—than those with blood types B or O when exposed in a controlled setting to an E. coli strain associated with traveler's diarrhea. It's believed that the nasty bacteria thrive better in the intestinal cells of people with type A blood.

What Does Your Blood Type Mean?

The blood is made up of components, including red and white blood cells, platelets and plasma, that help transport oxygen, fight off invaders and form clots in response to injury. One's individual blood type is determined by the surface marker, or antigen, it carries (A, B or A and B) on red blood cells—or, in the case of type O, does not carry. And the type we have is based on genetics. Type O is the most common, present in about 57%, 50% and 45% of the Hispanic, Black and Caucasian populations, respectively, in the US.

If you don't know your blood type, ask your doctor. If it's not already in your file, it's easily determined by a simple blood test.

WHAT YOU CAN DO

If you're wondering what all this means, it depends on who you ask. For scientists, the holy grail would be to come up with specific prevention strategies based on individual risks found among those with certain blood types. That's being worked on…but it will likely require years of additional research to achieve such a personalized approach.

In the meantime, you are not powerless. By being aware of your own blood type—and how it may raise your odds for certain health problems—you can take every possible step to minimize those odds. *What to do…*

•**Get serious about a healthy lifestyle.** This is important for everyone. But those with non-O blood types would be wise to adopt the healthy habits that all of us should already be practicing. This includes being physically active…maintaining a healthy body weight…not smoking…and eating a plant-focused, nutrient-dense diet. This matters even more to non-Os, since many blood type–related diseases impact blood vessel function, the mainstay of heart and brain health, both of which can be protected by a healthy lifestyle.

•**Know your numbers.** Routine screenings with your primary care physician provide a veritable smorgasbord of numbers and blood biomarker levels that you should carefully consider—especially in light of your blood type.

These include blood pressure (aim for a reading no higher than 120/80 mm/Hg)…cholesterol levels (total should be 125 mg/dL to 200 mg/dL and LDL "bad" cholesterol less than 100 mg/dL)…and glucose levels (fasting level of less than 100 mg/dL), since diabetes is also a major risk factor for cardiovascular problems. People with non-O blood type should keep an extra close eye on these numbers.

•**Speak up!** Talk to your doctor about what you've learned regarding your blood type and specific health risks. If you also have a family history that adds to your risk, you'll want to work aggressively to minimize your odds of developing that condition.

Marijuana Isn't as Risk-Free as You May Think

Deborah S. Hasin, PhD, professor of epidemiology at Columbia University, New York City, and lead author of the study titled "Cannabis Use, Attitudes, and Legal Status in the US: A Review," published in *Preventive Medicine*.

More than 75% of adult marijuana users age 50 or older believe that there's little to no risk in smoking a joint once or twice a week. After all, 33 states and the District of Columbia have legalized cannabis for medicinal purposes and 10 for recreational use. But perception isn't necessarily reality.

Experts caution that not enough is known to declare marijuana "risk-free." Rates of cannabis-use disorder are increasing in middle-aged and young adults. *Here's more about what is known…*

•**Overconsumption.** Marijuana is more potent than ever, with an increase in tetrahydrocannabinol (THC), the main active ingredient in cannabis, from 3% to 12% in the past decade, thanks to selective plant breeding.

Example: A baby boomer who hasn't had any cannabis since college could inadvertently consume too much and experience paranoia, acute anxiety and/or hallucinations. The psychoactive effects of inhaled marijuana are fast—usually within minutes. But the effects of edibles can take a half hour to two hours, meaning more could be consumed, leading to adverse effects when the edible THC finally has been absorbed.

•**Drug interactions.** If someone takes drugs or supplements to reduce blood clotting, marijuana may increase the risk of bleeding. Using cannabis while on an SSRI antidepressant may raise the risk for mania. It also can increase the drowsiness caused by some antidepressants (as well as alcohol). Discuss possible interactions with your doctor.

•**Falls.** Older users are at an increased risk for injury from falls not only because they may have weaker muscles and poor balance but also because marijuana can cause orthostatic hypotension (low blood pressure upon standing).

•**Heart attack.** Studies suggest an increase in risk for heart attack, especially in those who are older and who have cardiovascular disease, arrhythmias or other cardiac vulnerabilities. There's a higher risk for stroke, too.

The Latest in 3-D Medical Printing

Justin Ryan, PhD, a research scientist who leads the Cardiac 3D Print Lab at Phoenix Children's Hospital/Arizona State University and an adjunct faculty member at Arizona State University, where he specializes in the production of patient-specific 3-D models of hearts, brain tumors, bones and vascular anomalies. He is also cochair of Digital Imaging and Communications in Medicine (DICOM), which provides standards for the creation, storage and management of 3-D medical files.

This may sound like something from a sci-fi movie, but everything from hip implants to hearing aids…and artificial arms to prescription pills can now be produced with a printer. And 3-D–printed organs are on the horizon!

WHAT IS 3-D MEDICAL PRINTING?

Engineers and designers have been using 3-D printers for more than 25 years to make prototypes quickly and cheaply, but now 3-D printing is being used to revolutionize the medical field.

With 3-D printing, specialized printers don't use ink. Instead, they lay down layer after layer of plastic, powders, liquefied metal or other materials, even living cells, until the desired object is complete—often in a few hours or less.

When Arizona State University first started producing 3-D medical models in 2009, only a few hospitals (such as Mayo Clinic) were using the technology. Today, more than 100 hospitals have their own 3-D labs or are farming out projects to 3-D contractors. The technology has evolved so quickly that the FDA recently issued guidelines for companies that produce medical products ranging from 3-D–printed tissues to surgical scaffolds for bone repair.

3-D printing is less expensive than traditional manufacturing for individualized parts because it's fast and there's little waste.

Another advantage: 3-D products can be easily customized with a few clicks of a computer mouse.

HOW 3-D PRINTING IS USED TODAY

There's a good chance that you're already benefiting from 3-D medical printing. For example, dental implants, hearing aids and prescription eyeglasses are often made this way. *Other uses…*

•**Surgical planning.** The unique properties of 3-D printing, particularly the ability to add one thin layer after another, have made it possible to create exact replicas of body parts and tissues—including the intricate networks of nerves and blood vessels. Surgeons facing a challenging procedure will sometimes use 3-D models—created from CT or MRI scans of the patient—to plan their approach.

Example: Surgery for congenital heart defects is geometrically challenging. With a customized model, surgeons can see the unique intricacies—including the location of the coronary blood vessels, which vary from patient to patient—before the surgery.

•**Implants and prostheses.** 3-D printing makes it possible to produce implants and artificial limbs that precisely match each patient—for a fraction of the cost of traditional implants/prostheses.

Examples: A group called Enabling the Future works with thousands of volunteers worldwide who use 3-D technology to create prosthetic arms and hands.

A printed 3-D prosthesis might cost as little as $50, compared with thousands of dollars for a conventional device. This is particularly helpful for families who can't afford to replace prostheses when children quickly outgrow the old ones.

The majority of off-the-shelf hip implants used today are actually printed. Customized, patient-specific implants are the next step. Also, the surface roughness and natural porosity of bone can be recreated with 3-D technology so that the surrounding tissue grows into the implant (know as osseointegration), rather than just around it.

•**Printed medications.** This is now being done in research to improve drug production. And in 2015, the FDA approved the first 3-D–printed prescription drug, *levetiracetam* (Spritam), which is used for seizures. It's only a matter of time before patients can pick up a variety of printed drugs at the pharmacy.

With 3-D drug production, a pharmacist could analyze a patient's unique requirements—based on factors such as gender, age, race, drug response, etc.—before creating a customized dose and hitting the "print" button. And patients who have multiple chronic diseases could have their various medications printed in one tablet (or, at least, fewer tablets), which would provide convenience and could improve compliance.

•**Customized splints to aid healing.** In a widely publicized case, surgeons at University of Michigan took CT scans of an infant's damaged trachea. Sophisticated software and a 3-D printer soon produced a supportive splint, which was wrapped around the trachea. The infant gradually recovered—and the splint, made from layers of biodegradable material, eventually disappeared on its own. This technology will soon be tested in a clinical trial.

ON THE HORIZON

Printing new organs is the big goal for researchers. Producing organs with 3-D technology made from the patient's own cells would solve the problem of organ donor shortages and organ rejection. But it's a daunting challenge because organs are thick, complicated structures—they contain multiple cell types and require intricate pathways that permit blood circulation and the movement of oxygen between tissues.

An important advance in this area, known as bioprinting, is still in the early stages. With bioprinting, researchers apply living cells to a 3-D–printed scaffold. It's hoped that the cells will then multiply and grow to repair (or replace) damaged structures. For some types of cells, scaffolding isn't necessary—the cells figure out on their own where to go.

Possible uses: Skin transplants for burn victims…cartilage replacement for damaged joints…and the creation of complete organs.

Scientists have already produced printed skin…parts of a bladder…sheets of cardiac tissue that beat like a real heart…and functional liver tissue. It's likely that complete, working organs—starting with relatively simple ones, such as a bladder—will be 3-D printed within the next five to 10 years. More complicated structures, such as kidneys and hearts, are probably a few decades away. Interim steps, such as replacing parts of a heart or coronary artery, could be accomplished soon.

Lithium: Not Just for Bipolar Disorder

James Greenblatt, MD, chief medical officer and vice president of medical services at Walden Behavioral Care in Waltham, Massachusetts. He has been studying the effects of low-dose lithium for 30 years and is author of Nutritional Lithium: A Cinderella Story. He is also a clinical faculty member at Tufts University School of Medicine in Boston and Geisel School of Medicine at Dartmouth College in Hanover, New Hampshire. JamesGreenblattMD.com

Low-dose *lithium* may help prevent Alzheimer's…calm chronic irritability and anger…and ease depression.

Wait a second, you say to yourself—isn't lithium a serious drug for psychiatric conditions like bipolar disorder? Yes, in high doses of 150 mg to 1,800 mg. But in very low doses (say, 1 mg to 5 mg), lithium is a nutritional treatment, uniquely effective for a range of problems. *Here's what you need to know...*

ALZHEIMER'S DISEASE

It's becoming widely accepted by scientists that the neurochemical changes that lead to Alzheimer's develop over a period of decades—and that prevention is the goal.

In my medical opinion, lithium may be the most effective preventive agent. *Research is ongoing, but here are some key studies that support that statement...*

•**Low-dose lithium helps lower the risk for Alzheimer's.** A Brazilian study published in *British Journal of Psychiatry* involved 41 seniors with mild cognitive impairment, the memory loss and mental decline that often precedes Alzheimer's. Half were given low-dose lithium and half, a placebo. After one year, more of the people taking lithium had no mental decline, better memory, more focus and clearer thinking. Just 19% of those on lithium developed Alzheimer's compared with 35% in the placebo group.

•**Low-dose lithium helps treat Alzheimer's.** In another study, published in *Current Alzheimer Research*, 94 people with mild-to-moderate Alzheimer's were similarly divided into two groups. The lithium group had no cognitive decline during the 15 months of the study, while mental decline progressed by 20% in the placebo group.

•**Lithium improves sleep and eases agitation and psychosis.** In a case study report on three Alzheimer's patients with these symptoms, researchers from Columbia University Medical Center found that prescribing low-dose lithium led to dramatic changes in just two weeks—a normal sleep cycle and a marked decrease in symptoms.

How it helps: Lithium is a GSK-3 inhibitor—that means it blocks the enzyme GSK-3 to, in turn, stop the accumulation of plaques (beta-amyloid) and tangles, the changes that signal the development and advance of Alzheimer's. It improves the connections between neurons, triggers the growth of new neurons and boosts a protein that stops neurons from dying.

Lithium also protects against brain inflammation and oxidation and increases serotonin, which regulates mood and behavior.

IRRITABILITY AND ANGER

Because it improves problems with impulse control, nutritional lithium has a uniquely calming effect, demonstrated in research involving people with post-traumatic stress disorder (PTSD) and published in *Journal of Traumatic Stress.*

DEPRESSION AND SUICIDE

Lithium may be an effective way to combat the rise in suicide. Research done around the world has found that the lower the levels of lithium in the water and soil (it's a naturally occurring trace element), the higher the rate of suicide.

A study published in *Journal of Psychiatric Research* compared the suicide rate in 226 Texas counties with 3,123 lithium samples from the public water supply.

Finding: Lower suicide rates were linked to higher lithium levels in the water.

Research done in Lithuania and published in *Journal of Trace Elements in Medicine and Biology* found the same was true for men, in particular, and suggested that lithium may decrease suicide risk, which is two to four times higher among men than women.

BIPOLAR DISORDER

Pharmaceutical lithium is an effective treatment for bipolar disorder, but high doses can cause hand tremors, increased thirst, nausea, diarrhea, abdominal distress and even kidney disease. Low-dose lithium may produce positive results...without the health problems.

In fact, research published in *Experimental and Therapeutic Medicine* found that personalized dosing at lower levels than commonly prescribed can be helpful without causing the side effects of the typical prescription dose.

HOW TO USE LITHIUM

Besides drinking water, naturally occurring lithium is in vegetables, grains, eggs and milk, but you can't reliably get enough lithium from your diet to make a symptom-controlling difference.

My advice: I recommend 2.5 mg of over-the-counter lithium (see below) daily for prevention of cognitive decline or for chronic irritability… and 2.5 mg to 5 mg if you have symptoms of cognitive decline.

Also: If you have a personal or family history of bipolar disorder, substance abuse, suicide (or suicide attempts) or use prescription medication, see a physician before taking any lithium on your own.

Caution: Thyroid disorders and kidney disease can be caused by pharmaceutical lithium. If you have any health problem involving the thyroid or kidneys, talk to your doctor before using any lithium.

THE RIGHT LITHIUM…

For low-dose nutritional lithium, look for lithium orotate or lithium citrate, available over-the-counter. Avoid lithium aspartate, which can cause neurons to transmit impulses at a rapid rate and trigger headaches and brain inflammation in some people.

Timing Is Everything

Kenneth P. Wright Jr., PhD, professor of integrative physiology and director of the Sleep and Chronobiology Laboratory at University of Colorado Boulder. He has published more than 100 papers and chapters on the links between sleep, circadian rhythms and health.

You probably think of yourself as either a "morning person" or a "night owl"—and when it comes to your health and even your survival, the distinction might be crucial.

Emerging research on the body's circadian rhythms shows that everything from our gut health to our bodies' healing powers to our response to medications and even the outcome of surgery is directly affected by our biological clocks.

Sound far-fetched? It's not. The 2017 Nobel Prize in Physiology or Medicine was awarded to three American scientists for their groundbreaking research into the impact of the hundreds— even thousands—of ticking clocks buried deep inside our organs, tissues and cells.

Latest compelling evidence: A study published in *The Lancet* found that patients who undergo heart-valve replacement surgery in the afternoon are 50% less likely to suffer major cardiac events during the following 500 days compared with people who undergo the procedure in the morning—a huge difference in success rate. This finding builds on previous research showing that adults are most likely to suffer heart attacks in the morning rather than at night.

It's merely one example of the vast potential of the burgeoning field of chronobiology, the study of how living organisms respond and adapt to the daily 24-hour rhythms of life. Researchers have identified hundreds of genes that show a time-of-day pattern in heart tissue alone, and they appear to be important for healthy heart function.

Sleep, which is heavily impacted by natural light and darkness, also can be adversely affected when we alter our circadian rhythms. If you've ever traveled across multiple time zones, you've experienced what it feels like when the body's internal clocks are disrupted.

And that's only scratching the surface. *Other links are being discovered between circadian rhythms and…*

•**Gut health.** Trillions of bacteria in your gastrointestinal (GI) tract, known collectively as the microbiome, play a vital role not just in digestion but also in overall wellness. Now researchers are investigating whether circadian disruption adversely affects these bacteria.

The notion of the microbiome having its own circadian clocks comes from studies of late-night shift workers, many of whom are prone to developing GI problems related to sleep deprivation. In addition, multiple universities are researching rodents and humans to determine whether consuming probiotics (good bacteria) and prebiotics (plant fiber that feeds these probiotics) helps protect the microbiome from the effects of circadian disruption.

If confirmed, these studies might one day shield shift workers, members of the military (who frequently operate under sleep-deprived conditions) and typical night owls alike from digestive disorders—not to mention obesity, diabetes, heart disease and a host of other conditions linked to chronic sleep loss.

•**Wound healing.** Skin cells called fibroblasts that aid in healing are thought to function more efficiently during the day than at night because of circadian clocks in the skin that are more active during daylight hours.

A 2017 study published in *Science Translational Medicine* found that cuts and burns heal nearly 60% faster when the injury occurs during the day than at night. This may be an evolutionary advantage dating back to prehistoric times. Ancient humans were more likely to be injured during the day, when they hunted prey for that evening's dinner.

If chronobiologists can further pinpoint optimal times of day for different people's healing, patients may one day be able to schedule surgery at those particular hours, improving their odds of a speedy recovery.

•**Asthma symptoms.** For people with asthma, symptoms tend to worsen at night and in the early morning hours. Considering this, researchers have investigated the effectiveness of timing medication precisely to ease symptoms, an approach called chronotherapy.

Examples: Asthma drugs classified as leukotriene receptor antagonists, such as *montelukast* (Singulair) and *zafirlukast* (Accolate), are most effective at improving symptoms when taken in the evening, according to a 2011 study published in *Thorax*.

Similarly, taking a single dose of an inhaled corticosteroid at 5:30 pm was found in research published in 2013 in *Indian Journal of Pharmacology* to be nearly as effective as four doses spread throughout the day.

•**Diabetes.** Research suggests that the link between poor sleep and diabetes may have to do with the fact that if you're awake when your body's master clock thinks you should be sleeping, your body becomes less sensitive to insulin—a precursor to diabetes.

In a 2015 study published in *Current Biology*, five days with just five hours of sleep per night results in a 20% reduction in insulin sensitivity in otherwise healthy adults. That's because if you go to bed late, wake up early and eat breakfast, your pancreas will release insulin as

it should, but the body is less responsive to it because melatonin levels are still high, as if you were sleeping.

Result: Your blood sugar remains elevated, and your body continues overproducing insulin. This won't cause diabetes after just a few nights, but chronic poor sleep is certainly a risk factor.

•**Depression.** Daily early-morning exposure to bright light (also considered a type of chronotherapy) has been shown to rival the therapeutic benefits of antidepressants in people with major depression...and even to help major depression patients for whom such drugs have not been effective.

•**Cancer.** Decades' worth of clinical trials have found that strategically timed chemotherapy can shrink tumors more effectively and boost survival rates from certain types of cancer, including colorectal cancer and lung cancer—and even may reduce chemo's toxic side effects.

Important finding: Cancer cells tend to be less active at night than during the day, and it may be that evening chemotherapy sessions improve the odds of successfully targeting those cells because they are less active, according to research published in *Advanced Drug Delivery Reviews*.

"Yo-Yo" Cardio Danger

When blood sugar, blood pressure, cholesterol and weight fluctuate—go up and down—by more than 5%, it can shorten a person's life span, according to a new Korean study that followed 6.7 million people for five-and-a-half years. Those who had the highest fluctuations were 41% more likely to have a stroke...and 43% more likely to have a heart attack than those whose numbers did not fluctuate by more than 5%.

Seung-Hwan Lee, MD, PhD, associate professor of internal medicine, College of Medicine, The Catholic University of Korea, Seoul.

Lab-Grown Human Esophagus

Study by researchers at Cincinnati Children's Center for Stem Cell and Organoid Medicine (CuSTOM), Cincinnati Children's Hospital Medical Center, published in *Cell Stem Cell*.

A human esophagus has been grown in a lab. Researchers grew the esophagus from pluripotent stem cells, which can form any tissue type in the body. The first-of-its-kind organ grown this way is part of a long-term project to study and perhaps eventually treat birth defects and diseases affecting millions of people, such as gastric reflux and cancer.

Ketogenic Diet: More Than a Weight-Loss Fad

Tanya J.W. McDonald, MD, PhD, a practicing epileptologist and assistant professor of neurology in the department of neurology at the Johns Hopkins University School of Medicine in Baltimore. Her research interests include dietary therapies for adults with epilepsy, evaluations for seizure surgery and epilepsy in women. She is lead author of "The Expanding Role of Ketogenic Diets in Adult Neurological Disorders," a review article published in *Brain Sciences*.

The ketogenic diet has shaped up as the biggest weight-loss trend of the last few years.

What's not being talked about: Even though there are positive anecdotal reports on using this high-fat, very-low-carbohydrate diet for weight loss—and research is promising (see below)—few people know about its current and potential uses for neurological conditions and other chronic diseases…

NEUROLOGICAL CONDITIONS

•**Epilepsy.** Diet therapy was a common epilepsy treatment until the development of antiseizure drugs in the 1930s. Now researchers are taking a second look at the ketogenic diet because some patients with epilepsy are drug-resistant—that is, they have failed to respond to two different medications…and have less than a 5% chance of becoming seizure-free with the use of additional drugs.

Scientific evidence: Research has confirmed that 40% to 50% of adults with epilepsy will improve on the diet with the most benefits seen in patients who stick with it.

Among the many possible mechanisms, the diet is thought to dampen the brain-cell "excitability" that's associated with seizures. It also improves the balance of intestinal bacteria, which appears to provide seizure protection.

The ketogenic diet doesn't replace anti-epilepsy drugs—most patients will continue to take medication, although many will require fewer drugs and/or a lower dose. I advise a variety of epilepsy patients to try the diet for at least three months. If it's effective, they stick with it. If not, they slowly resume their consumption of carbohydrates, under the supervision of a medical professional or nutritionist.

•**Brain cancer.** Glioblastoma, a type of malignant glioma, is the most frequently diagnosed primary brain tumor. Early research suggests that a ketogenic diet could help patients with this type of cancer, particularly when combined with radiation and/or other treatments.

In laboratory studies, animals given a ketogenic-like diet showed improved survival times of 20% to 30%. Small studies—many of them case reports (descriptions of individual patients)—have shown improvements in disease progression and survival.

The diet may help because the cells that fuel cancer depend on glucose as an energy source. When you take away glucose with a ketogenic diet, cancer cells may lose the ability to proliferate.

My advice: If you or a loved one has been diagnosed with this type of cancer, ask your doctor if a ketogenic diet might help—and if he/she recommends participating in one of the clinical trials listed at ClinicalTrials.gov. (There are also trials that focus on the use of this diet for other types of cancer.)

•**Alzheimer's disease.** Like the cancer cells described above, the amyloid deposits that are the hallmark of Alzheimer's may depend on high levels of glucose in the blood.

In laboratory studies, animals given extracts that put their bodies into a ketosis-like state (see adjacent column) showed improved learning and memory. Studies involving Alzheimer's patients or those with mild cognitive impairment have shown that people given similar extracts had improvements in working memory and visual attention.

My advice: Because the research is too preliminary to conclude that the diet is—or isn't—effective for this purpose, I wouldn't advise Alzheimer's patients to try the diet without close medical supervision. But if you've been diagnosed with Alzheimer's—or have a high risk of developing it—you might want to discuss it with your doctor.

OTHER USES

•**Weight loss.** The ketogenic diet is a far cry from the plant-rich diets that most experts recommend for weight loss. In its most restrictive form, it limits many vegetables, fruits, beans and grains—all of the foods that can help you lose weight.

Yet people who switch to a ketogenic diet (the plans for weight loss are somewhat less restrictive than those used for some of the conditions described above) do lose weight—and they lose it quickly.

Caveats: Most experts agree that people who follow the diet can lose weight. But it doesn't appear to be any more effective than other, more conventional diets, and the drop-out rate is probably much higher.

•**Diabetes.** People with diabetes are usually advised to eat less fat because weight loss and a lower-fat diet have been thought to go hand in hand. But experts are taking another look at the ketogenic diet for diabetes control.

Reasons: Not only can the diet promote weight loss, but there's some evidence that it improves insulin sensitivity and lowers blood sugar.

Caution: People with diabetes who follow a ketogenic diet have an increased risk for diabetic ketoacidosis, a life-threatening condition due to elevated blood sugar and blood acids (ketones).

HOW THE DIET WORKS

The term "ketogenic" has become a catchall phrase for any high-fat, low-carbohydrate diet. But in the medical community, the diet calls for a severe restriction of carbohydrates and high amounts of fat. The requirements are so rigorous that the diet should be attempted only with the supervision of a doctor, as with any medical therapy.

How it works: Normally, blood sugar (glucose) from carbohydrates is your main source of energy. But when glucose is restricted, your body starts breaking down fat, a process that releases ketone bodies into the bloodstream. Cells use ketone bodies as an alternative fuel source until you start eating carbohydrates again.

If you stay on the diet long enough, the body enters ketosis. (You experience a mild form of ketosis when you've gone all night without food.) Ketosis mimics a starvation state—it triggers metabolic changes, including those that promote weight loss and improve insulin sensitivity.

The diet emphasizes foods high in fat, moderate in protein and low in carbohydrates (eggs, cheese, avocados, butter, olive oil, cream, bacon, steak, salmon, sardines, nuts, seeds, etc.).

An Implant That Helps Paralyzed People Move Again

The study "Recovery of Over-Ground Walking after Chronic Motor Complete Spinal Cord Injury" by researchers at the University of Louisville and published in *The New England Journal of Medicine*.

For the more than one million Americans paralyzed by a spinal cord injury, the dream of standing and walking again may soon be a possibility. Scientists at the Kentucky Spinal Cord Injury Research Center at the University of Louisville have developed a combination treatment using implants to stimulate the spinal cord, along with intense physical therapy to help paralyzed patients regain motor function. The implant itself has been used for the treatment of chronic pain. Its use in spinal cord injury patients is new and still experimental.

Epidural spinal cord stimulation involves surgically implanting nerve-stimulating electrodes into the lower spine, the area that controls movement of the hips, legs and feet. To trigger the electrodes, a stimulator is implanted in the abdomen.

The initial study of the technique involved four patients who had been unable to stand, walk or sit without support for between two and three years. Two of the patients had some sensation below the level of their injury.

The patients began with two months of physical therapy called locomotor training. Their weight was supported in an apparatus while therapists moved their legs on a treadmill for two hours a day, five days a week to rehabilitate their muscles.

The next step was to surgically implant the nerve-stimulating electrodes and the abdominal stimulator. After recovering from surgery, the patients started on months of near-daily locomotor training using the apparatus while getting constant stimulation from the device. Training sessions included standing, treadmill walking and, for those who could, walking on the ground. Over time, the support from the ap-

paratus was reduced to let the patients support more of their weight on their own.

All four patients gained some ability to move their legs, walk on the treadmill with support and stand using a walker. The two patients who had had some sensation were also able to walk on the ground, one with a walker and the other using poles or holding hands with physical trainers. Researchers believe the stimulation excites the healthy spinal cord below the level of the injury, making it receptive to information. Signals from the brain giving the intent to walk are able to cross the injury site. The spinal cord then integrates the command from the brain with sensory cues and generates the appropriate movement.

The length of time it took to reach these achievements was different for each patient, even between the two who were able to walk—it took one, a 23-year-old woman, 3.5 months and the other, a 35-year-old man, 18 months.

Overall, this research showed that the spinal cord stimulator, when combined with intense locomotor training and the intent to walk, led to the recovery of the ability to walk even years after a spinal cord injury.

With expanded research and improvements in stimulator technology, the scientists predict that more gains will be seen.

As of now, spinal cord epidural stimulation has moved into the trial phase, with a new 36-patient study supported by the Christopher and Dana Reeve Foundation under way at the University of Louisville. If you or a loved one is interested in participating in a future paralysis research trial, you can add your name to a database of potential research participants at https://victoryoverparalysis.org/participate-in-research-copy/.

CHAPTER 12

Medication Smarts

Are Your Medications Making Your Life Worse?

It happens for the best of reasons. Your cardiologist, say, prescribes one medication, then you see your endocrinologist and get another, and your rheumatologist gives you another—and the doctors don't talk to one another. Each is trying to help you—but collectively, they could be hurting you...possibly badly.

Polypharmacy—taking a combination of medications that does more harm than good—is a national epidemic, and it's getting worse. The truth is, our medical system is a lot better at prescribing medications than at stopping ones that are no longer needed—deprescribing. Yet doing so, carefully and under medical supervision, reduces the adverse side effects and often improves health. Would it help you to deprescribe?

A SNEAKY MULTIPLICATION

Polypharmacy can happen before you know it. *Case in point:* Many medications, regardless of the conditions they're prescribed for, can have depression as a side effect. They include certain blood pressure drugs...heart drugs... drugs for heartburn (proton pump inhibitors)... even painkillers. The more of these drugs you take, the higher your statistical risk of developing depression.

Polypharmacy also is associated with a host of other adverse effects including an increased risk for falls and cognitive impairment that can lead to emergency room visits and hospitalization. The problem often gets worse as you get older—you're not only likely to need more medications, but your body's ability to process those medications declines. A drug or dosage that was appropriate when initially prescribed might no longer be safe or appropriate. However, polypharmacy can happen at any age.

Barbara Farrell, PharmD, assistant professor in the department of family medicine and an adjunct assistant professor in the School of Pharmacy, both at University of Waterloo, Canada. She was named Pharmacist of the Year by the Canadian Pharmacist Association in 2011 and is cofounder of the Canadian Deprescribing Network. Deprescribing.org

A "MIRACULOUS" RECOVERY

You now understand polypharmacy. *For an idea of how deprescribing can work, consider this case study...*

The woman sat slumped over in her chair—and then slid out onto the floor when she tried to stand. She had been diagnosed with dementia and was on the waiting list for a long-term-care facility, where she seemed likely to live out her remaining days. Instead, 10 weeks later, she was walking and living an active life. Her long-term-care stay had been canceled—her doctors realized that she did not even have dementia!

What changed? A medical team reviewed this woman's case and discovered that she was taking 32 prescription medications each day—and together, the medications that had been prescribed to help this woman instead were ruining her life. The review team gradually eliminated 15 of those drugs and reduced the dosages of several others.

For most, polypharmacy's effects are subtler. And to determine whether it's happening to you, you probably will need to press your doctor or doctors. Most physicians are far more likely to write prescriptions than to review and eliminate them. That's slowly changing, but for now it's up to you to take the lead. *Here's how...*

•**Make a medications list.** It's a good idea to put all your prescription drugs, over-the-counter medications, vitamins and other supplements in a bag and bring them to your doctor and ask for a review. But also bring a list of each of these, including dosages, to help your doctor review them accurately and quickly. Group drugs together on the list by their purpose—heart drugs, pain drugs, etc.

•**Call your doctor's attention to medications that are likely to be problematic.** Certain kinds of prescription drugs, if used long term, are particularly likely to cause problems...

> •Sleeping pills
> •Blood sugar drugs (especially sulfonyl-urea drugs)
> •Blood pressure drugs (especially if they lead to low-pressure episodes)
> •Narcotic pain drugs

•Heartburn/GERD drugs (proton pump inhibitors)

•**Ask your doctor—or doctors—to review all your medications.** You might start a conversation this way—"I read an article about the dangers of polypharmacy, and I want to take a serious look at all of the medications I am taking..." For any particular medication, you might ask, "Is this prescription and dosage a problem to take for as long as I've been on it? Is it appropriate for my age? Could I be on a lower dose?" If you see several specialists, have this conversation with each one.

If you are prescribed medications after a hospital stay, follow up with your own doctor. According to a study of elderly patients discharged from 11 Veterans Affairs medical centers, 44% were prescribed one or more unnecessary drugs.

And even if the medications are appropriate for you at discharge, ask your doctor—or the hospital pharmacist—which ones you can stop taking a few weeks or a month later.

AVOID FUTURE UNNECESSARY PRESCRIPTIONS

To reduce your odds of being given unnecessary prescriptions in the first place...

•**If you develop a new health problem, raise the possibility that drugs are causing it.** Ask, "Could this be a side effect of any of the drugs I'm currently taking or the combination of drugs?" It might not be, but you'll ensure that your doctor considers that possibility.

•**Ask the following questions about any new medication**—how long should you take it...how will you know whether it's working... and what side effects should you watch for.

•**Explore lifestyle changes that can reduce the need for certain prescriptions.**

Example: Consider relaxation techniques before resorting to sleeping pills. Jot down your questions before you see your doctor.

•**Talk to your pharmacist.** With any new prescription, raise the question of polypharmacy with your pharmacist. If he/she has a concern that your doctor did not bring up, ask him to call your doctor's office to resolve the situation.

Helpful: Use the same pharmacy for all your prescriptions. That increases the odds that the pharmacist will spot potentially problematic drug interactions even before you ask about them.

•**Be aware of the risks of stopping certain medications too quickly.** Discontinuing certain prescription drugs can cause side effects—and some can be dangerous. This is especially true for certain classes of medications including antidepressants, blood pressure drugs called beta-blockers and sleeping pills. But there are others, too. So don't reduce or stop any drug without guidance from your doctor...and if a doctor does recommend ending a drug, ask whether it needs to be tapered and, if so, ask for detailed instructions on how to do that properly.

When Your Medication Makes You Gain Weight

Jack E. Fincham, PhD, RPh, professor of pharmacy administration at Presbyterian College School of Pharmacy in Clinton, South Carolina. He is a panel member of the FDA Non-Prescription Drug Advisory Committee and Peripheral and Central Nervous System Drugs Advisory Committee.

Medications that you take to improve your health—including, paradoxically, some of the same drugs that are used to treat obesity-related illnesses—could be adding inches to your waistline.

Shocking fact: It's estimated that more than 500 widely used medications have weight gain as a possible side effect. It doesn't happen to everyone, but be suspicious if you notice that you've gained a few pounds (or more) soon after starting a new medication. In some cases, the extra pounds drop off if the drug is stopped—but not always.

Take action: If the scales start creeping upward, tell your doctor. In many cases, switching to a different type of medication—or even another drug in the same class—can help. If the medication is working well, you can instead ask your doctor about taking a lower dose. In some cases, this may stem the weight gain but still have a therapeutic effect. *Among the common suspects...**

•**SSRI antidepressants.** The emotional and physical tolls of depression are widely recognized. But most people don't realize that the risk for obesity could jump by as much as 58% if you're depressed...and, in a cruel twist, the most popular drugs for treating depression can cause even more weight gain.

Up to 25% of patients who take antidepressants, including the selective serotonin reuptake inhibitors (SSRIs), notice that they've gained weight. It's common for drugs such as *paroxetine* (Paxil) and *sertraline* (Zoloft) to trigger weight gain that totals 10 pounds or more.

It is possible that the drugs' effects on serotonin, a neurotransmitter involved in mood, changes both appetite and the body's ability to metabolize nutrients. People who feel better after treating depression also may find that they're enjoying life (and food!) more than they did before. Weight gain mainly occurs in patients who have taken the drugs for more than six months.

My advice: Ask your doctor about switching to *venlafaxine* (Effexor XR) or *nefazodone* (Serzone). These antidepressants are effective but unlikely to cause weight gain. Another popular antidepressant, *bupropion* (Wellbutrin), can cause some people to lose weight.

•**Antihistamines.** You're unlikely to gain weight by taking an occasional antihistamine (for example, during allergy seasons—spring, summer and/or fall), but people who regularly take drugs such as *fexofenadine* (Allegra) or *cetirizine* (Zyrtec) often gain weight. It's believed that drugs used to block the effects of histamine may trigger brain changes that boost appetite.

Important finding: In a 2010 study published in *Obesity*, patients who took antihistamines daily to treat allergies had larger waist circumferences and higher insulin levels than those who didn't take these drugs.

*Always check with your doctor before stopping a prescribed medication or changing the dose. Making such changes without a physician's advice can cause serious side effects.

My advice: If you think an antihistamine is affecting your weight, ask your doctor about switching to a nonsedating antihistamine, such as *loratadine* (Claritin). You won't have the drowsiness that can occur with older antihistamines (such as Benadryl). You'll likely have more energy and might burn more calories.

•**Diabetes drugs.** If you've been diagnosed with type 2 diabetes, there's a good chance that you're taking one of the sulfonylureas, a class of drugs that includes *chlorpropamide* (Diabinese) and *glyburide* (such as Micronase). They're useful drugs because they stimulate the pancreas to secrete more insulin, but they may cause weight gain.

Patients who take these drugs, which also can change how the body metabolizes carbohydrates and sugar, gain, on average, a total of about four pounds.

My advice: Talk to your doctor about *metformin*, a biguanide medication that helps improve the body's sensitivity to insulin and lowers the amount of sugar produced by the liver. This drug is less likely to cause weight gain and even could help obese people lose extra weight.

As an alternative, consider one of the newer, self-injectable drugs that have similar effects. *Liraglutide* (Victoza) is taken once daily...another injectable drug, *dulaglutide* (Trulicity), is taken once a week. The drugs closely mimic the body's natural insulin responses—and make weight gain less likely.

•***Tamoxifen*** **(Nolvadex, Emblon, others).** It blocks the effects of estrogen on breast cells and is used for the treatment and prevention of breast cancer. Some studies have found that women who take it can gain a total of 20 pounds or more within one to three years.

When you're dealing with cancer, weight is probably not your greatest concern—but the extra pounds can increase your risk for diabetes and other health problems.

Important: It's not entirely clear if tamoxifen directly causes weight gain. Women with cancer often deal with depression, which could negatively affect their eating habits and activity levels. Other drugs that are used in cancer treatments, such as steroids, also can lead to weight gain.

My advice: As much as you can, try to make a healthy lifestyle—wholesome foods, regular exercise, etc.—part of your cancer care. If you're doing well on a brand-name version of tamoxifen, keep taking it. The drug has a narrow therapeutic index, which means that even slight variations in blood levels—which can occur when you switch to a generic—can decrease the effectiveness and/or cause weight gain or other side effects.

Tamoxifen usually is taken for five years, but some patients may be able to stop it after two to three years and use an aromatase inhibitor drug instead. Two of these drugs *anastrozole* (Arimidex) and *exemestane* (Aromasin) are associated with less weight gain.

•***Divalproex sodium*** **(Depakote).** This drug, also known as *valproic acid*, is commonly prescribed for seizures, bipolar disorder and migraine prevention. It often increases appetite as well as cravings for fast-food fats and carbohydrates.

Important finding: A 2007 study published in *Seizure* found that about 24% of men and 44% of women gained significant amounts of weight (14 pounds, on average) after taking the drug for a year or more.

Other antiseizure drugs may also be used as mood stabilizers. Two of these medications, *carbamazepine* (Tegretol) and *oxcarbazepine* (Trileptal), may lead to weight gain, but a third drug, *lamotrigine* (Lamictal), is less likely to have this side effect. In fact, it may result in weight loss.

Lithium, another drug used to treat bipolar disorder, might (or might not) cause less weight gain than Depakote.

My advice: If you're taking Depakote, ask your doctor if other mood-stabilizing medications will work for you. If there is no viable substitute, exercise and a healthy diet are essential while taking this drug.

•**Atypical antipsychotics.** They can be lifesaving medications for patients with schizophrenia or other psychiatric disorders, but they're known for causing serious weight gain. The drugs affect dopamine and leptin, substances in the body that impact both food cravings and appetite.

The older drugs for treating psychiatric conditions are known to cause dystonic reactions, such as involuntary muscle movements. The newer atypical drugs, including *clozapine* (Clozaril) and *olanzapine* (Zyprexa), don't generally have this unpleasant side effect, but about one-third of patients gain 10 to 30 pounds within the first year.

My advice: Never stop taking an antipsychotic drug without your doctor's advice—the mental health consequences can be severe.

Helpful: Talk to your doctor about how to control weight gain when you first start taking the drug. Research has shown that patients who talk to their doctors about their weight concerns when starting any new medication—and who follow up with healthier eating and other lifestyle changes—often can lose weight and/or keep it off during treatment.

However, with any drug that causes weight gain, you may need the medication to treat a specific medical condition. Once the condition is under control, you then can focus on weight loss if needed.

Very Common Drugs That Rob Your Body of Nutrients

Hyla Cass, MD, integrative physician in private practice in Los Angeles. She is author of several books, including *8 Weeks to Vibrant Health* and *Supplement Your Prescription: What Your Doctor Doesn't Know About Nutrition.* CassMD.com

If you're taking a prescription medication every day, it may be interfering with your nutrition—and your doctor may not know it. This problem is so common that I wrote the book *Supplement Your Prescription: What Your Doctor Doesn't Know About Nutrition.*

Fortunately, you can protect yourself. When I treat patients who are taking prescription medications, I almost always prescribe specific nutritional supplements to head off deficiencies that the drugs can cause.

Important: These are the minimum doses for my standard nutritional prescriptions. You may benefit from higher doses, which you should discuss with your health-care provider.

If you take metformin (Glucophage, Glumetza, Fortamet): This diabetes drug can deplete vitamin B-12. Metformin also may deplete the body of the antioxidant and cardiovascular protector coenzyme Q10 (CoQ10). A study published in *Archives of Internal Medicine* showed that people with diabetes taking metformin had B-12 levels that were, on average, less than half the levels of people not taking the medication. Metformin also depletes folate (vitamin B-9). You most often will see this vitamin supplied as folic acid, which is then metabolized in the body to folate. (It also can be supplied as methylfolate for poor metabolizers of folic acid.)

Daily supplements needed…

- **Vitamin B-12 (1,000 mcg)**
- **Folic acid or methylfolate (400 mcg)**
- **CoQ10 (100 mg)**

If you take a corticosteroid such as *prednisone, prednisolone, betamethasone, budesonide, triamcinolone, cortisone* or *methylprednisolone*: While these anti-inflammatory drugs often are prescribed for short-term use to manage conditions such as allergic rashes, people with certain autoimmune conditions such as rheumatoid arthritis, Crohn's disease, ulcerative colitis and lupus often take them indefinitely. The nutrients they can deplete include calcium, folate, magnesium, potassium, selenium, vitamin D and zinc.

Daily supplements needed…

- **Calcium (600 mg)**

Note: Most of your calcium should come from food.

- **Folate (400 mcg)**
- **Magnesium (400 mg)**
- **Potassium (99 mg)**
- **Selenium (100 mcg)**
- **Vitamin D (1,000 IU)**
- **Zinc (25 mg)**

If you take an ACE inhibitor blood pressure drug such as *benazepril* (Lotensin), *enala-*

pril (Vasotec), *lisinopril* (Prinivil) or *ramipril* (Altace). These medications can deplete zinc.

Daily supplement needed: Zinc (25 mg).

If you take a calcium channel blocker for high blood pressure such as *amlodipine* (Norvasc), *diltiazem* (Cardizem), *felodipine* (Plendil), *isradipine* (DynaCirc), *nicardipine* (Cardene), *nisoldipine* (Sular) or *verapamil* (Calan, Covera-HS, Isoptin, Verelan): These medications deplete potassium.

Daily supplement needed: Potassium—the average daily requirement is 4.7 grams (4,700 mg), best obtained through eating potassium-rich foods including bananas, cooked spinach and many other fruits and vegetables. Supplements top out at 99 mg (found in your multi), while pharmaceutical supplements are higher but also contain a lot of unneeded chemicals. Have your potassium blood level checked, and go by your health practitioner's recommendation.

If you take a beta-blocker for high blood pressure and/or heart disease: It can deplete CoQ10.

Daily supplement needed: CoQ10 (100 mg).

If you take a statin to reduce cholesterol: It can deplete the body of CoQ10, which is vital for heart health.

Daily supplement needed: CoQ10 (100 mg).

If you take an antibiotic even for a short time: It can deplete the nutrients biotin, inositol, vitamins B-1 (thiamine), B-2 (riboflavin), B-3 (niacin), B-5 (pantothenic acid), B-6 (pyridoxine), B-12 (cyanocobalamin) and vitamin K—and interfere with the beneficial bacteria in your gut.

Also: Fluoroquinolones (any antibiotic that has a generic name that ends with the suffix "-floxacin," including the well-known *ciprofloxacin*, aka Cipro), can deplete calcium and iron. Tetracyclines (ending with the suffix "-cycline") can deplete calcium and magnesium. Trimethoprim-containing antibiotics (Trimpex, Proloprim, Primsol) can deplete folic acid. Penicillins (ending with the suffix "-cillin") can deplete potassium.

Daily supplements needed...

•**You needn't worry about how to find and take all those nutrients!** The doses of magnesium, calcium and other nutrients con-

tained in a good multivitamin/mineral supplement should cover your needs for these nutrients during a course of antibiotic therapy.

•**Additionally, find a high-potency B-complex supplement that contains close to these ingredients and doses**—B-1 (25 mg), B-2 (25 mg), B-3 (50 mg), B-6 (50 mg), folic acid (400 mcg to 800 mcg), B-12 (10 mcg), biotin (50 mg) and B-5 (50 mg). A "B-50" formula generally will provide these levels.

•**B-12 (1,000 mcg), taken in sublingual tablets for better absorption.**

•**Vitamin K (30 mcg to 100 mcg).**

•**After a course of antibiotics, take a probiotic supplement** to restore the beneficial bacteria in your gut. Choose one that contains at least one billion live organisms per daily dose and includes both Lactobacillus acidophilus (L. acidophilus) and Bifidobacterium bifidum (B. bifidum).

8 Surprising Things Your Pharmacist Can Do for You

Mohamed A. Jalloh, PharmD, pharmacist, assistant professor of clinical sciences at Touro University California and spokesperson for the American Pharmacists Association.

If you still think of your local pharmacist as just the person who fills your prescriptions, you're shortchanging yourself. This medical professional can be a key member of your health-care team, offering valuable information and services without the cost of a doctor's office visit. *He or she can...*

•**Review your current medications.** Your pharmacist knows how each of your medications works and what you should expect from taking it, including side effects and ways to avoid them—tips that your doctor may not have given you when prescribing it. Take advantage of this knowledge by scheduling a "medication checkup"—a review of any and all meds you currently take as well as supplements and over-the-counter drugs. Your pharmacist will look for any potential negative interactions among the drugs you're taking. This is especially important if you're on medications prescribed by different doctors or on supplements those doctors may not know you're taking. (For example, St. John's wort, an over-the-counter herbal supplement, is often taken for depression but can decrease the effectiveness of some drugs such as blood pressure medications.) To save you time, your pharmacist can coordinate refills to reduce the number of trips you take to the drugstore.

•**Give more than the flu shot.** Pharmacists can also administer immunizations for pneumonia, shingles, tetanus, hepatitis A and B, human papillomavirus and vaccines for international travel.

•**Help you know when over-the-counter remedies aren't enough.** Whether you're suffering from cold and allergy symptoms, dry eyes, bug bites or constipation, talk to your pharmacist about your symptoms. He knows what questions to ask you…and can then advise you on whether an over-the-counter med will likely help or whether you really should see a doctor.

•**Show you ways to avoid medication side effects.** Beyond whether to take a medication with food or water, your pharmacist can tell you how to time different meds so that they'll work best without affecting your quality of life. For example, the common antidepressant drug *fluoxetine* has a stimulant effect, so if you take it close to bedtime, you may have trouble sleeping. A good pharmacist will advise you to take it in the morning.

•**Help keep you on track with taking your meds.** Sticking with a medication plan is a challenge for a large number of Americans. Your pharmacist may be able to help you choose the right pill organizer or a phone app to better manage or track your medications.

•**Give guidance when you're buying medical supplies.** Pharmacists are in the know about devices used to manage chronic conditions.

Example: If you're shopping for a blood pressure cuff, your pharmacist will tell you that the ones you place on the wrist may be easier to use but aren't as accurate as the upper-arm models. Before you buy any medical device, get your pharmacist's opinion.

•**Save you money on drugs.** Some medications are more affordable if you buy them straight from the pharmacy, so always ask your pharmacist to check whether a drug is cheaper through the pharmacy's special-pricing program, if available. And unless your doctor has specified brand-only, a pharmacist is legally allowed to substitute a less expensive, generic version without a call to your health-care provider.

•**Dispense emergency refills.** If you run out of or lose a supply of a drug that you've been taking for a long time, your pharmacist may be able to give you up to a 72-hour supply on an emergency basis while you wait to get a renewal prescription from your doctor. (This emergency refill practice varies state by state.)

Note: He won't do this for any controlled substances such as those with a high risk for abuse such as opioids.

Take note: While your pharmacist can't prescribe most medications, depending on your state, he might be able to independently dispense drugs that you and he agree might benefit you such as *naloxone* (Narcan) used to reverse an overdose of opioid pain medication…nicotine-replacement medications…and oral contraceptives.

Bottom line: Developing a relationship with your local pharmacist is simply good for your health and simple to start—all you need to do is ask.

How to Get Experimental Drugs

Charles B. Inlander, a consumer advocate and health-care consultant based in Fogelsville, Pennsylvania. He was the founding president of the nonprofit People's Medical Society, a consumer advocacy organization credited with key improvements in the quality of US health care, and is author or coauthor of more than 20 consumer-health books.

New legislation, known as the federal Right-to-Try bill, was passed by Congress and signed into law by the president in late May 2018. While the new federal law creates uniformity, it's important to know that 38 states* have passed Right-to-Try laws since 2014. These laws and now the federal law allow doctors with terminally ill patients to petition drug companies so that experimental drugs can be used under certain circumstances, even though those drugs have not been FDA-approved for use…and may never be.

What most people don't realize: A person with a terminal condition and no available treatment options has more than the new Right-to-Try law to turn to for assistance. An existing program, known as expanded access, has already been achieving the same purpose with greater safeguards and consumer protection.

The downsides of Right-to-Try: The state and even the new federal laws are complicated and often come with strings attached.

How these laws work: Doctors can ask pharmaceutical companies to give a terminal patient an experimental drug that has successfully gone through Phase 1 clinical trials, even if that patient is not enrolled in the formal clinical trial program. While patients seeking treatment under Right-to-Try laws can gain access to potentially lifesaving experimental treatments, they don't get the FDA's advice on dosage and safety (based on the information from clinical trials), as routinely occurs when using the existing expanded access program (described in more detail below).

Under Right-to-Try laws, a pharmaceutical company also can refuse to participate in the program. And in half the states with Right-to-Try laws, insurers can deny paying for hospice coverage should a patient require it after using a Right-to-Try drug. Some state laws also allow insurers to deny coverage for the costs to treat any complications that result from the drug.

Better alternative: In 2009, due to pressure to give patients access to experimental drugs, Congress amended the Federal Food, Drug and Cosmetic Act to create an expanded access (sometimes called "compassionate use") program so that patients could get experimental treatments when enrollment in clinical trials is impossible. This program is effective and efficient.

How it works: Patients and/or their doctors fill out a request form (taking less than an hour) and submit it to the FDA. In emergency situations, the FDA will reply within 24 hours. Overall, the agency approves 99% of all requests.

Note: Patients usually find out about experimental treatments from their doctors but also can research such drugs online at Clinical Trials.gov to see which ones have passed at least Phase 1 clinical trials.

But more importantly—and something that does not happen in Right-to-Try requests—the FDA will make safety changes before approving the request, adjusting factors such as dosage or frequency of treatment, based on the information already gleaned from testing and clinical trials. This is far safer for the patient and helps the doctor better use the drug. Unlike most state and the new federal Right-to-Try programs, the expanded access protocol typically

---

Does Your Doctor Get Drug Company Perks?

A report in *JAMA* found that about half of US doctors received industry payments (including gifts). And even though most doctors swear that they can't be "bought" for the price of a steak dinner or a sleek coffee cup, research shows otherwise.

For example, generic drugs are virtually identical to brand-name counterparts, and cost 80% to 85% less. Yet doctors who receive money and/or gifts from drug companies are less likely to prescribe the generics.

When hospitals impose restrictions—such as banning free meals and drug samples—brand-name prescriptions decline. This suggests that small gifts do matter.

Curious about your own doctor? To see whether your doctor receives money from industry sources, check the ProPublica database at Projects.ProPublica.org/docdollars. You may be surprised by what you find!

Rebecca Shannonhouse, editor, *Bottom Line Health*.

---

*For a list of states that have Right-to-Try laws, go to RightToTry.org.

includes the experimental drug free of charge to the patient.

Given the choice, I'd rely on the expanded access program to get a much-needed treatment!

Are You Addicted to Painkillers?

Mel Pohl, MD, chief medical officer of Las Vegas Recovery Center in Nevada, where he played a key role in developing the center's chronic pain recovery program. Certified by the American Board of Addiction Medicine and a distinguished fellow of the American Society of Addiction Medicine, Dr. Pohl is coauthor of several books, including *The Pain Antidote* and *Pain Recovery*. LasVegasRecovery.com

Here's a common scenario: You've had surgery...or you threw your back out carrying groceries. To help you get over that distressing hump, your doctor prescribes an opioid painkiller—a class of drugs that includes morphine, codeine and *hydrocodone* (Vicodin) and newer heavyweights such as *oxycodone* (OxyContin) and *fentanyl* (Duragesic).

But a few weeks or even months later, the pain is still nagging you. Your doctor agrees to refill your prescription. Considering the daily drumbeat of scary statistics related to painkiller use and abuse, you'd think it wouldn't be so easy to get a steady supply of these drugs.

But it often is, and the consequences are dire. In the US alone, more than 42,000 deaths from drug overdoses in 2016 were blamed on opioids. This translates into 115 Americans dying each day from an opioid overdose. A large percentage of these opioid users begin using the drug to treat pain.

DRIVING HOME THE DANGERS

Pain is a very real problem. More than one in four Americans have suffered from pain that lasts over 24 hours, according to the National Center for Health Statistics, and chronic pain is the most common cause of long-term disability.

But new research drives home the startling fact that opioids—once introduced—are habit-forming. A 2017 study involving 1.3 million noncancer patients showed that 12% of people prescribed an initial six-day supply of an opioid painkiller were still taking the drug a year later. Those odds doubled to 24% if a 12-day supply was prescribed. When a month-long course of opioid pain medication was prescribed, 30% were still taking a painkiller a year later.

Clearly, short-term prescriptions can create long-term problems if we don't pay close attention to our use of these medications. It's surprisingly easy for a person to inadvertently become dependent on these drugs...or even addicted.

DEPENDENCE VS. ADDICTION

In the world of addiction treatment, there are subtle but important differences between dependence and addiction. The distinction helps guide treatment decisions. *What each means...*

•**Dependence is the steady use of a drug that stops short of addiction.** It happens when you find yourself taking higher and higher doses of a painkiller over time to achieve the same level of relief from a physical condition. This is known as tolerance. As the cycle progresses, you become physically dependent on the drug...and can't stop taking it without experiencing withdrawal symptoms. People keep taking the drug to avoid the distressing withdrawal symptoms they suffer between doses.

Physical withdrawal symptoms include tremors, sweats, nausea, vomiting and diarrhea. People who are dependent on a drug also may become depressed and anxious, have trouble sleeping or feel withdrawn without the drug. But in the case of dependence alone (not addiction), you're not getting "high" or intoxicated by the painkiller and you don't crave it—you're just searching for continued pain relief. While dependence usually takes hold after 10 to 30 days, it can occur in as little as a week's time.

•**Addiction is more serious.** When you are addicted to a drug, in addition to tolerance and physical dependence, you will crave it when it's not being used—sometimes months or years after the drug was last in your system—even when you're not feeling pain. When addiction sets in, you'll use more of the pain medication than intended (a hallmark of addiction known as "loss of control") and/or continue to use it despite the occurrence of serious harm or consequences.

It's a disease involving the brain's reward pathways and a vulnerability to having an enhanced response to mood-altering drugs, including painkillers. Some people will use these medications for their effects on mood (for example, to feel energetic, less depressed and less anxious), while others are genetically or environmentally predisposed to this intensified response.

DO YOU HAVE A PROBLEM?

To be diagnosed with addiction or dependence, you need to be assessed by a professional such as a psychologist, psychiatrist, addiction physician or drug-and-alcohol counselor. But you can begin to consider whether you might have a problem by answering the questions below. The more questions you answer with "yes," the greater the odds that you've got a potential problem and should see a medical professional.

1. As time passes, do you find yourself needing to increase the frequency or dose of your medication before pain returns?

2. Are you increasingly preoccupied by thoughts of taking the painkiller between doses?

3. Are you experiencing mood changes or changes in your motivation level?

4. Are you noticing problems with your ability to think, concentrate or remember things?

5. Are you experiencing new sleep disturbances, such as the inability to stay asleep?

6. Have you gone to another doctor because the first wouldn't renew your prescription for more medication or increase your dose?

7. Have you ever lied to anyone about how much medication you're actually taking?

8. Have you ever run out of a prescription before you were supposed to because you used more than was prescribed?

HOW TO SEEK HELP

What should you do if you realize that you're in trouble? No one wants to be labeled an "addict," but fear of that diagnosis shouldn't keep you from seeking expert help. Do not attempt to stop taking your medication cold turkey—this approach may actually be physically dangerous because it will precipitate withdrawal, which can lead to changes in blood pressure, pulse and even cardiac function due to hyperactivity of the nervous system.

Depending on your individual situation, outpatient or inpatient care may be necessary to properly supervise your withdrawal process. A specialist can assess your situation and make a treatment referral—self-diagnosis and selection of treatment are rarely enough. Seek professional help. To find an addiction specialist, consult the American Society of Addiction Medicine at ASAM.org.

Most Powerful Opioid Yet—What You Need to Know

David Sherer, MD, anesthesiologist, based in the Washington, DC, area. He is author of the Bottom Line blog, "What Your Doctor Isn't Telling You," and lead author of *Dr. David Sherer's Hospital Survival Guide*.

When we're hearing so much about an opioid crisis, it would seem like the last thing we need is another such drug on the market. Yet the FDA has not only approved a new synthetic opioid—but the drug is 1,000 times more potent than *morphine*. You may be asking yourself, *Are they crazy?* Good question! *Here are some answers…*

•**Sufentanil (Dsuvia),** the newly approved drug, is a sublingual tablet. The drug has already been in use for several years as both an intravenous and epidural injection for anesthesia. The new tablet form will be available only in one strength and will be preloaded into a dispenser that releases the tablet under the tongue where it is left to dissolve. Dsuvia is intended to be used only for rapid relief of severe pain and only in medical facilities…and it should be dispensed only by a licensed or supervised health-care provider. It will not be available by prescription for home use. The only exception to the medical-facility restriction will be use on a battlefield.

As might be expected, the FDA's announcement of its approval has sparked considerable controversy…

•Critics, including consumer advocacy, public health and health-care professionals, say that this drug does not add any benefits that are not already available from other drugs—while warning that it does contribute very serious additional dangers to an already-overwhelming opioid crisis. They cite the example of fentanyl, another synthetic opioid, that was approved by the FDA in 1984. Fentanyl was developed to be used only as an anesthetic but is now a tragically popular street drug. In 2017 alone, *fentanyl* killed close to 30,000 Americans. Dsuvia is up to 10 times stronger than fentanyl. It is naive to think, the critics warn, that Dsuvia won't also eventually make its way to the street, where it will pose a new and more potent risk for addiction, overdose and death.

•In defense of its decision, the FDA argues that the potency of Dsuvia is deceptive. The only dose in which it will be available is very small—30 micrograms (mcg), equivalent to the common dose of intravenous morphine, 5 milligrams (mg). They also point out that Dsuvia does have the advantage of bringing pain relief more quickly than IV morphine—in as short a time as six minutes, with relief lasting about three hours. (Fentanyl also can provide relief in minutes, while morphine can take up to 30 minutes to take effect, and relief lasts for several hours with both drugs.) In fact, the Department of Defense worked closely with the drug developer, AcelRx Pharmaceuticals, Inc., and wants the drug for battlefield injuries.

The FDA further notes that Dsuvia will not be approved for more than 72 hours of use, with a maximum of 12 tablets in 24 hours. It will come in a disposable, single-dose applicator, which should reduce the danger of drug overdose or abuse.

Other advantages: Dsuvia can be used under conditions when an IV can't be started… when there isn't a vein that can be used for injection…or when a person is unconscious or unable to swallow. Although fentanyl and morphine also can be given sublingually, Dsuvia dissolves and is absorbed much faster than morphine or fentanyl. Dsuvia is expected to be available in 2019. You won't need to be injured in battle to get it—it may soon be the go-to drug for rapid pain relief in hospitals and emergency rooms, such as in cases where a person is injured or in severe pain and doing an IV is too difficult or time-consuming.

Don't Get Addicted to Xanax, Ativan, Ambien or Some Other Sedative

Cara Tannenbaum, MD, professor in the faculties of medicine and pharmacy at Université de Montréal. She is director of the Canadian Deprescribing Network and codeveloper of its website DeprescribingNetwork.ca, which provides information to seniors and health-care providers about reducing/eliminating drug prescriptions to minimize side effects and improve health.

Imagine that you've had a particularly bad year. Maybe you've lost a close friend…suffered from financial problems…or struggled with frequent insomnia.

A doctor—maybe a psychiatrist, but more likely an internist or a family physician—might suggest that a sedative will help you get through the rough patch. The drug will probably be a benzodiazepine, a class of "sedative hypnotics" that includes popular medications like *alprazolam* (Xanax), *lorazepam* (Ativan) and many others. Or it could be a related "Z" drug, such as *zolpidem* (Ambien) and *zaleplon* (Sonata).

You'll immediately start to sleep better and worry less. But every day that you take it, the risk for side effects—including addiction—increases. Experts now believe that the risks are so high that "benzos" should never be the first choice for insomnia and/or anxiety…and that their use should be limited to four weeks or less.

DANGEROUS DRUGS

Benzodiazepines are among the most popular drugs ever developed. A recent study found that about one-third of older patients who took a benzodiazepine did so for months, years or even decades—even though these drugs are intended for short-term use.

Why it's a problem: Benzodiazepines and the related "Z" drugs bind to brain receptors that cause sedation. They're highly addictive in patients of all ages…but the risk for side effects is much higher in older adults because of an age-related decline in kidney function and an increase in fat mass, both of which cause the drugs to accumulate in the body. A dose that would quickly be metabolized and excreted in a younger adult might stay active for days in older adults.

Older patients who take these drugs are at increased risk for a number of health issues. For example, they are five times more likely to suffer from memory/concentration problems… four times more likely to experience daytime fatigue…and twice as likely to fall, suffer hip or wrist fractures or have car accidents. There's even some evidence that benzodiazepines may increase the risk of developing Alzheimer's or other forms of dementia.

Important: When benzodiazepines are taken with opioid painkillers, the risk for opioid overdose increases significantly.

TOO MANY PRESCRIPTIONS

It's common in medicine to prescribe potentially risky drugs when the benefits clearly outweigh the risks. But for most patients, benzodiazepines do not pass this simple test.

For every 13 patients taking these drugs, 12 are not gaining benefit. Conversely, about one in five patients who takes benzodiazepines suffers from serious impairments (the "number needed to harm"), such as memory problems, lack of concentration and daytime drowsiness, that interfere with function.

For about 10% of patients, benzodiazepines are essential treatments. They're used, in some cases long-term, for seizures and some mental disorders, including disabling anxiety. They can be lifesavers when used short-term for patients who are withdrawing from alcohol or other drugs. But the vast majority of prescriptions are written for patients who would do just as well—or better—with nondrug treatments.

GOING DRUG-FREE

When I meet with patients who take these drugs, many say that they would like to stop because of side effects, such as fatigue, memory loss, incontinence, etc. But the drugs are addictive. People who try to quit often experience intense insomnia, anxiety and other symptoms during the withdrawal period, which typically lasts one to four weeks.

Good news: We conducted a study that looked at 261 patients who were taking these drugs for at least three months. After six months, 62% of those in an intervention group (who were given a patient-education brochure that discussed drug risks, nondrug treatments and advice on discontinuing drugs) had asked their doctors/pharmacists for advice about stopping…and 27% did stop, compared with 5% in a control group.

Caution: If you've taken a benzodiazepine for months or years and have developed a physical dependence, don't quit "cold turkey." (After two to four weeks, everyone develops a physical dependence.) Abruptly stopping the drug can cause confusion, heart palpitations, nausea and sometimes mental disturbances, including hallucinations.

About half of patients who quit a benzodiazepine will experience at least some side effects. To make the process easier (and safer), experts recommend gradually decreasing the dose—under the supervision of a doctor—over several months. Some patients might go four to five months before they're completely drug-free. *What to expect…*

•**Anticipate discomfort.** When you start reducing doses, you will experience withdrawal. I warn patients that they'll feel like they have jet lag for a week or two. Stick it out! If you absolutely can't function while you're tapering, it's OK to take the same dose for a while longer—but never go back to a higher dose.

•**To deal with daytime sleepiness,** I advise patients to avoid taking a nap and to keep active. Expose yourself to bright light (either outside or with bright indoor lamps). The goal is to get back on a natural energy and day–night wake cycle. This includes not going to bed until you're ready to sleep.

•**If you're taking one of these drugs to deal with anxiety,** talk to a health-care professional or a therapist to identify the root cause

of your discomfort and to help you get through stressful situations.

Support groups for anxiety-related disorders can help you learn to manage stress more effectively.

Relaxation techniques, such as stretching, yoga, massage or tai chi, can be worthwhile, too.

•**To deal with insomnia,** consider cognitive behavioral therapy for insomnia (CBT-I) and the use of a sleep diary. These are the most effective nondrug therapies for insomnia.

For more information on tapering off a benzodiazepine, go to DeprescribingNetwork.ca and click on "Essential Information."

How to Tell If You're Hooked on Antibiotics

David Hyun, MD, senior officer, Antibiotic Resistance Project, The Pew Charitable Trusts and coauthor of study titled "Comparison of Antibiotic Prescribing in Retail Clinics, Urgent Care Centers, Emergency Departments, and Traditional Ambulatory Care Settings in the United States," published in *JAMA Internal Medicine*.

Treating with unnecessary antibiotics accelerates the emergence of antibiotic resistance—the development of bacteria that are no longer sensitive to the antibiotics currently available.

This is an extremely dangerous situation: It's estimated that, every year two million Americans get an antibiotic-resistant infection and 23,000 people die from one.

It's also possible to have adverse reactions to antibiotics, ranging from minor symptoms such as rashes and gastrointestinal discomfort to severe complications including Clostridium difficile, a bacterial infection that can result when the drug kills off healthful bacteria in your body, and the potentially deadly epidermal necrolysis, a disorder that starts with a severe skin reaction.

ILLNESSES THAT DO & DON'T NEED TO BE TREATED WITH ANTIBIOTICS

Some bacterial illnesses are very unlikely to go away without antibiotics. Two common ones are bacterial pneumonia and urinary tract infections.

Conditions that are often inappropriately treated with antibiotics include…

•**Viral upper respiratory tract infections including the flu**

•**Viral pneumonia and bronchitis**

•**Asthma**

•**Allergies**

•**Sinus infections**

•**Sore throat**

•**Middle ear infections**

However, complicating things is the fact that sometimes sinus infections, sore throats and middle ear infections are caused by bacteria and do require antibiotics. But there is no good way to collect samples from the sinuses or the ears in a typical doctor's office to culture to find out whether bacteria are present. These are situations when prescribing antibiotics to be safe might make sense.

On the flip side, some scientists are reevaluating the common procedure of treating acute uncomplicated diverticulitis (inflammation of small bulging pouches that can form in the lining of the digestive system, especially the colon) with antibiotics. Two studies published in the *British Journal of Surgery* concluded that antibiotics didn't speed up recovery time or prevent complications or recurrence of the infection. With the growing concern over antibiotic resistance, some European guidelines have started to recommend managing acute uncomplicated diverticulitis without antibiotics.

Doctors in the US have not yet reached this conclusion. A review published in 2018 in *The American Journal of Gastroenterology* found that not treating diverticulitis with antibiotics appears to increase the need for elective surgery, and surgery carries its own set of risks. More study is needed before doctors should stop prescribing antibiotics for this infection.

HOW TO AVOID TAKING UNNECESSARY ANTIBIOTICS

It helps to recognize that your expectations and approach to your medical visit play a significant role in whether a health-care provider prescribes an antibiotic.

When an illness lands you in your doctor's office or at an urgent care center, go without the preconceived idea of needing an antibiotic. Ask questions about your diagnosis so that you can help make an informed decision about your treatment. If the doctor thinks that an antibiotic is necessary, ask why so that you're confident it's the right course of action.

If you have a condition for which it's not possible to confirm a bacterial cause, such as a sinus infection, you might work out a treatment-and-follow-up plan with your doctor that puts off taking an antibiotic while you wait to see if other remedies help.

To keep your need for antibiotics to a minimum, double up on efforts to stay well. Antibiotic use increases in the winter and throughout flu season because the flu can look like a bacterial infection or can lead to one. Take all the preventive steps you can, including getting vaccinations that are appropriate for you and frequent hand washing.

The OTC Painkiller Trap

Leslie Kernisan, MD, MPH, clinical instructor, division of geriatrics, University of California, San Francisco. Board-certified in both geriatrics and internal medicine, she is founder of BetterHealthWhileAging.net, a website that provides practical information for older adults and family caregivers. She has a geriatric consultation practice in the Bay Area and writes about geriatrics and new technologies at GeriTech.org.

Many people assume that over-the-counter (OTC) drugs are less likely to cause dangerous side effects than their prescription counterparts. But that's not always true—especially when it comes to pain-relieving medications.

Nonsteroidal anti-inflammatory drugs (NSAIDs), a class of painkillers that includes *ibuprofen* (such as Advil and Motrin), *naproxen* (such as Aleve) and aspirin, cause more than 100,000 hospitalizations and 7,000 to 16,500 deaths each year.

Acetaminophen, the active ingredient in products such as Tylenol, Panadol and others, is generally safer than NSAIDs. But even this drug, the most popular painkiller worldwide, can cause liver damage and liver failure at too-high doses.

The problem: It's common for people who have chronic pain—whether it's from a bad back, persistent headaches or a bum knee—to take multiple doses daily and continue using the drug month after month, greatly increasing the dangers. This is particularly true for older adults, who metabolize drugs differently than younger people and are more likely to have health conditions (such as impaired kidney function) that increase the risks even more.

A SAFER CHOICE

You've likely heard that acetaminophen isn't helpful for painful conditions that involve inflammation, such as arthritis and joint injuries. Studies generally find that NSAIDs are a bit more effective than acetaminophen for arthritis pain, which is one of the main reasons that older adults use OTC painkillers. Still, since acetaminophen is so much safer (when used at recommended doses) than NSAIDs, I almost always advise older adults to try acetaminophen first.

Important: Acetaminophen stops being safe when people exceed the recommended dose. This can happen when people think that they need a higher dose…or when they (often unknowingly) use other products that contain it.

Acetaminophen is an ingredient in dozens of OTC medications, including sleep aids (such as Tylenol PM) and cold and flu remedies (NyQuil and Theraflu). It's also used in some prescription painkillers (such as Vicodin). If you don't check ingredient labels, you could wind up taking far more than the recommended limit of 3,000 mg per day. (Aiming to take less than 2,000 mg per day is even safer.)

To prevent liver damage, people with a history of alcohol abuse—or those who drink alcohol frequently—definitely shouldn't take more than 2,000 mg daily. I advise patients who take daily doses of acetaminophen for long-term problems (such as arthritis) to ask their doctors if their liver enzymes should be checked—either occasionally or regularly.

USE CAUTION WITH NSAIDS

NSAIDs, such as ibuprofen and naproxen, are never my first choice because they frequently cause stomach/intestinal bleeding...increase blood pressure...and lead to kidney damage in those who already have impaired kidney function.

Sobering caution: In 2015, the FDA strengthened existing label warnings on non-aspirin NSAIDs to alert consumers about the increased risk for heart attack and stroke, which can occur even in the first weeks of using one of these drugs—especially when taken at higher doses...and in people with and without heart disease.

Caveat: Because some people get more relief from an NSAID than from acetaminophen, it's sometimes reasonable to accept the risks of using an NSAID for a short time, such as a few days to a week. But even then, I am cautious about recommending them for patients who take blood thinners (NSAIDs have a blood-thinning effect) or have impaired kidney function or other health problems.

My advice: It's probably OK for older adults to take an occasional NSAID if they feel acetaminophen doesn't provide enough relief...but these drugs are not safe for daily use. People with arthritis or other long-term conditions should talk to their doctors about nondrug ways to manage pain, such as weight loss, physical therapy, exercise and cognitive behavioral therapy—all of which have been proven to be effective.

WHAT ABOUT ASPIRIN?

Doctors today almost never recommend aspirin as a pain reliever. Even at low doses (81 mg), it increases the risk for GI bleeding and for cerebral hemorrhage...and the risks for complications are higher among older adults and those with high blood pressure or other chronic diseases.

Aspirin is most likely to cause bleeding and other side effects when it's taken at doses of more than 100 mg daily for months or longer. But even low doses, as mentioned above, can be risky. Because of these risks, I try to discourage patients from taking aspirin as a pain reliever.

Exception: If you've had a heart attack or stroke, your doctor might advise you to take a daily aspirin (typically 81 mg) to prevent blood clots and a subsequent heart attack/stroke. The benefits of this so-called secondary prevention are believed to outweigh the risks.

However, experts no longer recommend aspirin for primary prevention (preventing a first heart attack/stroke) except for certain high-risk patients—for example, someone who has received a stent or has diabetes and another risk factor such as smoking or high blood pressure. Unless a person is at relatively high risk for a cardiovascular event, the risk of bleeding from a daily baby aspirin is generally higher than the chance of avoiding a heart attack or stroke due to this therapy.

THE TOPICAL OPTION

If you feel that you need an NSAID for pain relief, using a topical cream or gel reduces some of the risks. Topical NSAIDs used for musculoskeletal pain are effective, according to a Cochrane (a nonprofit group that evaluates medical treatments) review.

My advice: If your stomach can't handle oral NSAIDs—and acetaminophen doesn't seem to work—a topical drug (including OTC topical aspirin, such as Bengay, Aspercreme and other products with salicylate listed on the label) might be worth a try. Some people may also get relief from capsaicin cream.

The Life-Threatening Drug Reaction You've Never Heard Of

Alan D. Kaye, MD, PhD, professor, program director, and chairman of the department of anesthesiology and professor in the department of pharmacology at Louisiana State University Health Sciences Center in New Orleans, and coauthor of "Clinical Considerations for Epidermal Necrolysis" published in *The Ochsner Journal*.

Y ou've probably heard of—and maybe even experienced—sun sensitivity from a medication, such as a burn after a slight sun exposure. But some common drugs in some people can cause so severe a skin reaction that it can turn life-threatening. Yes, it's rare, but it's also something that kills.

Known as epidermal necrolysis (literally skin that dies and falls off), this umbrella term includes two conditions that used to be considered separate entities, Stevens-Johnson syndrome and toxic epidermal necrolysis. They differ only in the severity of the reaction. With Stevens-Johnson syndrome, up to 10% of your skin dies and detaches from your body...with toxic epidermal necrolysis, it's 30% or more.

Overall each year, epidermal necrolysis affects just over 2,000 people in the US—Stevens-Johnson syndrome occurs in up to six people per million and toxic epidermal necrolysis, about one person per million. So they're rare—but a lot of people have greater risk than those stats indicate. Women and people of Asian descent are at greater risk than the general population... and so are people with cancer, a weakened immune system, HIV infection and certain genetic variations. (That's why your risk is higher if you have a family history of either condition.)

Also at higher risk: People who have had pneumonia, bacterial infections, such as strep, and certain viral infections.

Could a medication that you're taking trigger epidermal necrolysis? There's a good chance of that because more than 100 drugs have been implicated. *But the following account for about half of all cases...*

•**Aromatic anticonvulsants** for seizures.

•**Allopurinol** for reducing uric acid and kidney stone prevention.

•**Medications in the "oxicam"** class of nonsteroidal anti-inflammatory drugs for pain relief such as Mobic.

•**Lamotrigine** for seizures and bipolar disorder.

•**Nevirapine** for HIV.

•**Sulfonamides** for bacterial infections.

Important: Epidermal necrolysis triggered by a medication can sometimes occur as long as two weeks after stopping that medication.

The first signs of epidermal necrolysis are fever and other flulike symptoms. Within a few days, a flat, red rash appears and the skin starts blistering and peeling, resembling a hot water burn.

This usually begins on the face and chest and then spreads to other parts of the body, including the mucous membranes of the mouth, eyes and genitals. Arms and legs are largely spared, but the blisters can develop on the palms of the hands and the soles of the feet.

Because skin is the body's protective barrier, damage from epidermal necrolysis can lead to fluid loss and open the door for potentially life-threatening infections. The death rate from Stevens-Johnson is about 1% to 2% (some estimates are higher)...from toxic epidermal necrolysis, it's 25% to 30%. Blindness can result due to lesions in the eyes. That's why hospitalization is a must, either in the ICU, a burn unit or a specialized dermatology unit. Treatment is similar to that for severe burns and involves steps to prevent infection, replace fluids and electrolytes, help skin heal and control pain. If the eyes are involved, daily eye evaluations by an ophthalmologist and aggressive treatment of the inflammation are necessary—this might include saline rinses to keep the eyes and eyelids clean, lubrication, topical corticosteroids and antibiotics. If a medication is thought to be the trigger, of course it will be stopped immediately.

Affected skin usually grows back in two to three weeks—how it looks varies from person to person. A full recovery can take one to two months depending on how severe the symptoms were. Patients are at risk for a recurrence should they ever take the same medication again, but there have also been reports of recurrences triggered by different medications. Anyone diagnosed with either type of epidermal necrolysis should carry an allergy card or wear an allergy bracelet with the diagnosis.

Awareness is your best prevention. Because some drugs linked to epidermal necrolysis are common while others are rare, it's best that any time you take a new medication, you check to see whether there's a black box warning on the packaging or insert and, if so, whether epidermal necrolysis is listed as a known risk (this is a good step to take in general to be better aware of all potential serious reactions in a drug you're taking).

Note: Epidermal necrolysis may only be described as Stevens-Johnson syndrome on some package inserts. If you see either term listed, be alert for the early signs described above. Also, always make sure the dose dispensed by your pharmacy is the dose your doctor ordered—because high doses can increase the risk.

Should you develop epidermal necrolysis and can trace it to a drug, make sure that all your doctors know what happened so that you won't be given any drugs from the same class in the future. You can learn more about both forms of epidermal necrolysis at the Stevens Johnson Syndrome Foundation (SJsupport.org).

What If You Really Do Need an Opioid?

Jane C. Ballantyne, MD, FRCA, professor of anesthesiology and pain medicine, University of Washington, Seattle. Dr. Ballantyne is coeditor of *Expert Decision Making on Opioid Treatments* and president of Physicians for Responsible Opioid Prescribing, SupportPROP.org.

Every day, more than 115 people in the US die after overdosing on opioids. And the efforts now being made to curtail addiction and stem the shockingly high death and overdose rates are all over the news.

Under-recognized problem: While there's no question that opioid addiction is a serious problem in this country, there are some circumstances where patients need these drugs.

Opioids are powerful drugs that need to be monitored. They aren't likely to cause problems when they're taken for a few days for acute pain (after surgery, for example), but long-term use can cause serious side effects, including osteoporosis, digestive problems (such as constipation) and opioid-induced endocrinopathy—decreases in testosterone and other hormones.

I provide long-term opioid prescriptions only for select groups of patients (discussed below). Patients with acute pain—after a back injury, for example—might need opioids, but should take them for as short a time as possible…and only if they can't get adequate pain relief from safer approaches, such as exercise, physical therapy and/or over-the-counter (OTC) *acetaminophen* (Tylenol) or a nonsteroidal anti-inflammatory drug (NSAID), such as *ibuprofen* (Motrin) or *naproxen* (Aleve). Prescription antidepressants or anticonvulsants also can reduce pain regardless of its cause.

With some exceptions, I advise patients never to start treatment with *hydrocodone* and *acetaminophen* (Vicodin), *oxycodone* (OxyContin) or other opioids and to try other pain-relief methods first.

Exceptions: Patients who are terminally ill can have a much higher quality of life when they take high doses of opioids—and not just because of pain relief. Someone with a terminal cancer, for example, might feel more at peace when taking the drugs. Similarly, patients with intractable diseases that impair their ability to function—such as spinal cord injuries, severe multiple sclerosis, etc.—might do better when they take the drugs.

But for those who can do without an opioid, lifestyle approaches, including cognitive behavioral therapy or physical activity, can sometimes relieve pain more than prescription or OTC drugs. Only take an opioid when other approaches don't work…and only take a dose that's high enough to relieve pain but low enough to allow you to function normally. *Also important…*

•**Set limits.** Some doctors continue to write opioid prescriptions too casually.

My advice: Don't take an opioid for short-term pain unless you have a very clear injury—after a car accident, for example. Even then, take the drug for a few days at most.

Also: The safest way to take opioid medications—both for acute and chronic pain—is to use them only as needed to control severe or sudden pain…not around the clock, unless it's absolutely necessary.

•**Attend a pain clinic.** Patients with complex pain do better when they work with pain specialists at an interdisciplinary clinic (available at most major medical centers), where the medical team typically includes doctors, nurses, psychologists and physical therapists. Opioid medications may be prescribed carefully in these settings, but the emphasis is on other safer, longer-lasting methods of pain relief.

•**Talk to your doctor about dosing.** It's common for patients taking opioids to develop tolerance—they gradually require more medication to get the same relief. This is not the same as addiction. However, the higher doses will increase the risk for side effects, including addiction. Do not change your medication or dose on your own. Get your doctor's advice.

•**Ask about longer-acting drugs.** Patients with acute pain after surgery or an injury often need a fast-acting drug, such as nasal or sublingual (under-the-tongue) *fentanyl*. But patients with chronic pain usually do better with longer-acting drugs, such as extended-release *oxymorphone* (Opana ER) or a *buprenorphine patch* (Butrans).

Long-acting drugs provide a steady level of medication to stabilize their effectiveness—with fewer "letdowns" that can lead some patients into inappropriate addictive behavior. They're not a perfect solution because patients who take them may be given an additional prescription for a fast-acting drug to control "breakthrough" pain.

Addiction isn't likely to be a problem if you use these powerful medications only when needed and with the caveats described above.

Drugs That Can Damage Tendons

Robert E. Markison, MD, hand surgeon and clinical professor of surgery at the University of California, San Francisco. MarkisonMD.com

Some of the most surprising drug side effects don't make the top of the list on that insert your pharmacist hands you with your prescription. Yet they can be both more dangerous and less obvious than, say, nausea, constipation or dizziness. We're talking about soft-tissue injuries. Involving tendons, ligaments or muscles, these can be not only painful but also hard to heal. *Here are some of the drugs mostly likely to cause this damage...*

STATINS

These cholesterol-lowering drugs, including *atorvastatin* (Lipitor), *fluvastatin* (Lescol), *lovastatin* (Mevacor or Altoprev), *pravastatin* (Pravachol), *rosuvastatin* (Crestor), *simvastatin* (Zocor) and *pitavastatin* (Livalo), also block the formation of coenzyme Q10 (CoQ10), essential for synthesizing ATP, a chemical produced by mitochondria, the tiny powerhouses in every cell. ATP is the fuel needed for every body function, from thinking to moving to healing wounds.

By interfering with CoQ10 and ATP production, statin drugs may not only cause muscle pain, which is now well-known, but also can cause ruptures of the biceps and Achilles tendons, tendinitis in the wrist and trigger finger. With trigger finger, one or more fingers can lock or catch as you bend and straighten your hand. Some people must unlock their fingers manually with the other hand! Also, if you have an existing repetitive strain injury, such as carpal tunnel syndrome, statins can worsen it by causing tendinitis.

What's better: If you must take cholesterol drugs, ask your physician about alternatives to statins. If you must take a statin, ask whether the dosage could be reduced and also take a daily 200 mg to 300 mg supplement of CoQ10 to offset the drug's negative impact on mitochondria. The liquid form (Qunol) is best. Redoubling your lifestyle efforts to improve your diet and adding moderate exercise should also help reduce cholesterol in many people.

FLUOROQUINOLONES

These are drugs prescribed for acute illnesses such as bronchitis and sinus and urinary tract infections. The chief offender is *ciprofloxacin* (Cipro), but others include *gemifloxacin, levofloxacin, moxifloxacin, norfloxacin* and *ofloxacin*. These drugs can cause tendon problems because they interfere with collagen-regulating components (called matrix metalloproteinases) that maintain tendon integrity. (*Reminder:* Collagen cells are constantly replacing themselves.)

If you disturb this normal renewal process, the tendon may not have the strength to withstand the stress of repetitive motion and static posture. Some patients on Cipro for only one day have been brought to a standstill from the medication-induced aches and pains. Others experience tendinitis or nerve damage in the carpal tunnel system of the wrist or higher up in the neck and shoulder area.

What's better: Ask your doctor to prescribe another class of antibiotic based on the specific bug you are fighting.

AROMATASE INHIBITORS

Drugs in this group are used for treating hormone-positive breast cancer and include *anastrozole* (Arimidex), *exemestane* (Aromasin) and *letrozole* (Femara). When you "inhibit" aromatase, which turns androgen into estrogen, your body stops making estrogen, which can fuel the growth of cancer cells. But there's an association between using an aromatase inhibitor and developing trigger finger. Other side effects are joint stiffness and pain as well as bone loss and fractures.

What's better: Talk to your oncologist about taking *tamoxifen* instead of an aromatase inhibitor to help prevent a cancer recurrence.

CORTICOSTEROIDS

While *prednisone* and other drugs in this group can be absolutely lifesaving for people who otherwise couldn't breathe because of asthma or COPD, they can make your soft tissues very thin and weak and potentially rupture tendons.

What's better: If you must take steroids, be on as low a dose as possible for as short a time as possible.

LIFESTYLE HABITS THAT HELP

When you must be on any of the above drugs, double down on other health measures to help resist these side effects. These include getting restorative sleep, eating a healthful diet and making sure to get the appropriate daily amounts of vitamins A, B-6, B-12, C and D. Don't drink alcohol, don't smoke and don't eat gluten—gluten has been heavily hybridized and whether or not celiac disease (the intestinal wheat intolerance) is present, many patients experience gluten-related inflammation in a number of body systems.

While it's important to be as physically fit as possible, when exercising, avoid strenuous moves that could tax your tendons, specifically yoga's downward dog, the wrist-loading exercises such as the plank and strength-training with heavy weights—if you can't lift a weight for eight reps without straining, the weight is too heavy.

Beware These RX Mistakes

Frank Moriarty, PhD, senior research fellow, HRB Centre for Primary Care Research, Royal College of Surgeons, Ireland, Dublin.

In a review of 38,229 primary care patients age 65 and older, about half were prescribed potentially inappropriate medications, and the percentage was even higher among those who were hospitalized.

Examples of inappropriate prescribing practices: Receiving a higher dose of a current medication…and failure to stop or reduce a drug dosage after hospital discharge.

Self-defense: Carry a list of the medications you are currently taking (with dosages and reasons for use) whenever you see your primary care doctor or are admitted to the hospital—and review any changes with your doctor.

Apps for Saving on Prescriptions

Roundup of experts on medication costs, reported at WiseBread.com.

Easy Drug Card produces discounts of up to 80% if you do not have insurance or your insurance will not cover a medicine's costs—and it works for pet medicines, too.

•**FamilyWize** works whether or not you have insurance and reduces prescription costs by an average of 40%.

•**GoodRX** lists the price of any medicine at multiple pharmacies near you so that you can buy from the lowest-cost location and posts coupons that you can use to reduce prices further.

•**ScriptSave WellRX** does a similar price search and offers a savings card that can produce discounts up to 80%.

FDA Approval Doesn't Mean These Drugs Will Work Well

David Bearman, MD, a practitioner of cannabinoid medicine in private practice in Goleta, California. He is vice president of the American Academy of Cannabinoid Medicine and author of the forthcoming book *Cannabis Medicine*. DavidBearmanMD.com

The Food and Drug Administration has paved the way for drugs derived from the cannabis (marijuana) plant. But these won't work as well as they could.

Example: Epidiolex, the first such US prescription drug, treats the childhood seizure disorder Dravet syndrome. The active ingredient is cannabidiol (CBD), a compound that doesn't produce a "high," and it has only trace amounts of tetrahydrocannabinol (THC), which does. While CBD itself has therapeutic benefits, it often is more effective when combined with THC and other cannabis compounds. Studies show that's true for seizure disorders.

The CBD/THC combination is particularly important in treating a much more common medical dilemma—chronic pain. Consider *nabiximols* (Sativex), a spray medication with a 1:1 CBD/THC ratio. US clinical trials find that it effectively treats intractable pain, and it does it as well as the narcotic *codeine*. Sativex is legal for doctors to prescribe in 28 countries but not the US. Sativex only rarely causes patients to feel uncomfortably euphoric or "stoned." Many other cannabis formulations also reduce the amount of narcotics needed to relieve pain.

The truth is, cannabis has a wide range of therapeutic applications, including stimulating appetite, preventing nausea, bringing down chronic inflammation and even treating certain cancers.

What to do? While neither Sativex nor any other whole-cannabis medication is legal on a federal level, similar products are available in states where medical cannabis is legal. For some conditions, a high-CBD/low-THC formulation may be best. For others, a product with a 1:1 ratio may best serve you.

If you are considering using a medical marijuana dispensary, find a qualified cannabinoid medical practitioner who can guide you to the right formulation and who will adequately discuss the possible side effects of euphoria. To find one, go to the website of the American Academy of Cannabinoid Medicine (AACMSite.org), The Society of Cannabis Clinicians (CannabisClinicians.org) or the Association of Cannabis Specialists (Cannabis-Specialists.org).

CHAPTER 13

Men's Health

Myths About Male Sexuality

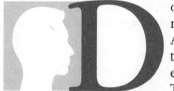

Do men crave sex more than women? Are they always in the mood? Do men enjoy the "chase"? The honest answers may surprise both genders.

In the movies, men always initiate sex—and like being in charge. Real life doesn't necessarily match that mystique. Male sexuality is far more complicated, and these myths not only hold couples back from finding deeper intimacy and connection, they can damage their sex lives with inappropriate expectations. When a man doesn't want sex, his female partner often feels alarmed. (He's supposed to want this, so there must be something wrong with me or our relationship.) And he may worry that his lagging interest is a sign that he's not masculine enough.

These are the most common misconceptions about men and sex—and the reassuring truths behind them that will help both of you connect in a more open way…

***MYTH #1:* Men are always in the mood for sex.** We have been taught that men have higher sex drives than women have. On the flip side, we're all familiar with the stereotype of a wife saying, "Not tonight, honey. I have a headache."

Reality: Research on men between the ages of 30 and 60 found that the guys were no more likely than their female partners to be the one with higher desire. While some research shows that 15% of men have had "problematic sexual desire" over the past six months, the percentage of men who have episodes of low desire is probably higher than that, according to my research. Ideally partners have a similar level of sexual interest, but when there is a discrepancy, it's just as common for the female as the male to be in the mood.

Sarah Hunter Murray, PhD, sex researcher and relationship therapist in private practice in Winnipeg, Manitoba. She is author of *Not Always in the Mood: The New Science of Men, Sex, and Relationships.* SarahHunterMurray.com

Problem: Because we believe the myth, women often squash down their desire, thinking, *I really shouldn't want sex more than he does.* They don't feel that it's their place to initiate it. A woman also may see his lack of interest as a sign that she's not attractive to him. Meanwhile, he may feel embarrassed or confused by his lack of desire. They're both left wondering, *Is there something wrong with us?*

New way of thinking: There's so much variability in sexual drive that there really is no "normal." Understanding that men have many of the same issues that women have—they're stressed, they're tired, they don't feel attractive—helps both partners feel understood. A man's desire at any given moment is not a marker of his partner's level of attractiveness. Your desires won't always be perfectly synced—leave a little space for each other to not be in the mood sometimes. Consider simply cuddling, since you don't need an orgasm to have intimacy. If "not tonight" starts becoming a pattern, try saying in a loving way, "I've noticed I've been in the mood a few times, and you haven't been. Is anything going on there?"

MYTH #2: Men's desire is driven solely by a woman's physical appearance. You've probably heard that male arousal starts with physical cues, such as seeing his wife's legs when she is wearing a short skirt.

Reality: When I ask men how important physical appearance is, they say, "Yes, I like it when she shows off her body, but if I'm not feeling emotionally connected to her, if we're not on the same page, then that isn't enough to do it for me." They feel most turned on when their relationship is running smoothly.

Problem: Believing the myth that all men want women with a 36-24-36 body completely ignores the depth of a man's sexuality. Women sometimes worry when they put on weight or get older that their partners will no longer be attracted to them.

New way of thinking: Yes, looks matter to some degree, but men have different views of beauty and are, in reality, most drawn to a woman's confidence and her ability to let him know, *I want to connect with you sexually.* Again and again, I have heard men talking about their sexual desire for partners who had a physical disability or who had put on weight after having children or who were in their 50s or older. It was her comfort in her own skin and willingness to share her body with him that was the real turn-on.

MYTH #3: Men are selfish in bed. The common stereotype is that a guy is looking out for only his own sexual needs—it's mainly about him climaxing and then rolling over and going to sleep.

Reality: Men want so much more than one-sided gratification. Men repeatedly told me how important their partners' sexual pleasure was to them. If she was acquiescing to sex—consenting but not really excited about it—that was a major turnoff. They would say, "I don't want to be having sex with somebody who isn't super-excited to be having sex with me." Bringing a woman pleasure and providing an orgasm feed into his feelings of masculinity. Men see their mate's enjoyment as a sign that they are on the same page. Pleasing her in the bedroom helps him feel connected to her outside the bedroom, too.

Problem: If a woman believes this myth— that he is looking only for his own sexual needs to be met—she might feel dismissive of him, thinking, *This is only for you. What's the point?*

New way of thinking: Recognize that he might want sex because he is longing to feel closer and that he truly wants to make you happy. This, in turn, will make you feel more receptive, which can lead to greater intimacy.

MYTH #4: Men like to be in charge in the bedroom. Society tells us that men should be the ones to initiate sex. Some of this goes back to college, when men tend to get socially rewarded for having sexual partners, while women are taught to be gatekeepers. ("Good girls don't have sex.") So a man still may feel pressure to pursue and make the first move.

Reality: Research tells us that men are getting tired of that standard. They feel enormous pressure to be the ones who make the first move, and they long for their partners to initiate, too. Why? It makes them feel good. It makes them feel wanted. And it makes them feel that some of that responsibility to take charge in the bedroom is off their shoulders. Also, it makes them feel vulnerable to always initiate sex and deal with the fear of rejection.

New way of thinking: While you may not be used to making the first move, it can be really empowering to step into a more assertive role. It's a mind-set of, *Hey I want closeness—so why not reach out instead of sitting passively waiting to see if he reads my signals?* Nonsexual overtures can be a good place to start—rubbing his shoulders or giving a little foot massage.

MYTH #5: **When men don't want it, something serious must be going on.**

Reality: The reasons that men might not be in the mood are the same as the ones that women report. It's been a long day. They're stressed. They're tired. We all have reasons to say no to sex that have nothing to do with our partners, and we need to be understanding about that.

Problem: While we're used to talking about what happens to a woman's sexuality after having kids, we don't discuss that a man's desire can take a nosedive, too. Research shows that dads today are more involved in their children's lives. They're changing diapers at night…they're coaching the hockey team…and they're feeling worn out and not always up for romance.

New way of thinking: Both sexes need time to recharge in order to be receptive to sex. It's essential to find pockets of time both separately and together. Allow for transition time after work—a little time to change clothes or read the mail. Ease into together time. Don't feel pressured to schedule special events—just going to bed at the same time can help you feel more in sync.

MYTH #6: **Men are confident and don't need compliments.** Have you noticed that women get complimented on their appearance much more than men do? They hear, "Your dress is so cute" or "I love your haircut." Men? Not so much.

Reality: Over the course of my research, I learned something startling—men wish they had this sort of attention from women. They want to be looked at by their partners. They want to be able to say, "Yes, I have been working out!" It's important to their desire, and it's

something that rarely gets talked about because it goes against that norm.

New way of thinking: How can a woman make her partner feel noticed? Giving him compliments such as, "I love how that shirt brings out your eyes," shows that you appreciate him in a physical way. Nonverbal cues (a peck on the cheek or a pat on the bum) also send him the reassuring message that he still does it for you.

Speak Up, Men! Don't Be Embarrassed by Incontinence

Study titled "Prolonged Duration of Incontinence for Men Before Initial Anti-Incontinence Surgery: An Opportunity for Improvement," led by researchers at The University of Texas Southwestern Medical Center, Dallas, published in *Urology*. For the study, researchers reviewed the records of 572 men who were evaluated for stress incontinence over a 10-year period.

Urinary incontinence is a women's problem, right? Not by a long shot! Men account for about 15% of the 13 million Americans who suffer from some degree of urinary incontinence.

When this annoying problem affects a man, it commonly comes in a form known as stress incontinence. With this condition, urine leaks when a man coughs, laughs, lifts something heavy or exerts himself during exercise. Men who have undergone prostate removal (prostatectomy) for prostate cancer are at increased risk.

Rates of stress incontinence following removal of a diseased prostate can be as low as 4% or as high as 42%. When a man is affected, it can dramatically impact his quality of life and increase his risk for depression. While some improvement comes with time, any residual incontinence left after a year is unlikely to go away on its own.

Considering the negative consequences of urinary incontinence, urologists at the University of Texas Southwestern Medical Center in Dallas wanted to find out just how long men tolerate the problem. The researchers' analysis focused on men who were evaluated by a urologic surgeon to determine how much time passed before they sought surgical treatment for their stress incontinence.

Study results: Most men put up with the problem for a median of more than two years, while one-third of them waited more than five years. Interestingly, younger men tended to wait less, but some men in their 80s waited a median of more than seven years before seeking anti-incontinence surgery.

A useful test for men: As part of this study, researchers recommended that both primary care doctors and urologists use a "standing cough test" as a simple, noninvasive method to determine the severity of a man's stress incontinence following prostate surgery. With this test, a man is asked to cough while standing. If he loses urine, he is suffering from stress incontinence. If he has minimal leakage, a surgically implanted "sling" procedure may be considered...if the leakage is more severe, he may need to replace his sphincter muscle with an artificial sphincter. The cough test is believed to be more reliable than asking a man how many incontinence pads he uses each day.

Bottom line: It's understandable that men would not rush into another operation quickly after prostatectomy, but if they are bothered by incontinence past the 12-month mark, it's time to talk with their urologist about possible surgical options.

When urinary incontinence is surgically treated, 73% to 90% of men report greater satisfaction and quality of life.

An "ED Gene"

Proceedings of the National Academy of Sciences.

The risk for erectile dysfunction (ED) is 26% higher in men with a particular gene variation. The discovery could lead to new, gene-based therapies to help the 50% of men who don't respond to Viagra or similar drugs prescribed for ED.

Considering a Late Shot at Fatherhood? Don't Toss Your Condoms Just Yet!

Michael Eisenberg, MD, director of the male reproductive medicine and surgery program at Stanford University School of Medicine in Stanford, California, and senior author of "Association of Paternal Age with Perinatal Outcomes Between 2007 and 2016 in the United States: Population-Based Cohort Study" published in *The BJM*.

While the health risks for babies of older moms have been known for some time, a study done at Stanford University suggests that a man's age can have a completely different set of concerns, not only for their babies but also for the moms as well.

The study tracked the maternal records of 40.5 million live births in the US and organized the babies' dads into five age groups, ranging from under age 25 to over 55. The researchers also controlled for factors such as smoking history, access to medical care and the mother's age—anything that might skew the results.

What they found was stunning. Babies born to men over age 45 were 14% more likely to be born prematurely, 14% more likely to have a low birth weight and 14% more likely to be admitted to an intensive care nursery for fetal monitoring than when the dad was under age 35.

Babies born to fathers age 55 and over were an additional 10% more likely to need a ventilator to help with breathing upon birth and an additional 28% more likely to be admitted to an intensive care nursery.

Surprisingly, the women giving birth to older men's babies were 28% more likely to develop gestational diabetes, a condition that's dangerous for both the mom and her unborn baby during pregnancy and possibly beyond, even when the gestational diabetes itself goes away.

The reason for all these risks is uncertain, but several likely possibilities exist. Along with wrinkles in their skin, older men get the equivalent of wrinkles in their sperm. Once a man begins to produce sperm, he begins to accumulate two new mutations to his DNA every year. Those mutations may accumulate in genes relevant to creating a baby.

What can you do? The connection between the dad's age and the baby's (and the mom's) health needs more study. But for now, older men should consider these findings and discuss them with their doctor and their partner before deciding if and when it's time for a child. And younger men and their partners should also weigh them as they start family planning—and perhaps not wait as long as they thought they might to have children.

Natural Ways to Reverse Erectile Dysfunction

Geo Espinosa, ND, LAc, IFMCP, CNS, naturopathic doctor, and clinical assistant professor in urology at New York University Langone Medical Center in New York City. He is author of *Thrive, Don't Only Survive: Dr. Geo's Guide to Living Your Best Life Before & After Prostate Cancer* and coauthor of *Bottom Line's 1,000 Cures for 200 Ailments: Integrative Medicine for the Most Common Illnesses. Disclosure:* Dr. Espinosa is cofounder of XY Wellness, LLC, that sells a combination ED supplement called XYVGGR. DrGeo.com

---

If you're a man reading this article, there's a reasonable chance that you have erectile dysfunction (ED)—you haven't been able to achieve and maintain an erection that is satisfactory for you and your partner. While it happens to some younger men, by age 40 22% of men have ED in some form, ranging from moderate/intermittent to severe, and by age 70, about 50% do. It's often progressive—it'll get worse if you don't do something about it.

But isn't the solution easy? After all, Viagra, Levitra and Cialis—prescription drugs that increase blood flow to the penis—are popular. They certainly help. But side effects can be severe, including headache, facial flushing, blurred vision, temporary hearing loss and back pain. Worse yet, these drugs actually can interfere with enjoyable sexual intercourse.

The good news is that in most cases ED can be prevented—or treated—without these drugs. *That's because the more natural interventions discussed below almost always work to restore erections…*

THESE SUPPLEMENTS MAKE A DIFFERENCE

There are four nutrients and herbs that I prescribe to prevent or reverse ED.

Important: Don't start taking these on your own. Do so under medical supervision (more on that below). You'll also need a little patience. These supplements work gradually, so they're best used on a daily basis, not right before sex. *Here they are…*

• **L-citrulline.** This amino acid converts in the body to L-arginine, which in turn boosts levels of nitric oxide, a gaseous chemical that relaxes the "smooth muscle" in the penis, opening up penile arteries and improving blood flow. These changes also are good for your cardiovascular system—L-citrulline can reduce high blood pressure, for example.

Scientific research: L-citrulline has been shown in clinical studies to improve erectile function in men with ED. In research at David Geffen School of Medicine at UCLA, it also has been shown to be effective when combined with other supplements. My typical prescription is to take L-citrulline twice a day on an empty stomach for a daily total of 750 milligrams (mg) to 1,500 mg.

Warning: If your blood pressure is low, either naturally or through treatment, L-citrulline can bring it down too low.

• **Horny goat weed** (Epimedium grandiflorum). This herb is rich in icariin, which, like the L-citrulline described above, boosts nitric oxide. It also helps normalize enzymes that control penile blood flow. My typical prescription is to take horny goat weed twice a day on an empty stomach for a daily total of 200 mg to 400 mg. Like L-citrulline, it may reduce blood pressure too low in people with low pressure.

• **Ashwagandha.** This herb from India boosts testosterone. Testosterone deficiency is a common cause of low libido and ED. Ashwagandha also is an adaptogen, an herb that helps the body deal with stress, a major factor in ED. It reduces the stress hormone adrenaline, which in excess tightens arteries, decreasing blood supply to the penis. My typical prescription is to take ashwagandha twice a day on an empty stomach for a daily total of 500 mg to 1,500 mg. It may cause stomach upset in some people.

Important: Don't take this supplement unless you have a testosterone deficiency—only a test done by your doctor can tell you that.

•**Rhodiola rosea.** This is another herbal adaptogen that helps restore physical and mental energy. Exhaustion, particularly at the end of a difficult day, is a common cause of ED.

Scientific research: Salidroside, one of the active ingredients in rhodiola, helps maintain the flow of oxygen to the corpora cavernosa, the spongy penile tissue that fills with blood to create an erection, according to a study published in *Evidence-Based Complementary* and *Alternative Medicine.*

HOW TO USE THESE SUPPLEMENTS

Seek out a complementary/integrative health professional, such as a naturopathic doctor, who can guide you. These supplements often work best in some combination depending on the patient's overall health profile. It's especially important to work with a complementary health-care professional if you already are being treated for ED—and even more so if you have another condition such as diabetes or heart disease and already take prescription medications or other supplements. A good integrative physician also will help you make essential lifestyle changes that are part of your journey back to sexual health.

THE GOOD-IN-BED DIET

Men with ED often have cardiovascular disease and/or diabetes, both of which impair blood flow. A diet proven to control and reverse those two deadly diseases also is effective for ED—the Mediterranean diet, rich in vegetables, fruits, beans, whole grains, fish, nuts and seeds, and olive oil, with a minimum of red meat, processed meat and refined carbohydrates.

Scientific evidence: In research published in *The Journal of Sexual Medicine,* Italian doctors studied more than 600 men with diabetes. Compared with men who ate the fewest foods in the Mediterranean diet, those who ate the most were 17% less likely to have any level of ED and 38% less likely to have severe ED (having erections infrequently or not at all). In another study, men newly diagnosed with type 2 diabetes ate either a Mediterranean diet or a low-fat diet. After eight years, those eating the Mediterranean diet were much less likely to have developed ED.

THE EXERCISE PRESCRIPTION

Exercise is a must in any approach to preventing and reversing ED. It improves circulation, boosts testosterone and reduces stress.

New scientific finding: In a scientific paper published in *Sexual Medicine,* researchers analyzed data from 10 studies on exercise and ED and found that six months of regular exercise helped reverse ED in men who were sedentary, overweight, had high blood pressure or had cardiovascular disease. *My recommendations...*

•**Interval training.** Compared with moderate aerobics, high-intensity interval training will help you shed more weight, get fitter faster and add more testosterone-triggering muscle.

What to do: Whether your aerobic activity is walking, running, biking or swimming, do it at a moderately easy pace for 60 seconds—and then as fast as you can for 15 to 20 seconds.

Caution: Men who have not regularly physically stressed their bodies should consider getting a cardiovascular evaluation that includes a stress test to confirm that their heart can handle the workout.

•**Dead lifts.** A circuit of strength-training exercises for all your muscles is great for you. One particular exercise should be part of your training, though—the dead lift. You lift a weighted bar off the ground to the level of your hips, then lower it slowly back. Dead lifts use the large muscles of the legs, buttocks and back, and the more muscle, the more testosterone. Safe, correct form is key, so learn from a trainer at a gym or by watching one of the many YouTube videos on dead lifts. Do the exercise as part of your strength-training program at least two to three days a week. A set is lifting the weight six times in a row. Work up to six sets, resting two minutes between sets. If you are able to do more than six repetitions without resting, the weight is too light.

REDUCING PERFORMANCE ANXIETY

If you're not confident before sex—if you're anxious about achieving or keeping an erection, an anxiety common in men who have experienced ED—it's more likely you will have erectile difficulties.

Smart idea: Just as professional athletes visualize their desired outcomes before performing, creating mental images of a successful performance such as getting a hit, making a basket or sinking a putt, you can visualize successful sexual performance. Take a few minutes to visualize yourself getting erect and enjoying intercourse. And then start sex with more confidence.

It's important to realize that no one thing alone reverses ED. But the right diet, exercise regimen, supplement combination and mental attitude can indeed reverse ED—close to 100% of the time.

Natural Ways to Boost Testosterone

Geo Espinosa, ND, LAc, IFMCP, CNS, naturopathic doctor, and clinical assistant professor in urology at New York University Langone Medical Center in New York City. He is author of *Thrive, Don't Only Survive: Dr. Geo's Guide to Living Your Best Life Before & After Prostate Cancer* and coauthor of *Bottom Line's 1,000 Cures for 200 Ailments: Integrative Medicine for the Most Common Illnesses. Disclosure:* Dr. Espinosa is cofounder of XY Wellness, LLC, that sells a combination ED supplement called XYVGGR. DrGeo.com

You know that testosterone—often referred to simply as "T"—is the main male sex hormone, responsible for a man's sex drive and performance. What you may not realize is that T does more than power his libido and penis.

Throughout the adult male body —in muscles (including the heart muscle)…bones…brain… and the immune system—there are receptors for vitality-giving testosterone. This means that low T doesn't only hurt a man's sexual wellness…it can hurt his overall health as well.

Good news: If you've been diagnosed with low T (see next page), you can stimulate your own production of testosterone—achieving optimal, disease-preventing levels—just by making a few lifestyle modifications.

T-BOOSTER #1: **Lose the belly fat.** Extra abdominal fat generates the enzyme aromatase, which turns testosterone into estrogen.

What to do: The best way to shed extra pounds (especially harmful belly fat) is to stop eating refined carbohydrates such as sugar and white flour. And one of the best ways to do that is to eliminate all processed foods, most of which contain sugar and/or refined carbs. Another common source of excess carbohydrates is alcohol. If your T is low, you're better off saying no to beer, wine and spirits.

T-BOOSTER #2: **Get your shut-eye**—particularly from 4 am to 7 am. The male body produces the most testosterone during these three hours, when rapid eye movement (REM) sleep usually occurs. Deep, restful sleep is essential for optimal T.

What to do: Difficulty falling asleep or getting back to sleep after waking up is often caused by worry—your mind is racing as you anxiously think about your health, your finances, your work or your relationship. To stop this unhealthy habit, keep a notebook on your night table and write down your thoughts before bed and/or if you wake up and can't get back to sleep—make a list of what you're worried about or what you think you need to do. Doing so will calm your mind, ease your worries—and let you fall asleep.

T-BOOSTER #3: **Lift a weight.** Regular exercise is a must for boosting testosterone—but it has to be the right kind of exercise. For T production, research strongly supports the use of weight-training.

Here's why: Using the biggest muscles of the body sends signals to the brain that the muscles need more testosterone—and the body starts producing more.

What to do: Deadlift a barbell or kettlebell. In this exercise, you bend over at your hips and bend your knees to lift the weight off the floor. Return to standing, hold the weight and then put it back on the floor. Repeat this lift until your muscles are fatigued. A dead lift uniquely targets your hamstrings, glutes, core, upper back and arms.

Learn the safe, correct way to do a dead lift (including the amount of weight that's right for you) from a trainer, exercise book or video, and then do dead lifts every other day, at least three times a week.

T-BOOSTER #4: **Take targeted supplements.** Some nutritional and herbal supplements are uniquely effective at helping your body produce more testosterone, preserving the testosterone your body is producing or making sure that your testosterone gets to its receptors. *Men with low T should consider taking…**

•Zinc, a mineral that stimulates the Leydig cells in the testicles that produce testosterone. Take 30 mg daily.

Caution: More is not better. Taking more than 30 mg of zinc a day lowers copper levels, which can be harmful.

•Vitamin D, which aids in the production of testosterone. The amount of vitamin D you take should be guided by a vitamin D test.

•Rhodiola and ashwagandha. Stress generates the hormone cortisol, which inhibits the production of testosterone. These herbs are adaptogens, which balance the body when it is under stress. Take 250 mg of rhodiola, twice daily…and 250 mg of ashwagandha, twice daily.

T-BOOSTER #5: **Make love, make T.** Sex stimulates the production of testosterone and is good for the health of your prostate.

What to do: Although many factors affect sexual frequency—including the desires of your sexual partner—I recommend sex at least twice per week to optimize testosterone. Many of my patients consider this my best advice!

Important: I recommend testosterone replacement therapy only as a last resort—for men whose T is so low that lifestyle changes don't adequately improve their levels and whose low testosterone is causing or complicating a chronic condition. In 99% of my patients, the right lifestyle changes do the trick.

DO YOU HAVE LOW T

A clinical diagnosis of low testosterone is made when the level of a man's total testosterone, as

*When considering the use of herbs and supplements, consult a naturopathic or functional medicine doctor for advice on dosage and potential interactions with medications. To find such a doctor near you, consult The American Association of Naturopathic Physicians, Naturopathic. org, or The Institute for Functional Medicine, IFM.org.

measured by a blood test, is 299 nanograms per deciliter (ng/dL) or lower. But an optimal level of total testosterone is 600 ng/dL to 800 ng/dL. Anything below 600 ng/dL puts you at risk for health problems and a lower quality of life. *If you answer "yes" to one or more of these questions, ask your doctor for a blood test to measure your "total testosterone" level to see if you have low T…*

1. Do you have extra belly fat? Abdominal fat is linked to low T.

2. Do you feel tired all the time? Daytime fatigue is a common symptom of low T.

3. Do you feel a lack of motivation—at work, in relationships and in your personal interests? Low T can make you apathetic and indecisive.

4. Are you a man in your 60s or 70s who feels that you just don't have the vitality and positivity you once had? If so, you may have low T.

5. Do you have little desire for sex—and when you try to have sex, do you have trouble achieving an erection? Those are each signs of very low T.

Enough Testosterone?

Study titled "Harmonized Reference Ranges for Circulating Testosterone Levels in Men of Four Cohort Studies in the United States and Europe," published in *The Journal of Clinical Endocrinology & Metabolism*.

Men who don't have enough testosterone, the primary male sex hormone, can experience reduced sex drive and low energy levels—but how much is enough? Surprisingly, no one knew until recently.

This knowledge gap changed in 2017 when a landmark study by the Endocrine Society and published in *The Journal of Clinical Endocrinology & Metabolism* found that the range of testosterone, even in healthy men under age 40, is amazingly wide. And that research informed the Society's 2018 guidelines for testosterone therapy for men—including those over age 65—which set "normal" levels in the blood at about 300 nanograms per deciliter (ng/dL) to 1,000 ng/dL.

This is a step toward making order out of chaos. Previously, whether a man's testosterone level was considered low depended on which lab analyzed his blood sample—each lab provided its own reference range. Plus, a man's testosterone level can fluctuate wildly even within a single day—around 30% of men who get a "Low T" reading on a blood test are in the normal range when retested. The best time to get tested is in the morning—when levels tend to be highest. Any lab used should be certified by the Centers for Disease Control and Prevention.

Should you get tested? Not if you feel fine—many men with below-normal levels report no problems with either energy or sex.

But if you have symptoms plus at least two blood tests showing levels below 300 ng/dL, treatment may benefit you. When you talk to your doctor, discuss risks, too.

Example: Men who have prostate cancer that has spread should not take testosterone.

To Avoid Prostate Cancer, Eat Soy

Catherine C. Applegate, MS, RDN, a graduate research assistant in John Erdman's lab in the division of nutritional sciences at University of Illinois at Urbana-Champaign and lead author of the study "Soy Consumption and the Risk of Prostate Cancer: An Updated Systematic Review and Meta-Analysis," published in *Nutrients*.

If eating a bowl of edamame and a tofu stir-fry each week could reduce your risk of prostate cancer, would you rethink your feelings about soy? According to a new research review, your answer should be a resounding yes.

Researchers at University of Illinois at Urbana-Champaign reviewed 30 studies, involving nearly 267,000 men in all, that specifically looked at the impact of soy foods on prostate health. Their analysis showed that eating soy foods reduces the risk of developing prostate cancer by nearly 30%, and all it takes is a few servings each week.

Men and Melanoma

Men taking aspirin daily for heart health have almost twice the melanoma risk of men not taking aspirin. But the benefits of taking aspirin likely outweigh the higher melanoma risk. Men taking aspirin should be sure to use sunscreen, avoid tanning beds and have regular skin checks. Women taking aspirin do not have increased melanoma risk.

Reason: Unknown, but it may be because men produce fewer protective enzymes than women.

Beatrice Nardone, MD, PhD, research assistant professor in dermatology, Feinberg School of Medicine, Northwestern University, Chicago, and senior author of a study published in *Journal of the American Academy of Dermatology*.

Because some of the studies asked patients to remember what they had eaten (rather than actually tracking what they ate), the suggested amount of soy can't be given to the ounce. However, researchers did find a clear distinction between the effect of unfermented soy foods, including tofu, soy milk and soybeans, and fermented soy foods such as tempeh, natto and miso. Unfermented soy foods had the most consistent beneficial effect…fermented soy foods neither reduced nor increased risk. No soy food was associated with a greater risk for prostate cancer.

Why eating soy may help: Soy contains phytoestrogens, which as their name implies have mild estrogen-like activity. Yes, men (not just women) naturally produce estrogens—and men need estrogens for their prostates to function normally, including fighting off cancer. So, by getting phytoestrogens in your diet, you're building your natural cancer defenses.

HOW TO MAKE SOY PART OF YOUR DIET

If you've turned up your nose at soy in the past, it's time to take another look.

A tasty way to develop a fondness for soy starts with snacks, such as having a bowl of edamame (steamed green soybeans—you'll find them in the freezer case of many stores) and soy "nuts" (roasted soybeans), which look and taste a lot like peanuts.

Next, replace some cow's milk in your diet with unsweetened and unflavored soy milk. An easy swap is in your coffee or tea, working up to cereal. If you cook, substitute soy milk for dairy in recipes. If you naturally like the taste of plain soy milk—as many people do—just drink some!

Tofu (soybean curd) comes in soft and firm varieties, and either way, it takes on the flavor of other ingredients in a dish, so if you don't naturally like tofu, try it in heavily seasoned foods like chili, curry and Asian stir-fries.

The caveat: Avoid highly processed soy foods such as soy-based hot dogs and burgers because they tend to contain little soy and lots of salt, fillers and preservatives.

The Right YouTube Videos for Prostate Cancer Advice

Study titled "Dissemination of Misinformative and Biased Information about Prostate Cancer on YouTube," led by researchers at New York University, New York City, published in *European Urology*.

While the Internet shouldn't be your primary source of health advice, it's hard to resist. There is a lot of good, useful health information online. Unfortunately, there's also a lot of garbage, and it's easy to be led astray by appealingly presented content that isn't reliable. Prostate cancer is a particularly popular search topic and an area that requires a lot of caution.

There are more than 600,000 YouTube videos that give advice on screening and/or treatment for prostate cancer. According to a new study from New York University, the information in most of them isn't trustworthy.

For the study, the researchers evaluated the 150 top YouTube videos that came up in a search for "prostate cancer screening" and "prostate cancer treatment," including the 75 most popular (up to 1.3 million views each). They rated the videos based on quality of information given, such as adherence to established guidelines and

evidence-based, understandable and actionable content…evidence of bias, such as favoring specific technology, complementary or alternative medicine or a commercial interest for monetary gain…and popularity. They also took into account information generated in reader comments, since that also gets widely read—and believed by readers.

Results: Most of the videos were out of date. Of the 150 videos evaluated, 115 (77%) contained potentially misinformative or biased content either in the video or comments…and 20% were rated as having a high level of misinformation. Worst of all, videos with the most misinformation were the most popular!

•**75% described the benefits of screening and treatment,** but only 53% also covered risks.

•**Only 50% promoted shared decision-making between patient and doctor,** which is what the current guidelines recommend. The rest of the videos ignored this recommendation.

•**25% were financially biased toward newer, expensive technology** without evidence of superiority over traditional methods.

It's important to know the risks of prostate cancer screening and treatment—which include false-positive test results and unnecessary additional testing and biopsies from screening…and treatment side effects such as bowel and urinary incontinence and erectile dysfunction. Presenting only benefits while ignoring risks does not offer viewers a balanced view of pros and cons so that they can have an informed discussion with their doctors.

The current guidelines state that screening and treatment decisions should be based on a man's individual risks versus benefits. This recommendation takes into account that a man's lifetime risk for prostate cancer is about 11%… that most men who get the disease do not die from it…and that studies have found that routine screening and surgery do more harm than good for many men.

Bottom line: If you're among the one billion viewers who like to get information from online videos, you don't have to give that up—but don't judge how good a video is by its popularity. The study found that the best prostate cancer advice comes from videos put out by national medical organizations. *Try…*

America Urological Association: https://www.youtube.com/watch?v=yA4JT3sW5Jg

Centers for Disease Control and Prevention: https://www.youtube.com/watch?v=jm8_OJ9xdIY

American Cancer Society: https://www.youtube.com/watch?v=5N-TYqmuNUk

---

Genetic Testing After Prostate Cancer

Jim C. Hu, MD, MPH, urologic oncologist and Ronald Lynch Professor of Urologic Oncology at Weill Cornell Medical College in New York City. Study titled "Evolving Intersection Between Inherited Cancer Genetics and Therapeutic Clinical Trials in Prostate Cancer: A White Paper From the Germline Genetics Working Group of the Prostate Cancer Clinical Trials Consortium," published in *JCO Precision Oncology.*

B eing diagnosed with prostate cancer is terrifying, and you understandably want to get treated as soon as possible. But there's an important step you should consider to be certain you'll get the most appropriate treatment for your type of prostate cancer—genetic testing. Available tests aid patients diagnosed with prostate cancer throughout the spectrum of the disease process. Knowing your DNA "profile" will not only guide your treatment (or active monitoring), but will also tell you whether other members of your family could carry a cancer risk.

What's involved: The latest innovation is called germline testing and is typically done when the cancer is an aggressive form. Rather than testing tumor cells, this is a blood test. It looks for mutations in DNA damage repair (DDR) genes. If you have these mutations, it is harder for your cells to repair DNA. Since cancer damages DNA, you may be at risk for a more advanced or aggressive type of cancer. Genetic testing may also find another type of germline defect called mismatch repair genes, which respond to a different kind of treatment.

Determining your DDR status is especially important if your cancer is advanced, metastatic (meaning it has spread) or considered high-risk based on the Gleason score. Cancer cells are examined under a microscope and are assigned a Gleason score (the old Gleason system used numbers between six and 10…the newer Gleason Grade Group assigns a number between one and five). A high score means your cancer is likely to be aggressive.

DDR testing is also valuable no matter what type of prostate cancer you have if you also have a personal history of prostate cancer before age 50 or if there's a history of breast, colon, endometrial, ovarian and/or pancreatic cancer in your family.

HOW GENETIC TESTING PINPOINTS TREATMENT

Two types of cancer drugs, PARP inhibitors and platinum chemotherapy, have been shown to work best on people with DDR mutations because they target DNA in cancer cells. People with mismatch repair genes respond better to cancer treatment called immunotherapy.

Another advantage to testing is that results may make you eligible to participate in a clinical trial testing a new treatment for advanced prostate cancer. Many trials look for patients with specific genetic defects.

HOW TESTING HELPS YOUR FAMILY MEMBERS

Your having germline defects can prompt your children and siblings to get genetic testing themselves to understand their cancer risk. Although prostate cancer is a male disease, it shares germline defects with other cancers including breast, colon, ovarian and pancreatic cancers. That means that your relatives could be at higher risk for any of these cancers. For instance, while the BRCA1 and BRCA2 genes are usually associated with breast cancer, they also have a strong link to advanced prostate cancer.

If a family member tests positive for germline defects, he/she can start cancer screenings at an earlier age. As an example, blood testing for prostate specific antigen (PSA) may be started at age 40 instead of the usually recommended age of 50.

Genetic counseling for men with prostate cancer is a field that is rapidly evolving. Leading groups such as the Prostate Cancer Clinical Trials Consortium, which includes prostate cancer researchers at leading cancer institutions across the country, recommend that men diagnosed with prostate cancer see genetic counselors promptly and discuss genetic testing. But for now, that's just a recommendation rather than the standard of care. So you might need to bring up the subject with your doctor and ask for a referral to a genetic counselor to discuss the benefits of testing for you.

Testicular Cancer Treatment's Surprising Long-Term Side Effects

Sarah Kerns, PhD, assistant professor, department of radiation oncology, University of Rochester Medical Center, Rochester, New York, and coauthor of the study titled "Cumulative Burden of Morbidity Among Testicular Cancer Survivors After Standard Cisplatin-Based Chemotherapy: A Multi-Institutional Study" published in *Journal of Clinical Oncology*.

Testicular cancer has an excellent five-year survival rate of over 95%. But, according to new research, the platinum-based treatment that cures it is also making patients ill—sometimes very ill—for decades to come.

There's no better alternative to the platinum treatment for most patients who need more than surgery alone. But there could be things you can do to spare yourself some of the long-term side effects.

A CURE THAT LINGERS

The problem is that platinum stays in the body for a very long time, and it's toxic. The level of platinum in cancer survivors can be up to 1,000 times above normal for 20 years after treatment. Knowing what its side effects are will help you get the continuing care you need as a cancer survivor.

THE STUDY

Researchers from 11 major cancer centers around the world surveyed more than 1,200 testicular cancer survivors who had been treated with the platinum-based chemotherapy drug *cisplatin*, asking about health problems they've

been experiencing. The participants ranged in age from 18 to 74, with 37 being the median age. The median time since treatment was just over four years. *The most commonly reported problems were...*

- **Obesity.**
- **Sensory nerve damage** causing tingling, numbness, and/or pain in the hands and feet.
- **Ringing in the ears.**
- **Hearing loss.**
- **Raynaud phenomenon,** which causes decreased blood flow to the fingers and toes leading to numbness and feeling cold.
- **Erectile dysfunction.**
- **Low testosterone.**
- **High blood pressure.**
- **High cholesterol.**

Platinum therapy was already known to have the long-term side effects of blood vessel damage and sensory nerve damage, with consequent effects on, for example, high blood pressure and cardiovascular disease. This study raises the possibility that cisplatin might contribute to all the commonly reported problems and characterizes the overall burden of multiple conditions, each with differing severities.

The researchers created a scoring system to measure the number and severity of adverse outcomes and measured how this score correlated with the men's quality of life. Close to 20% had high-to-severe scores, and 30% had medium-range scores. Only 5.4% had a score of zero. Importantly, a worse score correlated very strongly with worse self-reported health, indicating that the score reflects a health status perceptible to survivors.

Note: Cisplatin is given along with other chemo drugs, and these findings held true regardless of which of the two most commonly given combinations was used for treatment.

A promising finding: One individual factor was linked to having a lower score, meaning not a lot of negative impact on quality of life— engaging in vigorous exercise. This is promising because unlike certain factors such as one's age, exercise is something most people have a lot of control over. The type of exercise that seemed to help the most was vigorous, high-calorie-burning activity such as running, cycling and aerobics.

YOUR CONTINUING POST-CANCER CARE

Because testicular cancer tends to occur in younger men—18 to 39 is the typical age range—and because of the lingering effects of platinum treatment, survivors are at risk for adverse treatment effects for a much longer time than those who get cancer later in life. But at any age, if you've been treated with platinum-based chemo, taking a more rigorous approach to your health can limit its impact, says Sarah Kerns, PhD, MPH, one of the study's lead investigators. *To improve your quality of life, Dr. Kerns suggests…*

• **Let all your health-care providers know you are a cancer survivor who was treated with cisplatin.**

• **Watch your weight,** blood pressure and cholesterol, and take corrective actions if any of these gets out of a healthy range.

• **Stay active** with at least 75 minutes of vigorous activity each week as recommended by the CDC.

• **If you smoke, quit—**in the study, smokers suffered a greater decline in quality of life than nonsmokers.

Note: If you were treated with cisplatin for another cancer, including bladder, ovarian, oral, skin, brain or a metastatic cancer, you may also have some of these long-term side effects, and these care steps may help you as well.

Shorter Prostate Cancer Treatment

Amar U. Kishan, MD, assistant professor of radiation oncology, David Geffen School of Medicine, University of California, Los Angeles.

Prostate cancer treatment can be dramatically shortened. Undergoing an advanced radiation technique, called stereotactic body radiotherapy (SBRT), for four to five days was as effective as 45 days of conventional radiation, according to a seven-year study of more than 2,000 men with low- or intermediate-risk prostate cancer. SBRT is generally more precise, and while it uses higher doses of radiation per treatment, total exposure is less due to the condensed treatment plan. SBRT is now available at several medical centers across the US.

The Female Hormone That Gives Men Migraines

Study titled "Female sex hormones in men with migraine" by researchers at Leiden University Medical Center, OLVG Hospital, Elisabeth Tweesteden Hospital and Erasmus Medical Center, all in the Netherlands, published in *Neurology*.

Migraines aren't headaches just for women. Men also get these excruciating and often debilitating headaches. If you're one of them, listen up! For men, migraines could be a sign that something else is going on with your health…and your sex hormones.

It is well-documented that fluctuating levels of the female hormone estrogen are triggers for migraines in women. Women are three times more likely to get migraines than men during childbearing years (when estrogen levels tend to fluctuate greatly), and migraine attacks in females are most frequent during puberty, menstruation and pregnancy, when levels can spike like crazy.

Men have estrogen in their bodies, too, though far less of it, and it hasn't been known whether estrogen may trigger migraines in men, as well.

But now it is known, thanks to new research.

Study: Using blood samples, researchers from four medical centers in the Netherlands compared levels of estradiol (an estrogen) and the male sex hormone testosterone in 17 men who had migraines at least three times a month and 24 men who did not have migraines. Both groups also filled out two questionnaires used in diagnosing low testosterone (androgen deficiency). The men in both groups were age 47 on average and matched for age and weight.

Results: The men with migraines had significantly higher estrogen levels than the other men. Testosterone levels, on the other hand, were similar in both groups. Interestingly, even though their testosterone levels were not unusually low, 61% of the men in the migraine group reported symptoms of androgen deficiency (compared with 27% of the men in the control group)...and androgen deficiency symptoms were more severe in the migraine group. The culprit here, researchers said, was the ratio of testosterone to estrogen in the men with migraines—they had too little of the former to balance out their overabundance of the latter.

Bottom line: The sample size for this study was small—larger studies are needed to confirm these results.

Meanwhile, hormonal imbalances in men can have other wider-ranging health implications. For example, androgen deficiency is associated with risk for other health conditions, including heart disease and diabetes.

Natural Cures

20 Cures for 5 Embarrassing Problems

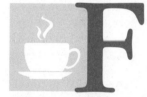

From dandruff flakes crowning our heads right down to corns on our toes, and other body parts in between, we all experience our share of minor but embarrassing health problems. A stye on the eye? Unsightly wart on the hand? A certain, well, odor that no one wants to claim? It's all part of being human, but you don't have to live with it.

Here we bring you wisdom from practitioners in a range of disciplines including conventional Western medicine, naturopathic medicine, Traditional Chinese medicine, herbalism and homeopathy (see key on next page).

Any health problem that could be a sign of something serious should, of course, be checked out by a doctor. But once you've ruled out anything serious and still are left with one of the embarrassing problems here, consult the options and choose the remedy that's right for you—or try several.

DANDRUFF

Many people mistakenly think the cause of their flakes is a too-dry scalp. It's not. Like all skin cells, dead scalp skin naturally sloughs off as new cells form underneath. With dandruff, the shedding is excessive, which can lead not only to visible flakes but also intense itchiness. The condition may be hereditary, and stress and anxiety can contribute.

•**Eat these foods.** Pears, celery, spinach, daikon radishes, carrots, brown rice, fish, oysters and mussels help prevent dandruff. **TCM**

•**Use grapefruit seed extract.** A few drops added to your shampoo can help tame an overgrowth of scalp fungus (dandruff may be the inflammatory response to the fungus). Leave shampoo in your hair for three to five minutes

Bottom Line's 1,000 Cures for 200 Ailments: Integrative Medicine for the Most Common Illnesses with Christine Gustafson, MD, Maura Sughrue, MD, Zhuoling Ren, TCMD, Beth MacEoin, MNCHM, RSHom and Geo Espinosa, ND, LAc, IFMCP, CNS.

KEY	
CM =	**Conventional medicine**
TCM =	**Traditional Chinese medicine**
N =	**Naturopathy**
HE =	**Herbalism**
HO =	**Homeopathy**

before rinsing. Antifungal shampoos with tea tree oil or selenium also can help. **N**

•**Take supplements.** B-complex (100 mg) and biotin (1,000 mcg to 3,000 mcg), taken together with meals, help treat dandruff. **N**

•**Soothe your scalp.** Research has shown that a 30% aloe lotion applied twice daily for four to six weeks improved dandruff. For inflamed patches, rub on a cream made from calendula and chamomile flowers. **HE**

WARTS

These benign tumors are caused by the human papillomavirus (HPV). Warts on the hands usually are near the nails or on the fingers and appear either solo or in clusters, shaped like tiny cauliflowers. They may itch and bleed.

•**Wrap in duct tape.** Cover the wart area with duct tape, and leave it on for a week. Remove the tape, soak the wart and debride it with a pumice stone. Wait a day, and repeat the whole process. Repeat as needed until the wart is gone. **CM**

•**Use 17% salicylic acid.** Purchase salicylic acid over the counter, and apply it twice a day to a clean, dry wart, then bandage the area. **CM**

•**Try a raw garlic patch.** Garlic has antiviral properties. Cover the wart and skin around it with a thin layer of castor oil or olive oil, top it with a thin slice of fresh garlic and tape it in place. Leave this on overnight. Repeat nightly for up to three weeks. (The wart will turn black as it dies.) **N**

•**Apply bittersweet nightshade.** The topical application of this plant as an ointment, available in health-food stores, has been shown to be effective in the removal of warts. **HE**

Immune-boosting tip: Avoid alcohol and convenience foods that are packed with chemical additives. Eat foods that are rich in antioxi-

dants such as tomatoes, strawberries, peppers, citrus fruit, blueberries and broccoli.

STYES

A bacterial infection that starts at the root of an eyelash, a stye forms an inflamed bump that looks like a small boil. It reddens and fills with pus and can be both itchy and sore. Usually styes come to a head and burst within seven days, but treatment can help a stye resolve faster. Try not to touch your eyes when you have one, as the infection is easily spread.

•**Apply a compress.** Using a sterile gauze pad soaked in warm water may help in the early stages. Or make an herbal compress—dilute five drops of tincture of eyebright or chamomile (both are infection fighters) or plantain or marigold (both are soothing) in one-quarter cup of water, and soak a gauze pad in the solution. Apply to the stye for 10 minutes three to four times a day. **CM, N**

•**Take Yin Qiao Je Du Pain.** This herbal pill can clear infection and is effective against styes. Find it in Traditional Chinese medicine stores. **TCM**

•**Supplement with zinc.** It's a known immune system strengthener and helps you heal faster. Take 30 mg to 50 mg daily. **N**

•**Use Pulsatilla.** This sublingual remedy may help if your stye is particularly itchy and crusty in the morning when you wake up. **HO**

CORNS

These harmless but often painful and unsightly yellowish bumps are caused by a build-up of hard, dead skin, usually on the toes and other parts of the feet. People with high arches are susceptible because of the increased downward pressure on the toes. Proper-fitting shoes are critical to prevent friction or toe cramping.

•**Find relief with moleskin.** Apply a patch to relieve painful pressure. **N**

•**Soften skin with calendula salve.** Apply this moisturizer/antiseptic two or three times a day. **N, HO**

•**Soak, then rub.** Soak the affected foot daily in a solution of Epsom salts and warm water for 10 minutes to soften the corn, then gently rub it with a pumice stone to remove the dead skin. If you cut the corn or it bleeds, you may need to see a doctor to prevent infection (pus or clear fluid is a sign of this). **N**

•**File, then apply salicylic acid.** Use a file or pumice stone to remove excess skin first. Afterward, apply 40% salicylic acid (available over the counter) to an area a bit larger than the corn and place a corn ring (also over the counter) on top to relieve pressure. Or apply essential oil of wintergreen, which contains salicylates, to the corn at night and wash it off in the morning to prevent irritating surrounding skin. Be sure to use natural, not synthetic, oil of wintergreen. **CM**, **HE**

Cautionary tip: Anyone with diabetes or circulatory problems in the feet should consult a medical provider before trying to remove a corn.

FLATULENCE

Everyone passes gas over the course of the day, but sometimes it happens too frequently.

Usual culprits: Having too much gas in the large intestine as bacteria act on undigested food, swallowing air while eating or chewing gum, consuming a lot of fiber if your system isn't used to it or a food intolerance. Flatulence also is a symptom of a number of diseases including irritable bowel syndrome, diverticulosis or diverticulitis, celiac disease and thyroid dysfunction. The remedies below are for the occasional normal bout.

•**Swallow a probiotic.** Take a combination of Acidophilus, Lactobacillus and S. boulardii daily for 30 days to improve your overall intestinal health. Or take 4 g of glutamine, an over-the-counter amino acid supplement, each day. **N**

•**Try an elimination diet.** There are a surprising number of foods that can upset the stomach and lead to gas. Start with the biggies—stop eating gluten, dairy, soy and processed foods for three weeks, and then reintroduce them one at a time to see if flatulence resumes. **CM**

•**Sip an herbal tea.** Peppermint tea can ease upper gastrointestinal gas and spasms. Ginger tea, brewed with fresh ginger slices, stimulates digestion and reduces gas. Or make fennel tea—pour a cup of boiling water over one to two teaspoons of freshly crushed, dried seeds, let it steep for 10 minutes, strain it and drink before or after meals. **HE**, **N**

•**Stimulate pressure points.** Try acupressure to move stomach and intestinal energy. While seated, exert pressure with a fingertip for one minute, then repeat.

Where to press: Use the Susanli point on the lower leg, one inch to the outside of and three inches below the kneecap, and the San Yin Jiao point on the inside of the leg, about three inches above the anklebone. Perform on each leg two to three times a day. **TCM**

Eating tip: Prevent flatulence by eating slowly and chewing thoroughly so that your saliva's digestive enzymes can mix with food and begin breaking it down.

Surprising Ways a Top Doctor Uses Nature to Stay Healthy

John La Puma, MD, FACP, board-certified internist and certified California naturalist, who runs an organic teaching farm in Santa Barbara, California. A *Lifetime TV* and *PBS* host, he is *The New York Times* best-selling author of *ChefMD's Big Book of Culinary Medicine* and *Refuel*, and coauthor with Michael F. Roizen, MD, of *The RealAge Diet*. DrJohnLaPuma.com

Jim, an executive in his 50s, believed that he thrived under pressure. But his blood pressure was too high and so was his blood sugar. He had become overweight. His wife thought Jim was caught up in an overly stressful cycle of working and commuting with no real break. He felt on edge all the time.

Jim knew that he should exercise, eat better, relax more and calm his anxiety. But he was, as his wife saw, essentially stuck. So he came to see me, his doctor. I'm a medical doctor, so I could have given him prescription medication for his blood pressure, anxiety and prediabetes. But instead I prescribed a specific trial of an ancient remedy—nature therapy.

For example, I told Jim to plant four small herb plants in a window box—parsley, sage, rosemary and thyme—and to spend five minutes tending to them daily, with his phone turned off. I instructed him to tell family or friends who thought he was slacking that the time was prescribed by his doctor. And I told Jim to ask his wife for support. He's now following his nature prescription, and he hasn't required any new medications to improve his health.

WHAT NATURE CAN DO FOR YOU

Nature can be your medicine, too. Here are some medical conditions that spending time in nature has been shown to improve—acute urinary tract infections…anxiety disorder…ADHD…cancer…cardiovascular disease…depression…diabetes…healing from surgery…musculoskeletal complaints…migraines…upper-respiratory-tract infections…and vertigo.

Example: In a pioneering randomized controlled study by Swedish environmental psychologist Roger S. Ulrich, PhD, post-op patients who had window views of nature from their hospital beds had improved moods, needed less pain medication, had fewer surgical complications and left the hospital sooner compared with similar patients whose rooms had no views. And these patients just looked outside.

Even just looking at pictures of plants has been shown by researchers at University of Essex in Colchester, UK, to reduce blood pressure, pulse rate and muscle tension after a stressful experience. Putting up beautiful pictures of nature—water, trees, forests or meadows—in your home (or if you are in a hospital, in your room) may sound trivial, but it's not.

Getting outside and into natural environments is even more powerful. People who spend just 30 minutes in a green outdoor space at least once a week are 7% less likely to develop high blood pressure, and 9% less likely to develop depression, than people who spend little or no time, according to a study published in *Scientific Reports*.

There's much more to nature as medicine. *Here are six more powerful ways to use nature to heal what ails you…*

TAKE A FOREST BATH

What forest bathers do is walk very slowly in a wooded area for two or three hours. They may cover only a quarter mile doing this. Whenever they feel like it, they sit for a few minutes, just to sense what is around them. A contemplative, sensual immersion, forest bathing has been part of Korean and Japanese disease prevention and treatment for decades. Dozens of peer-reviewed studies show that forest therapy reduces your blood pressure, heart rate and stress hormones…and then reduces the stress you experience for days afterward.

Trees play an important role, releasing essential aromatic oils called phytoncides that boost immunity and antiviral natural killer cells. MRI brain scans find that the longer a person is exposed to trees, the less activity there is in the amygdala, the part of the brain that controls distress and fear responses, contributing to anxiety disorders and depression.

What to do: Turn off your phone. Find a wooded area and comfortable sitting spot. Don't hurry.

Tune into the sounds first: Hear the closest sound and then the farthest.

Use your other senses: Watch the birds, feel the leaves, smell the breeze, appreciate the stillness. Get up and amble a bit. Become aware of your connection with the environment, which strengthens your concentration and focus.

Can't schedule two or three hours? Try meditating for shorter periods in a natural, electronics-free setting. If you already meditate, compare how you feel when you do it in nature versus in your usual spot.

GREEN THE INSIDE OF YOUR HOME

Gardening is excellent medicine for body and mind. Compared with others, gardeners tend to weigh less, are less susceptible to depression and anxiety, have greater self-esteem—and are between 36% and 47% less likely to develop dementia, research finds.

Of course, not all of us have the space to be outdoor gardeners. Plus, we spend up to 90% of our time indoors, often breathing indoor pollutants from household chemicals that can harm our lungs, heart and other organs.

Solution: Garden indoors! Greenery inside is beautifying, a psychological respite—and it literally purifies the air you breathe. Studies show that indoor gardeners get similar benefits to outdoor gardeners.

What to do: Choose houseplants that are especially good at removing toxins from the air. Examples include Dracaena Janet Craig (yes, that's the real name), Boston fern and spider plants.

EXERCISE OUTSIDE IN A GREEN SPACE

A recent Stanford study showed significantly reduced rumination—obsessive worrying—after a 90-minute walk in nature, compared with a 90-minute walk through an urban environment. Any exercise is better than none, of course, but "green" exercise appears to be better than indoor exercise at stimulating the release of endorphins, the body's feel-good chemicals, and triggering new brain-cell development.

It takes only five minutes of exercising in nature to boost mood and self-esteem, according to one British study. But like medications, there's a dose-response effect—the more you do, the greater the benefit…without any side effects, of course.

What to do: Exercise outside or in view of nature. Take a lunchtime walk to a park.

BREATHE THIS

Aromatherapy using plant essential oils smells good and is good for you, with proven clinical benefits. *Examples…*

•**Lavender blossom.** Reduces migraine pain and improves sleep quality.

•**Bergamot orange.** Lowers stress and improves fatigue.

•**Yuzu lemon.** Improves premenstrual emotional symptoms and lowers heart rate.

Caution: Whether you inhale, apply or massage essential oils, allergic reactions are possible. To minimize risk, wear gloves and wash your hands. Use a very small amount and see how you react. And buy certified organic products to make sure that you're not getting any pesticides. If you have a medical condition, talk to your doctor first.

THERE'S AN APP FOR THAT— AND WEBSITES, TOO

Can looking at your phone be "green"? Not if it replaces being in nature. But virtual nature experiences can be beneficial during your life indoors.

What to do: Try Calm.com (Apple and Android, $12.99 a month) to improve mood and Headspace.com (Apple and Android, $12.99 a month) to learn meditation. Find ambient sounds such as waterfalls on YouTube (free) or on an app such as Rain Rain, which is great for meditation and sleep (Apple and Android, free). Connect with amateur naturalists on INaturalist.org (free). Find more free resources at my website, DrJohnLaPuma.com.

TRY PET THERAPY

Most Americans already live with nature inside our homes. About two-thirds of all US households own pets, and dogs especially can provide unconditional love. Ironically, the dirt they bring into our homes may be good for our immune systems—and pets offer connectivity and emotional support to their owners, especially in times of crisis. That is powerful medicine. So, of course, is walking a dog. Dog owners have about one-third lower risk for heart disease than people who don't own dogs—a benefit that's especially strong in people who live alone.

What to do: If you don't have a dog, borrow one! Offer to walk a neighbor's dog, say, once or twice a week. Schedule walks in your calendar as if they were meetings. Your blood pressure will fall. So may your risk for heart disease.

A Brand-New Form of Medical Treatment: Helps Stroke, Depression, More

James Giordano, PhD, professor in the departments of neurology and biochemistry and chief of the Neuroethics Studies Program of the Pellegrino Center for Clinical Bioethics at Georgetown University Medical Center, Washington, DC. ClinicalBioethics.Georgetown.edu

Meredith Hutter Chamorro, a certified Yoga Tune Up teacher with advanced training in restorative yoga, Stroudsburg, Pennsylvania. SheSwingsOnAStar.com

Its name means "wandering," but it is far from aimless. It travels from the brain down each side of the neck, through the chest and deep into the gut. It helps regulate an astounding number of the body's essential functions—including breathing, heart rate, blood pressure, perspiration and digestion.

It's the vagus nerve, and it's turning out to be a key to wellness—and to fighting disease. Yogis call it the "Buddha Nerve" because the core benefits of meditation—calm and a sense of balance—stem from activating it. But it also now is the basis of cutting-edge medicine.

To understand the "vagus revolution," we reached out to two experts—James Giordano, PhD, a world-renowned neuroscientist at Georgetown University...and Meredith Hutter Chamorro, a restorative yoga teacher whose work focuses on improving vagus nerve function.

WHY THE VAGUS NERVE MATTERS

The vagus nerve plays a key role in stimulating the parasympathetic nervous system. This is your body's "rest-and-digest" response—a counterbalance to the "fight-or-flight" mechanisms of the sympathetic nervous system. An activated parasympathetic system means that we're calmer, have lower blood pressure, digest food better and produce less inflammation.

We need both systems, but health depends on how well we balance them. That's known as "vagal tone." If you have high vagal tone, you relax quickly after a stressful moment. In that state, your body is better at regulating blood glucose levels and cholesterol so that, over time, you're at less risk for cardiovascular disease, stroke and diabetes. You're also less anxious and better able to manage your emotions.

Conversely, low vagal tone is associated with increased risk for depression, gastrointestinal disorders and heart disease.

ELECTRIFYING MEDICINE

Vagus nerve stimulation (VNS) is fast becoming a new form of medical treatment. According to Dr. Giordano, it can be done in two ways—invasively, in which a device that is surgically implanted in the chest (with electrodes in the neck) sends very mild electrical pulses at regular intervals to the vagus nerve...or noninvasively, through the use of a handheld device that a patient applies to the neck. *Exciting research findings...*

•**Epilepsy.** VNS originally was developed to treat epilepsy patients who did not respond well to antiseizure medication. It gets more effective the longer it is used—in one study conducted at New York University Langone Medical Center, the frequency of seizures decreased by 36% in six months...58% in four years...and 75.5% in 10 years.

•**Parkinson's disease.** VNS allows some patients to get longer-lasting effects with lower doses of drugs. This is important because drugs used to treat Parkinson's tend to become less effective as the disease progresses, and increasing the doses can have debilitating side effects.

•**Migraines.** These headaches often begin in the back of the head where there's a branch of the vagus nerve. Several recent studies have found that by using a handheld stimulator over the nerve in the neck when symptoms begin, sufferers can decrease pain—and, in some cases, nip a migraine in the bud. In early 2018, the Food and Drug Administration cleared one such device—gammaCore—for home treatment of migraines. It's not cheap—$600 a month ($500 with an automatic discount) and may not be covered by insurance, although the company is working to expand coverage. The device requires a prescription.

•**Depression.** A landmark study published in *The American Journal of Psychiatry* followed 795 treatment-resistant depression patients for five years. Nearly half (43%) of those who used medication and therapy plus an implanted VNS device experienced remission of their depression—compared with only 26% of those who had only medication/therapy.

•**Anxiety, stroke and cognitive health.** VNS also is proving to be helpful in reducing anxiety disorders including post-traumatic stress disorder (PTSD). Some stroke patients benefit from VNS, as do some head-injury patients. Early research suggests that improving vagal tone (see below to learn how) may help people with cognitive issues improve alertness, focus, decision making and memory.

8 WAYS TO WORK OUT YOUR VAGUS

While medical advances are exciting for people with certain conditions, every one of us can take steps now to improve our vagal tone and vitality. Hutter Chamorro uses several approaches to improve vagal tone in her clients. *Try these every day…*

•**Deep diaphragmatic breathing.** Breathing through your nose, inhale deeply into your belly and exhale slowly. Control your exhale so that it lasts longer than the inhale—like letting air out of a tire. During the inhale, you'll massage the vagus nerve, and during the exhale the diaphragm releases around the vagus nerve, improving its functioning.

•**Massage.** Grab a squishy exercise ball—I use one that is about nine inches in diameter—and lay with your tummy on it. Don't use a firm ball because this exercise should feel comfortable with no pain. Do some diaphragmatic breathing, and try slowly rolling from side to side on the ball. This helps release tension in your core muscles, making it easier to take deep, diaphragmatic breaths.

•**Cold water.** Stimulate your vagus nerve simply by splashing cold water on your face. When your body adjusts to cold, your fight-or-flight response declines and your rest-and-digest system kicks in.

•**Singing and humming.** These vocal activities produce vibration in the neck, which stimulates the vagus nerve in a beneficial way.

•**Gargling.** Grab a glass of water each morning and gargle to contract the muscles in the back of the throat, which stimulates your vagus nerve and digestive tract. For the most benefit, gargle continuously until your eyes start to tear up—another vagus function.

•**Yoga.** Add "toning your vagus nerve" to your long list of reasons to do yoga. The practice incorporates diaphragmatic breathing, chanting and stress reduction.

•**Meditation.** All types of meditation are good for the vagus nerve. My favorite is compassionate, or "Loving-Kindness," meditation. Rather than letting your mind wander, you direct your good thoughts to other people. As positive emotions increase, so does your vagal tone.

•**Laughter.** Laughing reduces muscle tension in the face, neck and diaphragm that can cause bottlenecks in vagus signals. It also requires diaphragmatic movements and has been shown to improve vagal tone. Watch funny movies and comedy shows, and tell jokes with your friends—laughter really is great medicine!

These 4 "Super Spices" Have Hidden Benefits

Joshua Levitt, ND, a naturopathic physician and medical director at Whole Health Natural Family Medicine in Hamden, Connecticut. Dr. Levitt is a clinical preceptor for Yale School of Medicine and collaborates with the Integrative Medicine Center at Yale New Haven Hospital. He is author of *The Honey Phenomenon* and numerous other books and articles. WholeHealthCT.com

When it comes to "superfoods," fruits and veggies aren't the only heavy hitters. A handful of popular spices also have gained a rightful place on this list because of their own research-supported therapeutic effects.

Examples of the best known: Cinnamon for diabetes. Garlic for high cholesterol. Ginger for nausea. Cayenne for pain relief.

What you may not realize: Those same spices have even more benefits—little-known but powerful—that are also backed by scientific evidence. *How to use these spices for even greater preventive and curative effect…*

CINNAMON

A small daily dose of cinnamon has been proven in many studies to lower and help regulate blood sugar—crucial for those trying to prevent or manage type 2 diabetes.

Little-known benefit: Cinnamon also can lower high blood pressure.

Scientific evidence: In a recent study published in *Lipids in Health and Disease*, people who ingested 3 g (about two-thirds of a teaspoon) of cinnamon daily had a significant drop in blood pressure after four months—from averages of 136/88 to 122/80.

How to get more: Because cinnamon is so tasty, it's easy to include more in your diet. As a heavy cinnamon user, I buy organic Ceylon cinnamon (the highest quality) by the pound.

Note: Supermarket cinnamon is usually cassia (or Vietnamese), which contains a compound called coumarin that may damage the liver at high doses in susceptible individuals.

Cinnamon is great on roasted sweet potatoes and squash and adds delightful sweetness to pancakes and waffles. Plus, because it's such a powerful antioxidant, a sprinkle of cinnamon stops apple slices from turning brown—making the treat more delicious and more appetizing.

GARLIC

This potent spice—a rich source of many healing compounds—is proven to lower cholesterol, reducing your risk for heart disease.

Little-known benefit: Eating garlic regularly also may help reduce your risk for colorectal cancer.

Scientific evidence: When Italian researchers analyzed seven case-control studies on garlic consumption and colorectal cancer, they found that people who ate the most garlic reduced their risk for the disease by 37% compared with people who ate the least. These studies measured garlic intake in various ways, so there is no optimal intake. To be fair, there is also research showing no correlation between garlic and colorectal cancer risk, but even the potential benefit makes garlic a smart addition to one's diet.

How to get more: Lightly sautéed fresh cloves are likely the healthiest way to consume garlic, but you also can use garlic flakes or powder. I use garlic (usually combined with lemon) in nearly every cooking liquid, sauce and marinade that I make in my kitchen.

GINGER

Dozens of studies have proven ginger's usefulness in easing nausea and vomiting due to everything from chemotherapy to motion sickness to morning sickness.

Little-known benefit: Ginger also inhibits the COX-1 and COX-2 enzymes that play a role in the production of inflammation-causing compounds in the body. This means it works the same way as pain-relieving drugs such as *ibuprofen* (Motrin) and aspirin.

Scientific evidence: A study published in *Phytotherapy Research* found that ginger supplements are comparable to aspirin, ibuprofen,

naproxen (Aleve) and other over-the-counter painkillers in easing muscle pain caused by exercise and other types of strenuous activity.

Research also has shown that ginger is just as effective as the migraine drug *sumatriptan* (Imitrex).

How to get more: For a therapeutic, pain-relieving dose of ginger, take a 1,000-mg supplement, twice daily. For migraine, I recommend up to 1,000 mg at the onset of a migraine. If you want to use ginger to help prevent migraine, add fresh ginger to your daily diet or take a ginger supplement (250 mg to 500 mg daily).*

In the kitchen, add fresh ginger—finely diced or crushed—to sauces and marinades. Used three or more times a week, ginger in doses commonly consumed in the diet can have a mild pain-relieving and anti-inflammatory effect. Ginger is also great in smoothies.

CAYENNE

Cayenne is a powder made from dried, red chili peppers, and it's very hot when used to spice food. But the natural intensity of cayenne and its active ingredient capsaicin affect more than your taste buds.

It's the only natural compound that—when applied topically—can degrade substance P, a neurotransmitter that tells the brain to transmit pain signals. With less substance P, there's less pain—which is why capsaicin is a common ingredient in many creams, ointments and salves for pain problems such as arthritis, nerve pain, foot pain and back pain.

Little-known benefit: Cayenne can also help you lose weight. Capsaicin and other compounds in cayenne work because they have several effects that help you shed pounds—they suppress appetite…increase calorie-burning ("basal metabolic rate")…and burn up ("oxidize") body fat.

In a recent meta-analysis of nine studies on capsaicin and weight loss, published in *Critical Reviews in Food Science and Nutrition*, researchers concluded that the spice "could be a new therapeutic approach in obesity."

*If you take blood thinners such as *warfarin* (Coumadin) or if you have gallstone disease, talk to your doctor before using ginger supplements.

How to get more: For patients who want to lose weight, I usually recommend adding cayenne to the diet or using low-dose (2 mg) capsaicin supplements daily. (High-dose supplements can irritate the gastrointestinal tract.)

As a weight-loss aid, I recommend drinking one or more cups a day of warm water with a pinch of cayenne, juice from half a lemon, a teaspoon of honey and ground ginger (using a chunk of fresh ginger the size of half your thumb, from knuckle to tip). Cayenne is also excellent in marinades for fish and poultry and sprinkled on eggs. Plus, it adds a kick to salad dressings.

Essential Oils Make Cancer Treatment More Bearable

Cherie Perez, RN, CCRP, LMT, a licensed massage therapist with extensive training in essential oils. She is currently the manager of genitourinary research projects in genitourinary medical oncology at the University of Texas MD Anderson Cancer Center in Houston.

It's great that there are more cancer treatment options than ever before. Yet for all these advances, treatment side effects can still knock you off your feet and severely impact your quality of life. Surprisingly, relief can come from a centuries-old source…essential oils.

Derived from plant flowers, leaves, stalks and/or roots, essential oils contain unique chemical components that give each oil a distinct scent. Aromatherapy is the art of using these scents to improve well-being. Many essential oils stimulate your sense of smell in a way that can ease cancer treatment side effects, such as reducing stress and nausea.

To learn about the most effective essential oils for reducing specific cancer treatment side effects, we spoke to Cherie Perez, RN, CCRP, LMT, a researcher and a practitioner of aromatherapy for 25 years.

Perez emphasizes that different aromas have different effects on different people, and what smells good or at least acceptable to you may be intolerable to someone else. Therefore, you may

Hypnosis for IBS

Hypnosis improves irritable bowel syndrome (IBS) and other stomach issues. The brain and gut exchange chemical messages with each other, so when people are under hypnosis, targeted suggestions about abdominal and bowel discomfort help them develop coping mechanisms that reduce pain and improve quality of life. Cognitive behavioral therapy also helps, and both methods are recommended by the American Gastroenterological Association.

Megan Riehl, PsyD, a gastrointestinal health psychologist and assistant professor of medicine at University of Michigan, Ann Arbor.

want to try several different oils for relief of the side effects below to find the ones that create the best combination of pleasantness and effectiveness for you. It's worth spending time to find what you like because of the results—Perez says aromatherapy has been described as "red light meditation" because it can change your mood in the time it takes to stop for a red light.

HOW TO USE ESSENTIAL OILS

Essential oils usually are diluted because they're very concentrated—full strength on the skin, they can cause burns. Instead, they can be dispersed in the air with a diffuser and inhaled…or diluted in an odor-free oil, called a "carrier" oil, and massaged into the skin. Apricot kernel oil, jojoba oil and safflower oil are common carrier oils. For convenience with self-massage use, look for essential oils that already have been combined with carrier oils so that you won't have to worry about mixing the right concentration.

Another option that Perez frequently recommends is placing two or three drops of an essential oil or oil blend on a tissue and holding it two to six inches from your nose—no closer!—so you can inhale the vapor. (In terms of distance, placing the tissue against your upper chest is ideal.)

You might want to try each of these techniques to see which one you respond to best—some work better in certain situations, as you'll see on the next page.

Whichever method of inhalation you choose, to get the oil's benefits, take several slow, deep breaths every five to 10 minutes for as long as you like.

While you can try any oil whose scent appeals to you, here are specific ones that have been found to work to relieve the following cancer treatment side effects...

•**Nausea.** Ginger essential oil can help conquer nausea—and if you get rid of nausea, you can avoid its serious complications of dehydration and malnutrition. Orange and spearmint help some people, too. If you know that a cancer treatment brings on nausea, use an essential oil just before the treatment or at the first sensation of nausea. Perez says that the tissue method is very effective for nausea. Take two to five slow deep breaths, then flush the tissue in the toilet to avoid any chance of associating the scent with nausea later. Repeat this two or three times over a few hours.

Some people with treatment-induced nausea respond very well to essential-oil self-massage from the throat down to the abdomen. While gently applying oil, imagine that your stomach feels settled as your hands move downward, and picture your favorite vacation or relaxation place.

•**Sleeplessness.** Studies show that nearly half of all people with cancer suffer from sleep problems. Sleeplessness can be due to stress, extended hospital stays or side effects of treatment. Inhaling lavender, chamomile or vetiver essential oil—depending on your personal preference—can help improve sleep quality, especially when you add it to a good sleep-hygiene routine. Just before getting into bed, place a few drops of the essential oil you like best on a tissue and place the tissue on your pillow near your face or on your upper chest. You can use the tissue to help you get back to sleep if you wake up in the middle of the night. If you find self-massage more soothing, massage your upper chest and arms with a diluted oil or blend of oils.

•**Constipation.** Chemotherapy, pain medication, changes in diet and not drinking enough water can lead to constipation and related symptoms such as bloating, cramps and nausea. Essential oils such as ginger, peppermint, fennel and chamomile are good at helping when massaged clockwise on the abdomen once or twice a day.

•**Anxiety.** Being a cancer patient is stressful and creates anxiety. Perez favors the oils of neroli, frankincense, lavender and/or vetiver to promote calm and relaxation. While you can use any essential-oil technique anytime, if anxiety is making it hard to sleep, try taking a bath or shower with an essential oil bath gel.

Helpful: If you get anxious during a cancer treatment, exam or scan, take a tissue with a few drops of essential oil on it with you to the treatment area (even right into an MRI or a CT suite, where you can keep the tissue on your chest while the images are taken).

•**Fatigue.** Loss of energy and fatigue are common side effects of many cancer treatments, and often rest isn't enough to combat them. Try eucalyptus and bergamot oils for an invigorating boost of energy. A morning shower with an essential-oil body gel can be uplifting.

BUYING ESSENTIAL OILS

Because the FDA doesn't regulate the labeling or quality of essential oils, buying them from a person with aromatherapy training or a reputable online store is important.

The National Association for Holistic Aromatherapy (NAHA.org) has an online marketplace that can connect you to practitioners, including massage therapists, certified in medical massage who understand the needs of cancer patients. You'll also find listings of Internet and brick-and-mortar stores where you can buy essential oils.

Quality products should have the common and botanical names for the oil on the label, which helps better identify plant varieties. Avoid any brands with rubber eyedropper dispensers because the oil can cause the rubber to break down and contaminate the oil. Also, look for oils packaged in dark-colored bottles, such as amber or cobalt, to protect them from light.

ESSENTIAL OILS MAY BE EVEN MORE POWERFUL

Studies on additional benefits of essential oils during cancer treatment and recovery have been small but are promising. For instance, a 2016 study found that patients who sniffed a mixture of ginger and lemon essential oils had less salivary gland damage, a side effect of radioactive iodine therapy, compared with a group that sniffed distilled water.

Another study found that gargling with a mixture of one drop each of manuka and kanuka essential oils diluted in a glass of water eased pain and delayed the onset of mucositis, a painful side effect of cancer treatment, in people receiving radiation therapy for head and neck cancers. This can make it easier to eat, drink and stay hydrated.

More extensive research is needed to confirm these positive findings.

Essential Oils That Relieve the Common Cold

Jamison Starbuck, ND, a naturopathic physician in family practice, Missoula, Montana, and writer and producer of *Dr. Starbuck's Health Tips for Kids*, a weekly program on Montana Public Radio, MTPR.org. DrJamisonStarbuck.com

It might be hard to believe that something that's been used as medicine for literally thousands of years could be as effective as an over-the-counter (OTC) drug. But it's true. Essential oils—aromatic oils made from the fragrant parts of various plants—were first used by ancient cultures. But they are now popular among consumers of natural medicine—and for good reason.

Unlike OTC decongestants that can spike blood pressure and OTC antihistamines that can cause drowsiness and other unwanted effects, essential oils battle winter ailments safely and without adverse effects. Your best bet is to use essential oils in diluted topical applications that can be inhaled and improve circulation where applied. This form of aromatherapy works particularly well with respiratory complaints.

Caveat: Because essential oils are very concentrated, when used incorrectly they can irritate or burn the skin and mucous membranes (such as the inside of the mouth and nose) and even the stomach if swallowed. That said, es-

sential oils are high on my list of go-to natural remedies. *Some of my favorites for winter (with instructions for safety)…**

For the common cold: Spearmint. Spearmint is less irritating to sensitive, inflamed nasal passages than the more frequently used peppermint or eucalyptus.

What to do: Mix the spearmint essential oil in a carrier oil (such as almond or coconut oil), using a 1:10 ratio. Then put two drops of this mixture above your upper lip—one just below each nostril. This will reduce stuffiness and thin nasal mucus, allowing you to blow your nose effectively and to breathe more easily. Use spearmint oil in this way three times a day.

For sinusitis: Chamomile. Because bacteria are common causes of sinusitis, chamomile's antibacterial properties make it good medicine for this annoying and often painful condition.

What to do: Mix the chamomile essential oil with a carrier oil in a 1:10 ratio (as described above). Then put several drops of this mixture on your skin just below your cheekbones, rubbing it into the skin from beside your nose to the outer corners of your eyes near your temples. Be sure not to get this mixture in your eyes! Put another drop or two above each eyebrow—these are sinus points used for acupressure and the application of topical sinus medication.

Lie down with a hot, moist cloth over your face with your eyes closed (leave a little space for breathing through your nose). Cover with a dry towel for five to 10 minutes. You can do this several times a day. The essential oil vapor will reduce congestion and pain and will help you relax and rest.

For sore throat: Bitter orange. With its soothing citrus scent, bitter orange has antiseptic properties and promotes circulation of blood and lymph.

What to do: Mix bitter orange oil with a carrier oil in a 1:10 ratio (as described above), and then rub several drops into the lymph glands under your jaw and down your neck for relief of sore throat pain. Wrap a moist, hot towel

---

*To test whether you are sensitive or allergic to essential oils, put one drop of the diluted oil on the inside of your wrist and wait 24 hours. If you see a reaction, do not use the oil elsewhere.

around your neck, and then cover it with a dry towel. Leave in place for 15 minutes. Then gently stroke downward on your jaw and neck—this promotes lymph drainage. Repeat as often as desired throughout the day.

Natural Cures for a Leaky Bladder

Jamison Starbuck, ND, a naturopathic physician in family practice, Missoula, Montana, and writer and producer of *Dr. Starbuck's Health Tips for Kids*, a weekly program on Montana Public Radio, MTPR.org. DrJamisonStarbuck.com

Most women (and many men) have had that "oh, no!" feeling of leaking urine when lifting a heavy object or laughing a little harder than usual. The occasional incontinent moment isn't a big deal. But when it happens daily, it's a problem. Prescription drugs such as *oxybutynin* (Oxytrol) and *tolterodine* (Detrol) can relieve symptoms of this condition but often cause side effects, including dry mouth and constipation. Natural medicine is safer and can offer long-term relief. *The main types of incontinence…*

•**Stress incontinence and urge incontinence.** If you lose urine when the bladder is stressed—as with a big sneeze—that's stress incontinence. If you have a sudden urge to urinate and lose urine if you can't get to the toilet almost immediately, that's called urge incontinence. With both of these types of incontinence, weak pelvic-floor muscles are often to blame. *My advice…*

Urinate on a schedule: I suggest urinating every two hours while you are awake, whether you feel the urge or not. If your bladder is emptied more regularly, you're less likely to leak. If nighttime incontinence is a problem, stop liquids four hours before bed. Instead, have a piece of fruit—it's watery and refreshing but won't fill your bladder the way a beverage will.

Tone up: If your pelvic muscles are weak, Kegel exercises are the go-to solution…for both women and men.

What to do: While you're sitting or even standing, contract the muscles you would use if you suddenly wanted to stop the flow of urine. Do 10 contractions in a row, three times daily. You should notice a benefit within 10 days. If you hold a lot of tension in your lower abdomen or hip muscles—which often occurs in those who are sedentary—focus on gentle stretching, abdominal massage and deep breathing to help reduce incontinence.

Check for food allergies: Food allergies cause irritation and inflammation. When the bladder wall is irritated, it's more sensitive and reactive, and this can lead to incontinence. Dairy, wheat and eggs are common triggers. If you suspect that you have a food allergy, ask your doctor about IgG blood testing to check.

•**Temporary incontinence.** Excess caffeine, alcohol, smoking, a diet high in salt and even acidic and spicy foods can irritate the bladder and cause incontinence, along with such symptoms as urinary frequency and urgency. Avoid the potential irritants above one at a time until you find the culprit(s).

Try botanicals: Corn silk and gravel root soothe bladder tissue and calm the urge to urinate. A typical dose is one-quarter teaspoon (in tincture form) of an equal blend of these herbs, added to two ounces of water and taken three times daily (15 minutes before or after meals) until your incontinence improves. These herbs can be used for a long time, but it's best to talk to your doctor if you plan to take any herb for more than a month or so.*

Drink enough water: It may seem odd to drink more water if you're running to the bathroom all the time, but if you don't drink enough, your urine becomes concentrated, which aggravates the bladder and leads to incontinence. Drinking too much water can do the same. Use this formula—one-half ounce of water per pound of body weight daily. Your bladder will thank you!

*Consult your doctor before using corn silk if you take medication for diabetes, blood pressure or inflammation, or if you take *warfarin* (Coumadin) or diuretics…and before taking gravel root if you have liver disease or take a seizure drug or the antibiotic *rifampin* (Rifadin).

This Herb Combo Helps Urinary Incontinence

Andrew L. Rubman, ND, founder and medical director, Southbury Clinic for Traditional Medicines, Southbury, Connecticut. He is author of the Bottom Line blog "Nature Doc's Patient Diary."

Study titled "Urox Containing Concentrated Extracts of Crataeva nurvala Stem Bark, Equisetum arvense Stem and Lindera aggregata Root, in the Treatment of Symptoms of Overactive Bladder and Urinary Incontinence: A Phase 2, Randomized, Double-Blind Placebo Controlled Trial," led by researchers at University of Queensland, Australia, published in *BMC Complementary and Alternative Medicine*.

Urinary incontinence puts a damper on your whole life. Drugs don't always help…plus, they have daunting side effects. (Constipation, memory loss, reduced libido anyone?)

Promising news: A new study found that urinary incontinence can be reduced—maybe eliminated—without drugs. How? With a combo of three well-known herbs that have been used for centuries in traditional medicine.

Australian researchers tested an herbal blend called Urox that is a combination of three herbs—Crataeva nurvala (common name, varuna), Equisetum arvense (horsetail) and Lindera aggregata (Japanese evergreen spicebush). The herbs have been used separately to treat urinary symptoms in traditional medicines for centuries and have long-established safety profiles.

For the study, 150 men and women who had urinary incontinence were given either a daily capsule containing 420 milligrams (mg) of Urox…or a daily placebo capsule that looked identical. Both groups took the capsules for eight weeks.

Results: The group that took Urox reported significant improvement. *On average…*

•**Those in the Urox group needed to urinate four fewer times during the day and two fewer times during the night** than they had before the study. Meanwhile, there was very little difference (less than one fewer time on average for both day and night) in the need to urinate among those in the placebo group.

•**The Urox group had about two fewer episodes of urgency and two fewer episodes of incontinence per day** compared with less than one fewer episode of either for the placebo group.

Even better: For 60% of participants in the Urox group, urinary symptoms returned to normal—meaning they no longer had symptoms of urinary incontinence—while this result was seen in only 11% of the placebo group. No significant side effects were reported for either group, although a small number of participants in both groups experienced transient diarrhea or urinary tract infections.

Naturopathic doctor Andrew Rubman, ND, medical director of Southbury Clinic for Traditional Medicines in Southbury, Connecticut, and author of the Bottom Line blog "Nature Doc's Patient Diary," commented that each of these herbs also is effective alone…

•**Horsetail** has been a common remedy for incontinence and bed-wetting in Europe since Shakespeare's time. The plant contains silica, which is anti-inflammatory and acts as an astringent in the bladder to "tone" the bladder wall, which helps restore normal bladder function.

•**Varuna** is an Indian Ayurvedic medicine that increases tone and coordination in bladder muscle. It helps the bladder empty more completely.

•**Japanese evergreen spicebush** is a Traditional Chinese Medicine (TCM) remedy for frequent urination and incontinence. According to TCM, incontinence and frequent urination are caused by "cold energy," and this herb moves warm energy ("chi") into the bladder to disperse the cold energy. But whatever the scientific reason, the remedy often works.

Urox is manufactured in Australia but is available in the US online for about $40 for a one-month supply. It should be noted that this study of Urox was funded by the maker of Urox, but Dr. Rubman points out that the study appears to have been conducted according to acceptable research standards, the researchers shared all their data and the study was published in a peer-reviewed medical journal.

Natural Cures for Eczema, Rosacea and Dandruff

Alan M. Dattner, MD, a board-certified dermatologist and pioneer in integrating nutrition, holistic medicine and dermatology. He is author of *Radiant Skin from the Inside Out: The Holistic Dermatologist's Guide to Healing Your Skin Naturally*, as well as several professional articles and book chapters relating to holistic dermatology. HolisticDermatology.com

If you have a skin problem and go to a conventional dermatologist, you're likely to get a diagnosis and a prescription for medication that in actuality may only help keep your symptoms in check.

A different approach: In the world of holistic dermatology—where treatment is all about finding the root cause of a problem rather than just controlling the symptoms—the skin serves as a window to what's happening deep inside the body.

A LEAKY GUT

In healthy people, the inside of the small intestine has a cellular barrier that prevents incompletely digested food molecules and toxins from crossing through to the bloodstream. In a condition known as "leaky gut," the cellular bonds holding the intestinal lining together are broken, allowing these materials to slip through, activating the immune system to cause inflammation (see next page).

Leaky gut is often caused by an overgrowth of yeast (frequently from a high-sugar diet)… or from specific food components like gluten, a protein found in wheat, barley and rye. In fact, 40% of gluten-sensitive patients analyzed in a study published in 2017 in *World Journal of Gastroenterology* cited eczema or a rash as symptoms.

If you find that you're sensitive to gluten, a gluten-free diet can give a leaky gut time to begin healing. A diet that's low in sugars and simple carbohydrates can reduce the inflammation caused in the gut by yeast and also improve leaky gut. In addition, you should eliminate high-yeast foods such as bread (even gluten-free bread can contain yeast)…cheese…wine…and beer.

Also: Probiotic supplements and probiotic-rich foods like sauerkraut (eaten daily) can replace yeast in the gut with more diverse, healthy bacteria. *In addition to the steps described above, try the following holistic strategies to fight…**

ECZEMA

The rough, red, inflamed patches of eczema can cause itching so intense that it's nearly impossible not to scratch. *What to do…*

•**Stop the scratching.** Ice cubes in a wet towel applied to eczema patches for five or 10 minutes provide a satisfying sensation that calms the instinct to itch.

Helpful: The anti-itch supplement Nettle Quercetin from Eclectic Institute.

•**Cure infections.** Cracks, crusting and open scratch marks are vulnerable to infection. For protection, take an antimicrobial herb such as olive leaf. Check with a doctor who has experience prescribing herbal medicine for advice on dosage—it varies depending on the patient. Redness, swelling, tenderness, pus and honey-colored crusting are all signs that an infection should be treated by a doctor. At this point, the organism should be cultured to determine an appropriate antibiotic to use.

•**Ease inflammation.** Try a chamomile or chickweed anti-inflammatory ointment.

•**Try digestive enzymes.** These supplements can improve leaky gut by reducing the size of food molecules to simple building blocks like amino acids that do not trigger a reaction.

What helps: A digestive enzyme that contains dipeptidyl peptidase-4 (DPP-4).

ROSACEA

Rosacea is an inflammatory skin condition marked by facial redness, blood vessel enlargement and tiny pimples known as pustules. *What to do…*

•**Avoid problematic foods.** Certain foods dilate facial capillaries.

Common triggers: Spicy foods…hot liquids such as coffee…and alcohol.

*To find a holistic practitioner near you, consult the American Holistic Health Association, AHHA.org.

•**Watch out for extreme weather conditions.** Protect the skin from wind, cold and sun whenever possible—all can contribute to redness.

•**Get more vitamin C and the bioflavonoids that accompany it in fruits and vegetables.** Bioflavonoids reduce capillary fragility, which often manifests as broken blood vessels or easy bruising. Eat vitamin C–rich foods such as kale, spinach and broccoli (citrus fruit can aggravate rosacea)…or take a vitamin C supplement (500 mg twice daily).

•**Control your emotions.** Anger, anxiety and embarrassment can cause blood to rush to the face, intensifying rosacea.

What helps: Deep breathing and meditation.

DANDRUFF

This white and red scaling of the scalp, forehead, eyebrows or chest is caused by an inflammatory immune reaction to a specific type of yeast (called Malassezia) that normally lives on the skin.

Even though antidandruff shampoos containing *ketoconazole* (Nizoral), *selenium sulfide* (Selsun Blue) or *pyrithione zinc* (Head & Shoulders) are designed to kill Malassezia yeast, they won't fix dandruff at its root cause. *What to do…*

•**Reduce yeast.** With dandruff, it's crucial to cut sugar, use probiotics and take an antiyeast supplement such as caprylic acid.

•**Get the right oils.** Omega-3 fatty acids calm inflammation. Try eating two servings of cold-water fish, such as wild salmon, a week. Use cold-pressed, organic olive oil or safflower oil, and avoid oils heated to a high temperature.

Helpful: Supplementation with vitamin E as well as vitamin C, B-complex, zinc and magnesium will help the body keep inflammation-fighting oils in their more usable forms.

THE INFLAMMATION FACTOR

Even though chronic inflammation is widely known to fuel health problems ranging from heart disease and diabetes to cancer and rheumatoid arthritis, it also plays a crucial role in skin conditions.

Here's what happens: When the immune system becomes triggered—due to a variety of causes (see above)—it can attack cells, tissues or organs, as well as the skin, showing up as inflammation. That's why if you have a skin problem such as eczema, rosacea or seborrheic dermatitis (better known as dandruff), it's likely signaling a problem elsewhere in the body.

Natural Help for Bipolar Disorder Treatment

Andrew L. Rubman, ND, naturopathic physician and founder and medical director, Southbury Clinic for Traditional Medicines, Southbury, Connecticut. Study titled "Evaluating the Effect of Coenzyme Q10 Augmentation on Treatment of Bipolar Depression: A Double-Blind Controlled Clinical Trial" by researchers at Hamadan University of Medical Sciences, Iran, published in *Journal of Clinical Psychopharmacology.*

Could preventing depressive episodes be as simple as getting a daily dose of a dietary supplement? A new study has found that a powerful antioxidant and anti-inflammatory agent has a place in the complex treatment of bipolar disorder, characterized by manic highs and depressive lows.

Researchers in Iran have found that CoQ10 can help improve mood. They divided 69 patients with bipolar disorder into two groups—one group took 200 mg of CoQ10 a day in addition to their mood stabilizers and antidepressants…the other group added a placebo. After eight weeks, the CoQ10 group had greater improvement of depression symptoms than the placebo group.

The finding makes sense: CoQ10 is vital to every cell's energy-producing process. More energy means less fatigue and feeling down.

Important: CoQ10 alone may not be the answer to treating bipolar disorder and you should never take any supplements or substitute supplements for medication without consulting your health-care provider. It certainly can be a helpful complement to your treatment even if prescriptions are working well. (On the other hand, some doctors have successfully used CoQ10 to effectively treat certain cases of diagnosed bipolar disorder that are characterized primarily by depression without typical prescription drugs—don't be surprised if your provider is willing to give it a try as a solo therapy.)

HOW TO SUPPLEMENT WITH COQ10

Organ meats such as liver and kidneys are great sources of CoQ10 but not quite daily food choices people are likely to make. You'll find it in smaller amounts in beef, sardines, mackerel and peanuts, but not enough to get a significant amount in your system. That's why supplements are usually needed.

Once your doctor prescribes CoQ10, keep in mind that it's better to take 100 mg twice a day than a single 200 mg dose. Dividing the amount suggested by the study into two doses could prevent gastric upset, which is a rare but possible side effect. Also, more isn't better when it comes to CoQ10—more than 200 mg a day is often unnecessary and could invite more side effects.

Warning: If you also take a blood-thinner, some evidence suggests that CoQ10 may offset the blood-thinning effect of *warfarin* (Coumadin). Though other studies have not found this effect, if you decide to take CoQ10, ask your doctor to test your blood-clotting time to see if it has any effect on you.

MORE ABOUT COQ10

If you take statins to reduce cholesterol, taking CoQ10 can help you avoid some of the more unpleasant side effects of those drugs, notably muscle pain and weakness and possible tendinitis. CoQ10 use has also been linked to migraine relief and even high blood pressure reduction.

CHAPTER 15

Nutrition, Diet and Fitness

The Ultra-Healthy Foods You're Probably Not Eating

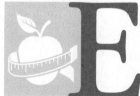

Eating right does not have to be complicated. By now, most of us know that the key is sticking with real foods—load up on veggies, along with some healthy fats. We also know that a food can be "low fat," "high fiber" or "gluten free" and still be pure junk.

Yet even the most knowledgeable eaters continue to miss out on plenty of ultra-healthy foods that fly under the radar.

To dispel some of the common myths that prevent so many people from benefiting from these lesser-known foods, we spoke with Mark Hyman, MD, a leading expert in nutritional wellness and director of the Cleveland Clinic Center for Functional Medicine.

MYTH #1: **Chicken is always a healthier choice than beef.**

The truth: There's nothing particularly healthy about America's most consumed meat—mass-produced chicken.

While the chickens raised in your grandmother's backyard ate a varied diet of grass, weeds, bugs and seeds, chickens raised on most commercial farms today get a steady diet of grains, corn and soy—often topped off with doses of antibiotics and arsenic.

This diet fattens them up quickly, but it produces poultry that's lower in inflammation-fighting omega-3 fatty acids and higher in inflammation-promoting omega-6 fatty acids. Grain-fed chickens also are lower in vitamins and minerals.

What to do: Choose chickens that are certified "100% organic" and pasture-raised (not free range—which only tells you that the birds got

Mark Hyman, MD, director of the Cleveland Clinic Center for Functional Medicine in Ohio. Dr. Hyman also is chairman of the board of the Institute for Functional Medicine and founder and director of The UltraWellness Center, based in Lenox, Massachusetts. He is author of several books, including *Food: What the Heck Should I Eat?* DrHyman.com outside, not what they ate). If you find that the cost of organic is an issue, "antibiotic-free" chicken is better than conventional but not ideal.

As for that beef: It does have a little more saturated fat than chicken, but 17 large reviews of the scientific literature on saturated fat found no link between saturated fat and heart disease.

That doesn't mean you should go crazy with saturated fat—we're still figuring out how much is healthy. But you should know that a nice grass-fed steak is more nutritious than the typical supermarket chicken breast.

MYTH #2: Liver is bad for you.

The truth: Even people who are comfortable eating steak, pork chops and pot roast may pause before trying that generations-old family recipe for liver and onions.

But liver is much more nutrient-dense than muscle meat—that's why when a lion takes down a zebra, it goes for the liver first. Liver contains ample amounts of vitamins A, B-12 and C, and minerals such as copper, iron, zinc, phosphorus and magnesium. It contains just as much protein as a beef roast or steak—and it's cheaper.

One reason liver fell out of favor is its high level of cholesterol. But research now tells us that eating cholesterol does not significantly raise our blood cholesterol (that's why we now know it's fine to eat eggs, too).

What to do: Whenever possible, choose liver from grass-fed animals.

And don't stop there: Try other organ meats, such as hearts, kidneys and sweetbreads. Even though they may not sound appealing, they usually taste good!

MYTH #3: Vegetables are boring.

The truth: If you think veggies are dull, you are doing them wrong. The most boring vegetables, such as iceberg lettuce and white potatoes, are the least nutritious.

The best choices are often the "weird" heirloom varieties you find from small farms—everything from purple carrots to knobby kohlrabi to dandelion greens.

As you surely already know, you should fill at least half of your plate with a wide variety of vegetables in a rainbow of colors, and I recommend aiming for seven or eight servings a day as a minimum. Go mostly for locally grown and organic veggies for the best flavor.

A good way to find more variety: Look to the sea. If you have eaten seaweed only as a sushi wrapper, you are missing out. Seaweed is not only rich in vitamin C and iron but also contains hard-to-come-by minerals, such as manganese and iodine, as well as anticancer compounds.

You can find several forms of seaweed, including wakame, kombu and nori, in Asian food markets. And some stores sell roasted, lightly salted seaweed snacks you can munch on like potato chips—without the guilt.

MYTH #4: Fresh fruit is always the best fruit.

The truth: Fruit that is flash frozen at the peak of ripeness can be more nutritious than fruit picked unripe so that it can then be shipped thousands of miles.

A frozen berry loses none of its antioxidants while it waits for you to open up your freezer and toss it into a smoothie or salad. A fresh berry does lose nutrients, and it can go moldy before you have a chance to use it. Frozen fruits are cheaper, too. If you buy frozen fruit, also opt for organic.

What to do: Regardless of the fruit you choose, it's important to not overdo it—especially if you are overweight or have diabetes or prediabetes. While fruit is a lot healthier than candy or juice, it still contains a lot of natural sugar and may raise your blood sugar. Two or three servings a day are plenty for anyone.

MYTH #5: Peanut butter is a great protein source.

The truth: Most commercial peanut butters are loaded with high-fructose corn syrup and industrial hydrogenated oils. Peanuts also can contain the fungus aflatoxin, which has been linked to cancer.

An occasional spoonful of peanut butter or handful of peanuts is fine, but this legume (it's not a nut) is not the nutritional powerhouse that tree nuts are.

What to do: If you like nut butters, go for almond, macadamia and cashew butters made without added oils, sugars or other ingredients.

See if you can find a store that grinds nuts into butter on the spot, but buy in small amounts so that the oils do not have a chance to go rancid. Store in the refrigerator.

***MYTH #6:* Soy foods are health foods.**

The truth: Many foods containing soy are among the worst in our diets.

The greatest offender is something you probably do not even know you consume—soybean oil, the oil of choice for most processed, packaged foods. It is the primary source of inflammatory omega-6 fatty acids in the typical American diet.

Processed soy protein is also found in many manufactured foods—for both animals and humans—that are not very healthy. Avoid foods, such as energy and protein bars, fake hot dogs, burgers and shakes, with "soy protein isolate" on the label.

Some fermented tempeh or simple tofu can be fine (if you buy organic to avoid pesticides and the GMO herbicide glyphosate) as well as steamed edamame, but there is no good reason to eat a soy hot dog. The soy protein isolate found in such products has been linked in some studies to allergies, cancer and dementia.

7 Surprising Foods That Beat Disease

William W. Li, MD, president of Angiogenesis Foundation, Cambridge, Massachusetts. He has served on the faculties at Harvard University, Tufts University and Dartmouth Medical School and is author of *Eat to Beat Disease: The New Science of How Your Body Can Heal Itself.*

Recently our society has been waking up to the fact that food and health are directly connected in both protective and destructive ways.

First, an overview: Our bodies contain five defense systems that not only protect us from illness but heal us when we're sick—angiogenesis, regeneration, the microbiome, DNA protection and immunity. In broad terms, they all help us fight off illness while keeping our organs healthy. Activating these systems can prevent many of the diseases we're most worried about, such as cardiovascular disease, cancer and type 2 diabetes. Research is proving that certain foods activate these systems. In fact, there are more than 200 foods that can intercept or even reverse certain diseases by boosting our health defenses. Of course, other foods that can damage our health have been shown to suppress the same systems, leaving us vulnerable to disease.

You may be thinking that you already know that barley, broccoli and dark leafy greens are good for you. You may be comfortable with your food choices, but challenging yourself to add the surprising foods identified here is well worth the effort. All are backed by extraordinary science…and none are in that "yuck, health food" category. You can easily add them to your meals to enrich and diversify your diet.

• **Chicken thighs.** Did you think white meat was the healthiest choice? Surprise!

Why it's so good for you: Dark chicken meat contains vitamin K-2 (also known as menaquinone), which has been shown to help control angiogenesis, one of our five defense systems. Angiogenesis is the process our bodies use to form and grow blood vessels. A healthy angiogenesis system regulates when and where blood vessels should grow and can prevent tumors from getting the blood they need to thrive.

Research at University of Illinois and Hiroshima University in Japan has found that vitamin K-2 can directly attack prostate cancer and colon cancer cells. Vitamin K also has been associated with a reduced risk for lung cancer. (See the section on Gouda cheese below.)

Keep in mind: Chicken thighs often are attached to chunks of fat, so trim off the fat before cooking.

• **Mangoes.** I call the mango a grand-slammer food because, from a health standpoint, it activates all five defense systems at once, hitting a home run for your health.

Why they're so good for you: Mangoes contain the bioactive compound mangiferin. Bioactive compounds modulate metabolic processes in the body. Mangiferin improves blood-sugar control and can prevent tumors from forming, according to research from several leading Chinese hospitals and universities.

Keep in mind: If you can't find fresh mangoes, frozen ones are just as nutritious. Even though they can help your metabolism, remember that mangoes are high in natural sugar, so people with diabetes or others who are limiting their sugar intake should ask their doctors about the recommended amount to eat.

•**Purple potatoes.** These strikingly hued potatoes are becoming more available and often are seen on restaurant menus.

Why they're so good for you: Research has shown that purple potatoes can kill colon cancer stem cells and reduce the number of tumors. Scientists at Penn State University fed the equivalent of one purple potato a day for a week to mice that were at high risk for colon cancer, and they found that they had 50% fewer tumors than mice not fed the potatoes. That is similar to the effect seen in prescription drug recipients.

Note: Ask at your grocery store if it carries the Purple Majesty variety—the kind used in the research. Purple potatoes can be prepared in different ways and still offer a health benefit.

•**Sourdough bread.** Remarkably, the element that gives sourdough bread its mildly sour taste is also what makes it healthful.

Why it's so good for you: The probiotics. Sourdough bread starter uses a natural, healthy bacteria called *Lactobacillus reuteri*, which has been shown in the lab to improve immunity, suppress tumor development, slow weight gain and speed up wound healing. The bacteria even can stimulate the brain to release oxytocin, the feel-good hormone. Scientists had long assumed that the health benefits of Lactobacillus reuteri were destroyed in the heat of an oven, but researchers at Massachusetts Institute of Technology found that even the fragments of killed bacteria can deliver the same benefits.

Keep in mind: Some sourdough bread does not actually use the right bacteria and is just flavored to taste tangy. Buy at bakeries where you can ask about the process. Eating bread loads you up with calories, so don't go overboard eating sourdough.

•**Gouda cheese.** It's surprising that cheese has health benefits, but it is indeed true when it comes to certain hard cheeses, such as Gouda.

Why it's so good for you: Just like chicken thighs, Gouda is high in vitamin K-2. Landmark research from Germany (the EPIC–Heidelberg study) examined the link between K-2 and cancer and found that eating between one and three slices (about one to three ounces) of hard cheese each day was associated with a 62% drop in risk for lung cancer. And eating the equivalent of two slices per day led to a 35% decrease in the risk for prostate cancer.

Keep in mind: Cheese is a source of saturated fat and high sodium, so less is more.

•**Kiwifruit.** This fruit—which is actually a large berry—came from China, where it was known for its benefits for digestion.

Why it's so good for you: Researchers at National University of Singapore showed that kiwi makes it easier for your gut microbiome to grow healthy bacteria, which can improve the state of your immune system. Meanwhile, scientists in Scotland found that kiwi can help prevent and repair damage to our DNA that is caused by the environment and linked to many serious diseases, including cancer.

Colorful Cauliflower

Regardless of color, cauliflower is low in calories—one cup cooked has about 27 calories—and high in nutrients, such as vitamins C, K and folate.

Colorful versions do provide a few special nutrients. Compared with white cauliflower, the orange variety has extra beta-carotene (about 480 mcg per cup versus about 9 mcg)...while purple cauliflower contains high levels of anthocyanins (about 7 g per cup), the same flavonoids that give purple carrots and asparagus and fruits like tart cherries, blueberries and blackberries their rich hues. Anti-inflammatory anthocyanins have been found to help reduce risk for a range of diseases, including cancer, heart disease and cognitive decline.

Lisa R. Young, PhD, RDN, a nutritionist in private practice and adjunct professor, department of nutrition and food studies, New York University, New York City. She is author of Finally Full, Finally Slim.

Keep in mind: Eating one kiwifruit a day is beneficial, but even more benefits were seen by researchers with three kiwifruits per day.

•**Concord grape juice.** OK, technically this is a beverage. But it's a powerhouse nonetheless.

Why it's so good for you: Besides being good for the heart as reported in previous studies, grape juice boosts your immune system, according to a study from University of Florida. Drinking one and a half cups of Concord grape juice every day for nine weeks was found to increase the level of T-cells, which play an important role in immunity and fighting cancer.

Keep in mind: Like all fruit juice, grape juice contains natural sugar, so if you need to control your blood sugar for any reason, check with your doctor before adding this to your diet. Also avoid juices with added sugars or artificial sweeteners.

Better Than Water! How to Stay Properly Hydrated

Dana G. Cohen, MD, an internist who practices integrative medicine in New York City. She is an adviser to the board of the American College for Advancement in Medicine, ACAM.org. Dr. Cohen is author, with Gina Bria, of *Quench: Beat Fatigue, Drop Weight, and Heal Your Body Through the New Science of Optimum Hydration.*

The mantra "Drink more water!" is heard so often that it seems like an obvious truth. Of course we should all drink water—preferably eight full glasses a day. Right?

Not so fast. It's true that many Americans don't drink enough water. According to some estimates, dehydration is a problem for up to 75% of adults. But chugging more water from the tap (or from an overpriced plastic bottle) is not the best way to stay hydrated.

New thinking: The water that you get from foods is more hydrating than "liquid" water. This gel-like form of water is about 10% more viscous than liquid water. Found inside all living cells, gel water moistens tissues better than liquid water…and contains more electrolytes, which enhance bodily functions.

What does this mean in practical terms? Simply put, eating your water is healthier than drinking it.

A HEALTHIER "DRINK"

Plant foods typically contain between 80% and 98% water, by volume. The electrolytes mean that gel water isn't merely moisturizing…it's a fuel that improves cognition, judgment and mood.

Of course, you still need liquid water. In fact, if you don't replenish the amount of fluid typically lost through sweating, urination and other bodily functions, it can cause a measurable loss of cognitive abilities…a decrease in the ability of blood vessels to contract/dilate…and an increase in cellular inflammation. But gel water does an even better job at keeping you hydrated.

HOW TO GET MORE

Instead of relying on liquid water alone, I recommend four steps that incorporate diet and exercise for healthful hydration. *To help stay properly hydrated…*

STEP #1: Drink two green, veggie-based smoothies a day. Even one smoothie (at least eight ounces) will increase hydration and improve energy, but two are ideal. Why vegetable-based smoothies? Because the gel water facilitates absorption by cell membranes…the fiber clears out toxins and cellular wastes…and the minerals (including natural sodium) improve hydration as well as flavor.

You can make a smoothie with virtually any combination of green vegetables, with a little fruit for flavor.

My favorite hydrating smoothie recipe: Blend at least one leafy green (such as spinach or kale)…a bit of apple, banana or carrot for sweetness…lime juice or apple cider vinegar if you like a little zing…herbs (such as parsley, cilantro or basil)…healthy fats (like avocado oil)…a sprinkling of nuts and/or chia seeds for thickening…and water as needed. Because of the gel water and minerals, a smoothie is much more hydrating than an equal amount of liquid water.

STEP #2: **Be sure to eat hydrating vegetables.** All plant foods contain healthy amounts of gel water, but some veggies are surprisingly good sources.

Examples: Cucumber (96.7%)...romaine lettuce (95.6%)...celery (95.4%)...radish (95.3%)... and zucchini (95%). Fruit is somewhat less hydrating—watermelon and strawberries are roughly 91% water...grapefruit and cantaloupe about 90%...and kiwi, apples and pears about 84%.

STEP #3: Use natural salt. Sodium often gets blamed for dehydration. But the real problem is processed salt that's been stripped of beneficial minerals. Natural forms of salt—such as sea salt, Celtic salt and Himalayan salt—contain iron, magnesium, calcium and potassium, in addition to sodium. The minerals improve hydration by increasing the electrical activity within cells.

Note: These salts typically contain very small amounts of iodine, so look for versions that are fortified with iodine if you're concerned about your iodine levels.

Also: I suggest avoiding—or at least limiting consumption of—processed foods. They're loaded with unhealthy salt and can be dehydrating because the body has to use water to metabolize them.

Important: Anyone with salt sensitivity can have sharp rises in blood pressure when they consume any form of salt, but most people can enjoy moderate amounts (more than the 1,500 mg daily recommended by many health groups) of natural salt without experiencing blood pressure changes. Consult your doctor for advice.

STEP #4: Move moisture with micromovements. It's easy to put more water into your body, but how does the water get where it's needed? It travels through fascia, the miles of thin, gauzelike tissue that lie beneath the skin and between and around organs and bones. The pulsing of fascia transports water droplets throughout the body. Even the smallest movements increase the pulsing action.

In addition to the standard exercise recommendation (150 minutes of moderate-intensity exercise a week), you can take advantage of micromovements—such as foot tapping, head turning and shifting your weight. Twisting motions—such as swiveling your body or moving your head in figure-eight motions—are par-

ticularly good because they squeeze moisture through the fascia, just like wringing a wet washcloth releases water.

The great thing about micromovements is that you can do them anywhere, anytime—in the car, at your desk, while watching TV, etc.

ARE YOU DEHYDRATED?

Many people suffer from some degree of dehydration, yet there isn't a reliable test to detect it. You probably know that normal urine should be clear or just slightly yellow. A dark yellow color (or a smaller volume than usual) could mean you're dehydrated.

Other important clues...

•**Your skin "tents" and holds the shape when you pinch it.** Healthy, hydrated skin—particularly on the backs of the hands—should snap back to its normal position.

•**You "fail" the fingernail test.** Press a fingernail for five seconds to flush out the color, then release. It should regain its normal color in one to three seconds. If it doesn't, you're probably dehydrated.

Beyond Peanut Butter

Sharon Palmer, RDN, a Los Angeles–based registered dietitian nutritionist and author of *The Plant-Powered Diet* and *Plant-Powered for Life*. Palmer also is editor of the newsletter *Environmental Nutrition* and nutrition editor for *Today's Dietitian*. SharonPalmer.com

What's so great about tree nuts and peanuts? They are filled with unsaturated fats, as well as vitamins, minerals, fiber and phytochemicals (plant compounds with antioxidant and anti-inflammatory activities).

Seeds, such as flax, sesame, sunflower, pumpkin, hemp and chia, may not have garnered quite the recognition for their health benefits at this time, but these tiny kernels possess similar nutritional powers as nuts.

Worth noting: Even though nut and seed butters are rich in the healthful variety of fat, they are still concentrated in calories. Most nut butters provide about 180 to 190 calories per serving (two tablespoons)—so a little goes a long way. That's why sitting down with a spoon and an open jar isn't the best way to enjoy these butters.

Instead, spread them on your favorite whole-grain breads…use as a dip with vegetable sticks or apple slices…add to smoothies…mix into your breakfast cereal…use them as a healthful fat source (instead of butter or margarine) in baking…and stir them into sauces and vinaigrettes.

Bonus: Nut and seed butters are a great plant-based protein option for vegetarians and people who want to cut back on their consumption of red meat—high amounts of which have been linked to increased risk for diabetes, heart disease and certain cancers. It's also a good idea to read the labels of nut and seed butters to avoid unwanted added ingredients, such as sugars and hydrogenated oils.

Nut and seed butters worth trying…

ALMOND

How to enjoy it: With its mildly nutty, sweet taste, almond butter is delicious when it's spread on avocado and tomato sandwiches. It also makes a terrific dip for fruit and veggies.

For a yummy, healthful surprise: Try adding almond butter to baked goods, such as oatmeal cookies and banana bread.

Special quality: Almond butter is a good source of calcium, providing about 8% of the Daily Value per serving (two tablespoons).

Nutritional value: In addition to being a reliable source of protein (5 g per serving), almond butter contains riboflavin, vitamin E, magnesium, phosphorus and manganese.

WALNUT

How to enjoy it: Try walnut butter in sauces to accent savory foods, such as seafood or lentil patties, as well as in wraps and on toasted whole-grain raisin bread.

Special quality: Walnuts have something unrivaled in the nut world—they have omega-3 fatty acids…and a lot of them. That's a big part of the reason why walnuts are good not only for the heart but also for the brain.

Nutritional value: Walnut butter has 5 g of protein per serving and is rich in magnesium, phosphorus, copper and manganese. With their

nutty and mildly astringent taste, walnuts also offer a high level of healthful phytochemical compounds.

PISTACHIO

How to enjoy it: To incorporate pistachio butter into your diet, add it to vinaigrettes for grain salads, biscotti dough and muffins.

Special quality: Pistachio butter is one-of-a-kind because of its color—a lovely shade of green! The green hue comes from lutein, a carotenoid that has antioxidant action, helping to lower blood pressure and fight chronic conditions such as heart disease and stroke, as well as protect eye health as we age.

Nutritional value: Pistachio butter is creamy and rich in protein (6 g per serving), fiber, thiamine, vitamin B-6, phosphorus, copper and manganese.

SUNFLOWER SEED

How to enjoy it: Spread sunflower seed butter on banana sandwiches, fill dates with it and stir it into butternut squash soup.

Special quality: This sweet, golden butter is a great alternative for people who might be allergic to tree nuts or peanuts. Sunflower seed butter is also a superstar for its impressive levels of vitamin E (it has 37% of the Daily Value in one serving). Research has linked this powerful antioxidant to improved immunity.

Nutritional value: It's packed with protein (6 g per serving), fiber, vitamin B-6, niacin, folate, pantothenic acid, phosphorus, zinc, copper, manganese and selenium.

SESAME SEED (TAHINI)

How to enjoy it: Sesame seed butter (tahini) is what gives hummus that earthy, nutty taste. But it's also delicious and nutritious in its own right. Try using tahini as a dip for falafels, as a spread in pita sandwiches, as a pasta sauce with noodles and as an addition when baking soft cookies.

Special quality: Tahini is a good source of plant-based calcium (providing 12% of the Daily Value). It also has cholesterol- and blood pressure–lowering effects.

Nutritional value: Pale in color, tahini is bold in nutrition, packing in protein (5 g per serving), fiber, thiamine, calcium, iron, magnesium, phosphorus, zinc, copper and manganese.

Give Cheesy "Nooch" a Try

Janet Bond Brill, PhD, RDN, FAND, a registered dietitian nutritionist, a fellow of the Academy of Nutrition and Dietetics and a nationally recognized nutrition, health and fitness expert who specializes in cardiovascular disease prevention. Based in Allentown, Pennsylvania, Dr. Brill is author of *Blood Pressure DOWN, Cholesterol DOWN* and *Prevent a Second Heart Attack*. DrJanet.com

I t may not sound appetizing, but hold on and give this hugely popular vegan food additive a second look. Nutritional yeast—referred to affectionately by many people as "nooch"—is a nonactive, cultured strain of the single-celled organism Saccharomyces cerevisiae (technically classified as a fungus). Saccharomyces cerevisiae is grown on molasses and then harvested, washed and dried with heat to kill or "deactivate" it. Because it's inactive, it is not like regular yeast, meaning it doesn't froth or grow like baking yeast does, so it has no leavening ability.

Note: If you have a known sensitivity to eating mold/yeast, try a small amount of this product. If you have a reaction, don't add it to your diet. Nooch is sold either as a yellow powder or flakes (larger grocery stores might have the Bob's Red Mill brand or Bragg brand in the natural-food section).

Why eat it? There are two simple reasons: Taste and nutrition. Nutritional yeast is added to foods to create a savory, nutty flavor that really does taste a lot like cheese. Nooch is a nourishing nondairy substitute for those who can't or choose not to eat dairy. But even if you're not vegan, nooch offers a load of nutrients with few calories and little saturated fat. It also has less sodium than real cheese.

Nutritional yeast is rich in B vitamins, folic acid, selenium, zinc, fiber and protein (a complete protein at that). It's gluten-free and contains no added sugars or preservatives. Most, but not all, commercially sold nutritional yeast has been fortified with B-12. Vitamin B-12 is found in animal foods, so prudent vegans must supplement their diets with a reliable source of B-12. Most healthy adults require 2.4 micrograms (mcg) of vitamin B-12 each day. Bob's Red Mill Nutritional Yeast, for example, contains 3.5 mcg of the vitamin in a two-tablespoon serving.

Best ways to enjoy nooch: Use it much like you would Parmesan cheese—sprinkle it on popcorn or roasted vegetables...add it to pasta sauce or salads...or mix into yogurt-based dressings and flours.

Omega-3s for Vegetarians

Sharon Palmer, RDN, a registered dietitian nutritionist and author of *The Plant-Powered Diet*. She also holds an MSFS degree, a master's of science in sustainable food systems. Read her blog at "The Plant-Powered Dietitian" at SharonPalmer.com.

M ost Americans don't get enough EPA and DHA in their diets, so they often take a supplement that contains these omega-3 fats in the form of fish oil.

But dietary preferences aren't the only reason that many people forgo fish. There also are increasing concerns about the sustainability of eating fish or taking fish oil supplements, based on the fact that about 85% of the world's fish species are overfished, according to the World Wildlife Fund.

For all these reasons, marine algae can be beneficial to many people. Like most plants, marine algae undergo photosynthesis—that is, they use sunlight, water and carbon dioxide to produce their own food. Though you may not realize it, the omega-3s found in fish oil mainly come from the marine algae that the fish consume—or from eating krill and other fish that feed on algae. So essentially the primary source of omega-3s is marine algae.

Marine algae can be consumed in food sources, too, including nori seaweed (typically found in sheets that are used in rolling sushi or as a crunchy, salty snack that can be added to rice bowls and soups) and kelp (available in sprinkles that can be used as a topping for salads and/or a substitute for salt). However, it can be difficult to get an appreciable amount of the long-chain omega-3s EPA and DHA from these food-based sources.

Bonus: Chlorophyll, the green plant pigment found in algae, also has potential health benefits, such as helping to boost immunity and reduce inflammation. The powdered supplements chlorella and spirulina are rich in chlorophyll and can be added to smoothies or juice.

In addition, marine algae are now grown in controlled environments and can be extracted and concentrated into supplements. Studies have found that the EPA and DHA in marine algae supplements have a similar ability to lower levels of blood lipids, including triglycerides, as fish oil supplements. It's important to note, however, that marine algae supplements may have variable levels of EPA and DHA compared with fish oil supplements.

Most healthy people should consider taking a supplement that contains 250 mg of EPA and DHA per day (roughly the equivalent of eating fish twice per week). If you have a known heart condition, your doctor may want you to have higher levels of EPA and DHA. To ensure that you are choosing a quality supplement, look for "third-party tested" or some other third-party certification on the label.

Try Coffee Flour

Jessica Dogert, RDN, nutritionist at Hi-Vibe Superfood Juicery, Chicago.

Coffee flour is made by drying and grinding the coffee cherry—the fruit surrounding the coffee bean that has traditionally been discarded. Unlike white or even whole wheat flour, coffee flour is packed with protein, iron, potassium, antioxidants and fiber. A tablespoon has 70 mg of caffeine, about as much as in a six-ounce cup of coffee.

Coffee flour has a mildly nutty, roasted fruit flavor and makes a great gluten-free and virtual-

ly fat-free substitute for some of the flour called for in a recipe. Replace 10% to 15% of your regular flour with coffee flour, and see how it affects your recipe. You also can add a tablespoon to a smoothie or sauces.

5 Vitamins Nearly Everyone Should Take

Hyla Cass, MD, integrative physician in private practice in Los Angeles, natural supplement formulator and consultant, and coauthor of several books including *8 Weeks to Vibrant Health.* CassMD.com

Joshua Levitt, ND, naturopathic physician in private practice in Hamden, Connecticut, a clinical preceptor for Yale School of Medicine and author of *The Honey Phenomenon: How This Liquid Gold Heals Your Ailing Body.* WholeHealthCT.com

Michael Murray, ND, author or coauthor of more than 30 books featuring natural approaches to health, including *The Encyclopedia of Nutritional Supplements* and *Bottom Line's Encyclopedia of Healing Foods.* He is based near Scottsdale, Arizona. DoctorMurray.com

Andrew L. Rubman, ND, director of Southbury Clinic for Traditional Medicines in Southbury, Connecticut, and author of the blog "Nature Doc's Patient Diary" at Bottom LineInc.com. SouthburyClinic.com

Jacob Teitelbaum, MD, holistic fibromyalgia and pain specialist in private practice in Kailua Kona, Hawaii, and coauthor of *Real Cause, Real Cure.* EndFatigue.com

Are there nutritional supplements that everyone should consider taking? We posed that question to five nutrition-savvy doctors who have served as experts for Bottom Line for years. Surprisingly, they not only all said "yes," but they all generally agreed on what these nutritional supplements are.

That consensus is even more surprising given the negative attention that multivitamin/mineral supplements have gotten lately. Some studies have failed to find that they protect against heart disease, for example. But that's not why most people even take multis—or should, our experts say.

Better reason: To ensure that you are getting adequate amounts of essential nutrients to function at your best day to day.

Many Americans don't get enough. According to the latest Dietary Guidelines report, common nutritional shortfalls include the B vitamin folate, vitamin D and magnesium. And deficiencies become more common for certain nutrients after age 50, when nutrient absorption often declines.

Important: Our experts agreed that in addition to the specific recommendations below, everyone should take a multivitamin/mineral supplement that supplies 100% of the Recommended Daily Intake (RDI) for most vitamins, minerals and trace elements (especially selenium, chromium and iodine).

Exception: Iron deficiency is rare in people over age 50, so iron should be part of your multi only if a doctor-ordered test shows that you are iron-deficient. Why? Too much acts as an unhealthy oxidant.

A healthy diet always comes first, our experts agree.

Example: Fruits, vegetables and beans provide fiber and potassium that supplements generally don't provide.

Does everyone need all these supplements? No. If you eat fatty seafood at least twice a week, for example, you could safely skip omega-3 supplements. But most of us would benefit from taking all of these supplements.

What follows are the amounts that our experts agree are safe and beneficial for everyone. They often prescribe higher amounts for certain patients.

Important: Share your supplementation plan with your health-care provider, who can offer individual guidance.

A good multi is just the beginning, our experts told us. *Here are four additional daily supplements that benefit nearly everyone...*

MAGNESIUM

Magnesium strengthens muscles, builds bone, energizes the brain, regulates the heart, reduces high blood pressure, balances blood sugar, aids sleep, eases pain, improves digestion, helps your body utilize calcium and more. Before processed food dominated the diet, Americans consumed 600 milligrams (mg) of magnesium a day on average. Today, that number is about 275 mg—well below the RDI of 420 mg for men and 320 mg for women.

Recommended daily dose: Our experts most often prescribe 200 mg twice a day—once in the morning, once in the evening—for a daily total of 400 mg.

Avoid: Magnesium oxide, which can sometimes cause loose stools.

Best: Magnesium glycinate.

B VITAMINS

B vitamins play important roles in the health of your brain and nerves, blood, digestive tract, muscles, skin and eyes. They help power every cell in the body. Our experts put a special emphasis on folate, B-6 and B-12.

Recommended daily dose: Take a "B-50-complex" supplement either once a day or in divided doses twice a day. This formulation, sold under a number of different brands, includes all the Bs. The name refers to the fact that the daily dosage is 50 mg or 50 micrograms (mcg) for many of the Bs. Those levels exceed the RDI in most cases but are safe to take daily.

Additional recommendation: If you are a vegetarian or a vegan or are over age 50, also take a separate B-12 supplement. While a B-50-complex supplement will have a small amount of B-12 (typically 50 mcg), taking an additional B-12 supplement is important because B-12 deficiency is particularly common as we age, in part because we produce less of the stomach acid needed to absorb it from food.

Tip: Look for a sublingual (under-the-tongue) product providing the most active form—methylcobalamin—at a daily dose of 1,000 mcg.

VITAMIN D

Vitamin-D deficiency is disturbingly common in the US. Indeed, most Americans have blood levels below a minimally healthy level of 30 nanograms per milliliter (ng/mL). Our experts agreed that blood levels above 50 ng/mL (but not higher than 80 ng/mL) are best for peak functioning of muscles, bones, digestion, immunity, hormones and circulation. Vitamin D also may help prevent breast and colon cancers.

Recommended daily dose: 2,000 international units (IU) of D-3, the form that's best absorbed. That supports a blood level of 50 ng/mL for most people and is safe to take daily long-term.

Important: Get your vitamin-D level tested. If it's very low, your doctor may prescribe higher doses, up to 10,000 IU daily.

FISH OIL

Fatty fish such as salmon and sardines are rich in the omega-3 fatty acids EPA (eicosapentaenoic acid) and DHA (docosahexaenoic acid). If you don't eat fatty fish at least twice a week, consider a daily omega-3 supplement.

It's true that recent studies have failed to find that these supplements prevent heart disease in healthy people. But omega-3s are key nutrients for every cell in the body, and most Americans don't get enough. And there is evidence that they are key to lifelong health.

Example: In a study from Harvard Medical School and several other leading institutions, researchers looked at 15 years of health data on more than 6,500 postmenopausal women and found that those with the highest levels of EPA and DHA were 11% less likely to die from any cause during the study than those with the lowest levels. Another recent study conducted at Tufts University on men and women found that higher blood levels of omega-3s were linked to healthier aging.

Reason: Omega-3 fatty acids make all cell membranes more flexible and youthful—and every part of the body benefits. They can ease arthritis, improve mood and ward off depression, protect against dementia, reduce high triglycerides (blood fats) and even slow skin aging.

Recommended daily dose: A supplement that supplies 1,000 mg of EPA and DHA combined. Higher doses may be prescribed to reduce high triglycerides.

Caution: Omega-3 supplements act as anticoagulants, so talk to your doctor before taking one if you already are taking a prescription anticoagulant.

The Clever Way to Cut Down on Sugar (It's Easier, Too)

Studies titled "Sleep Extension Is a Feasible Lifestyle Intervention in Free-Living Adults Who Are Habitually Short Sleepers: A Potential Strategy for Decreasing Intake of Free Sugars?" by researchers in the UK, Canada and the Netherlands published in *The American Journal of Clinical Nutrition*, "The Effects of Three Mindfulness Skills on Chocolate Cravings" by researchers at McGill University and published in *Appetite*, "Caffeine increases sugar-sweetened beverage consumption in a free-living population" by researchers at Deakin University and published in *The British Journal of Nutrition*, and "Temperature Affects Human Sweet Taste via at Least Two Mechanisms" by researchers at Yale School of Medicine and published in *Chemical Senses*.

You want to cut back on sugar, but simply telling yourself not to eat that slice of cake or bowl of ice cream just isn't cutting it. That's not a shocker, since you are probably addicted (like most people).

Solution: Trick your brain into wanting less sugar in the first place. *Here are the surprising, scientifically proven strategies that can do just that…*

1. Get more sleep. Following up on research that found that getting too little sleep leads to eating extra calories the next day, scientists have found that the reverse is also true—adults who increased the amount of sleep they got each night naturally ate 10 g less sugar each day and also chose better quality foods with more protein and less fat. And they didn't need to sleep their lives away, either. On average, they increased their nightly sleep by only 47 minutes.

2. Practice "disidentification." Mindfulness is a great tool for losing weight and improving diet in general, thanks to components such as awareness and acceptance, but the specific part of the practice called disidentification could have the biggest impact when you want to cut back on sugar. Mindfulness teaches you to think of your cravings as only thoughts you have—not as who you are—but with disidentification, you take it one step further and mentally distance yourself from these thoughts. According to a study published in the journal

Appetite, people who used these components of mindfulness had fewer cravings for chocolate than people who used another popular technique, distraction, to avoid eating it. Ways to learn mindfulness meditation range from an app, such as Stop, Breathe & Think, to online classes from organizations such as the pioneer in the practice, the Center for Mindfulness at the University of Massachusetts Medical School.

3. Drink up. Dehydration can masquerade as hunger. So you might think you need a cookie when all you really need is a glass of water. If you don't tend to drink a lot of water instinctively, set a schedule and keep it flowing.

4. De-link caffeine and sweet beverages. A study published in *The British Journal of Nutrition* found that people who drank high-sugar caffeine drinks had more of them than people who drank high-sugar but caffeine-free drinks. While it doesn't affect taste, caffeine causes a dependence that leads you to have more and more sugary beverages. You can still enjoy coffee, but skip the sugary flavored creamers and other add-ins.

5. Avoid sugary foods and drinks that are served cold. Cold decreases your perception of all tastes, including sweetness. You don't taste the sugar as acutely as if the food were at room temperature or warm, so you end up consuming more to scratch your sugar itch. Yes, this means you'll eat more ice cream than a warm pudding.

6. Be a sugar sleuth. There are 61 different named sugars that manufacturers slip into packaged foods. Some are obvious, such as high fructose corn syrup and sucrose, but others are more inscrutable such as barley malt and maltol. Check out the complete list from the University of California San Francisco (Sugarscience.ucsf.edu/hidden-in-plain-sight). Remember, just because a food sounds healthy doesn't mean it's not loaded with sugar. Read the label to be sure and to keep track of your intake. For women, the smart limit is 6 teaspoons or 25 g of sugar per day, and for men, it's 9 teaspoons or 36 g. (But those aren't targets—they're limits!)

Eating a Variety of Foods Might Make You Fat

Report titled, "Dietary Diversity: Implications for Obesity Prevention in Adult Populations: A Science Advisory From the American Heart Association," by Marcia C. Otto, MC, and others, published in *Circulation*.

Variety is the spice of…appetite. We may feel satisfied after eating a specific food, but a new food, flavor, even texture will fire our appetites right up again.

Example: Adult subjects were offered sandwiches to eat and then, about 20 minutes later, given an opportunity to eat more sandwiches if they were still hungry. Sometimes the second sandwich had the same filling as the first, sometimes different. When it was the same, they ate less.

So if you like the same healthful breakfast, lunch, even dinner every day, no worries! Indeed, limiting variety even may make it easier to keep calories—and weight—in check. Instead of going for variety, focus on eating the most nutritious foods.

When variety is a good thing: Other research has found that eating a colorful array of fruits and vegetables may help you get a wider array of vitamins and other protective phytochemicals. This kind of variety may make it easier to eat more—of the right stuff.

Are You Eating at the Right Time of Day?

Michael F. Roizen, MD, chief wellness officer at Cleveland Clinic and chief of its Wellness Institute. He is coauthor, with Michael Crupain, MD, MPH, of *What to Eat When: A Strategic Plan to Improve Your Health & Life Through Food*.

In the never-ending diet debates, people focus almost exclusively on what to eat. But when you eat may be nearly as important.

Your body's circadian rhythms—the daily cycles that dictate when you awaken, when you're alert, etc.—don't just influence your behaviors like sleepiness. The time-specific, daily release of hormones determines when you get hungry and how much you eat…as well as your body's metabolism—how efficiently you utilize fats, carbohydrates and other nutrients.

What scientists are now discovering: Chrononutrition—the concept that food habits should align with circadian rhythms for optimal health—can have a dramatic impact on your chances of developing a variety of serious conditions. *What you need to know…*

BENEFITS OF EARLY EATING

Most people get hungriest at night. But to realize the health-promoting effects of chrononutrition, the best time to eat most of your daily calories is before 2 pm.

Here's why: The body's cells respond more readily to insulin early in the day—important for food metabolism and healthy weight maintenance, as well as preventing diabetes.

Research has shown that insulin sensitivity is higher during the hours when you're most active. This makes sense because you need energy from your glucose reserve (which depends on insulin) when your muscles are moving. At night, when most people's energy needs are lower, you need less glucose.

THE "THREE-QUARTER" CHALLENGE

What happens when you eat earlier in the day? It's well-established that people who consume most of their calories during the daytime are less likely to be obese. That's why I recommend consuming three-quarters of your daily calories at breakfast and lunch.

Of course, changing your eating schedule isn't easy. People are naturally primed to eat more at night, probably because our ancient ancestors needed to store more calories to survive…and because they didn't live long enough to suffer the effects of harmful conditions such as arthritis, dementia and diabetes.

To get started: Try to get most of your daily calories between about 8 am and 2 pm for at least three days a week—more often if you can. As you become more accustomed to eating mainly during these hours, you can transition into this schedule seven days a week.

If you get hungry at night, have a healthy snack, like raw, crunchy vegetables (or roasted veggies if you prefer).

IMPROVE YOUR BLOOD SUGAR

As mentioned earlier, insulin resistance (the reduced ability of insulin to transport glucose into cells) is higher at night than during the daylight hours. Insulin resistance is a serious health problem because it increases the risk for diabetes, obesity—and even heart disease, cancer and dementia.

Animals given high-fat meals at night are more likely to consume more calories, gain more weight and have more insulin resistance than those that are given the same meals earlier in the day.

Similar changes occur in humans. The weight-management program at Cleveland Clinic encourages not only eating 75% of daily calories before 2 pm but also increased walking and a reduction of simple carbohydrates (such as chips, white bread and other processed foods). People with diabetes who follow the program for as little as two months often improve so much that they're able to discontinue one or two diabetes medications.

BOOST YOUR HEART HEALTH

A consistent finding is that daytime eating lowers high blood pressure, a leading cause of heart disease. The reduction is significant enough, in many cases, that it equals the effects of taking a blood pressure–reducing drug.

When you improve the metabolic state of the body by eating earlier (and healthier) meals, you also reduce the whole-body inflammation that can cause a gradual impairment of kidney function. Reduced kidney function can impair the renin-angiotensin system, a group of hormones that helps regulate blood pressure.

Other benefits: Daytime eating causes a decrease in triglycerides and LDL "bad" cholesterol…an increase in beneficial HDL cholesterol…and a lower risk of developing metabolic syndrome, a life-threatening constellation of symptoms that includes high blood pressure, high blood sugar and elevated triglycerides.

A HEALTHIER EATING PLAN

An optimal eating schedule can't overcome the effects of a poor diet. Everyone should avoid most processed foods and simple sugars (such as white flour) and eat more "whole" foods, including whole grains, beans, veggies, etc. *Also...*

•**Eat your breakfast!** There are surprisingly few randomized trials on the health benefits of eating breakfast, but research has shown that people who skip this meal are more likely to have higher LDL "bad" cholesterol levels. Those with diabetes often have higher blood sugar levels later in the day when they skip breakfast.

Make breakfast either the largest or the second-largest meal of the day. People who aren't normally breakfast eaters should at least practice "less-late" eating and get most of their calories at lunch.

•**Get some protein at breakfast.** A bit of protein reduces food intake later in the day.

Examples: Greek yogurt (with no added sugar), salmon, steel-cut oats and nuts or seeds. Aim to get about 25 g of protein at breakfast each day.

•**Skip the big suppers.** Get no more than about 25% of your total daily calories from snacks/supper combined. If you do eat at the regular supper hour (around 6 pm or 7 pm), have something like a small salad, accompanied by a small portion of a protein-rich food.

Easier Than a Diet...and Great for Your Health— Intermittent Fasting

Tina Marinaccio, RDN, integrative registered dietitian nutritionist and adjunct professor in clinical nutrition and food studies at Montclair State University in New Jersey. She leads the nutrition element of Dr. Dean Ornish's Program for Reversing Heart Disease. TinaMarinaccio.com

---

I am the first to admit that fasting sounds even worse than dieting. But some kinds of fasting can be easier than dieting—and have benefits that go well beyond weight loss. In fact, even people who are not overweight can get amazing benefits from fasting, including healthier hearts, stronger muscles and clearer thinking.

The technical term for what I'm talking about is "intermittent fasting," which means fasting for short periods—sometimes, just 12 hours—on a regular basis. Most intermittent-fast techniques are not daily, and many allow for some calories even on "fast" days. This is definitely not a hunger strike! Some researchers believe that these intermittent fasts are easier to maintain than daily "caloric restriction"—aka traditional dieting, which basically requires that you eat less than you want every single day forever. Intrigued? *Here's more on the benefits of intermittent fasting and how you could easily try it...*

WHY INTERMITTENT FASTING IS SO HEALTHY

Studies have shown that intermittent fasting can help people lose weight without losing muscle. Maintaining muscle is key to keeping weight off and healthy aging. People on intermittent fasts find it easier to control their appetite even on nonfasting days.

One reason: They are producing less insulin, a key "hunger hormone."

But there are many more benefits. These kinds of fasts have been shown to reduce blood pressure...reduce blood glucose levels and improve insulin sensitivity...reduce levels of triglycerides (blood fats) and improve the cholesterol profile...reduce inflammation...enhance muscle endurance...and even improve learning and memory. In animal studies, intermittent fasting can reverse type 2 diabetes, slow the progression of cardiovascular disease and prolong life.

Why is this kind of fasting so good for the body? One hypothesis is that our gut biome—the mix of gastrointestinal bacteria that's key to health—needs a rest to function optimally. In addition, fasting has been shown to help the body get rid of damaged cells and regenerate healthy new ones. Humans likely evolved eating this way—food was scarce, and we couldn't spend every day eating and snacking every few hours like we can now. Periodic fasting respects—maybe even resets—our internal body clocks.

CHOOSING A WAY TO FAST

The best fast is the one that fits into your lifestyle. *Here are three options supported by scientific evidence...*

•**Time-restricted eating.** This is the easiest fast to pull off. Every day, you simply restrict eating to a specific stretch of the day. You'll get the most benefits by limiting yourself to eating during just an eight-hour stretch—say, 10 am to 6 pm. But time-restricted eating is something you can ease into—for example, by restricting your eating to 12 hours...and then gradually scaling back to eight hours.

Eating at night, in particular, interferes with the body's natural day-night cycle, disrupting hormones in a way that favors weight gain. And there's psychology—choosing an endpoint to the day's eating helps eliminate nighttime eating.

Let's face it: No one is sitting in front of the TV at night eating carrot sticks. It's more likely to be ice cream or chips.

Tip: Get most of your calories early in the day, meaning you eat a big breakfast and a smaller lunch and dinner. It's fine to eat breakfast several hours after you wake up—that's healthy as long as it's not paired with late-night eating.

•**Periodic fasting.** On two consecutive days, you cut way back on calories—by 75%. The rest of the week, you eat in a normal fashion. The popular 5:2 Diet is an example of this approach.

•**Alternate-day fasting.** In this approach, you alternate days when you restrict calories—to perhaps 500 calories for the day—with days when you eat a normal, healthy diet. This way of fasting is one day on, one day off. It's effective, but some people find that they are too hungry on fasting days to sustain it.

Tip for periodic or alternate-day fasting: To meet your calorie goal and assure good nutrition on partial-fast days, make protein shakes with fruit and some form of healthy fat, such as ground flax or a no-sugar-added nut butter. A low-sugar plant-protein powder serves as the base. Two brands I like are Vega and Kashi GoLean (I'm fond of the Vanilla Vinyasa flavor).

Caution: Before you start any fast, discuss it with your health-care provider. That's especially important if you have a medical condition. For example, although fasting may help improve diabetes, people who take blood sugar–lowering agents need to be especially careful about low blood sugar. Plus, some medications need to be taken with food.

More tips for successful intermittent fasting...

•**See a registered dietitian (RD).** An RD can help you determine which of the eating patterns—if any—makes sense for you and help you put a plan into place. He/she can help you choose the most nutritious foods (especially important on days when you don't eat as much as you normally do)...and, if you need them, recommend nutritional supplements.

•**Be extra wary when you eat out on partial-fasting days.** Restaurants use more fat and sugar than you would at home, and portions are huge. It's easier to eat at home so that you know what you're taking in.

•**Consider professional metabolic testing.** How can you know what to eat to cut calories by, say, 75%? You start by calculating the calories you burn at rest—your resting metabolic rate, aka RMR—and then add everyday activities plus physical exercise. Online RMR calculators are notably inaccurate.

Better: An FDA-approved calorimeter, which measures your RMR when you breathe into it. These instruments are too expensive to make it worth buying one for home use, but many RDs have them in their offices.

•**"Cheat" with nonstarchy vegetables.** If you find yourself extra-hungry on a fasting day, don't suffer too much. The best way to "cheat" is with low-glycemic vegetables, many of which have lots of filling fiber and all of which have very little effect on blood sugar or insulin levels.

Examples: Salad greens, cruciferous vegetables (broccoli, cabbage, cauliflower, etc.), radishes, zucchini, summer squash, eggplant, tomatoes and mushrooms.

Bonus: These types of vegetables are especially good at feeding beneficial gut bacteria.

One caution, though: Don't pile on potatoes, winter squashes, corn, peas and the like—these are starchy vegetables that you shouldn't cheat with.

Want to Lose Weight for Good This Time? Don't Go It Alone!

Chyke A. Doubeni, MD, MPH, the Harrison McCrea Dickson, MD, and Clifford C. Baker, MD, Presidential Professor in the department of family medicine and community health and associate professor of biostatistics and epidemiology at Perelman School of Medicine, University of Pennsylvania.

If losing weight is so hard—which it is—why does almost everyone try to go it alone? People may be biased against working with a counselor for a number of reasons, such as not wanting to "admit" that help is needed or simply not wanting to spend the money. (*Tip:* Some health insurance companies pay for diet counselors, so ask yours.)

But know this: Just as getting assistance can help someone quit smoking or drinking alcohol, counseling could be your answer to permanent weight loss. *Unlike another fad diet, taking the following steps can help you reach that goal…*

•**Choose a counselor with the skills to address your unique situation.** A psychologist who specializes in eating disorders can help if you use food to ease stress, for instance. If you have a health condition, look for a counselor with additional credentials such as a registered dietitian if you need help reducing cholesterol or a certified diabetes educator if you have diabetes or prediabetes. Also consider logistics—the expert's schedule needs to work with yours. That might include online or virtual check-ins on your smartphone, tablet or computer to track your progress or to problem-solve with you between sessions.

•**Decide on an approach that feels comfortable to you.** Counseling can be one-on-one or in a group setting. If you don't like sharing personal details with strangers, choose individual counseling with a nutrition or health coach. On the other hand, a group setting allows for an exchange of tips that have helped others. It's also possible to have individual sessions and participate in a group.

•**Work with the counselor on improving your relationship with food.** He/she should help you identify what's getting in the way of achieving your weight loss goals, such as the triggers that set off mindless eating or obstacles to increasing your physical activity. More than just keeping a food journal, bring it with you to your sessions so that your counselor can assess your patterns and show you how to use the journal most effectively.

•**Have the counselor develop a plan tailored to your lifestyle.** For success, you need an eating and exercise plan, not a "diet" you go on and off of every time the scale moves. And that eating and exercise plan needs to be adapted to your likes and dislikes, health needs and schedule so it can be a permanent way of life. Your weight-loss counselor should be able to show you how to incorporate your favorite foods so that you don't give up because you feel deprived. If you eat out a lot, get a list of safe menu items. If you're too busy to cook every night, ask how to best stock your kitchen for quick, tasty and low-calorie meals that you will want to eat. Your counselor can also help you find forms of physical activity that are enjoyable and good for you so you're motivated to engage in them on a consistent basis.

•**Ask whether your goals are realistic.** Nothing sets you up for failure more than overreaching. Get help setting attainable weekly and monthly weight-loss goals. If you've barely gotten off the couch until now, don't ask how to train for a half-marathon in a month, but rather get tips to increase your activity in increments that you can reasonably stick with.

•**Keep going to sessions.** Meaningful behavioral changes don't happen overnight. Counseling generally needs to continue for at least a year. If you hit a weight-loss plateau, your counselor can give you tips to get back on track and keep you from going back to your old eating or exercise habits out of frustration. And when you hit your goal, a 15- to 30-minute follow-up phone call with your counselor once a week (perhaps scaling down over time to once a month) may be the best maintenance plan in the world to keep that weight off.

8 Surprising Diet Mistakes That Exercisers Make

Nancy Clark, MS, RD, sports nutritionist with a private practice in the Boston area and author of the bestseller *Nancy Clark's Sports Nutrition Guide Book*. NancyClarkRD.com

If you're trying to lose weight or simply avoid creeping weight, you're likely adding exercise to your daily routine—good for you! Yet you notice a problem...the weight's not coming off the way you want it to or worse, it's sneaking upward. What's that about?

Here's the truth about exercise and calories—plus eight other mistakes that may be keeping your exercise from bringing the results you want...

Mistake: **Overestimating the number of calories you burn** through exercise and, as a result, eating more than you need. Exercise has a ton of benefits ranging from boosting bone and brain health to warding off diabetes and heart disease, but unless you're working out at a very high level for a very long time, you're not burning through a large number of calories. As an example, walking at a brisk 4 mph for 30 minutes burns about 200 calories (depending on your height and weight) and that's the number of calories in just one ounce of some nuts—barely a handful.

Tip: Use a fitness chart or wearable fitness tracker to calculate what you're really burning off when you exercise, and factor that correctly into your diet strategy.

Mistake: **Counting on exercise alone for significant weight loss.** Using the same example as above, you can quickly calculate how many 30-minute walks it will take to burn off one pound, or 3,500 calories—yes, 17.5! For exercise to contribute significantly to weight loss, it needs to be coupled with cutting calories.

Tip: Although exercising more and eating less can combine to create the needed net calorie deficit, you really want to decouple the two things in your mind and put them into separate mental buckets. Exercising is vital for your health...and eating less is vital for losing weight.

Mistake: **Having a one-and-done approach to daily exercise.** If you work out for one 30-minute session per day and spend the rest of your waking hours at a desk or on the sofa, you aren't capitalizing on exercise as much as you should for weight loss and overall health.

Tip: Take a 24-hour view of activity and build on your formal workout. That could mean holding a walking meeting at the office instead of gathering around a conference table, adding an hour of gardening to your weekends, and jogging in place while you stream a TV show.

Mistake: **Working out too soon after a meal.** Exercise leaves many people hungry, and that can lead to eating more times during a day and taking in more calories than you had planned. Net result? You could end up with a weight gain, not a loss.

Tip: One way to account for post-exercise hunger is to make sure that your exercise session does not come soon after any meal—but rather, soon before a regular mealtime. That way you can satisfy your body's demand for fuel without adding extra calories (and in effect canceling out the calories you just burned). Just be sure to maintain—not add to—your food portion sizes.

Mistake: **Thinking you need to replace electrolytes with a sports drink**. Special "replacement" drinks are meant to boost fluid retention during heavy exercise, such as running a marathon. If you're exercising three hours or more in the heat, they may be helpful. Otherwise, they're not necessary. "Electrolytes" is essentially a technical term for salt. Chances are you're already getting plenty of that. (A slice of bread contains about as much salt as a 12-ounce sports drink.)

Tip: Water is all most people need to replace fluids after a typical workout, and it has no calories.

Mistake: **Eating the standard three meals a day.** Restricting yourself to breakfast, lunch and dinner is an old-fashioned way to fuel your body and can mean long stretches between meals. Instead, distribute your total daily calories somewhat evenly across four to six meals per day, depending on what works best for your schedule.

Example: Try a hearty breakfast at 7 am, lunch at 11 am, a "second lunch" (bigger and better than a snack) at 3 pm and a lighter dinner around 6 pm. You may find it helpful to work with a registered dietitian (RD) to design a food plan specifically for you, one that includes the most nutrient dense foods to keep you fueled and feeling full. The referral network at SCAN dpg.org can help you find a sports nutrition expert near you.

Mistake: Eating most of your protein at one meal. The body makes fast work of this essential nutrient. Protein in your food is best used to build and repair muscle in the first four hours after you've eaten, so you should include a serving of protein at every meal. Protein is filling, so it will help you curb your appetite, too.

Tip: Plan on 15 grams (g) to 30 g protein per meal (with larger people needing more than smaller people) if you're eating four meals a day…or 10 g to 20 g per meal if you're eating six meals a day. Healthy choices include two or three eggs (6 g of protein per one large egg)…turkey or chicken (3 oz/24 g)…fish (3 oz/19 g)…and black beans (½ cup/7 g). Looking for more nonmeat protein choices? Enjoy a banana with peanut butter, a handful of (high-calorie but healthful) nuts, cottage cheese or Greek yogurt.

What don't you need? Protein shakes, a source of unnecessary calories for the average person—even for people who exercise. What's more, packaged protein shakes are highly processed, commonly contaminated with heavy metals such as lead and arsenic, and they're missing many of the nonprotein nutrients found in whole foods.

Mistake: Eating a large meal close to bedtime. Remember to think of food as fuel. You need more fuel during daytime hours when you are active and less when you are sleeping.

Tip: Front-load your day by having more of your calories at breakfast. Resist the urge to eat after dinner—move any calories you're in the habit of eating at night into the next day's breakfast.

Is Your Workout Causing the Wrong Kind of Weight Loss?

Kristen M. Beavers, PhD, department of health and exercise science at Wake Forest University, Winston-Salem, North Carolina, and lead author of the study titled, "Effect of Exercise Type During Intentional Weight Loss on Body Composition in Older Adults with Obesity," published in *Obesity*.

Jacqueline Crockford MS, CSCS, an ACE (American Council on Exercise) certified personal trainer and exercise physiology content manager at ACE in San Diego.

A recent study shows that combining dieting with aerobic exercise can make people lose more muscle mass than if they didn't exercise at all!

The study: Researchers at Wake Forest University in North Carolina recruited 249 people in their 60s and 70s who were overweight and followed them for 18 months. Each participant was assigned to one of three programs—dieting with no exercise…dieting plus aerobic exercise (which, for this study, was walking)…or dieting plus weight training using weight machines. The two exercise groups worked out four days a week for 45 minutes.

The results: Diet plus aerobic exercise actually led to greater muscle loss than dieting alone. Among those who dieted only (no exercise), 16% of the weight they lost was muscle. Among those who dieted and did aerobic exercise, 20% of the weight they lost was muscle. On the other hand, among those who dieted and lifted weights, just 10% of the weight they lost was muscle.

Weight training won out in another way, too. Participants who dieted and weight trained lost 17 pounds of fat, on average, while those who dieted without any exercise lost just 10 pounds of fat. (The group that dieted and got aerobic exercise lost 16 pounds of fat.)

Now, no one, including the researchers, is saying that dieters should refrain from aerobic exercise—it's essential for heart health and for overall fitness. But this study shows just how important weight training is and why you should add it to your diet plan.

The benefits go beyond the scale: We all naturally lose muscle mass as we age, starting in our 30s. The additional muscle loss from dieting is greater in older people. So while losing excess weight is good for overall health, preserving as much muscle mass as you can with strength training will keep you strong and independent, prevent functional declines and help you avoid falls.

Important: If you're new to strength training, ask your doctor if it's OK for you to start. Once you get the green light, begin working out two days a week, and as you get stronger, you can work out every other day (muscles need about 48 hours between sessions to recover).

Are You Walking Fast Enough to Live a Long Life?

Study titled, "Self-rated walking pace and all-cause, cardiovascular disease and cancer mortality: individual participant pooled analysis of 50,225 walkers from 11 population British cohorts," led by researchers at University of Sydney, Australia, published in *British Journal of Sports Medicine.*

You know walking is good for you—no, great for you. Taking a walk is a pleasant, easy, no-cost way to exercise, and it produces a bounty of well-known health benefits—from helping with weight loss to reducing stress to keeping your memory sharp and your heart healthy.

It can even help you avoid premature death—but only if you move at more than a saunter, especially as you get older, new research reveals.

The good news: While you can't just piddle along and expect walking to do all its magic, you don't have to be a speed walker like Cary Grant in *Walk Don't Run* to get these long-life benefits.

THE SPEED OF LONGEVITY

It makes logical sense that regularly walking at a brisk clip might reduce your risk of early mortality. After all, the faster heart rate from that fast clip strengthens your cardiovascular system and stimulates health-improving physiological responses throughout your body. But while the overall benefits of exercise are well-documented, the role of walking speed hadn't been well-studied. In fact, the new research is the first study of its kind because it teased out walking speed's impact from the rest of someone's physical activity.

Scientists at the Universities of Sydney, Cambridge, Edinburgh, Limerick and Ulster examined results from the Health Survey for England and the Scottish Health Survey, two ongoing population-based studies that have tracked more than 50,000 men and women, age 30 and up, for an average of nine years. Their goal was to measure the influence of walking speeds against mortality from all causes as well as from cardiovascular disease and cancer. The participants reported their walking speeds—slow, average or brisk/fast. They reported how much walking in particular—and physical exercise in general—they engaged in on a regular basis.

Surprising results: Average walking speed, meaning just under three miles per hour (mph), was statistically linked to nearly the same health benefits as brisk/fast walking (3.5 or 4 mph). And compared with slow walkers (around 2 mph), average-speed walkers had a 20% reduced risk of dying over those nine years.

For brisk/fast walkers, the mortality risk reduction was only slightly greater: 24%. (Walking pace reduced mortality primarily by helping to prevent cardiovascular disease—there was no statistical benefit in terms of cancer prevention.)

But something much more powerful was discovered as well: The benefit of walking at an average pace—what fitness experts like to call "moderate intensity"—may get much greater as you age. For study subjects age 60 and older, walking at an average pace or faster was associated with a 46% lower rate of cardiovascular disease mortality compared with slow walkers. And brisk/fast-paced older walkers got the proverbial gold ring—a 53% reduction in cardiovascular mortality.

Now, this kind of observational study can't establish causality, so it doesn't prove that intentionally keeping up the pace in your walking style will help you avoid chronic illness or an early demise. Researchers noted the many cardiovascular benefits of walking at an average/moderate rate or faster—but they also acknowledged that some of the statistical differences in longevity between slow and average or brisk/fast walkers may come from the fact that people in declining health tend to walk slower.

In practical terms, however, the message is clear: If you can walk at a moderate pace or faster, do it! Strolling can be relaxing, but it isn't likely to do as much for your health.

HOW CAN YOU TELL IF YOUR PACE IS FAST ENOUGH?

To get the greatest potential life-extension benefits from walking, you want to make sure you walk fast enough.

An easy way to tell: Count the number of steps you take. Recent research suggests that you should aim for 100 steps a minute—a brisk pace that's easy to determine. For people with an average stride length, that pace will work out to just under three miles per hour—the "average pace" chronicled in this study.

Pump Iron for a Healthy Heart and Mind

Lift weights for heart health. Weight training improved cardiovascular risk factors, including high blood pressure, diabetes and elevated cholesterol, more than walking or biking, according to a study of more than 4,000 men and women.

Best: Combine weight training—often done at a higher (more heart-protective) intensity—with aerobic activity, which is also beneficial for heart health.

Maia P. Smith, PhD, MS, statistical epidemiologist and assistant professor, department of public health and preventive medicine, St. George's University School of Medicine, Grenada.

Strength training can beat the blues. A recent review of clinical studies suggests that strength training may benefit one in four adults with depressive symptoms. It is not known whether it has a preventive effect—or whether it is as effective on its own as when done in combination with aerobic exercise.

Brett R. Gordon, MSc, is postgraduate researcher, University of Limerick, Ireland, and lead author of a meta-analysis involving 1,877 participants, published in *JAMA Psychiatry*.

Use your watch or a stopwatch on your phone to count how many steps you take in 10 seconds and multiply that by six, or simply count your steps for a full minute.

Tip: It's about the same as the pace of the hit 1970s disco song "Stayin' Alive" by the Bee Gees—one step per beat. Get your pace set, and then head out for at least 30 minutes of moderate-intensity walking at least five days a week—as recommended by the Centers for Disease Control & Prevention—confident that you're taking a big step toward better health and longer life.

Want to aim for a brisk pace? That's 120 to 130 steps per minute. If you can, go for it!

See What's Missing from Your Workout...

Tom Holland, MS, CPT, an exercise physiologist, certified sports nutritionist and certified strength and conditioning coach. He is founder and president of Team Holland, a fitness-consulting company in Darien, Connecticut, and author of four fitness books, including *Beat the Gym: Personal Trainer Secrets—Without the Personal Trainer Price Tag*. TeamHolland.com

---

First things first: If you exercise regularly, pat yourself on the back. But if you're like most people and do just one exercise over and over again, listen up.

By simply varying your exercise routine, you can greatly improve the health benefits of your workout...overcome any boredom that might creep in...and even reduce your risk for injury.

The good news is, you don't need a lot of fancy equipment to vary your workout. *Here's how to mix it up if your favorite exercise is...*

WALKING

If you are a walker, add high-intensity interval training (HIIT). Whether you frequent your local outdoor track or use a treadmill, walking is arguably one of the best forms of exercise there is.

But to maximize the benefits, you need to ramp up your speed (and/or perhaps incline or resistance if you're using a treadmill). The best way to do this is to up the ante on your workout with some HIIT, which intersperses short bursts of increased intensity.

While your regular walking routine may feel like a five on a scale of one to 10, during HIIT intervals, you should feel like you're exercising at a seven or an eight. The variety makes a low-intensity, steady exercise like walking more interesting and fun, and people who have fun when they exercise are more apt to stick with it.

If you're trying to lose weight: HIIT burns extra calories both during and after the workout.

To try it: Walk or use a treadmill at a comfortable warm-up pace for three minutes, then alternate 60 seconds at a normal pace with 60 seconds at a faster pace or higher incline for the remainder of the workout. (Pumping your arms helps—use the safety cord if you're on a treadmill.) Be sure to do a three-minute cooldown at a slower pace. Try adding HIIT to your walking routine one to three times per week.

TENNIS

If you love tennis, add some foam rolling. Pulled muscles and strains are ubiquitous among tennis players in their 50s, 60s and beyond, thanks to the quick, sudden movements and direction changes. But just a few minutes of pre-tennis self-massage with a foam roller could be enough to keep you on the court.

Why foam rolling? Because this technique, which involves moving a foam roller back and forth along different parts of the body, enhances blood flow to different muscles, performing it preworkout can improve flexibility and range of motion, reducing one's risk for injury, according to research published in *International Journal of Sports Physical Therapy*.

Also: Foam rolling lower-body muscles prior to exercise alters perception of fatigue, so you won't tire as quickly.

To start rolling: Target your calves, quadriceps and iliotibial bands, the thick connective tissue running down the outside of each hip to just below the knee.

For calves, sit on the floor and place the roller perpendicular underneath your outstretched legs. While supporting most of your weight with your hands, lift your hips and slowly move the roller up and down your calves for 10 to 30 seconds.

Flip over to roll out your quads...and turn on your side for the iliotibial bands—roll these areas

for 10 to 30 seconds each. Try this rolling routine before tennis matches and a few times per week.

YOGA

If yoga is your thing, add cardio exercise. Mix things up with jogging or fast walking, biking, swimming or fast-paced aerobics classes. Just make sure that you're spending most of your time at your target heart rate for 30 minutes a day, five days a week. It's fine to do three 10-minute sessions to reach your goal.

Your target heart rate: Aim for 50% to 85% of your maximum heart rate, which is 220 minus your age. So if you're 55, your maximum heart rate is 165, and your target heart rate 83 to 140 beats per minute.

Exciting recent finding: Heart disease patients practicing yoga in addition to aerobic exercise had twice the reduction in blood pressure, cholesterol levels and body mass index compared with those who did either exercise alone.

Also: For all types of exercise, do strength training two days a week for a well-rounded regimen.

Smile to Make Exercise Feel Easier

Noel E. Brick, PhD, lecturer in sport and exercise psychology, Ulster University, Derry, Northern Ireland.

When volunteers smiled while they ran, their running economy (the volume of oxygen consumed during a workout) improved by a significant amount (2.78%) compared with when they grimaced...relaxed their upper bodies...or ran normally.

For the biggest boost: Grin at 30-second intervals.

Why smiling helps: It reduces the perception of effort...may relax the body...and offers a psychological boost.

Get One Hour of Fitness in 5 Minutes

Tom Holland, exercise physiologist and certified strength and conditioning specialist based in Darien, Connecticut. He is author of *Beat the Gym: Personal Trainer Secrets—Without the Personal Trainer Price Tag.* TeamHolland.com

You don't have to carve an hour out of your busy schedule to exercise—a five-minute workout one or more times per day can lead to noticeable improvements in your physical strength and cardiovascular fitness. *These very basic and well-known moves will work all the major muscle groups...*

1. Do a one-minute warm-up. You can jog in place or do jumping jacks to increase your heart rate and blood flow, raise your body temperature and improve your muscle elasticity. This will prepare your body for more vigorous exercise.

2. Do 30 seconds of squats. From a standing start, bend your knees, as if you're about to sit on an imaginary chair. Do not go any lower than a 90-degree angle where your thighs are parallel with the floor and your heels are down. Then return to a full standing posture. Hold your arms out in front of you for balance as needed. Repeat as many times as possible.

Beginner strategy: If you can't do deep squats, do more shallow squats—lower your body only a few inches. Then increase this depth as the days pass and you get stronger.

3. Do 30 seconds of push-ups. You probably already know how to do push-ups—with your hands positioned slightly more than shoulder width apart.

Beware of pitfalls: Keep your body straight, butt in line and your neck in a neutral position. Repeat this exercise as many times as possible in 30 seconds.

Beginner strategy: If you are not yet strong enough for a traditional push-up, do "knee push-ups," where your knees are on the ground instead of your toes.

4. Do a 30-second plank. Position yourself in the push-up position—body perfectly straight, supported by your toes and hands with arms extended, hands below your shoulders. Contract your abs, and hold this position for 30 seconds.

Beginner strategy: Support yourself on your toes and forearms rather than on your toes and hands...and/or try to hold the plank for less than 30 seconds.

5. Repeat steps two through four. Perform a second round of the three exercises above.

6. Do a one-minute cool-down. Jog in place for 30 seconds, then do 30 seconds of stretches. Stretch your quads by holding one foot up behind your backside for a few seconds (grasp a chair for balance if necessary), then repeat with the other foot. Stretch your shoulders by grasping your right elbow with your left hand and pulling your right arm across your body (keep your right shoulder down), then repeat on the left arm. If any other parts of your body feel tight, go ahead and stretch those, too.

CHAPTER 16

Optimum Aging

How Old Brains Stay Young—and How to Make Yours One of Them

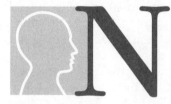

ot long ago, brain scientists believed that old brains didn't make many new connections. They thought that our brains slow down as we age because we don't make enough new neurons to replace those that naturally die.

In recent years, though, the results of some studies have challenged that theory, suggesting that even older brains continue to make many new neurons. Not all studies have found this, though, so it's been a controversial topic. Now, even more sophisticated research has settled the question—at least for a key part of the brain responsible for learning and memory.

And the answer is…yes, healthy older brains make as many new neurons as younger brains do in a key part of the brain that is responsible for learning and memory.

But there's a catch: Just making new neurons is not enough to keep our minds fit. The new research sheds a little light on that, too—and what you can do about it.

THE BRAIN'S LEARNING AND MEMORY CENTER

Researchers from Columbia University Medical School set out to determine whether new neurons continue to be generated in a specific region of the hippocampus, the part of the brain that is responsible for learning and memory. They examined brains from deceased patients that had been preserved quickly enough after death to not have undergone too many physical changes. The deceased patients ranged in age from 14 to 79. (To reduce any influence from disease, brain donors were confirmed to not have cognitive impairment or any neurologic or

Study titled, "Human Hippocampal Neurogenesis Persists throughout Aging," by researchers at Columbia University and elsewhere, published in the *Cell Stem Cell*.

psychiatric illnesses and to have no history of using medications that would affect reasoning or other thinking.)

Using specialized techniques and equipment, the researchers were able to "count" how many new blood vessels were being formed at the times of these patients deaths…and the quantities of different types of cells in several different parts of the hippocampus, each with different functions.

Results: The total volume of the dentate gyrus, the part of the hippocampus responsible for cognitive processing and making and recalling memories, was the same in brains that were in their eighth decade as in their second. Also, young neurons and specialized glia cells, which are essential to the function of neurons, were just as plentiful in older brains as in young ones.

The remarkably preserved specimens and the rigorous control of this study may account for why it found clear evidence of new neuron growth when some other studies haven't. But it's also worth noting again that the researchers excluded people with cognitive impairment such as dementia or neuropsychiatric illnesses such as depression. So it's not known whether everyone's brain keeps making so many new neurons and thus new connections. But it is evidence that our brains have the ability to keep significantly regenerating neurons, not only using old neurons—well throughout life.

WHAT OLDER BRAINS OFTEN LACK

What was different about older brains in the study?

One thing stood out: Older brains did not have as many new blood vessels compared with younger brains. To function optimally, neurons need the nourishment and oxygen that is carried to them through blood vessels.

A key takeaway: Your brain can keep refreshing itself with new neurons—but it's up to you to make sure that it gets the cardiovascular nourishment it needs. That means doing everything you can to stay physically fit and reduce your risk of heart disease and diabetes. If you keep the blood flowing, your brain might continue to help you remember well and learn new things for many, many years.

Look Younger Just by Doing These Face Exercises

Gary Sikorski, creator of Happy Face Yoga and co-author of a study published in *JAMA Dermatology.* You can buy or stream Happy Face Yoga at his website Happy FaceYoga.com.

When age and gravity cause your butt to droop or the backs of your arms to morph into floppy wings, you know what to do—get to the gym and up your squats or add an extra set of triceps moves.

But what about when your cheeks start to sag into jowls and your mouth seems stuck in a frown? Is it possible to exercise a few years off your face?

BUH-BYE JOWLS

Face-firming exercise is nothing new. The idea dates back at least as far as the 1960s when fitness guru Jack LaLanne led people through a series of "facenastics." And there have been dozens of face workouts since.

But none of them have been scrutinized by science until researchers at Northwestern University Feinberg School of Medicine decided to take a closer look at my program, Happy Face Yoga. Participants between 40 and 65 years old did two 90-minute training sessions in which I taught them 32 different moves targeting the face and the neck. (Don't worry—you don't need to learn 32 moves to make yourself look younger.) They then did the exercises at home for 20 weeks. For the first eight weeks, they spent a half hour each day flexing their facial muscles. For the next 12 weeks, they cut back to doing 30 minutes of exercises every other day.

Two dermatologists evaluated photographs of each participant taken at the beginning of the study…after eight weeks of facial exercise…and then after 20 weeks.

Results: The photographs showed a roughly three-year decrease in age appearance over the 20-week period. Not bad for just moving your face around at home, right? And it's possible that continuing to do the exercises could erase even more years off your look.

BEFORE YOU START

While changes to the structure of our skin play a large role in how we look as we age, changes to the muscles that underlie all that skin can have their effect, too.

I created 32 facial exercises so people have options, like when you go to a gym and there are so many types of equipment. But even if you do only a few of these exercises each day for 15 minutes, you can help yourself look younger.

Below I'll share three of the most effective facial exercises, but first, here are tips to help you get the most out of the overall program…

Because you'll be touching your face, wash your hands before you do the exercises.

Wash your face, too. You don't want your skin to be slippery with makeup or lotion.

Try to avoid touching the skin directly under your eyes, which is very delicate.

Use visualization when you are doing the exercises—imagine your muscles are moving and strengthening. This visualization tells your brain to send more signals to the muscles to get them working!

While you do the exercises, maintain good posture. Sit up straight. Good posture acts as an anchor and will allow you to focus on the facial muscles you are exercising.

Drink lots of water—at least six glasses a day. Water is the ultimate moisturizer. It helps carry nutrients and oxygen to your skin and muscles and helps flush out toxins.

Three face-firming exercises…

THE CHEEK LIFTER

The idea here is to strengthen the muscles in the cheeks—elevating droopy cheeks to more youthful heights.

1. Form a long/tall "O" shape with your mouth and fold your upper lip over your front teeth.

2. Smile to lift your cheek muscles. Place your index fingers lightly and directly on the top part of each cheek, directly under your eyes.

3. Relax your cheek muscles, allowing them to return to their original position (keep

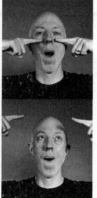

your mouth in an "O"), and then smile again to lift your cheek muscles. Visualize pushing the muscles up toward your eyes as you smile. You have just completed one "push-up." Repeat nine more times.

4. On the final push-up, hold your cheek muscles up as high as you can. Move your index fingers an inch away from your face, and raise them to scalp level while looking at them to help you visualize your cheek muscles lifting. Continue looking up at your fingers, and hold for 20 seconds. Release and relax.

Do the entire sequence of 10 cheek lifters three times per session.

THE HAPPY FACE LIFTER

This exercise strengthens the entire face and increases blood flow to the muscles of the face, neck and scalp. It's most effective when done standing up.

1. Form a long/tall "O" with your mouth, press your lips against your teeth, then slowly fold them over your teeth. Smile to lift your cheek muscles.

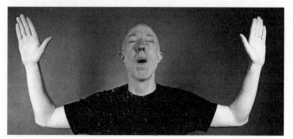

2. Close your eyes, and roll your eyeballs toward your scalp. Adjust your mouth to make the "O" as small as possible. Smile again to further tighten those cheek muscles, keeping the "O" small. Slowly tilt your head slightly back.

3. Tighten your abdominal muscles and buttocks, lift your chest and contract all your facial muscles. Keeping your eyes closed, slowly raise your hands up and over your head as you visualize lifting every single facial muscle off your body.

4. Hold the lift tightly for 30 seconds while taking long, deep breaths. On an exhale, allow your hands and head to drop toward the floor. Slowly inhale and relax.

Do this exercise one time every morning and every evening.

SCOOPING

This jaw-and-neck exercise firms sagging cheeks and droopy jowls and can diminish wrinkles on the sides of the chin.

1. Open your mouth, and make an "Ahh" sound. Fold your lower lip over your lower teeth and hold tightly. Extend your lower jaw forward.

2. Using your lower jaw only, scoop up very slowly, as if you're using your jaw to scoop up something very heavy, then repeatedly open it and scoop again. Each time you scoop, tilt your head back so that your chin rises about an inch, incrementally tilting your head farther and farther.

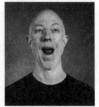

3. Do 10 scoops. By the final one, your face should be about parallel with the ceiling. Keep your chin extended and hold tightly for 20 seconds while visualizing the sides of your face lifting.

Repeat twice for a total of three sets.

The Secret Anti-Aging Agent You Should Be Eating

Paul Robbins, PhD, associate director of the Institute on the Biology of Aging and Metabolism at University of Minnesota, Minneapolis, and co-senior author of "Fisetin is a senotherapeutic that extends health and lifespan," published in *EBioMedicine*.

Move over, vitamin C. Step aside, collagen. There's a new micronutrient stealing center stage. It's the flavonoid *fisetin*, and it's starting to get its share of attention as a promising way to slow down aging.

Yes, that's what we said. Previously, lab studies on animals and on human cells had found that fisetin can reduce diabetes complications, protect against stroke and enhance memory. Fisetin also has been shown to relieve allergic reactions by inhibiting cytokine production.

But now we can add one more benefit: Slowing down the aging process and increasing

the prime-of-life years. When researchers from University of Minnesota and Mayo Clinic gave fisetin to older mice, the animals experienced a rejuvenation and longer-than-average span of time during which they were healthy (before any chronic diseases set in)—what researchers call their "healthspan." The study looked at 10 flavonoids in all, each with the potential to stop the aging process, but it was fisetin that stood out as the most potent.

FISETIN: FIGHTING CELL DAMAGE

In our bodies, cells go through an aging process known as cellular senescence, in which the cell stops dividing. These types of cells have been linked to many age-related diseases. Certain flavonoids have been shown to help the body remove these cells, with fisetin being the most effective.

So where can you get it and how much do you need? Clinical trials are under way to help find the best human dosages for fisetin's different benefits—it's likely that a higher amount is needed for antiaging than for enhancing memory, for instance. It's found naturally in (in order of richness) strawberries, apples, persimmons, lotus root, onions, grapes, kiwis, peaches and cucumbers, but current thinking is that it will take more food than you can comfortably eat every day to get enough fisetin to fully reap its antiaging benefits. You can already buy concentrated fisetin supplements, generally in 100 mg tablets, but there are no guidelines stating whether that's the ideal amount. To give an idea of what that amount translates to in food, you'd need to eat a pound of strawberries to get 100

Aging—It's All in the Mind

When brain scans were performed on adults (average age 71), those who reported feeling younger than their chronological ages had brains with structural characteristics that are more commonly found in younger people. The finding adds to the growing body of research into personal feelings about aging and their link to neurological changes.

Frontiers in Aging Neuroscience.

mg of fisetin—but at just 150 calories, that could be a wise choice.

In fact, despite the open questions on dosing, there's no reason not to choose fisetin-rich foods to get your recommended five to seven servings of fruits and vegetables each day…you'll also get the benefits of the many other nutrients in these foods.

Fight Aging with H2 Therapy

Sergej M. Ostojic, MD, PhD, professor of biomedical sciences at University of Novi Sad, and adjunct professor at University of Belgrade School of Medicine, both in Serbia. Dr. Ostojic has published numerous scientific papers on molecular hydrogen in many medical journals, including Sports Medicine, Annals of Medicine and Pharmacological Research.

Hydrogen (H2) is the most abundant element in the universe. In fact, we literally bathe in it (H2O). While tiny, scientists are discovering that the H2 molecule may have the powerful ability to help counter many of the effects of aging and related diseases with its purported antioxidant and anti-inflammatory effects. Although further research is needed to confirm the health benefits, ready-to-drink hydrogen-infused water and bath tablets are already widely available online.

WHY WE AGE

Research on the science of aging continues to evolve…

•**Free radical theory.** Free radicals are naturally occurring oxygen atoms missing an electron in their outer ring, making them unstable. Seeking stability, free radicals try to bind with other atoms and molecules. Too many free radicals can create what scientists call oxidative stress, a kind of cellular rust that ages us. Proponents of the theory claim that cellular rust is behind many of the conditions and diseases of aging, from arterial disease and arthritis to vision loss and wrinkles.

•**Telomere theory.** Telomeres are tips at the end of chromosomes that protect the genetic information within each chromosome. Through-out your life, every time a cell divides, telomeres become a little shorter. In telomere theory, the shorter the telomere, the more your body shows signs of aging. Scientific evidence links many of the ailments of aging—high blood pressure, diabetes, cancer, dementia—to shorter telomeres.

•**Mitochondrial energy theory.** Mitochondria are the energy factories in every cell. In this theory, broken-down mitochondria cause the body to work less efficiently, leading to accelerated aging and age-related diseases.

THE HOPE FOR HYDROGEN

Although hydrogen is essential to the formation of all matter, including life-giving water, it was thought to be biologically "inert," with no function in health or healing. But in 2007, Japanese scientists revolutionized the understanding of hydrogen gas. They showed in cellular and animal experiments that H2 could neutralize free radicals.

Some scientists also believe that H2 is a key signaling molecule, improving communication between brain cells and blood flow in arteries. It also activates health-protecting genes that promote the burning of fat and sugar. Plus, hydrogen may cool chronic inflammation, which fuels many diseases of aging.

In the last decade or so, there have been more than 400 cellular, animal and human studies on using H2 for health and healing, showing that hydrogen may help do many things, including…

•**Prevent muscle pain after exercise.**

•**Protect skin from sun damage.**

•**Protect the brain from stroke damage.**

•**Improve memory and cognition** in Alzheimer's disease patients.

•**Strengthen the heart in cardiovascular disease patients.**

•**Lower "bad" LDL cholesterol** and boost "good" HDL.

•**Balance glucose and insulin,** preventing or slowing diabetes.

•**Shield the retina from damage,** helping to prevent and control age-related macular degeneration and glaucoma.

•**Slow or stop the degeneration of cartilage,** which can lead to osteoarthritis.

Some of the latest studies that demonstrate just how powerful molecular hydrogen can be include…

•Heart health. In a study of middle-aged, overweight women, published in the *Iranian Journal of Medical Sciences*, Serbian researchers found that swallowing hydrogen-producing caplets significantly reduced body fat, insulin and triglycerides—risk factors for heart disease and diabetes—during the four-week study. They theorize that H2 makes cells more sensitive to insulin, thereby improving the burning of blood fats, leading to less body fat and cardiac stress.

In a study in *Circulation Journal*, patients who inhaled hydrogen gas when they arrived at the ER after a heart attack had less long-term heart damage.

In a study in *Vascular Health and Risk Management*, a team of Japanese researchers found that people who drank hydrogen-rich water had improved arterial health within 30 minutes—with 12% greater blood flow.

•Stroke. In a study published in *Journal of Stroke & Cerebrovascular Disease*, Japanese scientists studied people who had a stroke, dividing them into two groups. In the 24 hours after the stroke, one group inhaled hydrogen gas for one hour twice a day and one group received a placebo treatment. Those getting the H2 had less brain injury (as shown by an MRI), less severe stroke symptoms (such as facial palsy, the inability to use limbs and problems with speech) and more and faster benefits from physical therapy, as measured by function in daily living.

•Arthritis. In a study published in *International Immunopharmacology* on people with painful rheumatoid arthritis, researchers found that a month of hydrogen-rich saline injections administered intravenously reduced "disease activity" by about 29%—meaning less pain, swelling and tenderness. There was no change in a placebo group.

HYDROGEN-ATE YOUR BODY

Although most studies to date involve inhaled or injected hydrogen gas (which is not yet approved by the FDA), proponents of hydrogen suggest a much simpler and more accessible method of hydrogen-ating—drink or bathe in it…

•Hydrogen-infused water. Ready-to-drink hydrogen water is available. Popular brands include HFactor and Dr. Perricone. To make hydrogen water, manufacturers add odorless and tasteless molecular hydrogen gas to water, then package it in cans or aluminum-lined pouches. (The gas can escape from glass or plastic bottles.) You need to drink the water quickly—within 30 minutes of opening it—or the hydrogen levels will dissipate.

Note: Hydrogen water is different from alkaline water, marketed under brands such as Core and Essentia. Like hydrogen water, alkaline water has been associated with antioxidant properties, but it does not contain hydrogen gas.

You also can buy tablets or powders of electrolyzed hydrogen to dissolve in water (brands include Ultra H2 and AquaH2). Or you can generate hydrogen water by mixing a powdered magnesium supplement in water and letting the water sit for a few minutes.

Another option: Putting a metallic magnesium stick in your water bottle. The most tested stick is the Dr. Hayashi Hydrogen Rich Water Stick, which uses pure magnesium and is available at Amazon.com.

Optimal dosage of hydrogen-infused water is not yet known, but proponents say that you can drink as much as you want without harm. Start with two or three eight-ounce glasses a day.

•Hydrogen baths. You can put a hydrogen tablet or powder, available at Amazon.com, into your bath. Bathe in hydrogen-rich water for at least 10 minutes.

Limitations: There are no known side effects of drinking hydrogen-infused water, but more study is needed to determine the possibility of long-term side effects and health benefits. Because there are no dosing guidelines yet, drink in moderation. If using magnesium to make your hydrogen water, limit daily usage to the recommended daily amount of 350 milligrams.

Weak or Painful Hands? Try These Helpful Kitchen Hacks

Deborah Quilter, ergonomic design consultant and certified Feldenkrais® practitioner based in New York City. She is author of *Repetitive Strain Injury: A Computer User's Guide* and *The Repetitive Strain Injury Recovery Book*. RSIHelp. com

You may love cooking, or at least not mind it. But what happens if you have a hand injury or a chronic health condition, such as arthritis...or even just weak hands—so it is painful or even impossible for you to cook?

There are solutions! If you are frustrated with packaging that won't open easily, vegetable peelers that don't work for you, kitchenware that puts your hands in awkward positions, and so on, here are some of the special tools and techniques that can get you cooking again—and enjoying it...

KITCHENWARE THAT WORKS FOR YOU

If you've ever injured yourself trying to open hard plastic packaging with the wrong tool (e.g., a knife rather than scissors), you know that safe practices are important to protect your hands. But you may not realize that safety factors include the balance, weight and ergonomic design of your kitchen tools. Choosing well, especially if you have a chronic hand or arm issue, can protect you from cuts, scalds and serious kitchen accidents that could require months of rehab. *Use the following as a checklist for evaluating kitchenware...*

•**Weight.** When shopping for items ranging from knives and other utensils to casserole dishes, griddles, pots and pans and even storage containers, the absolute best thing you can do is pick up the item and notice its weight. If it feels heavy to you—especially if it's a vessel that's going to hold food—it weighs too much for your physical ability. Don't buy it.

•**Balance.** When you hold a skillet, pot or other kitchen item by the handle, how balanced does it feel? Is the length of the handle appropriate for the size of the pot? Is it easy for you to manipulate? This can often be the deciding factor between two equally attractive items.

Example: If you are buying a tea kettle, lift it and pretend to pour water from it. This will tell you how well-balanced it is and how well it works with your physiology or level of ability.

•**Handle design.** How easy and comfortable are an item's handles to grasp? How easy does it feel as you lift the item? When choosing between a lid with a knob and a lid with handle, the handle will most often feel more comfortable because it's a better match for the natural flexion of fingers. A knob is typically (though not always) small and harder to grasp because of the different type of grip you need to use.

•**Versatility.** Unless you're a gadget maven, choose products that can do more than one job well...rather than a lot of separate, very specialized tools.

Why: Having to rummage for the right item in a crowded drawer or cabinet can be just another stressor on your hands and arms, especially if you have to move other items out of the way to find them.

USEFUL TOOLS

Give your hands a break by upgrading the tools you use every day—look for specific features that will make it easier for you to accomplish a variety of tasks.

•**Spring-loaded scissors.** This tops the list of must-have kitchen tools for opening tough packaging, cutting off wire and plastic twist ties and other jobs that you might not even realize impact your hands, such as snipping grape stems, which requires a surprising amount of hand energy. When using traditional scissors, it's typically the movement needed to open them that exerts undue pressures on your hand, not the movement of closing them to cut. Spring-loaded scissors eliminate this pressure. You might find that having kitchen scissors in a variety of blade lengths is helpful—shorter ones for, say, snipping herbs, longer ones for cutting rounds of parchment paper for baking, etc.

•**Ergonomic knives.** These knives are better-shaped than most knives for the job you need to do with them—the blades are set lower than the handles to allow a more natural alignment of the hand as you cut. This is especially helpful when you need to use significant force to cut hard vegetables or thick or bony meat or when a food processor's blades won't do.

Caution: A sharp knife is easier to use and safer than a dull knife because you don't have to exert as much force with it. But if you buy new ergonomic knives, they're likely to be much sharper than the old knives you're used to—so be extra careful about not casually touching the blades, and store them with protective sheaths on (if they come with sheaths) or in a knife holder, not loose in a drawer.

•**Jar opener.** While there are electric jar openers available, an easier and essentially free trick is to use an ordinary bottle opener inserted under the lid of a new jar to break the vacuum seal...and to then twist off the lid with the grip-assistance of a dishwashing glove. As long as you don't bend the lid very much with the bottle opener, you'll be able to screw it back on easily. If this method doesn't work for you, you might find that it's worth buying an electric jar opener.

•**Plastic or silicone mesh sink mat.** Weak hands, nerve injuries and age-related loss of sensation can lead to poor grip and things slipping out of your hands. As insurance, buy a sink liner—the kind primarily made to prevent scratches to your sink's surface from utensils and dishes. It will help prevent glasses and plates from breaking if you drop them over the sink.

A special shopping note: "Ergonomic" kitchen items are big business these days, and you'll see lots of products labeled that way. But it's important to trust your assessment of a product and your instincts over the labeling. A product might be described as ergonomic or hand-friendly but might not be right for your unique situation. In fact, you might find that a run-of-the-mill item performs just as you need it to. For example, an "ergonomic" salad spinner with a top button you push down on might be great if you have arthritis, whereas someone with repetitive strain injury might find that same arm/hand movement painful. Try out numerous models of every tool to find the ones that answer your needs.

BETTER BIOMECHANICS

How you use your tools is as important as the tools that you choose...

•**Slide rather than lift.**

It might sound obvious, but it's not intuitive for many people: If you have, say, a heavy pot on the stove and need to move it to a different burner, slide it and use both hands. This enables your core muscles to do most of the work.

•**Store heavy objects between chest and waist level.** You might have gotten used to storing some of your heavy kitchen items up on a high shelf or down in a low cabinet earlier in life, when lifting things was easier, and just never thought to change that arrangement. Change it now! This way, you'll engage your core muscles to reach for them and not have to bend low or support weight on raised arms.

•**Transfer ingredients to smaller, easier-to-lift containers for storage.** This is especially helpful if you buy food in bulk to save money and time.

•**Keep your elbows near your torso when you're chopping.** You'll use the power muscles of your core and avoid straining your shoulders, which is more likely to happen when you work with your arms outstretched.

•**Get kitchen-prep help.** Instead of slicing and dicing yourself, see if your market will do it for you. Besides offering the services of a meat butcher and fishmonger, more and more markets now have a "produce butcher" who will take fresh, whole produce that you choose and slice or chop it for you (usually for a fee). Let this person know if you want your produce washed first—they don't always do that. This is a more nutritious alternative to buying pre-chopped produce that could be losing nutritional value over the hours, if not days, that it's been sitting already-cut in the market.

Gadgets That Make Driving Easier and Safer

Donna S. Stressel, occupational therapist at Sunnyview Rehabilitation Hospital in Schenectady, New York, a certified driver rehabilitation specialist and a driving instructor in the state of New York.

No longer being able to drive and losing your feeling of independence can be traumatic, and you're not likely to hang up your keys without a fight. Well, maybe you don't have to! If you're not as capable and confident behind the wheel as you used to be, whether due to a physical issue such as arthritis or to diminished vision, there are many devices that can help you stay on the road longer—safely. *Here are recommended products that can help remedy the most common issues facing older drivers, as well as drivers of any age with disabilities or mobility issues...*

•**Larger mirrors.** If you have trouble turning your head or are regularly vexed by blind spots in your side-view or rearview mirrors, clip-on or replacement mirrors can help. Blind-spot side-view mirrors that attach on top of existing side-view mirrors are a good choice. With these add-on mirrors, you can continue to use the mirrors you are used to but expand their view. $10 to $50.

•**The HandyBar.** For anyone who has a mobility issue or is recovering from an injury, this assistive device provides support as you get in and out of your vehicle. It's especially helpful for people who have difficulty getting out of a low vehicle, such as a sedan, or getting into a high vehicle, such as an SUV or pickup truck. $34.99. Stander.com/Handy-bar

•**Steering-wheel cover.** A soft foam or leather cover can help when arthritis or carpal tunnel syndrome makes it difficult to hold the steering wheel properly. The most important consideration is that it fits the steering wheel of your vehicle's make and model—this is not as easy as it used to be because today's steering wheels tend to incorporate lots of unique contours and buttons, so read reviews about fit before purchasing. $10 to $20.

•**Seat cushion for height.** On average, people lose a half-inch of height every decade after age 40 and even more than that after age 70. If you don't have much height to spare when it comes to seeing over the steering wheel and dashboard, a seat cushion can help...and ensure that the center of the steering-wheel air bag is safely facing your chest and not your face. Visibility—your sight line—should be at least three inches above the steering wheel. A firm foam wedge-shape cushion (higher in the back and lower in the front) can increase your height without raising your legs too close to the steering wheel or too far from the pedals. An orthopedic gel cushion also can help with back or hip pain. These kinds of cushions can be found for about $13 to $40.

•**Swivel-seat cushion.** This type of cushion makes it easier for people with stiff joints or limited mobility to pivot to get in and out of the driver's seat. $15 to $60.

ADAPTIVE-DRIVING EQUIPMENT

The following items are adaptive-driving equipment that should be prescribed by a certified driver rehabilitation specialist to be sure that you're getting the best equipment for your needs and can be trained in how to use it. This ensures that you'll be able to safely drive with the modifications and are compliant with all license-restriction procedures in your state. Only a certified mechanic specializing in installing adaptive equipment should make the modifications so that the equipment and installation meet all regulations. Note that not all vehicles can be modified in all ways, but if what you need is possible, the vendor will ensure that the appropriate equipment is used.

You can find a certified driver rehabilitation specialist through the Association for Driver Rehabilitation Specialists (ADED.net) or the American Occupational Therapy Association (AOTA. org)...and a certified installer through the National Mobility Equipment Dealers Association (NMEDA.com).

•**Swing-out swivel-seat replacement.** If a swivel cushion isn't enough of an accommodation, consider a swing-out or swivel-seat replacement. This involves completely replacing the seat that came with your car with a seat that stays anchored to the vehicle but moves in and out so that you can enter and exit without twisting or rotating. Cost can run several thousand dollars with installation.

- **Steering-wheel spinner.** This simple attachment, often a knob, is secured to a steering wheel to enable drivers with limited or no use of one arm to steer with their working arm. Price is about $100, including installation.

- **Left-foot accelerator.** People who have very limited or no use of their right leg, whether because of amputation, stroke or another condition, may be able to operate all the car pedals with their left leg. Prices range from about $500 to $2,000 depending on style (mechanical or electronic), including installation.

- **Pedal extenders.** If you can't comfortably reach the gas and/or brake pedal, professionally installed pedal extenders can help. They eliminate the need to sit too far forward in the seat, which can be dangerous. Price with installation is between $300 and $800 depending on the type of control (whether it is permanently fixed or one that tucks out of the way for other drivers).

- **Hand controls.** If you've lost the use of your legs from a condition such as paralysis, spinal stenosis or peripheral neuropathy, this device allows you to control the accelerator and brake using your hands. Prices start at about $1,500, including installation.

IF YOU'RE IN THE MARKET FOR A CAR...

Consider paying extra, if necessary, for certain features that will keep you more comfortable and safer on the road...

- **Power everything**—steering, windows, lift gate, door locks and seats that move up and down as well as forward and backward.

- **Tilting and telescoping steering wheel.**

- **Rearview camera** for backing up (now required on any new vehicle as of May 2018).

- **Factory-installed adjustable foot pedals** for the brake and accelerator.

- **Large dashboard controls with buttons,** which are easier to manipulate than knobs.

- **Warning systems to alert you to objects in blind spots,** especially while changing lanes, merging and parking.

- **Lane-departure warning system** to warn you if your car is veering outside your lane.

- **"Smart" headlights** with glare control that automatically pivot during turns and adjust the range and intensity of light based on oncoming vehicles.

- **Crash-mitigation systems** that sense when you might be in danger of a collision and automatically stop the car.

Editor's note: Unless noted, the products mentioned in this article are available on Amazon, at department stores and through specialty automotive and assistive-device sites such as IndependentLiving.com and LiveOakMed.com.

Also: The products typically are not covered by insurance but may be tax-deductible. See IRS Publication 502, Medical and Dental Expenses, for details.

Hearing Assistance at Prices You Can Afford

Abram Bailey, AuD, doctor of audiology, based in Austin, Texas, and founder of Hearing Tracker, Inc., which offers reviews and information about hearing aids and hearing professionals. HearingTracker.com

If you're among the more than 37 million Americans who have trouble hearing, hear this—there are ways to trim the high prices of hearing aids. For people with mild hearing loss, there are some alternatives to seeing the traditional hearing health-care provider—where the average price of a single hearing aid is about $2,300.

In fact, soon it will be possible to buy hearing aids over the counter—no ear exams or professional fittings required (see page 284). *In the meantime, here are some lower-cost options to get you back in the conversation...*

SOUND-AMPLIFICATION DEVICES

- **Personal sound-amplification products (PSAPs)** are comparable to hearing aids but much less expensive—often just a few hundred dollars. They are available online and over the counter, with no requirement that you see a state-licensed audiologist or hearing-aid specialist.

Downsides: PSAPs are not custom-fitted to the wearer's ear and provide limited amplification when compared with traditional hearing aids. PSAPs typically have limited fine-tuning capabilities, with most offering only a volume control or bass and treble adjustments. And most worryingly, some PSAPs actually can damage your hearing by overamplifying sound and boosting loud noises such as fire alarms and gunshots, which traditional hearing aids suppress.

If you have mild hearing loss and don't want to spring for a traditional hearing aid, there are a few PSAP models worth trying…

Best all-around hearing assistance without a prescription: Nuheara IQbuds Boost look just like a pair of wireless sports earbuds, and they are more sophisticated than your average PSAP. They suppress background noise and auto-calibrate to accommodate each individual's unique pattern of hearing loss with the help of the self-guided hearing assessment performed by their app (Apple iOS or Android). So you don't need a professional evaluation for the initial fitting, and you can tweak the sound to your heart's desire. Plus, they can stream audio from Bluetooth-enabled audio devices and TVs. Their rechargeable batteries provide up to 20 hours of Bluetooth streaming or up to 32 hours of hearing processing per charge.

Cost: $349 for a pair.* Nuheara.com

Best PSAP runner-up: BeHear Now is similar to the IQbuds Boost. It is a personalizable Bluetooth stereo headset with a wireless neckband.

Cost: $249. WearAndHear.com

For occasional hearing support: Williams Sound Pockettalker Ultra is a more affordable way simply to hear the occasional conversation or TV show. This shirt pocket–size gadget amplifies the sounds closest to the user while reducing background noise. It's effective, but its over-the-ear headphones are obtrusive.

Cost: $184. WilliamsSound.com

*Prices vary by retailer.

There also are apps that can transform a smartphone and its connected earbuds or headphones into a PSAP-like device. They're free, so it doesn't hurt to give them a try, but they are best used by those with only mild hearing loss. These apps are more common and typically more effective with Apple devices than with Android devices because the audio hardware is standardized across iPhones.

Best apps: EarMachine (Free for iOS)…Petralex Hearing Aid (basic functions are free for iOS and Android).

BUY AUDIO TECH THAT HELPS YOU HEAR YOUR TV

If your main hearing complaint is that you can't understand what they're saying on television—or your spouse says that you turn the TV volume up too high—a set of wireless headphones could be a cost-effective solution.

Examples: Sennheiser RS120 ($99.95), En-us.Sennheiser.com…Sony Wireless RF Headphones ($85), Sony.com.

If you don't want to wear headphones when you watch TV, a soundbar that can emphasize dialogue while de-emphasizing background sound on TV programs could help.

Example: ZVOX SB380 Sound Bar with AccuVoice Dialogue Boost. ZVOX.com.

Cost: $299.99.

BEST PRICES FOR HEARING AIDS

Two chains that offer hearing-aid bargains…

• **Costco** offers a range of hearing aids from top makers with prices of just $499.99 to $2,500 per pair, which includes professional fittings and exams. Even Costco's house brand Kirkland Signature hearing aids are produced by Sonova, a leading hearing-aid manufacturer. You must be a member of Costco to buy its hearing aids. Costco.com

• **Connect Hearing,** a hearing-aid retailer with more than 180 locations nationwide, offers the very capable NovaSense Elite behind-the-ear hearing aid for just $499 apiece (that's $998 for a pair), including fittings and exams. It's made by a division of Sonova, a leading hearing-aid manufacturer. ConnectHearing.com

If you don't have a Costco or Connect Hearing near you—or don't like the hearing aids they offer—you can buy effective lower-technology hearing aids from a licensed practitioner who unbundles its services, sometimes for as little as $500 per ear. To find discounted hearing-aid offers from nearby providers, check out my website, HearingTracker.com.

Consider an entry-level hearing aid made by one of the "big six" manufacturers—GN ReSound (which sells hearing aids mainly under the brand Resound)...Sivantos (sold under brand names including Signia and Rexton)...Sonova (brands include Phonak and Unitron)...Starkey...Widex...and Demant (brands include Oticon and Bernafon). A recent survey of audiologists found that Oticon and Phonak offer particularly good quality for the price.

These entry-level products typically offer all of the core features to ensure that you benefit and succeed with your hearing aids, but manufacturers typically reserve the most cutting-edge features for their flagship models.

GET HELP PAYING FOR HEARING AIDS

Only one of every four health insurance policies includes some hearing-aid coverage, so check with your insurer to see if you are covered. Insurance also may cover screenings and tests, but it depends on your plan. Three states—Arkansas, New Hampshire and Rhode Island—require that health insurance policies include hearing-aid coverage.

•**Medicare and Medigap** plans do not cover hearing aids, though a small percentage of Medicare Advantage plans do, at least in part.

•**Veterans' benefits.** If you are a veteran and your hearing loss is related to your military service, the Department of Veterans Affairs (VA) might cover the cost of your hearing aids and replacement batteries. Contact the VA for details (844-698-2311) or go to Prosthetics.va.gov and click on "Audiology."

Medicaid offers full or partial coverage of hearing aids in many states for qualifying low-income individuals. Some states have additional programs that can help those with low incomes afford hearing aids, too. Visit the website of the Hearing Loss Association of America at Hearing Loss.org and select "Financial Assistance" from the "Hearing Help" menu to find state agencies that offer such programs.

COMING SOON: OVER-THE-COUNTER HEARING AIDS

While sound-amplification products have been available online and over the counter for many years, there has been no such equal access to traditional hearing aids. That's about to change.

In October 2018, the Food and Drug Administration gave audio-equipment maker Bose the green light to begin marketing a "self-fitting" hearing aid intended for people who have mild-to-moderate hearing loss. It's the first FDA-authorized hearing aid designed to be fit, programmed and controlled by the user without the assistance—or expense—of a hearing health-care provider.

Bose has not yet announced when this new hearing aid will be available and how much it will cost (though some sites speculate less than $1,000 for a pair).

Within a few years, there likely will be many hearing aids designed to be sold without the help of an audiologist. The FDA is in the process of creating an "over-the-counter" hearing-aid classification, with draft regulations due no later than August 2020.

Stay Out of the Hospital

Elham Mahmoudi, PhD, assistant professor and health economist, University of Michigan Medical School, Ann Arbor.

In a study of 1,336 adults ages 65 to 85 with severe hearing loss, those who wore hearing aids had fewer visits to emergency departments and were hospitalized less often for any reason over a one-year period than those who didn't wear hearing aids.

Theory: Hearing aids may enable people with hearing loss to take care of their health with less costly doctor's office visits.

Fall in Love with Your Hearing Aids

Barbara E. Weinstein, PhD, professor of audiology and head of the Audiology Program at City University of New York Graduate Center in New York City, where she specializes in hearing loss in older adults, hearing screening, handicap assessment and evidence-based practice. She is author of the textbook *Geriatric Audiology*.

Why do so many new hearing-aid users falter? One underappreciated trap is that it can take weeks or even months to get accustomed to the sounds (and the feel) of new hearing aids. So it's crucial to not let the initial discomforts put you off.

Proper use of hearing aids can enrich your relationships and social life…possibly guard against accidents that can occur if you don't hear warning signals…and prevent falls that can be precipitated by walking while struggling to understand what someone is saying. Improved hearing may even help protect your brain health because you can better communicate with family and friends and remain engaged.

HEARING AND THE BRAIN

People cite a number of reasons for not wearing their hearing aids. Some complain that they hurt their ears. Others notice that the sounds they hear don't seem natural…or that they're bothered by sounds they hadn't noticed before.

While new hearing aids do take some getting used to, they are definitely worth the effort. For one thing, emerging evidence suggests that the part of the brain that processes spoken language (the temporal lobe) may be subject to

Diets Good for the Heart Help Hearing

People who ate a Mediterranean-style diet or the antihypertension DASH diet were about 30% less likely to develop moderate or severe hearing loss over a 22-year period than people whose eating habits were less healthful.

Analysis of 71,000 women in the Nurses' Health Study II by researchers at Brigham and Women's Hospital, Boston, published in *Journal of Nutrition*.

atrophy and volume declines when not stimulated. This means that people with an impaired hearing mechanism who wait too long to correct their hearing may not benefit as much from hearing interventions.

Even scarier risk: In a study by a group of researchers at Johns Hopkins who tracked 639 adults (ages 36 to 90), mild hearing loss was linked to twice the risk for dementia…and moderate-to-severe hearing loss increased the risk between three- and fivefold.

ADJUSTING TO CHANGE

It's easier to get used to hearing aids in your younger years, so don't wait until you're adjusting the TV volume to wall-shaking levels. The most important part of successful aging is staying socially engaged—and you can't do that when you can't hear or communicate with others. *Secrets to adjusting to your hearing aids…*

SECRET #1: **Wear them all day.** Depending on the degree/duration of your hearing loss, it might have been years since you've heard the sound of your own footsteps…water running in the sink…or the clatter of dishes. The "new" sounds can be distracting—even disturbing—until you get used to them.

My advice: Wear your new hearing aids all day, even when you first get them. We used to advise patients to use them for just a few hours a day at first, but we've found that people often do better with full-on exposure. Just know that it may take days, weeks or even months before background sounds truly fade into the background.

SECRET #2: **When it's too loud, make adjustments.** You'll probably find that most sounds—even the ones you want to hear—are uncomfortably loud at first. Some hearing aids have volume controls, which you can adjust, but it will take your brain time to adjust even to the lower settings. If sounds are too loud, be sure to return to your hearing-aid provider to make the necessary adjustments, as hearing aids have many features that can be adjusted.

My advice: As mentioned above, it's important to wear your hearing aids all day. You might want to make an exception, however, for unusually noisy environments—for example, in the subway, at a concert or at the airport. High-volume venues

285

won't always be an impediment, but they can be a turnoff during the adjustment period.

If the sound of your own voice is disturbing, ask your audiologist if the devices need adjusting. Turning down the volume might not do it. An audiologist can make adjustments—to the sound frequencies, for example, or the shape of the earpiece (known as the mold)—that will often help.

Important: To become comfortable with their hearing aids, most people require one or two additional visits for adjustments, which are typically included in the price of the hearing aids.

SECRET #3: Cut through the clutter. People with normal hearing may struggle to hear conversations when there's a lot of background noise, but it is worse for those with hearing loss. Even inexpensive hearing aids typically have a noise-cancellation feature that enhances higher frequencies (typical of speech) while suppressing lower frequencies (from background noise). The setting is often adjustable—learn how to use it.

My advice: If adjusting noise cancellation doesn't help, ask an audiologist to make changes in the "output" and/or "gain." Gain is the power of the signal that affects amplification, and output is the level of "sound pressure" that's produced by the combination of incoming sounds and the gain added by the hearing aid.

SECRET #4: Master the controls. Hearing aids keep getting smaller, which means that the controls also are getting smaller—too small, in many cases, for people (especially those with big fingers or limited hand mobility) to easily adjust.

My advice: Don't buy a hearing aid just because it has a zillion adjustable features. They won't do you any good unless you have the finger dexterity (and the technical savvy) to master them. An audiologist can help you decide which features you absolutely need—and those you can do without.

Helpful: Many hearing aids use Bluetooth wireless technology, which allows them to be adjusted by an app that appears on the screen of your smartphone. This is a great feature if you have one of these phones and you're willing to use it as a remote control. An audiologist talked my 93-year-old cousin into getting this feature…but in order to use it, she had to buy her first smartphone, which she didn't know how to use and actually found annoying.

SECRET #5: Learn how to fix whistling sounds. The squealing/whistling sounds that you'll sometimes hear are a type of feedback. It doesn't mean that there's a problem with the electronics. Most hearing aids have "feedback interceptors" that suppress whistles, but they don't eliminate them entirely.

My advice: Ask your audiologist if you need a tighter-fitting ear mold. Squeals and whistles occur when amplified sound from the hearing aid leaks out of the ear…gets picked up by the microphone…and then returns to the ear as a whistling noise.

SECRET #6: Don't put up with ear discomfort. Many people complain that their hearing aids are uncomfortable. They may find themselves constantly pulling/adjusting the ear mold to reduce discomfort, but the frequent back-and-forth adjustments only make the irritation worse.

My advice: You can get a hearing-aid lubricant/cream from an audiologist, online or at pharmacies. Brands include Westone Oto-Ease and Audiologist's Choice anti-itch cream. They're particularly helpful if you happen to have dryness in the ear canal.

Worth a try: If you continue to have problems, your audiologist might need to fashion an ear mold/tip that fits more comfortably. This is one advantage of buying locally. I don't discourage patients from buying hearing aids online, but this type of adjustment can be done only by a local professional.

Losing Your Sense of Smell?

Richard L. Doty, PhD, FAAN, director of the Smell and Taste Center and professor of psychology in otorhinolaryngology: head and neck surgery at the Perelman School of Medicine, University of Pennsylvania, Philadelphia. He is author or editor of 11 books, including *The Great Pheromone Myth* and *Smell and Taste Disorders*.

If you've noticed that your sense of smell (aka olfaction) isn't what it used to be, you're not alone. For some 20 million Americans, the ability to detect everyday smells, from baking bread to burning wood, is slipping away...or even gone.

Why this matters: Even though primary care physicians rarely ask patients about loss of smell, it can be an early red flag for certain chronic medical conditions.

A MULTITASKING SENSE

Few people appreciate the multitude of daily functions tied to their sense of smell. *This all-too-often neglected sense serves as...*

•**A key to appetite.** Smell is responsible for most of our sense of taste. People with a diminished sense of smell often have a poor appetite, remarking that food is tasteless or just doesn't taste the same. While taste buds can distinguish basic levels of sweet, sour, bitter, salty and umami (a savory, earthy taste), smell also plays an important but often underappreciated role in our ability to taste foods.

•**A harbinger of serious disorders.** A diminished sense of smell is often an early symptom of Parkinson's disease and Alzheimer's disease. In fact, smell dysfunction is the most common early symptom reported by Parkinson's patients even before they suffer motor-related symptoms, such as tremors or walking difficulties.

A HARD-TO-SPOT DEFICIENCY

Because few primary care physicians test for smell problems, you need to be alert for any suspected loss of this sense.

This can be challenging because the loss of smell that tends to occur with aging happens gradually, and most people with health problems don't recognize that they have lost their sense of smell. For example, loss of smell is present in about 90% of people with Parkinson's disease, but most don't recognize that they have a problem.

Self-defense: Even if you only suspect a change, you should report this to your doctor. If there is no obvious reason for the loss of smell, such as a cold, allergies or nasal congestion, then smell testing is recommended.

SMELL TESTING

A number of tests are available to assess one's ability to smell. These range from simple three-item scratch-and-sniff screening tests...the 16-item Sniffin' Sticks odor identification test that uses felt-tip pens to dispense odors...to longer tests, such as the 40-item University of Pennsylvania Smell Identification Test (UPSIT).* With the 15-minute UPSIT, you are asked to smell a series of odors (such as rose, pizza, cinnamon and mint) and identify each odor from a list of choices.

The UPSIT, which can be ordered by physicians online for a nominal cost, helps doctors to determine both the absolute and relative (to one's age and sex) degrees of smell loss.

TREATMENT OPTIONS

The first step in treatment is to identify the cause of the smell loss. Olfactory problems related to Parkinson's disease or brain damage are generally believed to be irreversible, but early detection is helpful in planning medical treatment.

There is strong evidence in a 2013 paper published in *JAMA Otolaryngology–Head & Neck Surgery* that regular exercise can help to maintain the ability to smell in later life, much like it can help to avert or delay the onset of dementia. However, it is not known whether exercise can reverse such impairment once it is present.

If the loss is due to simple inflammation, including that caused by chronic sinusitis, then treatment with powerful anti-inflammatories (such as corticosteroids) may bring back some sense of smell. Oral steroids typically restore smell function within about a week. Continued topical therapy with steroid sprays or washes can, in some cases, maintain the restored function. If nasal polyps are to blame, surgical removal can be helpful.

Promising therapy: Some evidence shows that the antioxidant alpha-lipoic acid may help one regain the sense of smell in certain cases, such as long-lasting dysfunction due to upper respiratory infections. The suggested dosage is 400 mg to 600 mg daily.

*Dr. Doty is president of Sensonics International, the manufacturer and distributor of the UPSIT.

Important: Before trying alpha-lipoic acid, talk to your doctor. This supplement has been shown to lower blood sugar, so people with diabetes need to use caution. It could also interact with some medications, including antibiotics, anti-inflammatories, tranquilizers, heart medications and chemotherapy drugs.

Another option: Small amounts of smell-restoring alpha-lipoic acid can be found in foods.

Good sources: Organ meats (such as kidneys and liver)…spinach…and broccoli.

ARE YOU AT RISK?

There are dozens of possible causes for smell loss. *Among the most common…*

•**Aging.** With age, the nerves that are involved in smell weaken, and odor-detecting membranes lining the nose become thin and dry.

•**Smoking.** Because it irritates nasal passages, smoking impairs one's sense of smell. The good news is that normal smelling function can return in less than a year after quitting in light smokers and over the course of several years in heavy smokers—providing another reason to quit.

•**Air pollution.** Research published in 2016 in *Environmental Health Perspectives* noted that the tiny particulates in polluted air enter the nose, cross through the olfactory bulb and actually enter the brain. There the stray microparticles, commonly found in diesel exhaust and air pollutants, can induce an inflammatory response that can lead to brain tissue damage, the development of Alzheimer's-like pathology and a loss of smell.

•**Certain medications.** More than 70 medications can affect one's sense of smell. The list includes heart drugs, such as the cholesterol-lowering medication *atorvastatin* (Lipitor) and blood pressure drugs such as *amlodipine* (Norvasc) and *enalapril* (Vasotec), and some decongestant nasal sprays. Unfortunately, there is not much data indicating whether stopping such drugs will reverse smell loss.

•**Head injury.** Even a relatively minor head injury, as might occur when one hits the back of the head on the pavement after slipping on ice, can permanently damage the delicate nerve connections to the brain that control your sense of smell.

See Better Than Ever! New Treatments for Cataracts and Glaucoma

Robert Abel, Jr., MD, an ophthalmologist at Delaware Ophthalmology Consultants in Wilmington. He is author of *The Eye Care Revolution: Prevent and Reverse Common Vision Problems.*

New advances are rapidly improving treatments for cataracts and glaucoma—especially when the problem is caught early.*

CATARACTS

Cataracts are caused by a clouding of the lens that results in such symptoms as blurry vision, cloudy vision, poor night vision and even double vision. The preferred treatment is cataract surgery—a procedure that's become increasingly effective in recent years. *Latest advances…*

•**Extended depth of focus lens.** With cataract surgery, a surgeon can remove the cloudy, vision-impairing lens of the eye in a matter of minutes and replace it with a clear corrective lens. But until recently, the replacement lens would only enhance either near or far vision in each eye.

This meant that doctors might treat one eye for near vision and the other eye for seeing at a distance…or they might use a "multifocal" implant that offered some improvement in both near and far vision. Most people simply choose to correct for far vision and use reading glasses the rest of the time.

The new extended depth of focus (EDOF) lens is an important advance because it can correct distance vision while also improving your ability to see up close. For eye surgeons, it's one step closer to the holy grail—the ability to completely reverse age-related vision loss without the need for glasses. With EDOF, you might actually see better than you ever did.

Drawbacks: The new lenses are expensive. If your insurance doesn't pick up the tab, you can expect to pay $1,500 to $2,500 more per

*The treatments included in this article may not be covered by insurance. Check with your insurer for details.

eye than you would for traditional replacement lenses.

Even though the new lenses are better for brightness, contrast and seeing colors—and they do improve vision at in-between distances—you still might need reading glasses in some cases.

Best for: Active middle-aged and older adults who want to avoid wearing glasses.

•**RxSight Light Adjustable Lens.** The FDA approved an artificial lens in 2017 that can be adjusted repeatedly after cataract surgery—important because slight errors in lens manufacturing (or eye changes that occur during healing) can skew the vision-correcting effects.

This adjustable lens contains a unique material that shifts in response to UV light. If your vision isn't optimal after the surgery, your doctor can fine-tune it with three or four laser treatments that modify the curvature of the lens, delivered about three weeks after the procedure.

The lens can provide vision improvements that are comparable to vision-correcting procedures such as LASIK. But for now (despite the FDA's approval), the lens has not yet become widely adopted and is mainly available for patients who are participating in ongoing studies.

Best for: Any cataract surgery patient who is looking for precise vision correction that is permanent.

GLAUCOMA

Glaucoma results from fluid buildup that damages the eye's optic nerve, potentially causing vision loss and even blindness. Depending on the extent of the disease, treatment has traditionally included medication (such as eyedrops or pills)…laser surgery (to help make sure that fluid drains out of the eye)…or conventional surgery (to create an opening for fluid to leave the eye). *Latest advances…*

•**iStent.** Because most types of glaucoma are accompanied by excessive fluid buildup (often leading to high pressure within the eye), one of the main treatments is to surgically install a stent (or a related device called a shunt) to improve drainage and keep eye pressure low.

The iStent is a game-changer. It's the first FDA-approved device that can be implanted during cataract surgery for patients who have

mild-to-moderate open-angle glaucoma, which accounts for at least 90% of all glaucoma cases. The device, which is about one-third the size of a grain of rice, creates a permanent opening to improve fluid drainage.

Previous devices worked similarly, but they required the surgeon to open a flap of skin from outside the eye, install the stent, then close things up. The iStent doesn't require a separate procedure when performed with cataract surgery.

Bonus: Patients who have the stent often can reduce their dependence on pressure-reducing medications, which tend to be less reliable and may cause side effects, including extremely low pressure. It's a phenomenal development!

Best for: Any glaucoma patient who is undergoing cataract surgery.

•**Pressure-reducing eyedrops.** More than 95% of adults with glaucoma use eyedrops (at least initially) to reduce glaucoma-causing fluid buildups.

About half of patients require two or more eye medications—and patients using multiple drugs are less likely to follow dosing instructions. The most commonly used medications are prostaglandin analogs (PGAs), which improve the functioning of the drainage pathway known as the uveoscleral outflow.

What's new: *Latanoprostene bunod ophthalmic solution* (Vyzulta), approved by the FDA in 2017. Unlike other PGAs, it increases the outflow of fluid through both the uveoscleral pathway and the trabecular meshwork (an area of tissue near the base of the cornea). In studies, it lowered intraocular pressure more than the older drugs…and the dual action means that some glaucoma patients can use only one eyedrop.

My take: All of the PGAs, including Vyzulta, can cause inflammation and red or puffy eyes. For this reason, I believe that glaucoma patients will often do better with other (nonPGA) eyedrops or laser treatments.

Best for: Vyzulta can be a reasonable choice for advanced glaucoma patients who must use eyedrops but are resistant to other products and are not significantly troubled by mild eye inflammation.

How Will Glaucoma Affect Cataract Surgery?

David F. Chang, MD, clinical professor of ophthalmology at University of California San Francisco. He is coauthor of *Cataracts: A Patient's Guide to Treatment*.

Most patients who do not have significant vision loss from glaucoma—a condition in which the internal pressure of the eye is so high that it damages the optic nerve—can expect good results from cataract surgery. In fact, eye pressure frequently decreases in glaucoma patients after cataract surgery, which gives them a bonus benefit along with improved eyesight. (It's important to realize that any vision loss due to advanced glaucoma is permanent, and that portion of vision impairment can't be restored with cataract surgery.) If you have glaucoma and cataracts and want to treat the cataracts, it's important to get the timing right.

WHY TIMING IS IMPORTANT

Cataract surgery is recommended when blurry vision from the cataracts starts to interfere with daily tasks such as driving. However, because cataracts are the normal aging of the natural lens, delaying surgery won't actually damage the eye. On the other hand, glaucoma, if it isn't controlled, damages the optic nerve causing permanent vision loss—so getting your glaucoma under control must never be delayed and takes priority over cataract surgery.

Once your glaucoma is under control, cataract surgery can frequently be done without any special precautions. Most people will continue using their pressure-reducing glaucoma drops immediately before and after cataract surgery. (Your doctor will let you know the specifics.)

If your doctor believes that it would be safer to reduce your eye pressure even further, he/she may suggest combining cataract surgery with a new type of glaucoma surgery to reduce your eye pressure.

Called minimally invasive glaucoma surgeries (MIGS), these procedures (there are several variations) are safe and usually don't lengthen the recovery time from the cataract operation.

Studies have shown that when combined with cataract surgery, MIGS devices reduce the eye pressure more than cataract surgery alone would have. Traditional "filtering" glaucoma surgeries reduce eye pressure the most, but these are more invasive than MIGS. They carry more risk, require a longer recuperation and are reserved for patients with more advanced glaucoma.

A MIGS procedure involves implanting a tiny drainage device, or stent, in the eye. Typical stents reduce eye pressure by increasing the fluid outflow through the eyeball's natural drainage system. Although they will not "cure" your glaucoma, a stent might reduce the number of glaucoma medications you need.

Cataract surgery is the ideal time for MIGS because the stent can be inserted through the same incision made for cataract removal.

Many glaucoma patients also wonder whether having glaucoma reduces their chances for successful cataract surgery. In general, the answer is that unless you already have significant vision loss from the glaucoma, you can expect good results from cataract surgery.

Glaucoma Usually More Advanced

Carlos Gustavo De Moraes, MD, MPH, medical director of clinical trials, department of ophthalmology, Columbia University Medical Center, New York City, and author of a study published in *JAMA Ophthalmology*.

Most people diagnosed with early-stage glaucoma actually have more advanced glaucoma than diagnosed. Thirty-three people were diagnosed with early glaucoma based on the common "24-2" vision test. Of those almost 70% had more severe cases as shown by the less common "10-2" vision test and "OCT" imaging test.

If you are diagnosed with early-stage glaucoma: Ask your doctor for a 10-2 test and an OCT to determine if more aggressive treatment is needed.

Muscle Weakness Increases Dementia Risk

Magdalena I. Tolea, PhD, a researcher at Florida Atlantic University, Boca Raton, Florida, and lead author of a study published in *Clinical Interventions in Aging*.

Adults with low muscle mass/strength, called sarcopenia, who also have a high percentage of body fat have poorer cognition than those with just one of those conditions. You can be at risk even with normal body weight—ask your doctor to check your body fat and strength. Maintaining strength while preventing fat gain may prevent cognitive decline.

Surefire Ways to Prevent Muscle Loss: Best Foods, Supplements and Exercises

Stuart M. Phillips, PhD, professor, department of kinesiology and Michael G. DeGroote School of Medicine, McMaster University, Ontario, Canada. He is director of the McMaster Centre for Nutrition, Exercise and Health Research and a fellow of the American College of Sports Medicine and the American College of Nutrition.

Loss of muscle mass and strength isn't just an inconvenience. It's one of the most accurate indicators—for seniors and the middle-aged and the young—that disease and death may be in your near future.

Scary findings: Study after study shows that people with less strength are more likely to be hospitalized or to die of any cause, including heart disease, stroke, cancer and pneumonia, within a given period. Scientists haven't figured out all the reasons that strength predicts health and well-being, but it's not only because unhealthy people get weaker—in fact, a reduction in strength is a better predictor of dying from cardiovascular disease than is high blood pressure.

If you've told your doctor that you're a bit weaker these days, and he/she said it's a "normal part of aging"—ignore him. You can and

should preserve and build muscle mass and strength at any age—it's as important to health and longevity as keeping your arteries free of plaque and your cells free of cancer.

BEST EXERCISES

Preserve and build the muscles in your arms, legs, hips and back that you need for everyday strength and activity by doing these three exercises two or three times a week at home or anywhere else…

• **Body-weight squat.** Stand directly in front of a stable, not-too-high chair with no armrest and with your back toward the chair seat and your feet shoulder-width apart. Slowly bend your legs, keeping your back straight and arms at your sides and knees over your toes, and lower yourself onto the chair. Then stand up slowly by reversing the motion. Do this 30 times. If you can't do 30 repetitions at first (and many people can't), start with what you can do, and over a period of days or weeks, work up to 30. (The same goes for the next two exercises.) If you can do even more, all the better—but 30 should be your minimum target.

• **Lunge.** While standing, keep your upper body straight and your shoulders back, and step forward with one leg, lowering your hips until both knees are bent at a 90-degree angle. Return to the standing position. Do 15 times on each side for a total of 30.

• **Push-up or modified push-up.** This oldie but goodie develops the upper back, shoulders, arms, chest and wrists. If you can't yet do "full" push-ups (with only your hands and toes on the ground), start with modified push-ups in which your toes and knees are on the ground… or even with easier "wall push-ups" where you stand facing a wall and place your hands on the wall at shoulder height. Your ultimate goal is at least 30 full push-ups.

Also important: Aerobic exercise to maintain fitness. You don't have to run miles and miles. A 25-minute jog or vigorous cycling just three times a week…or a 30-minute brisk walk five times a week will do the trick.

BEST FOODS

The most important dietary component for your muscles is protein, the material out of

291

which muscles are made. And believe it or not, despite the prevalence of meat in the typical Western diet, many Americans don't get enough protein for the best possible muscle strength.

The government's Recommended Dietary Allowance (RDA) for protein is 0.36 grams (g) of protein per pound of body weight per day. But that level is the minimum, not the optimum. For preserving and building muscle, we need at least 50% more—0.54 g of protein per pound of body weight per day. And some studies indicate that 0.73 g per pound of body weight is even better. (More than that doesn't build more muscle or strength.)

Problem: Most seniors get only two-thirds of the RDA, or about 0.24 g of protein per pound of body weight per day.

How much protein should you eat? Multiply your body weight in pounds by 0.54 to get the minimum number of grams per day…and multiply your body weight by 0.73 to get the maximum daily grams of protein likely to help your muscles. Then each day, aim to eat an amount in between those two results.

Example: A person who weighs 150 pounds would multiply 150 by 0.54 to get a minimum daily protein goal of 81 g…and multiply 150 by 0.73 to get a maximum useful daily protein amount of 109 g.

The best muscle-building protein has two features. It is digestible—the amino acids that are the building blocks of protein are easily absorbed. Protein from meat, poultry, fish and other seafood, eggs and dairy is far more digestible than protein from plants. And the best protein for muscles has a high level of the amino acid leucine, which kick-starts muscle-building. The digestible sources of protein mentioned above also have the most leucine.

To optimize muscle-building, you also need to get protein at every meal, because unlike unused carbohydrates and unused fat, unused protein is not stored by the body for later use.

Best strategy: Eat a highly digestible form of leucine-rich protein, chosen from the above sources, at every meal.

Examples: For breakfast, eat two eggs (12 g protein) and one-half cup of yogurt (6 g). For lunch, cut up four ounces of chicken breast (35 g protein) into a salad. For dinner, eat a six-ounce serving of high-quality (preferably organic) meat or fish (around 40 g protein) along with vegetables and whole grains. For a bedtime snack, have one-half cup of cottage cheese (12 g protein).

Grand total: 105 g of protein, or just about the perfect amount to help preserve strength for our 150-pounder.

Note: Some medical conditions, for example kidney disease, can make it dangerous to consume even moderate amounts of protein—check first with your physician.

CHAPTER 17

Pain Relief

Headache Sufferers: Are You Misdiagnosing Your Pain?

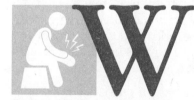When a headache comes on, sometimes you can just pop a pill and the pain goes away—end of story. But not all headaches quit that easily. If you've had a few that made you nauseous and foggy-brained, you might automatically assume that you have migraines. If you're congested, you might assume sinus headache. But the truth is that it's easy to misdiagnose the type of headache you're having. This guide will better help you interpret what you're feeling so you can take the right action.

THE GARDEN-VARIETY HEADACHE

A tension-type headache (TTH) is the most common headache, and more so among women than men. Typically, the pain is mild to moderate, feels like a tightness or vicelike sensation and affects your whole head—not just one side. This type of headache can last from 30 minutes to, quite surprisingly, a week. You might experience one only occasionally...or chronically—on 15 or more days a month!

While it's possible to experience nausea on occasion with a TTH, this type of headache typically doesn't interfere with ordinary activities—you can still go about your day, work, eat and even exercise. Still, easing the stress that often starts the chain reaction resulting in a headache can help you overcome it. And if you do need a pain reliever, *acetaminophen* or an over-the-counter nonsteroidal anti-inflammatory drug (NSAID) should do the job.

MIGRAINE: THE HEADACHE MISNOMER

A migraine isn't just a headache—it's a disabling neurological disorder with a strong genetic component, and it interferes with your

Nada Hindiyeh, MD, director of clinical research and clinical assistant professor of neurology and neurological sciences, Stanford University, Stanford, California, and principal investigator of many studies on migraine.

daily routine and your ability to concentrate. By definition, a migraine must last from four to 72 hours and have two of the following four pain characteristics—throbbing pain, moderate-to-severe intensity, pain on one side of the head and/or pain that gets worse with routine physical activity. It also must have at least one of these features—nausea (or vomiting) or sensitivity to light and sensitivity to sound.

So, for example, if you have a moderate headache that gets worse when you take a walk and find that it hurts to be in a brightly lit room, you meet the migraine criteria. About 25% to 30% of migraine sufferers also experience aura, a type of visual disturbance that precedes the actual pain.

The brains of people genetically predisposed to migraine are highly sensitive to stimuli. When you add in a trigger, such as a particular food, stress or a change in the weather, it seems to push the brain over the edge, leading to a migraine. Food triggers are very individual and include aged cheese, red wine, sugary processed foods, MSG and chocolate, among others. Dehydration or a change in barometric pressure, such as in the cabin of a jet, can set off a migraine. For women, the drop in estrogen right at the start of menstruation is a common trigger. (Three times as many women as men get migraines.)

Note: About two-thirds of women whose migraines are related to their menstrual cycle see an improvement after menopause, but it's also not unusual for a woman to get her first migraine after menopause.

Keeping a headache diary to track episodes and symptoms can help you pinpoint specific triggers to avoid. However, that alone may not be enough to prevent migraines.

There are abortive medications to reduce a current migraine and preventive ones to reduce headache frequency and severity. Depending on how often you get migraines and how disabling they are, you may need both. Until recently, drugs prescribed to prevent migraines had all been medications developed to treat other conditions. Then in 2018, the first migraine-specific drugs were introduced. They target a protein called calcitonin gene-related peptide (CGRP), which has been implicated in causing migraines.

But you can do a lot more than take medicine, starting with your posture. Next is engaging in regular, moderate aerobic exercise, such as a brisk 20-minute walk or cycling on a stationary bike. A healthy, protein-based diet that keeps your blood sugar steady, a regular schedule for eating and sleeping (going to bed and rising at set times) and stress-reduction techniques, such as meditation and biofeedback, all can help. Daily supplements, including magnesium, vitamin B-2 and CoQ10, have also been shown to reduce the frequency and severity of migraines.

PAINFUL YET RARE HEADACHES

Trigeminal autonomic cephalgias (TACs) represent a small group of distinct headaches. Best known among them are cluster headaches, so named because they come in clusters—say, three a day for two months—and then stop, often returning at the same time the following year. They cause excruciating pain, always on one side of the head, and can last anywhere from 15 minutes to three hours.

Notably, TAC headaches are accompanied by physical signs, such as tearing or red eye, facial flushing, a drooping eyelid or a feeling of fullness in the ear—in every case, on the same side of the head as the headache. Specific signs are key to identifying TAC headaches and distinguishing them from migraines. Each type of TAC has somewhat different symptoms, frequency, pain severity, underlying causes and treatment, and imaging tests usually are needed to make the right diagnosis.

THE HEADACHE THAT ISN'T

Yes, it's possible to get a headache when you have a sinus infection or other sinus-related condition, but most people who think they have sinus headaches actually have migraines. If you get successfully treated for a sinus condition and find that your headaches don't improve, see a headache specialist.

THE HEADACHE FROM HEADACHE MEDICATION

If you take pain relief medications for too many days in a row, you can get a rebound headache (also called "medication overuse" headache). The risk is that a rebound headache can lead to chronic headaches. Keep track of the amount of pain relievers you take, and limit your use to 10 days a month.

THE HEADACHE THAT'S A MEDICAL EMERGENCY

A headache that comes on very suddenly, feels like the worst pain you have ever had and is different from the headaches that you typically get should send you to the ER immediately, especially if you're over age 50. It could be an extremely dangerous condition, such as a stroke, other blood vessel problems such as an aneurysm causing a hemorrhage or a brain tumor. Other warning signs are neurological symptoms that are different from your normal headaches, such as weakness or numbness on one side of your body or slurred speech.

Bottom line: If head pain is interfering with your life, talk to your doctor. Once the underlying cause of the pain is found, you can start the appropriate steps to make it stop or at least keep it under control.

Safer, Faster Migraine Drug on the Horizon

Research presented by Sheena Aurora, MD, medical fellow and global launch leader, Eli Lilly and Company, Indianapolis.

Yes, there are medications for migraine. Unfortunately, they don't always completely relieve the symptoms…can take a long time to work…and cause side effects, including serious ones such as high blood pressure and increased risk for heart attack. Now a new drug—and the first in a new class of migraine drug in nearly 20 years—that promises safer, faster relief for this debilitating condition may soon be available.

Triptans have long been the go-to drug for acute treatment of migraine symptoms once they start. These drugs—such as *sumatriptan* (Imitrex), *zolmitriptan* (Zomig) and others—work by helping serotonin bind to sites in the brain called 5-HT receptors. Serotonin constricts blood vessels, and constricting blood vessels in the brain helps relieve migraine pain. Unfortunately, triptans constrict other blood vessels outside the brain, too, including heart vessels, which can cause chest pain, high blood pressure…and lead to heart attack.

The new drug, *lasmiditan*, also binds to 5-HT receptors—but only to those in the brain that are involved in migraine attacks. So the drug does not affect the heart or blood pressure. Lasmiditan is also very fast and effective—providing complete relief in as short a time as one hour.

Two clinical trials compared taking lasmiditan with a placebo among close to 4,500 people (average age 42) who reported three to eight debilitating migraines per month. Some but not all the participants had migraine aura, and most in both studies also had some risk factors for heart disease—and one study included people with known heart disease, arrhythmias and/or high blood pressure. The studies were conducted by Eli Lilly, the company that makes the drug, and the results were presented at the annual meeting of the American Headache Society in San Francisco.

Results: For migraineurs who took 200 milligrams (mg) of lasmiditan within four hours of a migraine attack, 32% in one study and 39% in the other were pain free—compared with 15% and 21% who took the placebo. Photophobia (pain associated with light) was about 41% to 49% relieved, compared with 30% to 33% for placebo. And even though they may not have had complete pain relief, 60% to 65% reported some pain relief, compared with 40% in the placebo group. (The researchers did not compare lasmiditan with triptans.)

Best: Cardiovascular side effects were not reported, even among migraineurs with known heart problems and/or high blood pressure. The most common side effects were mild-to-moderate dizziness, tingling or numbness, sleepiness, fatigue and nausea.

Lasmiditan is not yet available to the public (at this writing), but Eli Lilly applied for FDA approval in November 2018. Meanwhile, let your doctor know if you are interested in trying the drug so that he/she can let you know as soon as it is available.

The Confusing Migraine: Aura Without Pain

Nada Hindiyeh, MD, director of clinical research and clinical assistant professor of neurology and neurological sciences, Stanford University, California, and principal investigator of many studies on migraine headaches.

It's one of the scariest experiences you're likely to have—suddenly and for no apparent reason, you see a blank, black area in your vision. Then come black zigzag lines, sparklers, brilliant globes of color or some other sort of light show. Next, these strange visual disturbances start moving to your other eye. You might think you're losing your vision. But within an hour, the show is over, your vision is back to normal and you feel fine again.

WHAT'S GOING ON?

What you just experienced is the most common symptom of migraine headaches with aura...the aura itself. What's confusing—and can be scary—is that without the usual head pain that follows, you might be wondering whether there's something wrong with your vision or, worse, that you're having some sort of stroke, such as a TIA.

One difference: An aura can last anywhere from 15 to 60 minutes...the visual symptoms of a TIA generally last between three and 10 minutes. *Here's what else you need to know...*

THE RARE TYPE OF MIGRAINE

It's relatively common for migraine sufferers to experience an aura an hour or so before their head pain starts, and nearly all of the time it's the type of visual disturbance described above, says headache specialist Nada Hindiyeh, MD, of Stanford University. But these two phases don't always occur in every migraine episode.

Various studies have found that people who have "migraine with aura" experience an aura with no subsequent headache between 37% and 44% of the time. Among people with no history of migraine, it's estimated that about 13% have experienced aura alone. This can happen to anyone of any age, but it does seem to happen more often among people over age 50, primarily in those with a history of migraine with aura in their younger years but also, to a lesser extent, in some people who never had this type of head pain. Because it seemed as though only the eyes were affected, these events used to be called "ocular migraines," but Dr. Hindiyeh says that's a misnomer because the aura still originates within the brain, not within the eyes.

IF THIS HAPPENS TO YOU

If this was your first aura. Call your primary care doctor and describe your symptoms. He/she may want to see you to officially rule out more serious causes of visual disturbance, such as retinal disease, or confirm that you didn't have a stroke or TIA. If you have any sudden changes such as sudden weakness or numbness, especially on one side of the body, sudden confusion or sudden lack of coordination, immediately seek emergency care.

Look for a pattern. People with painful migraines typically keep a journal to spot any possible triggers such as a food or even bright lights. Even if you're not getting any head pain, keeping a journal will let you see any pattern to your auras and any subsequent changes in your pattern—from what the visual disturbances themselves look like to how long they last. If an aura lasts longer than your normal pattern, call your health-care provider.

Important: If you also experience new symptoms, such as sudden loss of vision or weakness or numbness on one side of your body, call 911. These can be signs of a stroke.

HOW TO WAIT OUT AN AURA

Although you may not be debilitated like you would if you had migraine pain, it's important to take safety measures as soon as you notice that your vision has been affected by migraine aura. For instance, if you're driving, pull off the road.

And because an aura can be stressful even though you know that it's not dangerous, you might want to practice your favorite relaxation method until it subsides.

Aimovig Gets FDA Nod as a Migraine Preventive Drug

The news release "FDA Approves Novel Preventive Treatment for Migraine," May 17, 2018.

The FDA has approved a new once-monthly injectable drug, *erenumab-aooe* (Aimovig), that helps reduce the number of days that migraineurs are affected by these debilitating headaches.

Even though medical experts still have not determined exactly what causes migraines, they have recently discovered that the levels of a molecule called calcitonin gene-related peptide (CGRP) rise in brain cells during migraine pain. Aimovig is the first drug that works by blocking the activity of CGRP.

Scientific evidence: To test the new treatment, three clinical trials, including 955 patients with different types of migraine, were conducted. Two of the trials enrolled people with episodic migraine (four to 14 headache days per month). Patients in the first study who used Aimovig over a six-month period reported one to two fewer monthly migraine days, on average, than those who received a placebo. Patients in the second study, which lasted three months, reported an average of one fewer migraine day per month than those in the placebo group. Put another way, that's 24 to 48 fewer hours per month without headache pain.

The third study enrolled patients with chronic migraine (15 or more headache days per month for three or more months). Over a three-month period, the Aimovig users reported an average of 2½ fewer monthly migraine days than those who used a placebo. That's 60 fewer hours per month without headache pain.

The Aimovig injection can be self-administered. The most common side effects reported by patients in the clinical trials were constipation, along with pain, redness, itching, tenderness or bruising at the injection site.

Important: Be sure to check with your insurer about coverage for Aimovig. Due to its high cost, insurers may require migraine patients to try other less expensive generic drugs before approving coverage for Aimovig.

Also: Check with your doctor and pharmacist about potential side effects and interactions with other medicines.

Avoid Neck Pain Without Giving Up Your iPad

Study titled "Gender and Posture Are Significant Risk Factors to Musculoskeletal Symptoms During Touch-screen Tablet Computer Use," led by researchers at University of Nevada, Las Vegas (UNLV), published in *Journal of Physical Therapy Science.*

Researchers surveyed 412 college students, staff, teachers and alumni about their tablet-using habits and any neck or shoulder distress. Stiffness, soreness, and aches and pains in the neck, upper back/shoulders, arms/hands or head were the most common complaints. A whopping 55% of those surveyed reported moderate discomfort…and 15% said that they had lost sleep because of the pain.

Surprising findings: Even though it's reasonable to assume that the more time you spend using a tablet, the more neck pain you'd have, the study suggests that's not the case. Instead, specific postures were at the root of most of the pain problems. *What helps…*

• **Sit in a chair with a supportive back.**

• **Use a stand for your tablet rather than placing it on a flat surface,** and attach an external keyboard so that you can maintain a more upright posture.

• **Wear a posture-reminder device,** which will beep or vibrate every time you slouch. These devices, sometimes called "posture trainers" or "posture coaches," are available online.

Also: Especially for women, who tend to be smaller and less muscular, strengthening the neck and back muscles through exercise helps prevent neck pain.

How to Really Recover from Whiplash

Robert Zembroski, DC, DACNB, MS, chiropractic neurologist, director, Darien Center for Functional Medicine, Darien, Connecticut.

Whiplash is the term for neck injury caused by quick, forceful back-and-forth snapping of the neck—typically from being in an auto accident, but you can also get whiplash from any kind of accident, physical abuse or trauma. Symptoms can include neck pain, neck and shoulder stiffness, headache and tingling and numbness in the arms. It's also common to feel dizzy and to have trouble sleeping.

Usually, whiplash symptoms resolve on their own within a few weeks or months. But for about one-third of people who get whiplash, it can be a long-term—even debilitating—disorder that never completely goes away. This is more likely to happen with repeated whiplash, especially when whiplash happens again before full recovery from the previous injury.

HOW TO RECOVER FROM WHIPLASH

There is no one-size-fits-all therapy, but whether you're treating your first episode of whiplash or your second (or third or fourth), these therapies can help…

•**Ice within the first 72 hours** of initial injury to reduce pain and swelling…after 72 hours, heat to improve circulation, improve motion and reduce pain.

•**Over-the-counter pain medications** such as *ibuprofen* (Motrin) or *acetaminophen* (Tylenol).

•**Gentle, assisted spinal manipulation from a chiropractor.**

•**Physical therapy.**

All of these potential treatments should be managed by a physician who examines you and tracks your progress—don't treat whiplash yourself.

It's generally best to wear a soft neck collar immediately after the injury for up to seven days to prevent excessive movement while the muscles and soft tissues heal enough to receive therapy. Wearing a neck collar longer immobilizes neck muscles, which can cause them to become stiff and weak. In fact, moving your neck and staying active is important for full recovery. But do avoid activities that have a greater-than-average chance of leading to another neck injury.

If dizziness persists, the cause needs to be determined. Neck trauma can cause orthostatic hypotension, a drop in blood pressure when rising from lying down or sitting that causes dizziness. Pain or other symptoms that last longer than a day or two should be checked by a medical or chiropractic neurologist to see if there is nerve damage.

Since inflammation is a big part of neck pain and other whiplash symptoms, an anti-inflammatory diet including lots of vegetables and fruit and omega-3 fatty acids from such foods as nuts, seeds and cold-water fatty fish can be very helpful.

Mysterious Neck, Shoulder, Arm or Hand Problems?

Ying-Wei Lum, MD, MPH, assistant professor in the department of surgery, division of vascular surgery and endovascular therapy at Johns Hopkins University School of Medicine, Baltimore. He specializes in the treatment of thoracic outlet syndrome, peripheral artery disease and abdominal aortic aneurysms.

Thoracic outlet syndrome (TOS) is a little-known condition that's tricky to diagnose and treat. This often painful and disabling disorder results from compression of nerves or blood vessels in the thoracic outlet, a narrow, bony, almost-triangular opening between the first rib at the top of the rib cage and the clavicle, or collarbone. It can cause a wide range of symptoms including neck, shoulder or arm pain…tingling or swelling in an arm, a hand or fingers…weakness in a shoulder, an arm or a hand…and/or impaired circulation in a hand.

Many other conditions (such as diabetes, carpal tunnel syndrome, Raynaud's disease, fibromyalgia or even a heart attack) can cause similar sensations, making it difficult to diagnose. But with the development of a clear set of criteria, vascular surgeons and other specialists can now identify TOS from a careful medical history, basic imaging tests and an in-office physical exam.

TOO CLOSE FOR COMFORT

Two major blood vessels, the subclavian artery and vein, pass through the thoracic outlet. So does the brachial plexus, a bundle of nerves that travels to the shoulders, chest, arms and hands. The scalene muscles in the neck border the thoracic outlet.

Anything that crowds the blood vessels or nerves going through the thoracic outlet can cause TOS. This can include an extra rib that protrudes from the neck part of the spine (a cervical rib)…repetitive overhead motions—from activities such as swimming or house painting…and intense weight lifting, whiplash injuries or even weight gain. The symptoms usually affect only one side of the body but can sometimes affect both sides.

NERVES VS. BLOOD VESSELS

Nerve-related TOS symptoms are different from those caused by pressure on an artery or vein…

•**Nerve pressure accounts for more than 90% of TOS cases.** These patients can have pain, numbness or tingling (or all three) that starts in the neck and radiates down to a hand. The discomfort may come and go but usually worsens when an arm is elevated. Patients will continue to have disabling symptoms without treatment.

•**Pressure on a vein or an artery** can restrict blood flow and cause swelling and discoloration of the fingers, hand or arm…or feelings of coldness in the hands. This type of pressure also can increase risk for blood clots in the shoulders or arms, which could potentially lead to a pulmonary embolism (a blood clot in the lungs).

A DIAGNOSTIC CHALLENGE

If your doctor suspects TOS, you'll probably be given a chest X-ray to detect rib abnormalities, including the presence of a cervical rib. You'll also be given an ultrasound to help identify blood-vessel abnormalities and clots. But in many cases, doctors can't actually see what's causing the pressure, even with these imaging tests. A thorough medical history, along with an in-office physical exam, are among the best ways to diagnose TOS.

The doctor will take the patient through a variety of maneuvers. Patients with nerve-related TOS will usually notice an increase in pain/other symptoms when they rotate their head or tilt it from the ear to the shoulder. And raising the arms will usually cause an increase in symptoms within 30 to 60 seconds.

Also helpful: An injection of local anesthetic into one of the scalene muscles in the neck. In patients with nerve-related TOS, this will often stop pain almost immediately. The pain relief lasts only for about a day, so it's not a treatment—but it's a good diagnostic test.

A doctor also will look for physical signs like abnormal skin color and cool skin, which indicate severely restricted blood flow or a clot.

NEXT STEPS

Surgery (see next page) is often advised for vascular-related TOS, while more conservative treatment can often be used to avoid (or delay) surgery for nerve-related TOS…

•**Stretches and/or physical therapy can often help patients with nerve-related TOS.** The movements stretch and strengthen muscles, restore normal posture and relieve compression of affected nerves.

Note: Be sure to get a physical therapist's consent before trying stretches on your own.

Sample stretch: Make an "OK" sign with your thumb and forefinger…turn your hand upside down…raise your elbow in the air…and place the circle over your eye. Your palm will be facing toward your face and your other three fingers will be touching your cheek. Hold the stretch for about 30 seconds. Other stretches can be found online (try YouTube) or from a physical therapist.

•**Massage and acupuncture seem to help** some patients with TOS caused by nerve pressure, and there's no downside to trying them, even though there's little evidence to prove these approaches work. But do get checked out by your doctor first to make sure you're not overlooking another problem.

•**Botox injections** in the scalene muscles will shrink these muscles and potentially open up the space in the thoracic outlet to relieve pressure. For about 10% of my patients, the injections provide long-term relief—sometimes for many years.

But more often, an injection gives relief for only two to four months and repeated injections are needed. Most patients aren't willing to keep getting injections, particularly because they tend to get less effective over time. If your symptoms have not improved after three or four attempts, the injections are probably not going to work for you.

•**Blood thinners** are an essential component of therapy when TOS presents with a blood clot in a vein. These patients are at risk for recurrent deep vein thrombosis (DVT) and pulmonary embolism if not treated with surgery (see below). Blood-thinning medications, such as *enoxaparin sodium* (Lovenox) or *rivaroxaban* (Xarelto), can be used until the clot is surgically removed.

IF SURGERY IS NEEDED…

In some cases, surgery is required to treat TOS.

For nerve-related symptoms, the goal of surgery is to remove the tissue—either bone or muscle—that's causing the pressure. For clot-related symptoms, surgery is a standard treatment. It's used to remove clots…reconstruct or replace damaged arteries…or remove bone/muscle that's pressing on the affected area.

These procedures typically require a one-to-three-night hospital stay, and patients should do physical therapy as part of their rehab.

Is a "Slipping Rib" Causing Your Pain?

Cassidy Foley Davelaar, DO, FAAP, CAQSM, division of orthopedics and sports medicine, Nemours Children's Hospital, and assistant professor, University of Central Florida College of Medicine, both in Orlando. She is also clinical care provider for the United States Tennis Association.

The cause of abdominal pain can be hard to figure out, with so many key organs, muscles and skeletal parts located between the shoulders and hips. But if your belly, back or chest hurts when you move certain ways—

and other conditions have been ruled out—you might have slipping rib syndrome. Here's what happens…and what to do about it.

You probably think that your ribs expand enough to allow breathing, but they basically stay in place. And that's mostly true. However, your eighth, ninth and 10th ribs are not attached directly to your sternum (the flat bone at the center front of the chest, aka the breastbone). Instead, they are attached to cartilage that attaches to the sternum.

The cartilage itself can weaken because of trauma from activities that involve major movement of the rib cage. Or the cartilage attachments can weaken from unknown causes. The weakening allows one of the ribs to slip from its proper position during normal movements of the abdominal muscles.

Most often, the slipping rib is the 10th one… and 90% of the time it occurs on just one side of the body. The slippage compresses and irritates the intercostal nerve that runs through the tissue between the ribs. This causes pain that comes and goes, often worsening with exercise or certain movements. (More on that below.)

WHO'S AT RISK?

Slipping rib syndrome first came to medical attention about 60 years ago. While the condition is not considered common, it is so often missed or mistaken for other conditions—such as an ulcer, gallbladder disease, kidney stones or appendicitis—that it's hard to know exactly how common it really is. For instance, 54 cases were found at one sports medicine clinic between 1999 and 2014. And a recent study published in *Clinical Journal of Sports Medicine* found that the average person with this condition sees more than two specialists and takes more than 15 months to get a correct diagnosis.

Slipping rib can happen at any age and afflicts more women than men, particularly during reproductive years. (In the sports medicine clinic study mentioned above, 70% of cases were in women.) Certain sports, such as running, rowing, swimming and weight lifting… and conditions that cause chronic coughing, such as asthma or bronchitis, can make slipping rib syndrome more likely. Being hypermobile (the medical term for "double-jointed") also increases risk. About 20% of patients with slipping rib syndrome are hypermobile.

SYMPTOMS AND DIAGNOSIS

Upper-abdominal pain unrelated to an obvious injury is the most common symptom of slipping rib. The pain usually starts gradually and is described as sharp, severe or cramping...although over time it may fade to a dull ache. The pain usually is triggered by activities that involve upper-arm movement. However, coughing, getting up from a chair or just rolling over in bed also may cause pain.

Once other conditions have been ruled out and slipping rib is suspected, it's actually not hard to diagnose. This is often done with a simple test performed in the doctor's office called a "hooking maneuver." The doctor hooks his/her fingers under the edge of the lower rib cage and pulls upward and outward to see if that triggers pain. Ultrasound also can confirm the diagnosis.

TREATMENT OPTIONS

Depending on the patient's age, activity level and disability from the condition, treatment usually starts with less invasive treatments—nonsteroidal anti-inflammatory drugs (NSAIDs), Lidoderm patches, chiropractic treatment and acupuncture. Generally, noninvasive treatments are about 30% effective at relieving pain, although some work better than others. Diclofenac gel was found to be 60% effective, and osteopathic manipulative treatment (OMT) was 71% effective at relieving pain.

If these methods aren't effective or don't help enough, physical therapy and special home exercises can be beneficial for roughly half the patients who try these therapies.

For patients who still aren't getting adequate pain relief, an ultrasound-guided nerve block can be tried. Injections of numbing medication and/or steroids can provide full relief for several months...and may resolve the pain permanently.

For severe cases of slipping rib, surgery to remove the affected cartilage attached to the problematic rib can relieve the pain. Once healed, pain usually goes away permanently—and the patient can return to normal activities, including sports.

Gender Bias with Pain

Study in which 264 adults were asked to rate the pain of a child during a doctor's finger-prick test, by researchers at Yale University, New Haven, Connecticut, published in *Journal of Pediatric Psychology*.

Boys' pain is taken more seriously than the same pain felt by girls. Women, in particular, rated boys' pain higher—while men rated boys' and girls' pain more similarly. The reason is unknown, but researchers hope that the findings will add insight into the role of gender bias in pain management and health care.

Your Wrist Pain May Not Be Carpal Tunnel Syndrome

Robert E. Markison, MD, hand surgeon and clinical professor of surgery at the University of California, San Francisco. MarkisonMD.com

Jane Bear-Lehman, PhD, OTR/L, FAOTA, FNAP, clinician and researcher in hand and occupational therapy.

Ann Porretto-Loehrke, DPT, CHT, COMT, CMTPT, therapy comanager at the Hand to Shoulder Center of Wisconsin. *Soft Tissue Injuries*, Chapter 8: "Forearm, Hand and Wrist," by Stephen Southern and John Sloan (*Emergency Medical Journal*, EMJ.BMJ.com).

Don't take wrist pain lightly! Our lives have become increasingly technology-centric, and this puts the vulnerable wrist joint at great risk for repetitive strain injury (RSI). Even nontech activities like riding a bike, playing a musical instrument, knitting or gardening and other hobbies can make your wrist hurt all the time—and many people don't realize just how debilitating wrist pain can be. They don't take their symptoms seriously early on, when they could do something about them—and then the condition could become permanent.

Another mistake: Assuming that any chronic wrist pain is carpal tunnel syndrome and treating it that way. It's often not. *Here's how to know what's going on with your wrist...*

UNDERSTANDING WRIST PAIN

Carpal tunnel syndrome is only one type of issue that can affect the wrist. It is (or should be)

a very specific diagnosis involving compression of the median nerve at the wrist (the nerve itself starts in the neck and travels all the way down the arm to the fingers—its branches feed through the thumb, index and middle fingers and half of the ring finger). If you have carpal tunnel syndrome, you might experience not only pain in the thumb and index, middle and ring fingers as well as the hand but also numbness and tingling in your fingers, and symptoms might persist all day and even wake you up at night.

But other ailments could be causing your wrist pain. For instance, pain on the thumb side of the wrist, especially when you make a fist, twist or grasp an object forcefully, could mean de Quervain's tenosynovitis, an inflammation of the tendons that straighten the thumb and move the thumb away from the palm. Another possibility is ulnar tunnel syndrome, sometimes called Guyon's canal syndrome, which happens when the ulnar nerve (running from the neck down into the hand) is compressed at the wrist. This syndrome affects half the ring finger and the pinky, can make them numb and tingly, and can result in weakness in your hand grip or finger pinch.

WHEN TO SEE A DOCTOR

If you have numbness, tingling, swelling, weakness and/or pain in your hand or wrist that either persists for longer than a month or that repeatedly comes and goes, don't assume it's carpal tunnel syndrome…don't assume you can treat it with a drugstore splint or other device marketed for carpal tunnel syndrome…but instead, get yourself to a doctor for a real diagnosis. If you don't, you may miss the opportunity for a full recovery.

See a hand surgeon, a physician who has specialized training in the evaluation and treatment of hand, wrist and arm conditions. But don't be afraid that he or she will automatically recommend surgery. Hand surgeons are hand doctors first, and they don't perform surgery on everyone they see—far from it. Occupational medicine doctors or physiatrists can also diagnose RSI.

When surgery isn't necessary, healing will most likely involve working with an occupational or physical therapist, such as a certified hand therapist (CHT). You want a health-care professional with intricate knowledge of hand

anatomy and hand conditions and your type of injury in particular. (These therapists can also help you postoperatively.)

What about the original cause of the injury? Your doctor and hand-therapy specialist will discuss with you which kind of movements provoke symptoms, how to limit these motions, how to reduce the pain…and then stay as symptom-free as possible. (You can find a certified hand therapist through the American Society of Hand Therapists, ASHT.org)

BE YOUR OWN BEST HEALER

What you do on your own, not just in therapy sessions, is also an important part of your recovery, and nutrition, including supplementation, can play a big role in success. *Robert E. Markison, MD, a hand surgeon and clinical professor of surgery at the University of California, San Francisco, often recommends these nutrients to his patients…*

•**Liquid vitamin D3,** which is more easily absorbed by the body than D3 in capsule form, to maintain musculoskeletal health. A periodic blood test can help you maintain your blood vitamin-D level between 50 and 80 ng/mL.

•**Vitamins B6 and B12,** preferably from food. These vitamins actively support central and peripheral nerve system function. Supplemental vitamin B6 can cause neuropathy (nerve pain) if you take amounts over the safe upper limit of 100 mg per day (the recommended daily allowance is only 1.3 mg), but high intake of this vitamin from food has not been shown to have adverse effects. Foods with generous amounts of B6 include chickpeas, chicken breast, yellowfin tuna and bananas. The recommended daily allowance of vitamin B12 is 2.4 µg. Foods high in B12 include beef liver, fish, meat, poultry, eggs and milk. Your doctor can monitor your levels of both vitamins with a blood test. For B6, the healthy range is between 5 and 50 µg/L, and for B-12, it's between 200 and 900 ng/mL. Dr. Markinson suggests aiming for at least the middle of the ranges.

•**Stay well-hydrated.** Microcirculation carries nutrients and oxygen to the cells and takes away waste. Regularly drinking water also ensures that you get up periodically to use the bathroom—sometimes that's the only break from computing that people get.

These ergonomic pointers can help, too…

•As much as possible, use a voice-recognition program, not a keyboard or touch screen, for computer work. For texting, use voice-to-text, not your thumbs.

•When you must type at your computer, use a split-and-tilt keyboard. It allows you to adjust the keyboard to fit your body, rather than having to contort yourself to a molded plastic keyboard. Also, use a light touch—don't pound on the keyboard.

•If you use a mouse, alternate it between your left and right hands to balance out the workload.

•Sit tall and avoid a forward-head posture. Relax your shoulders and keep your arms near your torso.

•Keep your hands warm to improve circulation, important for avoiding RSI.

A note about pain relief medication: Discuss options with your care providers before taking anything so that you don't mask symptoms and jump back into activities before you've truly healed.

When to Be Concerned About a Bruise

Eric H. Kraut, MD, hematologist, professor of internal medicine, The Ohio State University, director of benign hematology, Hemostasis Thrombosis Treatment Center, The Ohio State University Wexner Medical Center, both in Columbus.

Different people have different healing times when it comes to bruises. Some people's bruises disappear within two or three weeks, while others' linger longer. Age can be a factor. Bruises tend to last longer for people older than 65 because of changes in the skin.

Tip: As with swelling, you can speed the healing of a bruise by elevating the area above the heart, icing it for about 15 minutes every hour for the first 24 hours, and resting the injured area.

There are certain signs that any bruise, regardless of location, warrants a trip to the doctor.

WHEN TO SEE A DOCTOR

•You have swelling and pain. If you had an injury and there's swelling and pain at the bruise site, you could have a sprain or a fracture that needs evaluation and treatment.

•You have other signs of a bleeding disorder. You'll experience more bruising and other types of bleeding if you have a disorder that impacts your blood's ability to clot. Besides easy bruising, other signs to look for include having frequent nosebleeds, bleeding excessively after getting a cut or having dental work done, having heavy menstrual periods or bleeding at unusual spots, such as around your joints.

•You have symptoms of anemia. Anemia, a problem with red blood cells, deprives the body of oxygen. If you have abnormal bleeding and bruising, you may have anemia. Other symptoms of anemia include shortness of breath, dizziness, a faster heartbeat, cold hands and feet, weakness, chest pain, pale skin and headaches.

•You have a large bruise on your torso. Small bruises or bruises on your arms or legs don't usually point to an underlying issue. A large bruise on your chest, back or stomach, especially if you haven't fallen and don't know what caused it, should be examined. This could be a sign of abnormalities in clotting due to low or abnormal platelets in your blood and or an inherited bleeding disorder. This should be evaluated by a physician since blood tests may explain the problem.

•There's a sudden change in your bruising pattern. A good rule of thumb is to pay attention to what's common for you. If you suddenly experience more bruising for no known reason, get checked out by your doctor.

Better Movement = Less Pain

Patricia A. Buchanan, PhD, a movement-improvement expert focusing on the Feldenkrais Method in Toledo, Ohio. She previously was an associate professor in the physical therapy program at Des Moines University. DrPatBuchanan.com

Many people have never heard of the Feldenkrais Method, but there are plenty of reasons why it should be on your radar. It can be used to resolve chronic musculoskeletal pain, speed recovery from injuries and/or surgery and provide relief from chronic conditions such as fibromyalgia. So what exactly is it…and how can it help you?

IT'S HOW YOU MOVE

The Feldenkrais Method (developed by Moshe Feldenkrais, DSc, an Israeli physicist, mechanical engineer and martial arts expert, after he suffered a serious knee injury) helps people become aware of the habitual movements that could be causing pain or discomfort and teaches them to replace these motions with movements that are less stressful to the body. With practice, the new movements become ingrained and automatic, and discomfort or pain is greatly minimized—pain medication can often be reduced or even stopped.

Example: If you have hip pain, you might unconsciously contract the large muscles that surround the hip joint in an effort to protect the painful area from more injury or pain. You might start to keep these muscles tight all the time—whether you're standing, sitting, walking or sleeping. This forces other muscles to over-compensate…causes imbalance in the body… and eventually increases pain and stiffness.

Research on this treatment's effectiveness for pain relief continues to mount. In a small study published in *Journal of Occupational Rehabilitation,* industrial workers who had Feldenkrais therapy showed significant reduction in neck and shoulder complaints compared with the physical therapy group. And research at California State University, Northridge, found that Feldenkrais was effective in reducing pain and decreasing disability in men and women (average age 52) with chronic low-back pain.

Important: The Feldenkrais Method is not a substitute for medical care but is often used to complement conventional medical treatment. If you have acute or severe pain, see your doctor for an evaluation before starting this treatment.

LEARNING THE METHOD

Certified Feldenkrais practitioners often have a background in physical therapy or massage, but all undergo a three-and-a-half-year accreditation program. They conduct both individual lessons (known as Functional Integration) and group sessions (Awareness Through Movement).

During individual lessons (sessions last 30 to 60 minutes), the practitioner will first ask what the client hopes to achieve—typically it will be relief from back, neck, hip or shoulder pain or recovery of mobility/function after an injury or surgery.

The practitioner will observe the client's movements/posture and use hands-on touch to discover where he/she is tight and how his movements are painful or inefficient. During a session, the client will be guided through a variety of movements, which could include everyday actions such as bending, walking or getting up from a chair.

The practitioner will then develop a lesson plan that's tailored to specific goals—for instance, how to climb stairs or raise arms with less pain or how to sit at a computer with less muscle tension.

During group sessions, the practitioner will lead a class through a series of slow movements. As in the one-on-one sessions, clients discover which movements can be done without pain and movement options for various functions such as reaching, getting up from a chair, etc. A movement that feels right for you might not work for the person next to you. These sessions last about an hour.

Some people get relief in one session while others need more. Some have lessons every week, like going to a regular yoga or Pilates class.

Feldenkrais sessions are not usually covered by insurance, but check with your provider. Individual sessions can run $100 or more, but group sessions typically cost $15 to $25. There are about 1,200 Feldenkrais practitioners in the US. To find a practitioner in your area, consult the Feldenkrais Guild of North America, Feldenkrais.com.

It is best to work with a practitioner who can give you customized instruction, but CDs, DVDs and MP3 downloads (available at Felden kraisResources.com) can give you an overview of the process.

Not just for pain: As mentioned earlier, people often try the Feldenkrais Method because they suffer from chronic pain, but it's also popular among athletes, musicians and other physically healthy people who want to learn how to move with more efficiency and less tension. It can benefit people with multiple sclerosis as well.

10 Moves to Prevent Knee, Hip and Joint Pain

Marilyn Moffat, PT, DPT, PhD, professor of physical therapy, New York University, New York City, past president of the American Physical Therapy Association and coauthor of *Age Defying Fitness: Making the Most of Your Body for the Rest of Your Life.*

C reaky, achy joints and nagging back pain aren't an inevitable part of aging. There are dozens of exercises that target thighs, glutes and core, the muscles that support the knees, hips and back, the three most-common pain spots. Here are the ones that work best.

Important: Start slowly and at low intensity if you're new to exercise. You shouldn't feel any pain when doing these exercises. If you experience pain—or you have known physical problems—consult a physical therapist for customized exercise advice.

STRENGTHENING EXERCISES

Add these exercises to an existing workout routine or use them as the basis of a new one. With each exercise, be sure to listen to your body. Take as much time as needed between any repetitions and build any hold time or repetitions gradually.

•**Bridging.** *Primary targets:* Core, gluteus maximus, hamstrings, quadriceps and adductor muscles. Lie on your back, knees bent, thighs parallel and feet facing forward with heels directly under your knees. Keep your arms flat on the floor, slightly out to the sides with elbows bent and palms up. Place a small pillow between your knees and press your knees together as you slowly lift your buttocks and back off the ground. Now press shoulders, upper arms and feet into the floor and straighten your right leg out at the level of the left knee to form a straight line from your right shoulder to your right foot. Hold for up to 30 seconds. (If it's too difficult to hold for that long, start with five to 10 seconds and gradually build up to 30.) Then bend your right knee, returning your right foot to the floor and repeat the move with your left leg.

Note: Thighs stay aligned throughout the exercise. Repeat up to three times with each leg if holding for 10 seconds…or do just once if holding for 30 seconds.

•**Plank with leg extension.** *Primary targets:* Core, gluteus maximus, quadriceps, shoulder and arm muscles. Start on hands and knees, with hands directly under shoulders and knees directly under hips. Straighten one leg back behind you so that you're supported on your toes…then straighten the other leg to support yourself on the toes of that leg. You will now be in a full plank or push-up position. Hold the position for 10 seconds. Then raise one leg about six inches, keeping the knee straight. Hold for 10 seconds. Lower that leg back to the push-up position and raise the other leg for 10 seconds. Slowly build up to repeating the entire sequence three times.

Helpful: If this is too strenuous, start on your forearms rather than with your arms extended. To add difficulty, gradually increase hold time for each phase to up to 30 seconds, at which point one full repetition is enough.

•**Half-side half planks.** *Primary targets:* Core, glutes, shoulder and lower leg muscles. Lie on your right side. Prop yourself up on your right elbow, which should be directly below your right shoulder. Bend your right knee toward your chest and straighten your left leg out directly in line with your body (like a dart). Lift your hips off the ground and reach your left hand toward the ceiling and hold for 10 seconds. Switch sides and repeat. Repeat the entire sequence up to three times.

Note: Slowly increase hold time until you reach 30 seconds for each side. At that point you can progress to full side planks—with both legs positioned in a straight line with the upper body, the lower arm straight and your weight supported by your hand, not your forearm.

•**Wall slide.** *Primary targets:* Quadriceps, core. Stand with your back flat against a wall and your chin tucked so that the middle of your neck is as close to the wall as is comfortable. Keeping your entire back against the wall, raise your arms into a goal post position (upper arms at shoulder height, elbows bent at a 90-degree angle and backs of hands against the wall if you have sufficient flexibility in your shoulders). Position your feet shoulder width apart and in front of the wall at about a distance roughly equal to the length of your thighs. (This is so that your knees will be positioned in line with your ankles when you're in the "seated" position.) Slowly slide your back down the wall until your hips and knees are nearly at a right angle. Hold for 10 seconds, then slowly slide back up. Extend hold time as you grow stronger, working up to 30 seconds. Repeat up to two times. For additional challenge, increase the hold up to one to two minutes.

Warning: To avoid unnecessary stress on your knees, your knees should never be farther from the wall than your ankles during this exercise.

•**Side steps.** *Primary targets:* Gluteus medius, core and leg muscles. Grab one end of an elastic resistance band in each hand and stand on the band with both feet close together in the middle of it. Cross the ends of the band and shorten it up so that it is fairly taut with your hands at approximately waist level. Keeping your foot on the band, step to the left with your left foot, taking as big a step as you can…then return your foot to starting position. Repeat the step up to five times with the left foot…then do the same number of steps to the right with the right foot. Start with up to three repeats of the entire sequence…building up to three repetitions of 10 steps in each direction.

STRETCHES

Do these stretches after any workout or after five to 10 minutes of light activity such as walking. Ideally stretches should be held for 30 to 60 seconds.

•**Hip and knee stretch.** While lying on your back, bring your right knee to your chest and wrap your hands around your right knee, then slowly extend your left leg straight along the floor. Gently push the back of your left knee toward the floor and hold for 30 seconds. Return your left knee to the starting position and lower your right leg to the starting position. Repeat reversing leg positions.

•**Hamstring stretch.** Lie on your back with both knees bent and your feet on the floor, holding one end of a resistance band (or a yoga strap, bathrobe belt or even a dog leash) in each hand. Loop the strap under the arch of your left foot and raise that leg toward the ceiling, keeping your knee straight. Your upper arms should stay flat on the floor against your sides, elbows bent. Use the band to pull your toes gently toward you, lifting your leg as high as you comfortably can, ideally until the sole of your foot is parallel to the ceiling. (*Note:* Raise your leg only as high as you can while keeping your knee perfectly straight.) Hold for 30 seconds, then bend your knee and return your foot to the starting position. Repeat the stretch with your right leg.

•**Hip and back stretch.** Lie on your back with your knees bent and your feet flat on the floor (place a thin pillow under your head for comfort if desired). Place your left heel on your right thigh just above your knee. Now link your hands together under your right thigh to bring your right knee toward your chest…or if you are very tight, use a band or strap under your right thigh to bring your right knee toward your chest. Make sure your head stays flat on the floor. Hold for 30 seconds, then switch sides.

•**Back-hips-knees stretch.** Get on your hands and knees, then drop your buttocks back toward your heels without moving your hands. Arms should be extended out straight in front of you with your head tucked between them, face toward the floor. Hold for 30 seconds. Your knees can be either together or spread apart during this stretch, depending on what's most comfortable for you.

•**Lunging hip flexor stretch.** Kneel on your left knee, left toes pointed behind you, and your right knee bent so that your right foot is flat on the floor and as far forward in front of you as possible. Make sure your right knee is directly over your right ankle, not in front of it. Your left knee should be far enough back to feel a stretch in the front of your left hip. Position your hands wherever comfortable for balance. Hold for 30 seconds, then switch legs and repeat.

Collagen Supplements for Joint Pain

Mark A. Stengler, NMD, naturopathic medical doctor, founder and medical director, Stengler Center for Integrative Medicine, Encinitas, California. He is author of several books, including *The Natural Physician's Healing Therapies* and *Bottom Line's Prescription for Natural Cures.* Dr. Stengler offers a collagen supplement on his website that is not listed in this article. MarkStengler.com

Collagen supplements are the new "it" nutrient. In fact, if Ponce de Leon were alive today, he might stop searching Florida for the "fountain of youth" and take them instead. Is there anything to all the wonderful claims—or is it just hype and wishful thinking? *Here's the answer...*

•**Collagen is found throughout our bodies.** It's a protein that gives strength to our bones and keeps our connective tissue strong and elastic. There are more than 16 types, but about 90% is Type I, II or III. Types I and III are mainly found in skin, tendons, bones, muscles and ligaments, while Type II is a component of joint cartilage. As we age, collagen production slows—hence the wrinkly, saggy skin and achy joints. Eating too much sugar and highly processed food, too much exposure to UVA and UVB rays, and smoking also deplete collagen.

However, swallowing collagen to replace our bodies' declining stores is not a straightforward solution. There is no high-quality research showing that run of the mill collagen supplements have any benefits at all. On the other hand, there is recent research suggesting that collagen that has been specially processed for enhanced absorption can.

•**Reduce joint pain and inflammation.** Several studies have found joint benefits from taking a patented Type II collagen called UC-II. (UC-II is "undenatured"—not processed using heat or chemicals—rather than hydrolyzed.) For instance, in a clinical trial conducted by the University of Houston College of Pharmacy and other universities (and supported by a pharmaceutical company that makes nutritional supplements), participants with knee osteoarthritis who took 40 mg of UC-II daily for 90 days reported greater reductions in stiffness and pain in their knees than those who took glucosamine and chondroitin, a popular supplement combination for arthritis. The collagen group reduced their pain score by 40% versus 15.4% for the glucosamine/chondroitin group.

HOW TO CHOOSE A SUPPLEMENT

You already know the best proven ways to fight off the effects of aging—eat plenty of antioxidant rich fruits and vegetables, don't smoke and use sun protection even on cloudy days. But if you want to give collagen supplements a try, they're not very expensive (about $25 to $40 for a month's supply), are considered safe—and you may find that they do make your skin smoother and your joints less achy.

Make sure to get the right product: Look for supplements that contain Type II collagen, such as BioCell collagen type II or UC-II collagen. Brands I prescribe for my patients include Olympian Lab, Health Logics, NOW and Life Extension.

HOW TO TAKE COLLAGEN

Collagen supplements should be taken on an empty stomach—that means at least two hours after or half an hour before eating. If you take a powdered form of collagen, you can stir it into water, tea, coffee or juice—and it's OK to add one or two tablespoons of cream, milk or half-and-half and/or sweetener. But don't add collagen supplements to other foods or beverages, especially those that contain protein, because protein interferes with collagen's absorption. As for snack bars and smoothies that have collagen added to them, there is no evidence that collagen in these forms gets absorbed into the bloodstream.

Risk for side effects from taking collagen supplements is low. Some people might have an allergic reaction, primarily to collagen that is made from fish if they have a fish allergy. Collagen made from fish can also raise calcium levels, increasing the risk for hypercalcemia, a potentially deadly condition. But taking the amounts recommended on supplement labels is unlikely to raise calcium to dangerous levels. (Or you can stick to supplements sourced from cow, chicken or pig, which don't carry the risk.) As always when taking a new supplement, it's smart to check with your health-care provider first.

7 Natural Ways to Relieve the Pain of Rheumatoid Arthritis

Harris H. McIlwain, MD, a board-certified rheumatologist, founder of the McIlwain Medical Group in Tampa, and former chair of the Florida Osteoporosis Board. He is coauthor of *The NEW Arthritis Diet: A 5-Step Plan to Lose Weight, End Pain and Be Active Again!* and *The NEW Arthritis Diet Recipes: Recipes and Super Foods to Help You Lose Weight, End Pain and Be Active Again!*

If your rheumatoid arthritis (RA) pain has you reaching for medications more and more often, it's time to investigate natural ways to ease your symptoms.

Certain lifestyle habits can support the disease-modifying antirheumatic drugs (DMARDs) that you take to stop the disease's progression without increasing side effects and health risks. What's more, many bring overall health benefits, such as reduced risk for cancer and improved heart health.

EASE RA THE NATURAL WAY

•**Practice range-of-motion (ROM) exercises.** An active lifestyle is the single most effective way to keep joints bathed in soothing synovial fluid. It might be challenging—or even impossible during a flare-up—but done regularly, exercise can decrease pain and fatigue. RA responds particularly well to range-of-motion exercises.

These stretching moves, such as shoulder shrugs and circles, wall pushes and bending and straightening each leg while lying on your back, increase flexibility and keep your muscles strong. Work with a physical therapist to create a program tailored to your specific needs.

Bonus: Improved flexibility from ROM exercises translates into fewer falls, which are common among people with RA.

Tip: For extra pain relief, do as many of these exercises as possible while in a warm tub or shower or after applying heat directly to any painful joints with a hot, wet towel or heating pad for 15 minutes.

•**Rub on capsaicin.** Yes, the same compound that makes your mouth burn when you eat chili peppers can counteract the feeling of pain in your joints when applied to the skin surface. Capsaicin blocks substance P, a chemical responsible for transmitting pain signals to your brain. You'll likely feel a mild burning sensation that lessens over time. After a few days of thrice-daily applications to the affected joints, the capsaicin should begin curbing painful RA sensations. Once RA pain subsides, you may continue to apply capsaicin for maintenance or as needed, up to three times daily.

Good over-the-counter products: Zostrix and Capzasin. These are available as creams and gels and in different strengths—try a low-dose version first. If you don't get enough relief after a few days, step up to a higher concentration.

Caution: Use medical gloves when applying to avoid getting it directly on fingertips, and be sure not to get any near your eyes, nose, mouth or genitals. Also, don't combine capsaicin topicals with a heating pad—doing so can cause burns. Skip capsaicin if you have psoriasis, eczema or any other skin condition or rash, and stop using it if it causes a skin reaction, such as redness or swelling.

•**Work toward a healthy weight.** The more overweight you are, the more inflammatory chemicals are coursing through your body and the greater your risk for pain. One such chemical, C-reactive protein, is also associated with diabetes, heart disease and cancer. Extra weight is also harder on weight-bearing joints, such as hips, ankles and knees. Losing as little as 10 pounds can make a big difference in symptoms, especially when combined with an anti-inflammatory, plant-based diet—lots of legumes and produce. This one-two punch creates changes at the cellular level, decreasing inflammation and reducing pain, stiffness and disability.

•**Load up on fruit with deeply colored skins.** Purple grapes, blueberries, blackberries, raspberries and dark cherries all contain anthocyanins, pain-relieving plant compounds that are anti-inflammatory.

•**Consider cupping.** This centuries-old technique involves applying suction to the skin via glass cups filled with hot air (the treatment lasts five to 20 minutes). Despite the marks made, cupping doesn't hurt and seems to work well for localized RA pain. Exactly how cupping helps isn't known for sure, but one theory is that the suction may improve circulation and aid in tissue repair in the skin and muscles. For this reason, it may also help ease RA-related spasms and muscular pain. Seek out a certified acupuncturist, physical therapist or licensed massage therapist with training in the technique.

•**Calm the mind to calm the body.** Stress is a well-recognized pain trigger. It doesn't cause pain, per se, but the way your mind and body respond to stress can increase your interpretation of and response to pain.

Stress-relieving techniques include deep abdominal breathing, which oxygenates the blood, triggering the release of morphine-like pain-relieving chemicals called endorphins. Tai chi, a series of slow, graceful movements practiced while standing, increases balance, flexibility and strength while easing emotional stress. Beginners can call their local arthritis foundation for a nearby class recommendation. Music therapy, visualization and meditation also can help. Just be sure to choose a method that works for you. Set aside 10 to 15 minutes a day to practice it.

•**Slash caffeine.** RA fatigue can be more limiting than the pain itself, but consuming caffeine for energy can backfire. The stimulant mimics the body's natural stress response and, especially at higher amounts, might cause a short-term rise in heart rate and blood pressure

and set up an inflammatory cascade that can ultimately lead to more pain. And while caffeine is sometimes added to pain medications, which can temporarily improve energy, caffeine also can heighten the side effects of pain medications, including anxiety and trembling.

Helpful: Green and black tea have beneficial antioxidant and anti-inflammatory effects but less caffeine than coffee.

Try holistic sleep strategies for fatigue, such as a warm bath before bed, keeping your bedroom cool and dark, and avoiding evening exercise.

Tip: Make sure your mattress is firm—a soft mattress puts extra stress on your joints.

It may take a week or two of practicing these therapies to notice a difference, but many RA patients ultimately discover a significant degree of relief.

The High Risks of Low-Dose Steroids for Rheumatoid Arthritis

Study titled "Association Between Glucocorticoid Exposure and Healthcare Expenditures for Potential Glucocorticoid-related Adverse Events in Patients with Rheumatoid Arthritis" by researchers at University of Pittsburgh, published in *The Journal of Rheumatology*.

Yes, steroids can block damaging inflammation from this disease, but they are not a long-term answer because, in addition to side effects, they don't change the course of rheumatoid arthritis. In contrast, a more recent class of drugs called "DMARDs" are a better ongoing treatment because they can actually slow or halt joint destruction.

You might sometimes also need a steroid to ease symptoms—such as when first starting a DMARD (because it can take weeks for it to take effect versus mere days for steroids) or when changing from one DMARD to another as you try to find the best one for your condition.

KNOW THE RISKS

In a recent study, researchers reviewed two years of medical records of 84,000 people with rheumatoid arthritis—they tallied the amount of steroids taken during the first one-year period and then looked at side effects during one year of follow-up.

They found that 48% of patients had taken oral steroids. Even though they were on a so-called low daily dose of 10 mg, many of them had taken this dose for relatively long periods—with terrible consequences. For example, patients who took steroids for between 80 and 180 days in the year had a higher risk for osteoporosis, fracture and infection than those who did not take steroids.

Even worse, those who took low-dose steroids for a total of six months out of the year or more were at risk for an even longer list of complications that additionally included aseptic necrosis (bone loss from lack of blood supply), type 2 diabetes, heart attack or stroke.

Knee Arthritis Pain Reduced by Whole-Body Massage

Adam Perlman, MD, MPH, director of integrative health and well-being at the Mayo Clinic in Jacksonville, Florida, and lead author of a study published in *Journal of General Internal Medicine.*

Osteoarthritis limits movement and diminishes quality of life, but few treatments are effective for pain relief. A recent study showed that weekly whole-body Swedish massage, which involves kneading, friction and vibration, significantly reduced knee pain and stiffness and improved function.

Could You Have Rheumatoid Arthritis and Not Know It?

Faizah Siddique, MD, assistant professor, department of rheumatology, Stritch School of Medicine, Loyola University, Chicago.

Are you frustrated because your joints are stiff, painful and swollen and you're tired all the time...yet your doctors can't tell you what's wrong? You may have a hard-to-diagnose form of rheumatoid arthritis. The longer it stays undiagnosed—and untreated—the greater your risk for permanent disability. You need to read this now.

Rheumatoid arthritis (RA) is an autoimmune disease. Antibodies produced by the body's immune system attack joint tissues, causing pain, swelling and stiffness in multiple joints. These antibodies, called rheumatoid factor (RF) and anti-CCP antibodies, are detectable in blood tests and help to diagnose RA.

However, up to 20% of people with RA have a form of the disease that doesn't show up in blood tests—seronegative rheumatoid arthritis. In the past, doctors thought that seronegative RA was a milder form of regular (seropositive) RA. It may be that patients with seronegative aren't producing enough antibodies to show up in current blood tests. Recent studies show that seronegative RA is just as serious as the regular kind...and for some patients can be hard to treat.

GETTING SERONEGATIVE RA DIAGNOSED

To diagnose seronegative RA, imaging studies, such as X-ray and ultrasound, may be taken to look for joint changes. However, such changes may take time to develop. Blood tests, such as C-reactive protein (CRP) and erythrocyte sedimentation rate (ESR), also may be done to look for evidence of generalized inflammation. But without the confirmation of antibodies, diagnosing seronegative RA is mainly based on a physical exam and symptoms.

Unlike with osteoarthritis, which usually causes symptoms in a single joint, RA causes pain and stiffness in multiple joints all over the body—including hands, knees, elbows, hips, feet and ankles. Joints, especially knuckles but also throughout the body, are evaluated for swelling and stiffness...and then monitored over at least six weeks or longer for any progression of swelling and stiffness. *In addition, doctors check for...*

•**Morning stiffness that lasts longer than 30 minutes after waking and gets better with movement.**

•**Joint swelling or redness throughout the body.**

•**Unusual fatigue that can't be explained by other causes.**

TREATMENT AND PROGNOSIS

In most ways, seronegative RA acts just like regular RA and is treated the same. For mild cases, treatment may start with steroids to reduce inflammation and nonsteroidal anti-inflammatory drugs (NSAIDs) to reduce inflammation and pain. For more severe cases, drugs called disease-modifying antirheumatic drugs (DMARDs) may be used to try to halt or slow disease progression. Recently, new DMARDs called biologics have been found to be very effective for moderate-to-severe disease. To help reduce symptoms, doctors sometimes keep patients on steroids or NSAIDs while waiting for DMARDs or biologics to take effect, and then taper off the NSAIDs and/or steroids. The American College of Rheumatology guidelines support a "treat-to-target" strategy for medication, with the target being remission.

There are also nondrug approaches that can help ease RA symptoms, such as range-of-motion exercises, deep abdominal breathing and capsaicin creams.

CHANGING DIAGNOSIS

Seronegative RA can change over time. Some patients will start to produce enough antibodies to become seropositive. Seronegative RA can also evolve into other seronegative diseases, such as psoriatic arthritis, spondyloarthritis, polymyalgia rheumatica or osteoarthritis. That is one reason why it's important to check with your doctor regularly if you have seronegative RA. If your diagnosis changes, your treatment may need to change.

And if you think you might have seronegative RA but confirmation is proving elusive, don't give up! Getting diagnosed and starting treatment as early as possible can prevent long-term disability. If your symptoms have lasted longer than six weeks without a diagnosis, ask your primary care doctor to refer you to a rheumatologist. This kind of specialist is best at diagnosing seronegative RA and at developing a treatment plan.

How to Exercise Despite Pain

Marilyn Moffat, PT, DPT, PhD, a practicing physical therapist and professor of physical therapy at New York University, New York City. She is author of two books for the lay audience and four professional books in the field. Steinhardt.nyu.edu/faculty/Marilyn_Moffat

Exercise is the magic elixir. It protects the heart, strengthens bones, lifts mood, increases energy, improves memory, boosts metabolism and prevents disease. But how can you get these benefits if your body hurts?

That is the problem for millions of Americans with chronic pain, especially knee pain or back pain. You want to exercise, but getting over that "pain hump" while you exercise is just too tough.

The irony is that pain not only makes regular exercise tougher—it also makes it more important. Why? It's a path toward less pain and a greater ability to do everyday tasks.

To learn how to get exercise when jogging or even walking is painful, we spoke with physical therapist Marilyn Moffat, PT, DPT, PhD. She homed in on two of the biggest obstacles that keep most people away from pain-relieving exercise—knee pain and back pain. *Her recommendations…*

FINDING YOUR OWN PATH

I'll provide exercises below that almost everyone can do. But no single exercise is perfect for everybody, and your unique limitations and physical condition will dictate your ideal activity. Many people with chronic joint or back pain benefit from a detailed individual plan developed with a physical therapist. Ask your healthcare provider for a recommendation or go to the website of the American Physical Therapy Association (MoveForwardPT.com), and click on "Find a PT" at the top of the page. It's always a good idea to check with your doctor before beginning a new exercise program.

When trying these exercises, start slowly, be cautious and pay attention to doing them correctly.

Important: Many people may need to build up to the "hold" times. For example, if an exercise calls for you to hold a pose for 30 seconds and that's too hard, try doing it for 10 seconds. If even that's too hard, just hold it as long as you can. You'll get stronger over time.

Stop immediately if any particular movement causes sharp pain, especially in a joint area. On the other hand, muscle fatigue (even burn) should be expected, especially with strengthening exercises. It's a good thing!

Let's get moving…

IF YOU HAVE KNEE PAIN

The best way to reduce knee pain is to increase the strength and flexibility in the muscles that support your knee. The key is to find exercises that permit pain-free range of motion. That means taking the load off the joint as much as possible. Walking in waist-deep water is a great way to do this—but not everyone has regular access to a pool. *Alternatives…*

•**Seated straight-leg raises** build up the quadriceps, which help support the knees.

What to do: Sit on the floor with your back against a wall. With one knee bent and the other leg straight out in front of you, wrap your hands around your bent leg, then slowly raise the straight leg up, keeping the knee as straight as possible—hold for 30 seconds. Then slowly lower the straight leg back to the floor. Do the exercise two or three times on each side,

•**Bridges** strengthen the hamstrings and quadriceps (key knee muscles), as well as the glutes and both the front and back of your body's core.

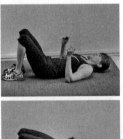

What to do: Lie on your back with your knees bent, and your feet and upper arms on the floor. Bend your elbows to a 90-degree angle, with your fingers pointing to the ceiling. Lift your glutes (butt muscles) off the floor, then straighten one leg out in the air at the level of the

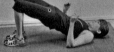

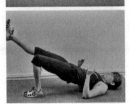

opposite knee and hold for 30 seconds. Bend the knee down, put your foot back on the floor and lower your butt. Alternate legs. Do this exercise two or three times per leg.

IF YOU HAVE BACK PAIN

People with spinal stenosis (narrowing of the spaces within the spine) or other degenerative changes in the low back have a hard time with many exercises. Even walking can be difficult with spinal stenosis because each step slightly extends the spine, which narrows the spinal canal, exacerbating the pain.

What helps: Increasing flexibility and core strength. Yoga planks with the spine straight or slightly rounded are especially beneficial—they strengthen the core muscles that support the back as well as the arm and leg muscles. Pay attention to good form.

•**Basic front plank.** Start on your hands and knees with your hands directly under your shoulders and your knees directly under your hips. Straighten one leg all the way back, then the other leg, and you should be in perfect position. (If weight bearing on straight arms is too difficult, do a plank on your forearms.) Tuck your chin in so that your neck is straight and you are looking at the floor. Your spine should be in a straight line and not arched. Maintain as straight a line as is comfortable from your head through to your ankles. Hold for 30 seconds. Do two or three times.

•**Side plank** also strengthens the core muscles and the arms and legs. Start by lying on your right side and with your right hand directly under your right shoulder. Ideally your feet should be stacked one on top of the other, but it's fine to start with the bottom knee bent. Lift your hips off the floor, and keep a straight line from your head through your shoulder, hips and feet. As you lift your hips, push your right hand into the floor. (Again, if weight bearing on a straight arm is too difficult, do the side plank on your forearm.) Hold for 30 seconds. Alternate sides. Do two or three times on each side.

AEROBIC FITNESS FOR ANYONE WITH PAIN

Whether you have pain in your knees or back (or hips or somewhere else), getting aerobic activity to improve your circulation and protect your heart can be challenging. But it's vital! *Here are ways to do it...*

•**Recumbent exercise bikes (the kind where you are seated against a backrest)** and seated stepper machines allow you to build your aerobic capacity. Being seated while doing aerobic exercise usually is easier for your back and reduces the forces on your knees that would occur if you were using a treadmill. The seated stepper, which resembles a recumbent elliptical machine, engages your arms as well as your legs. Many gyms have these machines.

•**Walking—and you can do it comfortably.** To absorb impact, wear sneakers that have good cushioned bottoms, add gel inserts into the sneakers and wear padded socks.

When walking on a treadmill: Use the handrails for support and to off-load some of the force of the body weight on your back and knees.

When walking outside: Choose school tracks or nature paths if possible—they're a little easier than paved sidewalks and roads—and you might consider walking poles. They help to absorb some impact, engage your upper body, help intensify your workout and improve stability. They are available at sporting-goods stores and online. Be sure to use two poles for the best balance and posture.

How to Talk About Pain with Your Doctor

2018 survey led by researchers at California State University in Northridge.

During doctor visits, the manner in which patients describe their pain affects how they are viewed by the doctor, according to a recent survey. *Advice to follow at your next office visit...*

•**Try your best to maintain a relaxed and pleasant demeanor.** Think of your doctor as a teammate who can help you reach the goal of pain relief.

•**Describe your pain by combining words and numbers.** For example, use descriptive words (such as stabbing, aching or throbbing) and a number scale (such as zero to 10, with zero meaning no pain and 10 meaning excruciating pain). You also can compare your current pain with a pain you've felt in the past, such as a broken ankle or passing a kidney stone.

•**Describe your family history of pain—** especially if any other family members have a pain-related condition or are highly sensitive to pain.

•**Be as specific as possible in conveying the duration of your pain**...the circumstances when it started...and anything that makes it better or worse.

Helpful: Keep a "pain diary" in which you record your symptoms and their severity.

•**List some activities you enjoyed in the past but now avoid because of the pain.**

Better Care for Back Pain That Just Won't Go Away

Christine Goertz, DC, PhD, CEO, The Spine Institute for Quality, Davenport, Iowa.

In a recent study, researchers found that adding chiropractic care to traditional medical treatment, including pain relievers and physical therapy, reduced pain better than traditional treatment alone. Chiropractic care included spinal manipulation plus hot/cold packs, exercise recommendations and other treatments. The chiropractic care participants were less likely to use prescription drugs and had significantly greater improvements in pain, disability and treatment satisfaction than those who received medical care alone. Specifically, 58% of those receiving chiropractic care reported at least a

30% improvement at six weeks, versus 32% of those in the medical care–only group.

For Relief from Common Aches and Pains, Change the Way You Sleep

Matthew O'Rourke, PT, DPT, CSCS, OMT, adjunct professor of physical therapy at Simmons University in Boston and a physical therapist in the outpatient clinic at Lahey Hospital & Medical Center in Burlington, Massachusetts.

Whether you like to curl up on your side or sprawl flat out on your stomach, you probably have a favorite sleeping position. But did you know that if you suffer from common aches and pains, this familiar position might be aggravating your pain?

Here's how to adapt your preferred sleeping style for pain relief and better sleep…

NECK PAIN

Back-sleeping is often said to be the best position for neck pain. But back-sleeping can actually increase neck discomfort when using a pillow that's too thick (which causes the head to flex forward) or too thin (which causes the head to flex backward).

For back-sleepers: Be sure to use a pillow that keeps the neck in a neutral position, in line with the spine. When viewed from the side, the ear should be in line with the shoulders or slightly above them.

For side-sleepers: Add a thin pillow or rolled-up bath towel between the neck and the mattress in addition to your regular pillow to provide neck support and prevent the spine from bending to either side.

For stomach-sleepers: This position is the worst for neck pain because you'll need to turn your head to one side or the other, which puts strain on the neck. It's best to try another position, if possible.

LOW-BACK PAIN

Many people say that their backs feel better when they sleep on their backs, particularly if they use a pillow or two to slightly elevate the knees. But side-sleeping often feels more natural.

For side-sleepers: Lie on one side in a "stacked" position, with your shoulders, knees and hips in up-and-down alignment and knees slightly bent.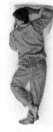

Helpful: Place a pillow between your knees. This helps to prevent the top leg from rolling over the bottom, which can twist the spine.

For stomach-sleepers: This position can strain your lower back. However, if you find it difficult to try the positions above, place a pillow under your stomach to reduce excessive spinal extension.

KNEE PAIN

With knee pain, back-sleeping can be painful because the knees are extended all night…but side-sleeping can cause irritation where the knees touch.

For back-sleepers: Try placing a pillow under the knees to prevent them from over-straightening.

Note: This position can be painful for some people.

For side-sleepers: Sleep with a pillow between your knees or use cloth knee pads (such as those that volleyball players wear), turning them sideways so that the area where the knees touch is well padded.

For stomach-sleepers: This position can put painful pressure on your knees. But if it's tough for you to switch to one of the above positions, put a pillow under your stomach to take some pressure off the knees.

HIP PAIN

For back- or stomach-sleepers:
People with arthritis-related hip pain often have more pain when sleeping on their back or stomach. It's best to try side-sleeping (see below). However, a small pillow under the knees (when lying on your back) or under the stomach (when lying on your stomach) may provide some relief.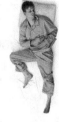

For side-sleepers: Side-sleeping is usually best for arthritis-related hip pain.

Helpful: Keep your knees slightly bent and use a pillow (a body pillow works well) between the knees and thighs to keep the hip in a more neutral position. If lying on one side is more painful than the other, switch sides.

YOU CAN CHANGE HOW YOU SLEEP

When you get into bed, start in the position in which you would like to sleep. Then spend about a minute visualizing yourself staying in this position for the night. If you wake up and are out of position, calmly go back to the position you are trying to change to. In most cases, good progress can be made in four to six weeks, but it's something you'll need to keep working on—it's easy to fall back into old habits.

New Diet for Chronic Pain

Panagiotis Zis, MD, PhD, honorary senior lecturer, University of Sheffield, UK.

Some people with a gluten sensitivity (confirmed by a blood test) suffer from "gluten neuropathy," which can cause nerve pain or numbness that generally affects the hands and feet. In a study of 60 adults (average age 70) with gluten neuropathy, researchers found that those following a strict gluten-free diet (no wheat, barley or rye) were 89% less likely to have pain than those who consumed gluten.

Shoe Inserts Do Not Relieve Plantar Fasciitis

Nadine Rasenberg, PhD student, Erasmus Medical Centre, Rotterdam, the Netherlands, and leader of a study published in *British Journal of Sports Medicine*.

Inserts known as orthotics often are recommended for this common foot problem that accounts for 15% of foot symptoms requiring medical attention. But in a recent clinical test, the inserts gave no more relief than a placebo—and custom-made orthotics had no more effect than mass-produced ones. It is possible that orthotics may help some people with heel pain and not others, and using them does not cause further harm. But there is no need for people who want to try orthotics to pay for expensive custom-made ones.

Could You Use a New Ankle?

Roundup of experts on ankle replacement, reported in *The Wall Street Journal*.

Ankle replacements are becoming more common. They can relieve the pain of ankle arthritis. Patients often live with the arthritis pain for decades until medication and rest no longer are enough to allow them to function.

Now a device called the STAR (Scandinavian total ankle replacement) system, available in the US since 2009, is increasingly being implanted surgically—in some 10,000 patients in 2017, twice as many as in 2011.

The device has proved durable and long-lasting, although 25% of 761 recipients studied needed some sort of additional surgery within 15 years—usually to replace the device's plastic parts, which wear out faster than the metal ones.

The replacement is not intended for all uses—recipients cannot run or jump—but it restores everyday function and relieves pain.

Cost: $19,000 to $30,000 or more, usually covered at least in part by insurance.

Pain-Relieving Stretch for Peripheral Artery Disease

Neel P. Chokshi, MD, MBA, assistant professor of clinical medicine, Perelman School of Medicine, medical director, Cardiology and Fitness Program, University of Pennsylvania, Philadelphia. Study presented at the American Heart Association's Arteriosclerosis, Thrombosis and Vascular Biology/Peripheral Vascular Disease 2017 Scientific Sessions.

For people with peripheral artery disease (PAD), a buildup of fatty deposits in arteries that prevents sufficient blood and oxygen from reaching muscles, exercise is not just good for cardiovascular health—it can mean the difference between keeping their legs and needing amputation. That's because exercise increases vital circulation to the limbs. There's a catch-22, however. Having PAD can make activities such as walking, climbing stairs and just moving around so painful that many of the 8.5 million American adults who have the disease avoid exercise as much as possible.

In a small study from Florida State University College of Medicine in Tallahassee, patients with PAD who stretched their calf muscles for 30 minutes a day, five days a week for a month improved both blood flow to their calves and their walking ability. They were able to walk farther during a timed period (six minutes)…and they were able to walk for a longer distance without needing to stop and rest because of discomfort.

While it's premature to suggest any specific stretching protocol based on just this small study, it does suggest that if you have PAD, calf stretching can help you better manage the condition. For the study, participants stretched using a special splint that flexed their ankles about 15%, pulling their toes up toward their legs. But you don't need splints to stretch your calf muscles. A physical therapist can show you how to do it—and recommend for how long and how often you should do it.

CHAPTER 18

Women's Health

What Matters Most When It Comes to Breast Cancer Risk

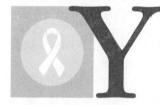

You probably know the odds—one in eight women will be diagnosed with breast cancer at some point in her life.

What you may not realize: In spite of all the focus on genetic testing and BRCA genes, most cases of breast cancer are not genetic. There's a lot of emphasis on family history when it comes to all forms of cancer, but 87% of women diagnosed with breast cancer do not have a single first-degree relative (mother, sister, daughter) with breast cancer. The older you are, the more likely it is that breast cancer is caused by things you eat or do, not your genes. This means there's a lot that's within your control! *An ever-growing body of research has shown what the myths are and what matters…*

THE MYTHS

The following have zero to do with breast cancer…

Bras: Myths abound about underwires, cup size and how old you were when you started wearing a bra, but there is no research to support any increase in breast cancer risk due to bra usage.

Antiperspirant: Multiple studies have failed to find any conclusive links between the aluminum chlorohydrate in antiperspirants and breast cancer.

Hair relaxers: No association has been found between breast cancer and how often relaxers or straighteners are used, the number of burns experienced or the type of relaxer. Still it's always a good idea to choose products without parabens and phthalates, which have been linked to cancer.

Mobile phones and power lines: While much debate surrounds mobile phones and

Kristi Funk, MD, board-certified breast surgeon and co-founder of Pink Lotus Breast Center in Los Angeles. She is author of *Breasts: The Owner's Manual*. PinkLotus.com brain health, they do not emit the right type of energy—or a high enough amount—to damage breast cell DNA. The same goes for living near power lines. Multiple studies have debunked the idea that the electromagnetic fields (EMFs) generated by high-voltage power lines increase breast cancer risk.

Breast surgery: If you have had breast-reduction surgery, numerous studies support the finding that your risk for breast cancer actually decreases. On the flip side, research shows that most implants—no matter what type, the positioning or how long you've had them—do not cause breast cancer. They do make cancer harder to detect, however, so you should have more rigorous screening—such as an ultrasound along with your mammogram.

Note: Some new concerns have been raised about textured implants possibly causing a form of lymphoma, but not breast cancer. Additional research is ongoing.

Coffee: No link between coffee consumption and breast cancer has ever been found, and there even is some evidence that drinking coffee may have a protective effect.

Note: Artificial sweeteners have not been linked to breast cancer, but they have been associated with obesity and insulin-resistance (so have no more than two servings a day).

HERE'S WHAT DOES MATTER

The good news is that there are many positive steps you can take to lower your risk for breast cancer. *Not surprisingly, they involve diet, exercise and other lifestyle choices, such as…*

•**Watching your weight.** Being overweight or obese is the single most preventable cause of breast cancer worldwide. Having more fat tissue raises your estrogen and insulin levels. Extra weight increases your risk by anywhere from 50% to 250%. The research is very clear that the risk for breast cancer is much higher if you are overweight postmenopause, although the exact reason for that is not known.

•**Lowering the amount of alcohol you drink.** Alcohol is the other big enemy of healthy breast tissue. All types of alcohol increase estrogen levels, and estrogen is a potent fuel for cancer cells. One drink a day increases your breast cancer risk by 10%…two drinks, by 30%…three drinks, by 40%—you can see where this is going. However, one drink a day does ostensibly provide heart-health benefits. To keep the heart-health benefits and minimize breast cancer risk, stick to no more than one drink a day (or seven over a week) and make it red wine with its breast-friendly resveratrol and anti-estrogen effect.

•**Colorizing your plate.** Aim for a meal that's 70% fresh fruits, vegetables and leafy greens. Fruits and vegetables are loaded with phytonutrients, plus anticancer and anti-inflammatory properties that directly target cell mutations and put the brakes on cancer development. They prevent and repair DNA damage, destroy harmful cells, inhibit blood supply to tumors and protect against cell damage from environmental toxins.

•**Going meatless more often.** Animal protein, including fish, can increase your risk for breast cancer. Think of it as a side dish, not the main star of your plate. Even egg consumption should be limited to two a week. In one large-scale UK study, a high intake of meat (red meat, white meat, processed meat, poultry) showed increases in breast cancer risk when compared with vegetarians. Red meat was particularly flagged—the study found a 41% increased risk. But even poultry increased participants' risk by 22%. Yes, fish contains omega-3s that generally are beneficial, but fish—like meat and poultry—causes the body to produce insulin-like growth factor-1 (IGF-1), which has the primary job of promoting cell growth. That's great when you are a child. Once you're an adult, you need some IGF-1 to repair cells after exercise, for example, but an excess is going to send cell production into overdrive, including production of cancer cells. (See box on next page for surprising alternative sources of protein.)

To make matters worse, conventional meat in the US and Canada contains a growth hormone (zeranol) that has been banned in Europe for decades because of its link to early puberty, which increases breast cancer risk. In fact, zeranol has been shown in labs to turn healthy breast cells to cancer in only 21 days.

Meatless Monday All Week Long

Trying to go meatless more often, but worried about getting enough protein? You know to eat beans and nuts, but here are five lesser known foods that are full of protein...

- **⅓ cup seitan*** = 21 grams protein (avoid if you have celiac disease or are gluten-intolerant)
- **1 cup green peas** = 8 grams protein
- **1 cup cooked wild rice** = 6.6 grams protein
- **¼ cup dry steel-cut oats** = 5 grams protein
- **½ cup cooked of either spinach, broccoli, brussels sprouts, organic corn, avocado** = 2 grams protein

*Seitan is a popular vegetarian meat substitute made from wheat that has the look and texture of meat when cooked.

Note: Even if you choose organic or grass-fed meat, be careful how you prepare it. When meats are well-done or char-grilled, cancer-causing compounds can form on the surface. Women who consistently eat well-done hamburgers, bacon and steak have a 362% higher risk for breast cancer than women who consume meat cooked rare or medium.

•**Moving your body more.** Women who get just three to four hours a week of moderate-to-vigorous physical activity have 30% to 40% lower risk for breast cancer than women who are inactive. Work out more than four hours a week, and you'll enjoy a 58% decrease in risk. Activity reduces estrogen levels, improves insulin sensitivity and maintains weight loss.

• **Finding alternatives to hormone replacement therapy.** Decades of evidence show that hormone replacement therapy (HRT) can increase risk for breast cancer. According to the Women's Health Initiative, there are 25% more breast cancers in HRT users than nonusers. To relieve the symptoms of menopause, try topical vaginal estrogen and laser treatments for vaginal dryness. For hot flashes, try herbal remedies such as black cohosh, evening primrose oil and soy. Acupuncture, biofeedback and yoga also may be beneficial. If you do decide to try HRT or bioidentical hormone replacement therapy (BHRT), take the lowest possible dose for the shortest amount of time necessary.

•**Avoiding environmental toxins.** Minimizing your exposure to endocrine disrupting compounds (EDCs) such as BPA, phthalates and parabens, which lurk in many household products, can help lessen your breast cancer risk. Choose organic and locally grown foods when possible, filter all water sources, fill your home with houseplants that act as potted air purifiers and pass on personal-care products that list EDCs on the label.

•**Finding time for daily stress relief.** Acute or chronic stress impairs the immune system, which gives diseases the opportunity to flourish, so take 20 minutes a day to do something that centers you, such as yoga or meditation.

Why Your Screening Mammograms Should Be in 3-D

Susan Harvey, MD, director of breast imaging in the Russell H. Morgan Department of Radiology and Radiological Science at Johns Hopkins Medicine in Baltimore.

While a 3-D mammography machine looks like a 2-D machine and compresses your breasts just as a 2-D does, there's a big difference. The top of the 3-D machine moves in an arc above each breast taking multiple images—think of each one as a thin slice—from many angles. A computer then takes all those thin slices and arranges them into a set of highly focused 3-D images for a radiologist to read. This imaging technology is called tomosynthesis.

The 3-D images make it easier to distinguish normal overlapping breast tissue from tumors, so it's harder for cancers to hide. That means not just better detection but also fewer false positives and fewer callbacks, when you're asked to come back because of a potentially abnormal finding. In other words, fewer scary moments waiting to get another test to know if something is wrong—though it's often a false alarm, who wants a day or even a few hours of anxiety while waiting to find out?

It's true that 3-D mammography exposes you to more radiation than 2-D does, but the extra amount is small and the total amount is small—and certainly less dangerous than having an early cancer go undetected.

Another advantage to 3-D: Because 3-D mammography is better than 2-D mammography not only at finding abnormalities but also at characterizing abnormalities, women are less likely to need follow-up biopsies, which are invasive. And if you are recalled after a 3-D mammogram, there's a greater chance than with a 2-D mammogram that a follow-up, noninvasive breast ultrasound will provide all the additional information needed.

In women with dense breasts, having a 3-D mammogram makes tumors easier to see.

Note: If you have dense breasts, you might also need a breast ultrasound as an extra screening, but you may be able to schedule both tests for the same day—and have both tests covered by insurance as wellness screenings if having dense breasts is listed in your medical records. Ask your insurance provider in advance.

Also: When 3-D first became available, most insurance companies wouldn't cover it. Now most do.

Less Side Effects for Breast Cancer Treatment

Lyndsey Kilgore, MD, a researcher and resident, department of surgery, University of Kansas Cancer Center, Kansas City, and leader of a study presented at the annual meeting of the American Society of Breast Surgeons.

Painful breast cancer treatment side effects can be reduced. The new technology Bioimpedance spectroscopy (BIS) is a noninvasive test that detects lymphedema—arm swelling that often results from standard treatment such as lymph node surgery or radiation. Early detection with BIS enables the use of home therapy, including compression sleeves and massage. In a study of 146 women, BIS identified 49 women with lymphedema—and home therapy greatly reduced symptoms in 40 of them.

Breast Cancer Diagnosis? How to Get Needed DNA Testing

Steven J. Katz, MD, professor of medicine, health management and policy, University of Michigan, Ann Arbor, and lead author of the study "Association of Attending Surgeon with Variation in the Receipt of Genetic Testing After Diagnosis of Breast Cancer," published in *JAMA Surgery*.

In a new study that's likely to shake up breast cancer treatment, researchers at University of Michigan surveyed 5,000 women who had undergone surgery for breast cancer as well as 377 breast cancer surgeons and found that almost half the patients who should have received genetic testing before surgery to help determine the best treatment did not get it.

As a result, neither these women nor their surgeons had all the information they could have had to know whether a lumpectomy, mastectomy or double mastectomy would be the most beneficial type of surgery to have for their cancer.

Genetic testing can be a game changer for breast cancer treatment. As an example, most women who test positive for either the BRCA1 or BRCA2 genetic mutation choose a double mastectomy because that particular surgery significantly reduces the likelihood that the cancer will recur. (*Note:* The BRCA1 and BRCA2 mutations are highly linked to risk for both breast cancer and ovarian cancer.) Women who don't have these gene mutations might choose a breast-sparing lumpectomy. Meanwhile, new types of tests that look for a wider set of gene mutations with ramifications for choosing the best treatments are becoming more available—but if surgeons aren't even looking to the older, well-established tests for guidance, they may not put these newer tests to use for women's benefit, either!

It's hard to understand why, with the kind of advantage that genetic testing offers, so many breast cancer surgeons are unlikely to order it. The surgeons who responded to the survey were not amateurs. They are highly trained specialists with, on average, 20 years of experience under their belts.

How can you make sure that you get genetic testing before breast cancer surgery? *Here are the two steps you must take…*

•**Have your primary care physician or ob-gyn step up to the plate.** Ask him/her to refer you to surgeons who are most familiar with genetic testing before surgery. Your doctor may have to do some legwork and ask around. But that could be a good thing not only for you but for other patients—because it will likely encourage discussions among primary-care physicians and surgeons and get them to think more deeply about the proper role of genetic testing in treatment (something University of Michigan is already promoting).

•**Specifically tell your surgeon to order the genetic test.** After the test results are in, if it's not possible for you to see a genetic counselor in a timely manner, you and your surgeon can discuss the test results, and he can go over their meaning and the surgical options with you. That doesn't negate the role of counseling—you can still meet with a counselor anytime one is available to discuss future ramifications of the test results for you and other family members (including, possibly, your children) who may have inherited the same mutations. Once that's done, both you and any relatives with the gene mutation can be referred to a medical oncologist, a specialist who will watch over all of you and guide your care in the years to come.

A Healthy Diet Delays Menopause

University of Leeds.

A healthy diet can delay menopause by nearly three years, while a refined-food diet can start it a year and a half sooner. Later menopause—associated with a diet high in oily fish, beans, greens, etc.—may reduce risk for osteoporosis and heart disease.

Breast Cancer Treatment: Opting Out of Chemo

Joseph A. Sparano, MD, professor of medicine and obstetrics, gynecology and women's health at the Albert Einstein College of Medicine, New York City, and coauthor of the study titled, "Adjuvant Chemotherapy Guided by a 21-Gene Expression Assay in Breast Cancer", published in *The New England Journal of Medicine*.

Chemotherapy is the most dreaded part of breast cancer treatment for many women because of the horrid side effects. But what if you didn't have to have this chemical cocktail to cure your cancer or keep it from coming back?

That was the focus of a study involving women with early-stage hormone-receptor-positive breast cancer, the type of cancer that uses the hormones estrogen and progesterone to grow and represents about half of all breast cancers. The goal was to see whether the guideline to give chemotherapy to almost all women with this form of breast cancer did indeed cut the risk of it coming back…or was unnecessary, at least for some.

Nearly 10,000 participants were given a genomic test called Oncotype DX. The test looks at 21 genes to create an estimate of how likely a woman's breast cancer is to return and of how beneficial chemotherapy will be.

Some results of this test are cut and dried. A high "recurrence score" (26 and up) strongly suggests that chemotherapy would be beneficial, and a low score (0 to 10) strongly suggests that chemotherapy isn't needed. But what about the majority of women, whose scores fall somewhere in the middle? They were the ones, 6,711 women in all, who the researchers zeroed in on.

These women had surgery to remove the cancer, either a mastectomy or breast conservation surgery plus radiation, followed by hormone therapy to block the cancer's fuel source, but only half received chemotherapy as well. After nine years of follow-up, the researchers found that the two groups had similar outcomes—83%

of the women who hadn't had chemo were still in remission…and so were 84% of the group that had had chemo.

The researchers concluded that overall, when you add back in women who score very low on the Oncotype DX test, the test could point to up to 85% of women with early hormone-receptor-positive breast cancer as being able to be spared chemotherapy without increasing their chances of a recurrence.

Within that broad percentage of women, there are two key groups that emerged: Women over 50 years old with scores of 25 or lower on the test…and women 50 and under with scores of 15 or lower. (Treatment decisions tend to be more aggressive in younger women.).

Women: Avoid These Heart Attack Traps

C. Noel Bairey Merz, MD, director of the Barbra Streisand Women's Heart Center, Linda Joy Pollin Women's Heart Health Program and Preventive and Rehabilitative Cardiac Center at the Smidt Heart Institute, all at Cedars-Sinai Medical Center, Los Angeles.

Common medical mistakes are putting millions of middle-aged and older women at risk for a heart attack, the number-one killer of American women, with nearly 300,000 deaths every year.

A common scenario illustrates the problem women face. Let's say a woman sees a doctor and complains about persistent chest pain. The doctor orders an angiogram, a test that detects the plaque in the major arteries of the heart that can decrease or stop blood flow, triggering a heart attack. But the angiogram shows no blockages, so the doctor tells the woman she doesn't have heart disease. A week later, she has a heart attack.

Many women experience angina, which is marked by frequent and intense chest pain, even when they do not have blockages in the major arteries of the heart—the leading cause of heart attack in men. In women, the pain also can be caused by coronary microvascular dysfunction in the tiny arteries around the heart.

This condition poses a similar threat to a woman's heart as a blockage in the major arteries. But standard heart tests—such as an angiogram or an electrocardiogram (which detects abnormal heart rhythms and poor blood flow)—don't detect coronary microvascular dysfunction.

Troubling recent finding: Researchers from the Barbra Streisand Women's Heart Center, Smidt Heart Institute at Cedars-Sinai in Los Angeles asked 340 women who complained of chest pain but had no blockages in major coronary arteries to have a cardiac MRI, a highly detailed imaging scan of the heart.

Result: Nearly one in 10 (8%) of the women had already suffered a heart attack—in most cases, previously undetected.

Other sobering research: In a study conducted by researchers at the Yale School of Public Health, 62% of women having a heart attack were found to have three or more non–chest pain symptoms (see box below)—and more than half of those women said their healthcare provider did not think the symptoms were heart-related.

Red Flags Women Should Watch For…

Most women who are having a heart attack don't experience crushing chest pain, the "classic" heart attack symptom found in most men. *Instead, a woman might have…*

- **Sharp or burning pain** or pressure in the chest.
- **Pain or pressure** in the neck, jaw, throat, abdomen or upper back.
- **Shortness of breath.**
- **Indigestion and heartburn.**
- **Nausea and vomiting.**
- **Extreme fatigue.**
- **General upper-body discomfort.**

Doctors frequently fail to recognize these symptoms as red flags for heart attack. The result—heart disease and heart attacks are often misdiagnosed in women.

7-STEP PLAN

Because women with heart disease are routinely undertreated, it's crucial to develop a strategy to effectively diagnose the condition—and, if it's present, to effectively treat it. To do this, partner with your physician. *Here's what you need to know...*

***STEP #1:* Take heart disease seriously.** It kills more women than any other disease—more women than all cancers combined. If you've got one or more risk factors for heart disease, ask your primary care physician for a cardiovascular workup (see below). Those risk factors include high blood pressure, high LDL cholesterol, smoking, excess body weight, a sedentary lifestyle, a poor diet (one that emphasizes sugary, fatty processed foods) and a family history of heart disease.

***STEP #2:* Get a second opinion.** Perhaps your physician has conducted tests and told you that you don't have heart disease—but you have symptoms that make you suspect you do, such as shortness of breath or unexplained chest pain or pressure. Get a second opinion from a doctor who will listen to your concerns. It could be an internist or a cardiologist. Second opinions are covered by most health insurance and—given the seriousness of heart disease—it's a prudent action.

***STEP #3:* Get the right stress test.** If your risk factors put you at high risk for heart disease, your doctor may order a stress test, also called a treadmill test, exercise electrocardiogram, graded exercise test or stress electrocardiogram. This test—in which you exercise at increasingly intense levels while hooked up to electrodes that measure the electrical activity of your heart—determines blood flow to your heart and can detect abnormal heart rhythms.

Other options include a stress echocardiogram or nuclear stress test, both of which also generate images of the heart and can more accurately determine blood flow...and the *dobutamine* or *adenosine* stress test, a drug-based test used in people who are unable to exercise. If you have any questions about the right stress test for you, consult a cardiologist.

***STEP #4:* Ask about a stress cardiac MRI or cardiac PET scan.** These tests have become more widely available only in the last 10 years. They are more sensitive, so they improve the detection of more subtle and female-pattern abnormalities in smaller hearts—which means they help women more than men. Either test would be particularly important in women with persistent chest pain and an abnormal stress test.

***STEP #5:* If you're having unexplained heart symptoms,** ask your doctor to investigate less common forms of heart disease. One uncommon condition is spontaneous coronary artery dissection, a tear in the artery wall. This condition, which can lead to heart attack, is more often detected in younger women (half the time during or shortly after pregnancy), who have symptoms such as unexplained chest pain.

The other is stress-related cardiomyopathy (also known as "broken heart syndrome"), which can cause chest pain and shortness of breath. It is caused by severe mental stress or shock, such as the death of a spouse, or a near-miss automobile accident. The condition is usually treatable, and most patients recover, although recurrence can happen in 5% to 10% of cases.

***STEP #6:* Demand standard therapy.** Studies show that women with diagnosed heart disease are significantly less likely than men to be treated with standard therapy. If you've been diagnosed with heart disease, talk to your physician about lifestyle changes (including smoking cessation, diet and exercise), along with the drugs you may need—such as low-dose (81 mg) aspirin to prevent artery-clogging blood clots, a statin to lower high cholesterol and medication to reduce blood pressure.

***STEP #7:* Go to the ER.** If you're having any of the symptoms of a heart attack that are common in women (see page 322), the emergency room is where you belong. And once you're there, don't let anyone tell you that you're not having a heart attack. Instead, insist on getting the troponin test, which detects protein in the blood generated by damaged heart cells...in other words, by a heart attack. This simple test—a sample of blood is all that's required—generates results in 15 to 20 minutes and provides incontrovertible evidence as to whether you are or aren't having a heart attack.

Important: Call 911 instead of driving yourself, and take a low-dose aspirin if you suspect that you are having a heart attack.

Stroke Risk for Women Is Different

Kathryn M. Rexrode, MD, associate professor of medicine, Brigham and Women's Hospital, Boston, and senior author of the study titled "Stroke Risk Factors Unique to Women," published in *Stroke*.

Stroke is not an equal-opportunity health issue. Even accounting for women's average longer life spans, more women than men in the US die of stroke—it's the fourth-leading cause of death for women but only the fifth for men. And women with diabetes and abnormal heart rhythms are more likely to have strokes than men with these conditions. While doctors have long known these facts, their cause has not been clear. Now new research sheds light on what could be driving women's increased stroke risk.

Recent research: In a review of the scientific literature on ischemic stroke (when blood flow through an artery in the brain is blocked) the researchers found that the most common causes of stroke for both men and women were conditions such as smoking, high blood pressure, diabetes and abnormal heart rhythms. However, they also found specific hormone-based risk factors unique to women that could be contributing to their higher stroke rates. Some of these factors are already known to raise stroke risk—early menopause (before age 45)…use of oral contraceptive pills that contained synthetic estrogen…being pregnant…and taking oral synthetic estrogen hormone therapy for menopausal symptoms. However, researchers also found two unsuspected factors associated with stroke—having begun to have monthly periods early (before age 10)…and having a low level of DHEA-S, a naturally occurring hormone that is a building block of testosterone and estrogen and that decreases with age and stress.

While not much can be done about some risk factors, such as when periods begin or menopause starts, knowing more about unique risks they face reinforces for women—now maybe more than ever—why it's good to take charge of what is within their control. According to the American Heart Association and the American Stroke Association, 80% of strokes are preventable, and recommendations for everyone to reduce their stroke risk include maintaining healthy blood pressure, blood sugar, weight and cholesterol, eating a healthy diet that includes at least five daily servings of fruits and vegetables, getting adequate exercise, limiting alcohol and not smoking.

Women: Don't Hesitate to Call an Ambulance for Yourself

Findings from the Polish Registry of Acute Coronary Syndromes (PL-ACS) presented at Acute Cardiovascular Care 2019, a European Society of Cardiology (ESC) congress.

New research shows that women who suffer heart attacks may be undermining their own survival.

Study details: In research presented at an Acute Cardiovascular Care conference of the European Society of Cardiology in Malaga, Spain, researchers tracked 7,582 men and women who suffered a heart attack caused by a major artery blockage. When treating this type of heart attack, known as an ST-elevation myocardial infarction (STEMI), the goal is to resolve the blockage as promptly as possible—restored blood flow means less heart tissue death…a lower risk for future heart failure…and a lower overall risk for death.

It's recommended that treatment (opening the blocked artery with a stent) begin within 90 minutes of diagnosis. The quickest way to diagnose a heart attack is via an electrocardiogram (ECG) that is administered in an ambulance as the patient is being transported to a hospital. In this study, 45% of patients were treated within that crucial 90-minute window, but fewer of them were women (41% compared with 47% of men).

The research also showed a disparity in the use of ECG during the ambulance transport. While 40% of men of all ages received an ECG, on average, only 34% of women age 54 and under got tested in the ambulance (45% of women age 75 and older were tested).

The treatment delay in women was due, in part, to women hesitating to call an ambulance for themselves. Women put off making that call because they believed they minimized the seriousness of their symptoms and/or had too many responsibilities, including their work and childcare duties. The researchers noted that this is especially true of younger women (under age 55).

Women may also fail to recognize their own symptoms as those of a heart attack. Chest pain and tingling in the left arm are the classic symptoms, but they may have pain elsewhere, such as the back, shoulder or stomach.

Takeaway: Don't wait! Call 911 if you or anyone around you experiences possible heart attack symptoms, such as pain in the chest, but also in the jaw, throat, neck, shoulders, back or stomach for 15 minutes or longer.

Ease Endometriosis Pain...Naturally

Andrew L. Rubman, ND, founder and medical director, Southbury Clinic for Traditional Medicines, Southbury, Connecticut, and author of the Bottom Line blog "Nature Doc's Patient Diary." SouthburyClinic.com

Endometriosis can be extremely painful, so the enthusiasm for the newly FDA-approved drug to treat the pain, Orilissa, is understandable. However, the drug comes with a serious potential side effect.

Alternative: A natural protocol that reduces the pain and inflammation of endometriosis (when tissue from inside the uterus grows outside the uterus)—but doesn't compromise the rest of your health.

Orilissa—its chemical name is *elagolix*—is a pill that is taken once or twice a day and has just been approved for moderate-to-severe endometriosis pain. Studies show that it reduces endometriosis menstrual pain, pain between periods and pain during sexual intercourse. However, it can be taken for only two to six months, depending on the dose, because it creates a risk for irreversible bone loss.

Why would a pain drug cause bone loss? Orilissa works by blocking the effect of gonadotropin-releasing hormone, which stimulates the ovaries to produce estrogen and progesterone. Since the inflammation and pain of endometriosis are triggered by estrogen, blocking its production results in less pain. However, estrogen is also important for bone health—which is why extended use of the drug can cause bone loss. Other side effects of low estrogen include night sweats, hot flashes and mood problems such as anxiety and depression.

The good news is that inflammation can be reduced naturally without the side effects of medications. This is especially important for women who are trying to get pregnant...who already are pregnant (Orilissa cannot be taken during pregnancy)...or whose pain is not severe enough to require medication. Natural inflammation reducers also won't interfere with medication if it becomes necessary.

Diet changes that can reduce the pain of endometriosis...

• **Eat an egg every day.** Eggs have cholesterol, the source material for the steroidal hormone cortisol, a hormone that helps control inflammation. (You may think of cortisol as an inflammation producer, but that's because as levels of cortisol increase, another hormone called cortisone, which needs to stay in balance with cortisol, decreases—encouraging inflammation.)

Best: Boil the egg or poach it in water because frying the cholesterol produces oxides, which are inflammatory. And don't worry about creating any heart issues by adding this bit of cholesterol to your diet because inflammation is the trigger that makes cholesterol form plaques on artery walls.

• **Eat wild-caught cold-water fish such as salmon and sardines,** rich sources of anti-inflammatory omega-3 fatty acids. You can also get omega-3s from fish oil supplements. A typical recommended daily dose is 1,000 mg of combined *eicosapentaenoic acid* (EPA) and *docosahexaenoic acid* (DHA). (Interestingly, my patients who move to Florida and stop eating fish from cold water start having more inflammation issues.)

•**Get some seeds into your diet,** especially the inflammation-fighters chia and flaxseeds. Both also are high in omega-3 fatty acids.

•**Get plenty of antioxidants from brightly colored fruits and vegetables,** especially dark blue and purple berries…beets…and green, leafy vegetables. Also include cruciferous vegetables such as broccoli, cabbage and kale.

•**Take three supplements that can help the liver bind and remove inflammatory compounds**—vitamin B, dandelion root extract and methylsulfonylmethane (MSM). These are generally safe for most people, but check with your doctor if you are being treated for a medical condition or have allergies (such as to ragweed in the case of dandelion supplements). Dosages should be prescribed by your doctor based on the severity of your endometriosis.

Typical daily amounts: 50 mg vitamin B complex, taken twice a day…2 grams (g) to 6 g of MSM, divided into two or three doses…about 30 drops (1 milliliter) dandelion root extract once a day.

Exercising regularly to reduce body fat and limiting intake of caffeine and alcohol also help keep estrogen levels lower.

If natural therapies and drugs fail to relieve your pain, endometrial tissue outside the uterus may be surgically removed. Women who have this surgery often find that their bodies respond better to anti-inflammatory foods and supplements afterward.

Beware Vaginal Bleeding

Megan A. Clarke, PhD, MHS, postdoctoral fellow in the division of cancer epidemiology and genetics at National Cancer Institute, Rockville, Maryland, and coauthor of a meta-analysis published in *JAMA Internal Medicine*.

Vaginal bleeding after menopause can be an early sign of cancer. About 9% of women with postmenopausal bleeding are diagnosed with endometrial cancer, which is curable in its early stages. If you have bleeding, be sure to have an ultrasound or biopsy to rule out cancer.

The Endometriosis/ Cancer Connection: What You Need to Know

Oskari Heikinheimo, MD, PhD, professor in the Department of Obstetrics and Gynecology, Helsinki University Hospital, physician in chief at Helsinki University Hospital and coauthor of the study titled "Risk of Gynecologic Cancer According to the Type of Endometriosis," published in *Obstetrics and Gynecology*.

You already know the basics about endometriosis. Tissue that's usually found inside the uterus grows outside of it, causing pain for most women with the condition and fertility problems for many. *But you may not know that there are three different types of endometriosis based on the location of the growth…*

Peritoneal endometriosis: The most common type. Growths develop anywhere in the pelvic cavity.

Deep infiltrating endometriosis: The rarest type. Growths develop within the pelvic cavity but also extend deep into tissues.

Ovarian endometriosis: Just as it sounds, growths develop within the ovaries.

THE STUDY

Researchers in Finland analyzed the hospital records of women who had had surgery to treat their endometriosis to look for associations between the three types of the disease and various types of cancers of the reproductive organs.

The good news: None of the types of endometriosis raised the risk for endometrial cancer or other uterine cancers, cervical cancer or genital cancer. Surprisingly, there was a decrease in the risk for squamous cell cervical cancer among women with endometriosis, though it's unclear why.

Women with peritoneal or deep infiltrating endometriosis did not have a higher overall risk for ovarian cancer than the average woman, though the researchers did say that longer study is needed to better understand whether deep infiltrating endometriosis could have a cancer association over the long-term.

The not-so-good news: Women with ovarian endometriosis had a higher risk for ovarian cancer than the average woman, particularly for two rare types of cancer—clear cell ovarian cancer and endometrioid ovarian cancer. The number of women with ovarian endometriosis who got ovarian cancer was relatively small at 2%, but that risk was higher than earlier studies had found and higher than the 1.3% risk for ovarian cancer among women in general. These women also had a higher-than-usual risk for borderline ovarian tumors, growths that begin along the outer edges of the ovaries, meaningful because these are thought to be starting points for ovarian cancer due to endometriosis.

WHAT THIS MEANS FOR YOU

The study authors said that even though the absolute risk for ovarian cancer remained relatively small, knowing about this risk could help women make decisions about treatment of ovarian endometriosis—in particular, whether to opt for ovarian conservation (keeping the ovaries) versus removing the ovaries. (Once the ovaries are removed, the risk for ovarian cancer drops substantially.)

Bottom line: Each woman with endometriosis should talk with her doctor about the type she has…any resulting effect on her risk for ovarian cancer…and her treatment options based on this risk. Also consider getting a second opinion from an oncologist who specializes in gynecologic cancers to make the most informed decision.

Minimally Invasive Surgery for Cervical Cancer? Not So Fast!

Studies "Minimally Invasive versus Radical Hysterectomy for Cervical Cancer" by an international group of researchers and "Survival after Minimally Invasive Radical Hysterectomy for Early-Stage Cervical Cancer" by researchers at leading cancer centers across the US and both published in *New England Journal of Medicine.*

Two new blockbuster studies on treating cervical cancer serve as a warning—when it comes to medicine, newer is not always better.

Background: Radical hysterectomy—the complete removal of the uterus and cervix as well as some surrounding tissue—is the gold standard for treating early stage cervical cancer, with an expected cure rate well over 80%. Before 2006, most radical hysterectomies were done through a large, open incision. But since then, many surgeons have moved to minimally invasive laparoscopic surgery with its small key-hole incision, sometimes using robotic arms to control the laparoscopic tools.

Minimally invasive techniques for many types of surgery have become popular because they offer shorter recovery and a slightly reduced risk for complications such as bleeding, swelling in the legs and sexual or bladder dysfunction. The benefits for cervical cancer in particular led the National Comprehensive Cancer Network, an alliance of 27 outstanding US cancer centers, to change its guidelines to state that both minimally invasive laparoscopic surgery and open surgery were appropriate. And in short order, laparoscopic became the dominant choice. However, there were few large or long-term studies at the time to support this preference.

Both of the new studies set out to compare results of the old and new surgeries. One, led by researchers at MD Anderson Cancer Center in Houston, looked at disease-free survival (meaning no signs or symptoms of the cancer) and overall survival. Participants included 600 women with early-stage cervical cancer. Half had minimally invasive surgery, the other half had open surgery. After 4.5 years, the open group had a 96.5% disease-free rate compared with 86% for the minimally invasive group. They also had a higher overall survival rate—99% compared to 93.8% after three years.

The second study analyzed the mortality rates of women undergoing cervical cancer surgery at leading cancer centers and university hospitals using two time frames. First, they used a large cancer registry to track women for four years. They looked at about 2,500 women with early cervical cancer evenly divided between open and minimally invasive surgery during 2010 and 2013. Once again, open surgery was better for survival—the four-year mortality rate was 5.3% among open surgery patients, but 9.1% among the minimally invasive group.

These researchers also took a longer view, going back to mortality rates between 2000 and 2010. They found that before 2006, when open surgery dominated, survival rates remained stable. But after 2006, when minimally invasive surgery became dominant, they saw a gradual drop in the survival rate of close to one percentage point.

While these studies may not result in the end of minimally invasive surgery for cervical cancer, it's important to be aware of their significant findings when considering surgery choices and to discuss them in depth with your oncologist.

Beware: Uterine Cancer Is on the Rise

Centers for Disease Control and Prevention, Morbidity and Mortality Weekly Report, "Uterine Cancer Incidence and Mortality–United States, 1999-2016," December 2018. Cancer.net

While many cancers, including lung and colon cancers, have been decreasing in the US, the opposite is true of uterine cancer.

New cases of this cancer (also called endometrial cancer because it starts in the endometrium, the lining of the uterus) are up 12% since 1999 and deaths are up by 21%!

What's going on? These trends follow the rise in obesity among women in the US. Women who are overweight or obese are two to four times more likely to develop uterine cancer than women who are at a healthy weight. The connection is the female hormone estrogen, which stimulates this cancer and is overproduced in fat cells. In fact, about 40% of uterine cancer cases are linked to obesity.

Other uterine cancer risk factors include having diabetes and eating a diet high in animal fat (two factors also associated with being overweight or obese), being over age 50 and having a family history of uterine cancer. Black women are twice as likely to die from uterine cancer as women of other races. This may be due to a higher rate of obesity and being diagnosed at a later stage of the cancer than other women.

To lower your risk for uterine cancer, the Centers for Disease Control and Prevention suggests eating a healthy diet and being physically active in order to maintain a normal weight.

Because screening tests for uterine cancer are not done routinely, it's important to know the warning signs, most commonly vaginal bleeding after sexual intercourse, between periods or after menopause. This is often the first and most important sign that can lead to an early diagnosis—90% of women with this cancer have abnormal vaginal bleeding, so don't ignore it. Other signs include pain after sexual intercourse, lower-belly pain and pain after passing urine.

Note: The test called transvaginal ultrasound is available for screening women at high risk for uterine cancer. It is also used to help diagnose cancer in women who have symptoms.

Early diagnosis and treatment are the keys to survival. When treated at an early stage, survival rates after five years are 80% to 90%. Once this cancer has time to spread, the five-year survival rate drops to under 30%.

Five Surprising Causes of Post-Menopausal Bleeding That Aren't Cancer

Frederick "Ricky" Friedman Jr., MD, associate professor, Icahn School of Medicine at Mount Sinai, director, division of obstetrics and division of generalists, department of obstetrics, gynecology and reproductive science, Mount Sinai Health System, New York City.

If you've reached menopause, you probably thought that your days of any bleeding down there were over—but then you saw blood. You might have even panicked because you know that can be a sign of cancer.

While there is a link between bleeding and cancer in the uterine lining (endometrial cancer), in 90% of postmenopausal women when bleeding occurs, it's something else.

Note: Even if it is just spotting, any postmenopausal bleeding should prompt a visit to your doctor to figure out what is going on. If you can see your doctor while you are actively bleeding, it is easier to identify the cause.

That being said, here are some of the surprising reasons a postmenopausal woman can have bleeding...

YOU HAVE AN STD

You might not realize that you're at risk for a sexually transmitted disease during this chapter of your life, but if you're not in a longstanding, monogamous relationship, you are. There's been a dramatic rise in STDs among older Americans in recent years. A lot of this can be traced to increased sexual activity because of drugs, such as Viagra, that make men more able to have sex, but that's not the only reason for the increase—there's a female connection, too. After menopause, vaginal tissue grows thin due to the lack of the female sex hormone estrogen, making it more prone to tearing, which can leave you more vulnerable to an STD. Gonorrhea, chlamydia, herpes and syphilis can all cause bleeding, especially early on. Other symptoms that may suggest your bleeding is an STD include discolored cervical mucus and pain during urination. Your doctor will ask for a urine sample or swab your cervical discharge and send it off to the lab for a diagnosis.

IT'S REALLY A BLADDER INFECTION

You may think the bleeding is coming from your vagina, cervix or uterus, but it may be trickling down from your bladder. That's because bladder infections or the bladder condition interstitial cystitis can sometimes cause bleeding. Other clues include needing to go to the bathroom often and urgently and/or pelvic pain. A urine sample will identify a bladder infection. Additional testing may be needed for suspected interstitial cystitis including a biopsy of tissue from the bladder wall.

YES, IT CAN BE A POLYP

Polyps inside the uterus or cervical canal are fairly common, but the amount of blood they cause can be scary, especially after menopause. As your uterine lining thins due to the drop in estrogen, these polyps also grow thin, and your body may shed the surface of the polyp—causing the bleeding. It's usually light spotting or staining, but at times it can be surprisingly heavy.

Your doctor will run a series of tests including a sonogram to locate the polyp and likely remove it to make sure it's not cancerous.

HORMONES GONE HAYWIRE

While vaginal or endometrial thinning can lead to postmenopausal bleeding due to atrophy or too little estrogen, being on hormone replacement therapy can do so for the opposite reason—the lining of the uterus (the endometrium) thickens, and then bleeds. In peri-menopause, many women are still making some estrogen, which causes the lining to thicken due to cell growth. However, they might not be ovulating. Since progesterone is generally made by the ovary only after ovulation, the "unopposed estrogen" causes a very thickened lining of growing cells. This is called endometrial hyperplasia, this condition often occurs when a woman has too much estrogen and not enough progesterone to balance it out (hormone replacement therapy that includes both estrogen and progesterone can help avoid this). The uterine lining may shed in this circumstance for several reasons. If the lining is too thick, the buildup may outgrow its blood supply and be shed. Similarly, as the hyperplasia develops, the attachment of cells to each other weakens. It's important to find out whether hormone replacement is causing your bleeding because endometrial hyperplasia has been linked to the development of endometrial cancer.

IT'S REALLY A HEMORRHOID

If you see blood on toilet paper or in your toilet bowl, it could actually be rectal bleeding from hemorrhoids. Other possible causes of rectal bleeding include a fissure or cut, a bacterial infection or inflammatory bowel disease. If the source of your bleeding turns out to be rectal, your doctor will likely suggest a stool test and, if it could be more than a hemorrhoid, possibly an imaging test such as a colonoscopy to find the cause.

Every one of the above causes of postmenopausal bleeding is far more common than uterine cancer, so again, if you've seen blood, don't panic...but do see your doctor right away.

Licorice Root for Hot Flashes

Laurie Steelsmith, ND, LAc, medical director of Steelsmith Natural Health Center in Honolulu. She is author of Natural Choices for Women's Health, Great Sex, Naturally *and* Growing Younger Every Day *and writes the "Natural Healing Secrets for Women" blog at BottomLineInc.com. DrSteelsmith. com*

Probably the most well-known use of licorice root is as a sweetener in candies (it's also often used as a sweetener in herbal tea formulas). But you might not know that this herb has been used for medicinal purposes for centuries—including for the relief of hot flashes.

As women go through the transition of menopause, estrogen levels fall, which is thought to trigger hot flashes. Up to 80% of women experience hot flashes during menopause, and a study found that the uncomfortable symptoms can last for up to 14 years. Licorice root can help reduce both the frequency and severity of hot flashes because it's a phytoestrogen, which means that it contains very weak estrogens.

Recent finding: In one small study, women who took a 330-milligram licorice root capsule three times a day reported a decrease in the frequency and severity of hot flashes over eight weeks. And no significant side effects were reported.

If you would like to try licorice root for hot flashes, be sure to consult a naturopathic doctor to get the dosage that's right for you.

Caution: Licorice root can cause high blood pressure, irregular heartbeat and low potassium levels in some people. A chemical called glycyrrhizic acid is responsible for these effects, so choose a deglycyrrhizinated licorice supplement, which has this chemical removed.

Drinking a daily cup of licorice root tea is another way to help mitigate hot flashes, but this also can increase blood pressure in some people, due to the glycyrrhizic acid. If you're prone to high blood pressure, choose other teas rich in phytoestrogens such as red clover or evening primrose.

Additional alerts on licorice: Besides the blood pressure caution above, if you have a hor- mone-sensitive condition, such as breast, uterine or ovarian cancer, endometriosis or uterine fibroids, you should avoid phytoestrogens such as licorice. And a recent study found that several compounds in licorice supplements can potentially interfere with the way the liver processes both prescription and over-the-counter drugs, so if you take medication, check first with your doctor before taking a licorice supplement or drinking licorice root tea.

Depression During Perimenopause

"Guidelines for the Evaluation and Treatment of Perimenopausal Depression: Summary and Recommendations," from The North American Menopause Society, National Network on Depression Centers Women and Mood Disorders Task Force, and International Menopause Society, published simultaneously in Menopause *and* Journal of Women's Health.

Hot flashes, night sweats and sexual dysfunction are synonymous with menopause and perimenopause—the three- or four-year period just before menopause. Such symptoms often emerge for the first time as a woman's hormone levels begin their life-changing decline.

An underrecognized threat: A woman's risk for depression also increases during perimenopause. Unfortunately, depression in perimenopausal women often falls under the diagnosis radar because these symptoms tend to get lost amidst other menopause-related changes.

Good news: A task force of clinicians and scientists recently published the first-ever guidelines for recognizing and treating perimenopausal depression. The new guidelines have been endorsed by the International Menopause Society.

According to the guidelines, perimenopause should be viewed as a "window of vulnerability" for the development of depressive symptoms, and clinicians are encouraged to look for signs of psychological distress in perimenopausal women. Red flags for triggers that can lead to depression include bereavement (women may experience more losses of loved ones during this time than in previous years)…and body changes associated with reproductive aging (such as weight gain and vaginal dryness).

Takeaway: Because each woman experiences perimenopause differently, it's important to schedule regular doctor's visits and discuss any symptoms with the physician.

The most appropriate treatment will depend on the woman's particular distress. For example, if she has low energy due to poor sleep caused by night sweats, hormone therapy may help. If a woman has a history of depression and perimenopause is making it worse, an antidepressant might be most effective. Cognitive behavioral therapy—with or without medication—may be the best choice if a woman finds herself ruminating over family and career burdens.

How Drinking Can Weaken Your Muscles

Study titled "Associations between high-risk alcohol consumption and sarcopenia among postmenopausal women," by Hee-Taik Kang, MD, Chungbuk National University College of Medicine, Republic of Korea, and colleagues, published in *Menopause: The Journal of the North American Menopause Society*.

You knew that alcohol could hurt your liver—but shrink your muscles?

A new study finds, in fact, that drinking is strongly linked to worsening sarcopenia, the age-related loss of muscle mass and strength. Sarcopenia is increasingly recognized as an important contributor to falls and fractures as well as many chronic diseases.

How much you drink is the key. A little bit—not to worry. If you're still drinking like you did when you were younger, however, it's time to ask yourself, *Is my drinking setting me up for a fall?*

Background: The US Centers for Disease Control and Prevention recently recognized sarcopenia, a combination of low muscle mass and weakness in older adults, as a diagnosable medical condition. It can affect balance and walking and interfere with the ability to take care of the activities of daily living that allow for independence. Muscle mass is also key to metabolic and cognitive health—sarcopenia is linked with increased risk for heart disease, diabetes and cognitive impairment. In short, minimizing or preventing sarcopenia can help you remain healthy, functional and independent at older ages.

We naturally start losing muscle mass in our 40s. By the 50s, the average man or woman loses 1.5% a year. After age 60, that goes up to 3% a year. Sarcopenia, as opposed to just normal age-related muscle loss, is defined as a substantial loss of both muscle mass and strength—so much so that walking is affected. While statistics vary, it is estimated that as many as 15% of Americans age 60 and older and 50% of those age 80 and older have sarcopenia.

A healthy lifestyle that includes regular exercise and a good diet helps prevent sarcopenia. But too little has been known about the role of alcohol, which is what researchers set out to address in the latest study.

Study: Using data from a large national patient registry, South Korean researchers pulled medical records on about 2,400 postmenopausal women. (The issue affects men, too.) The records included measurements of lean body mass (aka, muscle). The women filled out questionnaires about their frequency and quantity of alcohol use, whether they drank alcohol in the morning (a sign of problem drinking), guilt or concern about drinking and known alcohol-related injuries. Based on their responses, they were classified as either at low, medium or high risk for alcohol problems. On average, the women were 62 years old. About 8% had sarcopenia.

Results: Women who were at risk for alcohol problems were at substantially increased risk for sarcopenia. *Here are the percentages of women who had sarcopenia associated with their drinking habits…*

- **Low risk**—7.6% had sarcopenia.
- **Medium risk**—11%.
- **High risk**—22.7%.

Heavy drinkers, of course, also tend to have otherwise less healthy lifestyles than light drinkers or teetotalers. But even after adjusting for age, weight, blood pressure, cholesterol levels, blood sugar, smoking and exercise habits, high-risk drinkers in this study were more than four times more likely than those in the low-risk group to have sarcopenia.

A Woman's Guide to Overcoming Opioid Disorder

Leslie A. Hayes, MD, a family medicine practitioner who specializes in women's health and addiction at El Centro Family Health in Española, New Mexico. The study titled "Women and Opioids: Something Different Is Happening Here" by researchers at Yale University School of Medicine, New Haven, Connecticut, was published in *The Lancet*.

O pioids are an equal-opportunity health threat, yet women aren't getting their fair share of help to overcome this form of substance abuse. If you're a woman with an opioid addiction (or know someone who is), take these steps now. They could save your life.

WHY WOMEN ARE AT GREATER RISK

Many people don't realize that the opioid epidemic is hitting women as hard as it is men, with troubling distinctions. Women are more sensitive to pain than men and, as a result, are more likely to start taking opioids and get hooked on them sooner than men. Women also are prescribed opioid pain pills more often than men are. In addition, women in general have a telescoped course for substance use disorder—with almost every substance, women get more complications sooner.

Women also are more likely than men to receive prescriptions for other medications such as benzodiazepines, tranquilizers with side effects that, when taken along with opioids, dramatically increase the chances of an overdose.

Yet because the "profile" of an overdose victim still is thought of as a young man, women often don't get the help they need in this kind of emergency. For instance, according to a report on opioid-related deaths in Rhode Island, EMTs were three times less likely to administer the overdose antidote *naloxone* (Narcan) to women.

This all translates to an alarming statistic: According to researchers from Yale University, the rate of overdose deaths from opioids among women jumped by 583% from 1999 to 2016, compared with a 404% increase among men over the same period—that means, women accounted for 50% more deaths than men.

HOW TO HELP YOURSELF NOW

Take the following steps to save your life…

•**Don't wait any longer to get help for addiction.** Because of responsibilities at home and at work, many women wait too long to seek treatment for opioid abuse—well after they acknowledge that they have a problem. Every three minutes, a woman in the US arrives at an emergency room for prescription painkiller misuse or abuse. Don't put off getting treatment.

•**Choose a treatment program sensitive to the needs of women.** Look for a program that offers Seeking Safety with a trauma-based approach. It is not designed specifically for women, but since so many women with opioid use disorder have a history of trauma, it is a good option. Effective treatment often combines medical-assisted therapy with counseling. Ask your doctor or therapist for a recommendation if you're having trouble finding one on your own.

•**Keep lifesaving naloxone in your home.** Given as an injection or nasal spray, naloxone (Narcan) can reverse an opioid overdose. It's available in many states without a prescription at most major pharmacies. Everyone in the house should know where it is and how to use it.

Important: It does not replace getting immediate medical attention—call 911 right after using it.

Note: If you're still experiencing the condition that first led you to opioids, work with your doctor to control it, ask about alternative medications and consider other steps to conquer pain.

Index

A

Abdominal pain, 118, 119, 120, 121, 128
ACE inhibitors, 205
Acetaminophen (Tylenol), 85, 214–15, 217, 298
Acetic and butyric acids, 100
Acetylcholinesterase inhibitor (Aricept), 27–28
Active hexose correlated compound (AHCC), for flu, 169
Acupressure, 147–48, 237
Acupuncture, 124, 299
Adderall, 163
ADHD (attention-deficit/hyperactivity disorder), 29–30, 162–64
Afatinib (Gilotrif), 38
Aging, 273–92
    alcoholism in seniors, 143–44
    anti-aging flavonoid, 276–77
    anti-aging hormone, 16
    attitude about aging, health and, 276
    better biomechanics, 280
    caregiver abuse, 152
    caregiving, dementia patient, 150–51
    car features, driving gadgets, 281–82
    cognitive exercises, 17–18
    comfort at the end of life, 154
    depression and seniors, 139–40
    face exercises, 274–76
    flu risks, 170
    hands, weak or painful, 279–80
    hearing aids, 26, 283–86
    hearing assistance, 282–84
    hearing loss, 26, 284

    how old brains stay young, 273–74
    hydrogen therapy, 277–78
    kitchenware and useful tools, 279–80
    maldigestion and, 127
    muscle loss, 10, 19–20, 291–92, 331–32
    omega-3 supplements, 261
    protein and diet, 291–92
    safer driving for seniors, 151–52
    sedatives, addiction caution, 211–13
    sense of smell and, 286–88
    suicide and seniors, 140
    surrogate health decisions, 149–50
    theories about why we age, 277
    vitamin D and, 22–23
Air filters, 62
Air quality, 11–13
    indoor gardening and, 238–39
    sense of smell and, 288
    VOC's and, 85–87
    wildfire areas and, 159
Alcohol consumption, 168, 214, 318, 331–32, 326
Alcoholism, 101–3, 132, 143–44, 159
Alectinib (Alecensa), 38
Allergies, 1–4, 6–7, 31–32, 164, 185, 213
Aloe lotion, 236
Alpha-lipoic acid, 287–88
Alprazolam (Xanax), 211
ALS (amyotrophic lateral sclerosis), new help for, 30
Alzheimer's disease, 15, 19, 20, 22, 194, 195, 198–99, 268
Amlodipine (Norvasc), 288

Anaphylactic shock, 2–4
Androgens, 219, 233–34
Anemia, 112, 124, 185, 303
Aneurysm, 295
Anger, 119, 133, 134, 147, 151, 156, 194, 195, 249
Angina, 64, 65, 322
Angiogenesis, 253
Ankle replacements, 316
Antacids, 127
Anthocyanins, 111, 254, 309
Antianxiety agents, sedatives, 134, 212–13
Antibiotics
    autoimmune diseases and, 173–74
    fluoroquinolones, 218–19
    microbiome and, 122–23
    nutrients depleted by, 206
    resistance, 180
    unnecessary, 213–14
Anticoagulants. See Blood thinners
Antidepressants, 134–35, 145, 203
Antifungal medication, 5–6
Antihistamines, 203–4
Anti-inflammatories
    drugs, 43, 69, 78, 85, 123, 172, 205, 214, 216, 217, 287, 288, 293, 311
    natural or dietary, 85, 111, 124, 126, 189, 242, 247, 248, 249, 254, 256, 277, 298, 301, 309, 318, 325, 326
    See also NSAIDs
Antioxidants, 54, 111, 116, 168, 169, 205, 236, 242, 249, 252, 256, 257, 259, 277, 278, 287, 307, 309, 326
Antipsychotic agents, 134, 204–5
Anxiety, 130–33

benzodiazepines and, 212–13
brain-gut connection and, 119
DIY acupressure for, 147–48
essential oils for, 244
finding a psychiatrist, 132–33
marijuana and, 193
nature therapy for, 237–38
non-drug approaches, 130
VNS for, 240
Appetite, 115, 116, 140, 144, 145, 172, 203, 204, 220, 242, 262, 268,287
Aromatase inhibitors, 204, 219
Aromatherapy, 239
Arthritis, 124, 125–26, 214, 261, 310. *See also* osteoarthritis; RA
Artificial sweeteners, 117, 255, 318
ASCs (ambulatory surgery centers), 77–78
ASD (autism spectrum disorders), 135–37
Ashwagandha, 225–26, 228
Aspirin, 43, 55, 69, 70, 72, 214–15, 229, 242, 323, 324
Assistive technologies, 28
Asthma, 4, 5, 6, 7–8, 9, 11, 78, 80, 84, 159, 164, 169, 170, 171, 197, 213, 219
Atezolizumab (Tecentriq), 37, 45
Atorvastatin (Lipitor), 218, 288
ATP (adenosine triphosphate), 218
Atrial fibrillation (AFib), 7–8, 65, 68–69, 80
Autoimmune diseases, 115, 119, 123, 173–74, 187,188, 205, 310
Avelumab (Bavencio), 45
Avocado, 16, 19, 199, 255, 257, 319

B
Back pain, 281, 312, 313–14
Bad breath (halitosis), 126–27
Baking soda remedy, 117–18
Baloxavir marboxil (Xofluza), 169
Barefoot, 54
Beans, 16, 64, 87, 99, 100, 111,112, 128, 199, 226, 269, 264, 268, 319, 321
Beef, 97, 126, 250, 251, 252, 302
Beef liver, 252
Belching, 117, 121
Benzodiazepines, 211–13
Berberine, 97
Beta-blockers, 58, 64, 130, 203, 206
Beta-carotene, 254
Bioflavonoids, 249
Bioimpedance spectroscopy (BIS), 320
Biotin, 206, 236
Bipolar disorder, 194–95, 204, 249–50

Bittersweet nightshade, 236
Bladder cancer, 44–46
Bladder infection, 329
Bleeding
hemorrhoids and, 329
post-menopausal, 326, 328–29
post-op problems, warning signs, 80
Bloating, 25, 119, 121, 125, 128, 154, 244
Blood clots, 57, 70, 71, 107, 157, 191, 193, 215, 299, 323
Blood pressure, 192
ankle-brachial index test, 71
caffeine and, 61
CKD and, 82
dementia risk and, 20
diuretic and skin cancer, 38–39
exercise to lower, 271
HEPA air filters and, 62
herbs, spices, or foods to lower, 54, 97, 241, 250, 258
indoor thermostat setting and, 60
intermittent fasting to lower, 264
measuring, 61–62
medications, 202, 205
nature therapy for, 237–38
readings considered high, 62
safe cooking to lower, 60–61
salt sensitivity, 126, 256, 301
testicular cancer and, 232
Blood sugar
alpha-lipoic acid and, 287–88
CGMs and, 97–98, 104
cinnamon to lower, 241
circadian rhythm and, 197
diabetes medication and, 95–96
fiber to control, 99–101
fruit, juices, and, 252, 255
high glucose spikes, 98
hot baths to lower, 98
lifestyle changes to control, 96–97
mangiferin and, 253–54
medications, 202
OGTT for, 100
when to eat and, 263
Blood thinners
AFib and, 69
alcohol consumption and, 144
CoQ10 caution, 250
HAS-BLED score, 69
NSAIDs caution, 215
omega-3 caution, 261
TOS and, 300
Blood type, 190–92
Body odor, 126, 127, 301
Botox, 300

Bowel movements, 125, 127, 128
BPD (borderline personality disorder), 133–34
Brain cancer, 46, 198
Brain fog, 25–26
Brain-gut therapy, 119–20
Brain health, 15–32
ADHD help, 29–30
adult dyslexia, 28–29
ALS and, 30
attitude toward aging and, 276
blood pressure and, 20
brain-building breakfast or lunch, 19
cardiovascular nourishment for, 274
cognitive exercises, 17–18
concussion treatment, 32
dancing for, 17
exercise and, 16, 24–25
glucose metabolism and, 19
herbs, spices, supplements, and foods for, 15, 16, 19, 21–23, 254
how old brains stay young, 273–74
inflammation and, 22, 173
iNPH and, 20–21
learning and memory center, 273–74
one-week plan for, 15–17
microglia and toxin removal, 16
MS and, 30–32
picture books and brain function, 164
sedative agents, negative effects, 172
"skinny fat" risk, 19–20
sleep and, 16
stress and, 16–17
VNS for, 240
See also Alzheimer's disease; dementia; Parkinson's disease
Brain tumor, 295
Breast cancer, 36
alcohol consumption and, 318
animal protein and, 318–19
aromatase inhibitors, 219
beta-blocker drugs and, 130
BRCA genes and, 36, 232, 317, 320
CEA test, 34
chronic stress and, 319
diet and, 318
dinner timing and risk, 35
DNA testing and, 320–21
ductal carcinoma in situ, 75
environmental toxins and, 319
exercise to lower risk, 319
genetics and testing, 33–34, 317

growth hormone and, 318
HRT and increased risk, 319
lumpectomy, 320
mammograms, 3-D, 319–20
myths about, 317–18
nongenetic factors, 317, 318–19
obesity or being overweight
and, 318
Oncotype DX test, 321–22
opting out of chemo, 321–22
reducing risk, 318–19
side effects of treatment, 320
tamoxifen and other drugs for,
204
Breast implants or reduction, 318
Breathing exercises, 10, 241, 249
Brigatinib (Alunbrig), 38
"Broken heart syndrome," 323
Bronchitis, 213
Bruises, 303
"Bruit," 71
Bug repellents, 173
Bunions, bunionectomy, 77–78
Bupropion (Wellbutrin), 203
Butterbur, 85

C

Caffeine, 16, 61, 68, 158, 262, 309,
326
Calcium, 22, 205, 206, 256, 257, 258
Calcium channel blocker (CCB),
206
Calendula salve, 236
Calorimeter, 265
Canakinumab, 56
Cancer, 33–52
anthocyanins to reduce risk, 254
blood tests, 34–35
blood type and, 191
"cancer susceptibility genes," 34
chemotherapy side-effects,
avoiding the ER and, 49–51
childhood cancer and health,
47–48
circadian rhythm and, 197
clinical trials and, 36–37
ctDNA testing, 34, 36
diabetes and increased risk,
98–99
dinner time/bed time and risk,
35
eight types most often fatal, 36
genetics and, 33–34, 43
germline testing for, 34–35
HPV and, 51–52
hydration and risk reduction, 44
inflammation and, 147, 249
"late effects," 48
liquid biopsy, 34, 38
massage and, 52

new drug treatments, 43–44
nutrition for preventing, 44
palliative care, 51
pathologist and, 74–76
psychological issues of, 129–31
sex after, 48–49
support groups, 130, 131
supporting someone with,
152–54
treatment breakthroughs for,
37–38
Caprylic acid, 6, 249
Capsaicin, 215, 242, 243, 308, 311
CardiaX (caffeine sensitivity test),
61
Caregiver abuse, 152
Carotid endarterectomy, 72
Carotid ultrasound, 72
Carpal tunnel syndrome, 218, 298,
301–2
Cataracts, 288–89, 290
Cauliflower, colorful, 254
Cayenne, 241, 242–43
CBD (cannabidiol), 220
C. difficile, 123, 183, 185
Celecoxib (Celebrex), 123
Celiac disease, 127, 160, 219, 237,
319
Cell phones, 18, 139, 183
Cellular senescence, 276
Ceritinib (Zykadia), 38
Cervical cancer, 176–78, 327–28
CGMs (continuous glucose
monitors), 97–98, 104
Chemotherapy
avoiding the ER and, 49–51
BRCA mutations and, 36
cisplatin, 231, 232, 233
opting out of chemo, 321–22
side effects, nasal spray for, 52
Chest pain, 57, 65–66, 80, 174,
295, 303, 322, 323, 325
Chewing, 118, 124, 126, 127, 237,
301
Chicken, 126, 128, 251–52, 253,
254, 268, 292, 302
Chickweed, 248
Chiropractic care, 298, 313–14
Chlorophyll, 259
Chocolate, 16, 61, 116, 262, 294
Cholesterol, 192
heart health and, 55–56
LD, how low to go, 62–63
nondrug ways to lower, 54, 63,
218, 242, 258, 264, 271, 277
statin drugs and, 55–56, 63,
206, 218
testicular cancer and, 232
when to eat and, 263
Chronobiology, 59, 196, 263

Cimetidine (Tagamet), 144
Cinnamon, 88, 241–42, 287
Ciprofloxacin (Cipro), 218–19
Circadian rhythm, 59, 190, 196–97
when to eat and, 262–64
CIS (clinically isolated syndrome),
31
CKD (chronic kidney disease),
80–82
Clinical trials, 36–37, 43–44, 198
Clonazepam (Klonopin), 14
Cocoa, 116
Coffee, 61, 68, 116, 126, 154, 158,
230, 248, 262, 301, 307, 309, 318
Coffee flour, 259
Cognitive behavioral therapy
(CBT), 119–20, 145, 213, 331
Colds, 144, 161, 168, 182, 245–46
Collagen, 89, 218, 307–8
Colon and colorectal cancer,
33–34, 36, 41–43, 242, 254
Colonoscopy, 41–43, 51, 128
Conjunctivitis (pink eye), 162
Constipation, 27, 44, 112, 117,
118, 119, 121, 125, 128, 207, 217,
218, 244, 246, 247, 297
Consumer health alerts, 73–94
banned artificial flavors, 88
best kidney checkup, 80–82
bone broth choices, 89
doctor-patient relations, 73–74
drug recall awareness, 90–91
environmental toxins, 84–85
eyeglass lens options, 82–84
hospice warning, 92–94
household products and air,
85–87
nursing home evictions, 94
older surgeons and death
rates, 78
painless IV's, 76–77
pathologist and you, 74–76
post-op problems, 79–80
prescription drug savings,
91–92
radon testing concern, 89
safer food, beverage containers, 87
simple surgeries turn deadly,
77–78
sun protection and sunscreens,
89–90
weed killer in cereal, 87–88
well water caution, 85
COPD (chronic obstructive pulmonary disease), 7, 8–9, 54, 72,
162, 219
Copper, 252, 257, 258
CoQ10, 205, 206, 218, 249–50
Corn silk, 246, 246n

Coronary artery calcium scan, 56
Corticosteroids, 205, 219, 287,
    309–10
    PCP risk and, 173–74
Cortisol, 142
Cosmetic surgery, 77
COX-2 inhibitor (Celebrex), 78
C-reactive protein (CRP), 63, 308,
    310
Crizotinib (Xalkori), 38
Crohn's disease, 127, 185, 205
Cupping, 309
Curcumin, 21–22, 85, 124

D
Dancing, 17, 48
Dandelion root, 326
Dandruff, 235–36, 249
DASH diet, 285
Daylight saving time, 58–60
Dehydration, 256, 262
Dementia, 9, 20–22, 261, 291
    caregiving and, 150–51
    hearing loss and, 285
    iNPH and, 20–21
    "skinny fat" risk, 19–20
Dental care, 52–53
Depression
    antidepressants, 134–35, 203
    circadian rhythm and, 197
    diabetes and, 101–3, 141
    as drug side-effect, 140, 201
    exercise to help, 145
    finding a psychiatrist, 132–33
    heart disease and, 141
    inflammation and, 147
    lithium and, 194, 195
    obesity and, 203
    omega-3s for, 261
    pain-isolation-depression cycle,
        137–39
    perimenopause and, 330–31
    physical symptoms, 140
    PPIs and, 124–25
    as response to a diagnosis,
        130–31
    SAD and, 144–46
    seniors and treatment, 139–40
    VNS for, 240
    walking to alleviate, 141
    weight training for, 270
    See also bipolar disorder; suicide
De Quervain's tenosynovitis, 302
DHA (docosahexaenoic acid), 15,
    258–59, 261, 325
Diabetes (type 1), 187
Diabetes (type 2), 95–114, 185, 298
    berberine supplement for, 97
    cancer and increased risk, 98–99
    cinnamon for, 241–42

circadian rhythm and, 197
CKD and, 82
depression, suicide, or
    alcoholism, and, 101–3, 141
drugs for, heart health and,
    95–97
drugs for, weight gain and, 204
ED and, 226
exercise for, 96–97
eye screening for, 110
fasting and, 101, 108
fiber and, 99–101
foot problems and care, 105–7
hot baths to lower risk, 98
inflammation and, 147, 249
ketogenic diet and, 108–10, 199
kidneys and, 105
lifestyle changes for, 96–97
low iron risk, 112
Medicare coverage and, 101
nutrition and, 99, 110–11, 253
pancreatic cancer risk, 114
risk factors, 99
screening for, 97–98
SGLT2 inhibitors risk, 107–8
sleep and, 97
smoking and, 107
testing for, high-tech devices,
    104–5
two-one-two formula for meals,
    97
uterine cancer and, 328
walking to lower risk, 103–4, 105
"Diabetes distress," 102
Diabetic retinopathy, 110
Diarrhea, 119, 121, 123, 191
Diet drink–stroke link, 70
Digestive disorders, 115–28
    bad breath, body odor, and,
        126–27
    brain-gut connection, 119–20
    circadian rhythm and, 196
    depression and PPIs, 124–25
    diverticulitis, 127–28, 213, 237
    first aid for, 117–18
    GERD surgery, 122
    gut microbiome and, 115–17, 123
    joint pain and, 125–26
    keeping digestion working
        great, 118
    SIBO testing, 121
    stomach acid and, 125–26, 127
    stress and, 125
    viruses and, 118
    when to see a doctor, 118
    worst drugs for gut health,
        122–24
Disidentification, 261–62
Divalproex sodium (Depakote), 204
Diverticulitis, 127–28, 213, 237

D-lactic acid, 25
DMARDs, 308, 309, 311
DNA protection, 253, 254–55
Dogs
    dog bites, 181–82
    health benefits, 104, 166, 239
    marijuana danger to, 166
    saving money on pet care,
        164–66
    "sniffer" dogs for disease, 200
DPP-4 inhibitors, 95
Dravet syndrome, 220
Driving gadgets, equipment, 281–82
Driving safety for seniors, 151–52
Drug abuse, 132, 133, 142–43
Drug recall awareness, 90–91, 219
Dulaglutide (Trulicity), 204
Durvalumab (Imfinzi), 37, 45
DVT (deep vein thrombosis), 80
Dyslexia (in adults), 28–29

E
Ear infections, 162, 213
Ear ringing, 232
Eating disorders, 146–47
Echinacea, 161
E. coli bacteria, 117, 123, 124, 191
Eczema, 65, 248, 249, 308
ED (erectile dysfunction). 224–26,
    232
Eggs, 32, 108, 126, 195, 199, 246,
    252, 268, 292, 302, 325
Elderberry, elderberry tea, 161, 169
Electrocardiogram (ECG), 324–25
Electronic devices
    ergonomic tips for using, 303
    neck pain and, 297
    wrist pain and, 301–3
Emotional health, 129–48
    alcoholism in older adults,
        143–44
    autism, ways to connect, 135–36
    BPD diagnosis, treatment,
        133–34
    depression and seniors,
        139–40
    DIY acupressure for anxiety,
        147–48
    eating disorder relapse and,
        146–47
    fear of illness and, 129–31
    finding a psychiatrist, 132–33
    jealousy, 135
    opioid drugs, 142–43
    pain-isolation-depression cycle,
        137–39
    SAD and, 144–46
    self-compassion, 131
    walking for depression, 141
    See also Anxiety; Depression

Emulsifiers, 116–17
Enalapril (Vasotec), 288
Endometrial cancer, 326, 329
Endometrial hyperplasia, 329
Endometriosis, 325–27
Endoscopy, 78
Enoxaparin sodium (Lovenox), 300
Environmental toxins, 84–85, 319
Enzymes, digestive, 126, 301, 248
EPA (eicosapentaenoic acid), 55,
    63, 258–59, 261, 325
Epidermal necrolysis, 215–17
Epidiolex, 220
Epilepsy, 198, 240
EpiPen, 2–4
Epsom salts, 161–62, 236
Erenumab-aooe (Aimovig), 297
Erlotinib (Tarceva), 38
Esketamine (Spravato), 134–35
Esophageal cancers, 36
Esophagus, lab-grown, 197
Essential oils, 243–46
Estrogen, 61, 64, 75, 227, 229, 318,
    319, 326, 329, 324, 325, 326, 328,
    329, 330
    breast cancer and, 204, 219,
        318, 321
    migraines and, 233–34, 294
Exercise
    aerobic, 233, 268, 270, 313
    back pain and, 312
    for bowel movements, 128
    for brain health, 16
    breast cancer risk and, 319
    calories burned and, 267
    cardio exercise, 24–25, 271
    for childhood cancer survivors,
        48
    circadian rhythm and, 59
    dead lifts, 226, 227–28
    for depression, 145
    for diabetes, 96–97
    diet mistakes and, 267–68
    for easing RA pain, 308
    endorphins and, 141
    for the face, 274–76
    foam rolling, 271
    heart health and, 56
    HIIT, 270–71
    immune system and, 7, 168
    interval training, 226
    knee pain and, 312
    memory retention and, 24–25
    one hour in five minutes,
        272
    outdoor, nature therapy and,
        239
    pain, exercising with, 311–13
    for pain relief, 308
    pregnancy and, 157–58

preventing knee, hip, and
    joint pain, 305–7
preventing muscle loss, 10,
    291
push-ups and heart health, 58
to reduce endometriosis pain,
    326
reversing ED and, 226
smiling and, 271
sports drinks, 267
target heart rate, 271
testicular cancer treatment,
    lowering side effects, 232–33
testosterone levels and,
    227–28
triglyceride lowering with, 64
varying your workout, 270–71
weight loss and, 268–69
weight training, 268–69, 270
    See also walking
Eyeglass lens options, 82–84
Eyes
    cataracts, 288–89, 290
    diabetic retinopathy, 110
    eyelids and sun protection, 39
    glaucoma, 289–90
    hydrogen therapy, 277
    sleep apnea symptom and, 13

F

Family health matters, 149–66
    ADHD medication concerns,
        162–64
    caregiving for dementia, 150–51
    comfort at the end of life, 154
    help after a suicide attempt,
        154–57
    kids and healthy food, 159–60
    kids and toothpaste, 164
    kids' anti-flu program, 160–62,
        160n
    marijuana danger to dogs, 166
    new info about pregnancy,
        157–59
    pacifier cleaning, 164
    picture books and brain func-
        tion, 164
    protection from caregiver abuse,
        152
    safer driving for the elderly,
        151–52
    saving money on pet care,
        164–66
    supporting cancer patients,
        152–54
    surrogate health decisions,
        149–50
    tonsil and adenoid removal, 162
    wildfire areas and air quality,
        159

Fasting, 54, 101, 108, 264–65
Fat, body, 242, 278, 326
    belly fat and testosterone, 227
    dementia risk and, 19–20, 291
    waist size and, 56, 103, 203
Fatigue, 4, 7, 13, 41, 44, 59, 84,
    140, 170, 171, 172, 185, 186, 212,
    228, 244, 295, 309, 311, 312, 322
    help for, 41, 52, 54, 120, 148,
        239, 244, 249, 271, 308, 309
Fats, dietary, 16, 19, 63, 64, 108,
    127, 168, 199, 204, 251, 252–53,
    255, 256–58, 263
    See also omega-3 fatty acids
FDA fast-tracking approvals, 66–67
Fecal transplants (FMT), 184–85
Feet
    amputation risk, 107–8
    corns, remedy for, 236–37
    diabetes and care for, 105–7
    orthotics and, 315
    plantar fasciitis, 315
    socks and shoes for diabetes,
        106
    ulcer, 105–7
Feldenkrais Method, 304–5
Fennel tea, 237
Fentanyl, 209, 211, 218
Fermented foods, 6, 26, 116, 229,
    253
Fever, 9, 42, 50, 78, 79, 118, 123,
    128, 171, 174, 175, 182, 184, 216
    flu and, 161, 162, 169, 170
Feverfew, 124
Fiber, dietary, 26, 85, 99–101, 117
    foods for, 100, 128, 256, 257,
        258, 260
    to prevent diverticulitis, 127–28
    supplement, 85, 100, 117
Fibromyalgia, 298
Fidgeting, 53
Fisetin, 276–77
Fish, 16, 126, 158, 301, 318, 325–26.
    See also Salmon
Fish oil, fish oil supplements, 126,
    161, 164, 258, 261, 301, 325
5-hydroxytryptophan (5-HTP), 295
Flaxseed, 54, 100, 326
Flu, 161–62, 167–71
    shots, 9, 167–68, 170, 173, 174,
        214
Fluoroquinolones (Cipro), 206
Fluvastatin (Lescol), 218
FODMAPs, 117
Folate, 164, 205, 257, 258, 260
Food allergies, 3, 32, 159, 246
Food cravings, 109, 144, 204, 261,
    262
FOS foods, 116
Fournier's gangrene, 107

Fruits
amount of per day, 252
antioxidants and, 326
colorizing your plate, 318
dietary fiber and, 100, 128
fiber, potassium, and, 260
flash frozen vs. fresh, 252, 254
hydration and, 256
potassium-rich foods, 206
raw foods and, 126, 301
types high in anthocyanins, 309

G
Gardasil 9 vaccine, 178–79
Gargling, gargles, 169, 175, 241, 245
Garlic, 26, 54, 116, 126, 236, 241, 242
Gas, flatulence, 118, 121, 125, 127, 237
Gaviscon, 123
Gefitinib (Iressa), 38
Gene-modulating drugs, 38
Genetics
BRCA genes, 36, 232, 317, 320
cancer and, 34–35, 43
DDR testing and prostate cancer, 231–32
DNA testing and breast cancer, 320–21
ED, genetic link, 224
NLRP12 and obesity, 189
Oncotype DX test, 321–22
test for caffeine sensitivity, 61
Genital warts, 179
GERD. See heartburn/GERD
Ghee, 116
Ginger, ginger tea, 124, 162, 237, 242
Glaucoma, 289–90
GLP-1 agonists, 95, 97
Glucomannan, 118
Gluten-free diet, 117, 219, 248, 315
Gouda cheese, 254
Grapefruit seed extract, 235–36
Grape juice, Concord, 255
Gravel root, 246, 246n
Grounding or earthing, 54
Gut bacteria, gut microbiome, 253
antibiotics and, 122–23
best and worst foods for, 115–17
cardiovascular risk and, 125
circadian rhythm and, 196–97
dietary fiber and, 100, 101, 117
gluten-free diet and, 117
H2 blockers and, 123
intermittent fasting and, 264
kiwis for, 254
NSAIDs and, 123
omega-3 fatty acids for, 118
PPIs and, 25, 123
processed foods and, 125

H
H2 blockers, 123, 125
Hands
grip and pulmonary function, 10
weak or painful, help for, 279–80
Hand sanitizer, 168, 183
Hand washing, 171, 173, 183, 214
Headaches, 293–95
medical emergency, 295
painful yet rare (TACs), 294
rebound headache and, 294–95
remedies, 124
sinus infection and, 294
Hearing aids, 26, 283–86
Hearing assistance, 282–84
Hearing loss, 26, 232, 284, 285
Heart attacks
actions to take if one occurs, 324
blood type and, 191
chest pain evaluation, 65–66
circadian rhythm and, 196
coldest months and, 60
daylight saving time and, 58–60
diet drinks and, 70
ECG and, 324–25
HEART scoring system for, 66
hydrogen therapy for, 278
lifestyle changes and, 323
marijuana and, 193
MINOCA risk, 56–57
risk factors, 323
scuba diving risk, 56
stroke risk after, 70
symptoms, 80, 298, 325
symptoms in women, 57, 322, 325
troponin test, 323
women's health and, 322–24
"yo-yo" danger, 197
Heartburn/GERD, 119, 122, 123, 124–25, 126, 127, 202
home remedy, 25
low stomach acid and, 125
medications, alcohol warning, 144
PPIs and, 25, 123–25, 127, 201, 202
surgery and, 122
when to see a doctor, 125
Heart devices, 66–67
Heart health, 53–72
air filters and, 62
anthocyanins for, 254
aspirin and, 55, 70, 215
berberine for, 97
CAC scan and, 56
cholesterol and, 55–56
depression and, 141
diabetes and, 95–97
disease prevention myths, 55–56
eczema and, 65

ED and, 226
EPA supplement (Vascepa) for, 55
exercise and, 56, 270, 271
gut health and, 125
healthy habits, 56
hydrogen therapy and, 277
indoor thermostat setting and, 60
inflammation and, 56, 147, 249
MRIs and pacemakers, 68
nutrition and, 253
push-ups and, 58
stem cell therapy for, 188
ten changes for, 52–54
triglycerides and, 63–65
walking and, 103, 269
when to eat and, 263
Hemorrhoids, 329
Hepatitis C, 185–86
game-changing drugs for, 185
Hibiscus tea, 54
High-intensity interval training (HIIT), 270–71
Hip pain, 281, 304, 315
HIV/AIDS, 180, 181, 216
Homeopathy, 160n, 161, 235–36
Honey, 19, 47, 243
Horny goat weed, 225
Horsetail, 247
Hospice warning, 92–94
HPV (human papillomavirus), 51–52, 176–79
HRT (hormone replacement therapy), 319, 329, 331
HTLV-1, 179–81
Hydrochlorothiazide (HCTZ), 38–39
Hydrogen for anti-aging, 277–78
Hypersensitivity pneumonitis, 6
Hypnosis, 243
Hypnotherapy, 120

I
IBS (irritable bowel syndrome), 117, 119, 120, 121, 125–26, 185, 243
Ibuprofen (Advil, Motrin), 85, 123, 214–15, 217, 242, 298
Immune system, 253
exercise for, 7, 168
foods to boost, 7, 253–55
hydration for, 7
immunoglobulin A (IgA) and, 7
light-therapy for, 168
pacifier cleaning and, 164
self-compassion and, 131
sleep for, 7, 160–61, 168
stress and, 319
Immunizations, 174–75, 207. *See also* flu shots; pneumonia
Immunotherapy, 5, 37–38, 45
IncobotulinumtoxinA (Xeomin), 14

Indigestion, baking soda for, 117–18
Indomethacin (Indocin), 43
Induced pluripotent stem cells (iPSCs), 189, 198
Infectious diseases, 167–86
    C. difficile, 183, 184–85
    doctor's office hot spots, 182–84
    dog bites and, 181–82
    flu, 160–62, 167–71
    hepatitis C, 185–86
    HPV, 176–79
    immunizations for, 174–75
    mosquito-borne, 173
    PCP, 173–74
    petting zoo danger, 180
    sepsis, 171–73
    STDs, 175–81
    steroids and, 173–74
    strep throat, 175
Inflammation
    brain health and, 22, 173
    cancer and, 147
    CRP and, 63, 308, 310
    diabetes and, 147
    foods that promote, 7
    foods that reduce, 325–26
    ginger for, 242
    heart health and, 56, 147
    hot baths to lower, 98
    immunotherapy as cause of, 45
    intermittent fasting to lower, 264
    joint pain and, 125–26
    obesity and, 189, 308–9
    sadness, anger, and, 147
    skin conditions and, 249
    supplements to reduce, 326
    symptoms of, in the gut, 125
    vitamin D to lower risk, 22
Injuries, 199–200
    concussion treatment, 32
    falls, causes of, 193, 201, 212
    head injury and smell loss, 288
    whiplash, 298
INPH (idiopathic normal pressure hydrocephalus), 20–21
Insomnia, 27, 41, 59, 130, 145, 148, 172, 189–90, 211–12, 213
Insulin, 20, 100, 203, 318
    as "hunger hormone," 264
    hydrogen therapy and, 278
    olive oil and, 116
    resistance, 263
    saving money on, 113–14
    sensitivity, 100, 197, 263, 264, 319
    storage danger, 112
    when to eat and, 263
Insulin-like growth factor-1 (IGF-1), 318
Insulin pens and pumps, 105

Iodine, 39, 245, 252, 256, 260
Iron, 112, 124, 206, 252, 256, 258, 260
Irritability, 147, 148, 194, 196

J
Japanese evergreen spicebush, 247
Jealousy of adult child, 135
Joint pain, 125–26, 305–8

K
Kegel exercises, 246
Ketogenic diet, 108–10, 198–99
Kidney disease, 80–82, 196
Kidneys, NSAIDs caution, 215
Kiwifruit, 254
Klotho, 16
Knee pain, 310, 311, 312, 314–15

L
Lachnospiraceae, 189
Lactose intolerance, 127
Lactrectinib (Vitrakvi), 43–44
Lasmiditan, 295
Latanoprostene bunod ophthalmic solution (Vyzulta), 289
Laughter, 241
L-citrulline, 225
Leaky gut, 126, 248
Leg cramps, 79
Levodopa (Sinemet), 27
Licorice root, 330
Light, sunlight, 22, 41, 60, 82–84, 144–45, 151, 168, 173, 196, 197, 212, 215, 282, 289, 294, 295, 296
Light-therapy, 145, 168
Liraglutide (Victoza), 204
Lithium, 194–96, 204
Liver cancer, 36, 46–47
Liver health, 185, 186, 214
Longevity, 269–70, 291
Lorazepam (Ativan), 211
Lovastatin (Mevacor or Altoprev), 218
Lung cancer, 36, 37–38, 43, 254
Lung health, 9
    air quality and, 11–13
    grip strength and, 10
    popcorn lung, 10–11
    spirometry test and, 9
    vaping, e-cigarettes and, 10–11
Lupus, 173, 174, 205
Lymphedema, 320

M
Magnesium, 99, 205, 249, 252, 256, 257, 258, 260
Malaria, 200
Maldigestion, 127
Mammograms, 319–20

Manganese, 257, 258
Mangoes, 253–54
Marijuana, 166, 192–93, 220
Marine algae, 258–59
Massage, 52, 241, 244, 299, 310
MCI (mild cognitive impairment), 15, 20
Meals, mealtime
    breakfast, 19, 263, 264, 268, 292
    circadian rhythm and, 59
    early eating, benefits, 263
    dinner, 35, 59, 126, 262, 265, 267, 268, 292
    drinking beverages with meals, 118, 124, 126, 127, 301
    lunch, 19, 126, 137, 262, 263, 264, 265, 267–68, 292
    meatless meals, 319
    muscle-building meals, 292
    raw foods and, 126
    "three-quarter" challenge, 263
    two-one-two formula for meals, 97
Medical care
    chemotherapy side-effects, ER and, 49–51
    diabetes, doctor knowledge gap, 96
    doctor-patient talks, 73–74, 313
    doctor's office hot spots, 182–84
    hospice warning, 92–94
    nursing home evictions, 94
    painless IV's, 75–76
    pathologist and, 74–76
    pharmacist and, 206–7
    prescription drug savings, 91–92
    second opinion and, 75
    surgery, 77–78
    telemedicine and, 109–10
Medical news alerts, 187–200
    blood test for best bedtime, 189–90
    blood type and health risks, 190–92
    circadian rhythm and health, 196–97
    ketogenic diet benefits, 198–99
    lab-grown esophagus, 197
    low-dose lithium, new uses, 194–96
    marijuana risks, 192–93
    obesity and genes, 189
    spinal cord injury implant, 199–200
    stem cell therapy, 187–89
    3-D medical printing, 193–94
    "yo-yo" cardio danger, 197
Medicare, 101, 105, 284

Medications, 201–20
  apps for saving on, 220
  deadly skin reaction, 215–17
  depression as side effect, 201
  discontinuing drugs, 203, 204n
  drug company perks for
    doctors, 208
  drug interactions and alpha-
    lipoic acid, 288
  drug interactions and marijuana,
    193
  drug recall awareness, 219
  drugs and nutrient loss, 205–6
  drugs likely to cause
    problems, 202
  drugs that damage tendons,
    218–19
  experimental drugs, 207–9
  FDA approval, cannabis drugs,
    220
  making a medications list, 202
  new synthetic opioid, 210–11
  NSAIDs, dangers of, 214–15
  opioids, 209–10, 217–18
  polypharmacy, problems of,
    201–3
  rebound headache and, 294–95
  Rx mistakes, avoiding, 219
  sedatives, addiction caution,
    211–13
  sense of smell loss and, 288
  3-D medical printing and, 194
  unnecessary antibiotics, 213–14
  unnecessary prescriptions,
    202
  weight gain and, 203–5
  what your pharmacist can do,
    206–7
  See also antibiotics; opioid drugs;
    specific drugs
Meditation, 56, 163–64, 241, 249
Mediterranean diet, 16, 19, 56,
  126, 226, 285, 301
Melanoma, 34, 38–39, 185, 229
Melatonin, 59–60, 190
Meloxicam (Mobic), 123
Memory, 264
  blood type and problems, 191
  exercise and new motor skills,
    24–25
  glucose-rich foods for, 19
  hearing loss and, 26
  hippocampus and, 273–74
  hydrogen therapy for, 277
  pink noise for, 23
  simple strategy for, 21
  sleep and, 13, 16, 25
  stress and, 130
  tip-of-the-tongue moments, 21
Meningococcal meningitis, 173

Menopause, 319, 321, 324, 326,
  328–29, 330
Men's health, 221–34
  ED, 224, 225–27
  good-in-bed diet, 226
  incontinence, 223–24
  melanoma, 229
  migraines and sex hormones,
    233–34
  prostate cancer, genetic testing
    following, 231–32
  prostate cancer advice, 230–31
  prostate cancer risk, 229–30
  prostate cancer treatment, 233
  prostate surgery, 224
  sexuality myths, 221–23
  sperm of older men, 224–25
  testicular cancer, 232–33
  testosterone and, 227–29
Metabolic syndrome, 100, 103, 263
Metabolism, 262–63, 265
Metformin (Glucophage), 20, 95,
  96, 204, 205
Micromovements, 256
Midazolam (Versed), 172
Migraines, 204, 233–34, 240, 242,
  250, 293–94, 295–97
MIND diet, 16
MINOCA heart attack, 56–57
Mold, toxic mold, 4–7
Monolaurin, 168
Mood, 249–50, 261
MRIs, pacemakers and, 68
MS (multiple sclerosis), 30–32, 305
MSM (methylsulfonylmethane), 326
Muscles
  intermittent fasting to benefit,
    264
  loss of, 10, 19–20, 291, 331–32
  pain after exercise, 277
  preventing loss, 10, 291–92

N

Nabiximols (Sativex), 220
N-acetyl cysteine (NAC), 168
Naproxen (Aleve), 85, 123, 214–15,
  242
Nasal irrigation, 6
Nasal spray, 52
Nasal vestibulitis, 52
Natural cures, 235–50
  for bipolar disorder, 249–50
  for corns, 236–37
  for dandruff, 235–36, 248, 249
  for eczema, 248
  essential oils, 243–46
  for flatulence, 237
  hypnosis for IBS, 243
  for rosacea, 248–49
  for styes, 236

  "super spices," 241–43
  top doctor's choices, 237–39
  for urinary incontinence, 246–47
  vagus nerve and, 239–41
  for warts, 236
Nature therapy, 237–39
Naturopathic physicians, 1, 7, 97,
  117, 126, 161, 226, 228n, 235,
  247, 301, 330
Nausea, 9, 27, 42, 44, 49, 50, 52,
  57, 66, 78, 86, 97, 119, 128, 135,
  147, 154, 175, 186, 195, 209,
  212, 218, 293, 294, 295, 322
  help for, 118, 148, 220, 241,
    242, 243, 244
Neck pain, 297, 314
Nefazodone (Serzone), 203
Nettle Quercetin, 248
Neurofeedback, biofeedback,
  29–30, 163
Nitric oxide, 225
Nivolumab (Opdivo), 37, 45
NSAIDs (non-steroidal anti-
  inflammatory drugs), 43, 69, 78,
  85, 123, 214–15, 311
  alternatives to, 123–24, 215
Nursing home evictions, 94
Nutritional supplements
  AHCC, 169
  alpha-lipoic acid, 287–88
  antifungals, 6
  anti-yeast, 249
  ashwagandha, 225–26, 228
  berberine, 97
  biotin, 236
  calcium, 205
  collagen, 307–8
  CoQ10, 205, 206, 218, 249–50
  curcumin, 22, 124
  dandelion root, 326
  digestive enzymes, 126, 301
  echinacea, 161
  elderberry, 161
  feverfew, ginger combination, 124
  fiber, 85, 100, 117
  fish oil or omega-3s, 15, 55, 69,
    126, 161, 164, 258, 261, 301, 325
  folic acid, folate, 205
  horny goat weed, 225
  iron, 124
  L-citrulline, 225
  licorice root, 330
  liquid vitamin D3, 302
  magnesium, 205, 249, 260
  melatonin, 59–60
  monolaurin, 168
  MSM, 326
  multivitamin/mineral, 206, 260
  NAC, 168
  Nettle Quercetin, 248

olive leaf extract, 168
potassium, 205, 206
probiotics, 85, 123, 206, 248, 249
pulsatilla, 236
rhodiola rosea, 226, 228
Robuvit, 169
selenium, 205
turmeric, 6, 16
Vascepa, 55, 63
vitamin B-6, 260
vitamin B-12, 205, 206, 260
vitamin-B complex, 206, 236, 260, 326
vitamin C, 249
vitamin D, 22–23, 205, 228, 260–61
vitamin E, 249
vitamin K, 206
vitamins for everyone, 259–61
zinc, 205, 228, 236, 249
Nutritional yeast, 258
Nutrition and diet
banned artificial flavors, 88
best and worst foods for gut bacteria, 115–17
best foods for dandruff cure, 235
best foods for muscles, 291–92
body's defense systems and, 253
bone broth, consumer alert, 89
breakfast, 19, 264, 268
breast cancer risk and, 318
cancer-fighting foods, 44
cauliflower, colorful versions, 254
coffee flour, 259
colorizing your plate, 318
cruciferous vegetables, 44
DASH diet, 285
dinner timing and cancer risk, 35
elimination diet, 237
fasting and, 264–65
foods high in vitamin B6, 302
foods high in vitamin B12, 302
foods that beat disease, 253–55
foods that increase liver cancer, 47
foods that promote inflammation, 7
foods to reduce diabetes risk, 99
foods to reduce endometriosis pain, 325–26
foods to reduce inflammation, 325–26
food variety, 262
fruits, vegetables recommendations, 16, 252
fruits high in anthocyanins, 309
glucose-rich foods, 19
gluten-free diet, 117, 219, 248, 315
good-in-bed diet for men, 226
healthier eating plan, 264

healthy eating for kids, 159–60
high-fiber foods, 100, 128
high-iron foods, 112
hydration from vegetables, 255–56
immune system boosting and, 7
increasing HCL production, 126, 301
ketogenic diet, 108–10, 198–99
low-FODMAP diet, 117
meatless meals, 319
Mediterranean diet, 16, 19, 56, 126, 226, 285, 301
menopause and, 321
MIND diet, 16
mushrooms, benefits, 16
nut and seed butters, 252–53, 256–58
nutritional yeast and, 258
nuts and cancer protection, 42
omega-3-rich foods, 16, 126, 301
omega-3s for vegetarians, 258–59
organic foods, 84, 87–88
organ meats, 252
potassium-rich foods, 206
prebiotic foods, 26
probiotics and, 128
protein, 10, 54, 97, 108, 111, 115, 126, 127, 252–53, 257–59, 261, 264, 265, 268, 291–92, 294, 301, 307, 318–19
raw foods, 126, 301
rice types for diabetics, 110–11
salt, natural, 256
soy foods, 229–30, 253
sugary foods, 16, 63, 127, 249, 261–62
"superstar" foods, 16
"three-quarter" challenge, 263
two-one-two formula for meals, 97
ultra-healthy foods, 251–53
uterine cancer and, 328
vegetarian diet, 258–59, 318
vitamin C-rich foods, 249
weed killer in cereal caution, 87–88
weight loss counselor, 266
when to eat, 262–64, 268
Nuts and seeds, 42, 100, 264, 326
butters, 252–53, 256–58

O

Oats, 117, 264
Obesity, 141, 185
breast cancer and, 318
circadian rhythm and, 196–97
depression and, 203
diseases related to, 189
flu and, 170–71

genetics and, 189
inflammation and, 189, 308–9
testicular cancer and, 232
triglycerides and, 63
uterine cancer and, 328
Olive leaf extract, 168
Olive oil, 116
Omega-3 fatty acids, 54, 118, 126, 134, 164, 301, 318, 325–26
food sources, 16, 126, 249, 257, 301
supplement, 15, 55, 69, 118, 261
for vegetarians, 258–59
Oncotype DX test, 321–22
Opioid drugs, 25, 26, 77–78, 202
addiction vs. dependence, 209–10
fentanyl, 209, 211, 218
medical need for, 217–18
naloxone (Narcan), 332
new synthetic, powerful, 210–11
overdose, survival and, 142–43
woman's guide for addiction, 332
Oral glucose tolerance test (OGTT), 100
Oregano oil gargle, 169
Organic foods, 84, 87–88
Orilissa, 325
Oseltamivir (Tamiflu), 169
Osimertinib (Tagrisso), 38
Osteoarthritis, 277, 310
Ovarian cancer, 33–34, 36, 320, 326–27

P

PAD (peripheral artery disease), 315–16
Pain, pain relief, 54, 293–316
acupuncture, 124
ankle replacements, 316
anthocyanins for, 309
back pain, 281, 312, 313–14
bruises and, 303
cayenne or capsaicin for, 215, 241, 242, 308
curcumin for, 124
diet for, 315
doctor-patient communication, 313
exercise and, 305–8, 311–13, 315–16
Feldenkrais Method for, 304–5
feverfew, ginger combination, 124
ginger for, 242
headaches and migraines, 293–97
healthy weight and, 308–9
holding hands for, 314

joint pain, 125–26, 305–8
lower leg pain, 79–80
massage for knee pain, 310
natural choices, 85, 308–9
neck pain, 297, 314
opioid drugs, 217–18
orthotics and, 315
pain clinics, 217
physical therapy, 123–24
post-op problems, warning signs, 79
RA pain, 308–9, 311
rib, 300–301
saunas and, 54
sleep position and, 314–15
steroid risk, 309–10
TOS and, 298–300
whiplash injury, 298
wrist pain, 301–3
yoga for, 123–24
See also NSAIDs
Pancreatic cancer, 33–34, 36, 99, 114
Pancreatitis, 64
Panic attack, panic disorder, 133
PAP test, 176–77
Parkinson's disease, 22, 27–28, 268, 240
Paroxetine (Paxil), 203
Pathologist, 74–76
PE (pulmonary embolism), 80
Peanut butter, 252–53, 256
Pecans, 42, 99, 116
Pembrolizumab (Keytruda), 45
Penile injections, 49
Peppermint tea, 162, 237
Perimenopause, 330–31
Periodontal disease, 52–53
Pet care, 164–66
Pet therapy, 239
Petting zoo danger, 180
Phosphorus, 252, 257, 258
Phytochemicals, 256, 257
Phytoestrogens, 229
Pimozide (Orap), 30
Pink noise, 23
Pitavastatin (Livalo), 218
Plague, 173
Plantar fasciitis, 315
Pneumonia, 8–9, 213
    pneumocystis pneumonia, 173–74
    vaccination and, 170, 173, 174
Polyphenols, 116
Polyps, 329
Potassium, 205, 256
Potatoes, purple, 254
PPIs (proton pump inhibitors), 25, 122, 123, 124–25, 127, 201
Pravastatin (Pravachol), 218

Prebiotics, 26
Prediabetes, 100, 237–38
Pregnancy, 157–59
    baby's crib, safest, 158
    bed rest and, 157
    caffeine and, 158
    dad's age and baby's health, 224–25
    epidurals and, 157
    exercise and, 157–58
    labor progress, speed of, 158
    sushi and fish, safe choices, 158
    vaginal birth after cesarean, 157
    weight gain and, 158
Prescription drug savings, 91–92
Probiotics, 25–26, 118, 237, 248, 254
    food sources, 128
    supplements, 85, 123, 206, 248, 249
Processed foods, 16, 116–17, 125, 126, 256, 260
Prostaglandin analogs (PGAs), 289
Prostate cancer
    dinner timing and risk, 35
    genetic testing after, 33–34
    Gouda cheese to lower risk, 254
    PSA test and, 232
    soy to lower risk, 229–30
    stereotactic body radiotherapy, 233
    surgery and incontinence, 224
    testing for, 34
    testosterone caution, 229
    YouTube videos for advice, 230–31
Protein, 54, 111, 115, 127, 252, 257, 258, 307
    from beef and liver, 252
    blood sugar control and, 294
    breast cancer and, 318–19
    growth hormone in meat, 318
    healthy choices, 126, 268, 301, 318
    including with every meal, 264, 268
    ketogenic diet and, 108, 199
    meal suggestions, 292
    for muscle strength, 291–92
    nonmeat, 257–58, 259, 268, 318–19
    sleep improvement and, 261
    soy protein, 229–30, 253
    two-one-two formula for meals, 97
Protein shakes, 265, 268
Psychiatrists, psychotherapy, 132–33, 134, 140
Pulsatilla, 236

R
RA (rheumatoid arthritis), 205, 249, 278, 308–11
Radiation treatment, 35, 36, 48, 49, 52, 75, 198, 233, 245, 320, 321
Radon testing, 89
Ranitidine (Zantac), 144
Raynaud's disease, 232, 298
Regeneration, 253
Registered dietitian (RD), 265
Resveratrol, 318
Rhodiola rosea, 226, 228
Riboflavin, 257
Rib pain, 300–301
Rice, 110–11
Rifaximin (Xifaxan), 121
Ritalin, 163
Rivaroxaban (Xarelto), 300
Robuvit, 169
Rosacea, 248–49
Rosuvastatin (Crestor), 218

S
SAD (seasonal affective disorder), 144–46
Salicylic acid, 236, 237
Salmon, 126, 158, 199, 249, 261, 264, 301, 325
Salt sensitivity, 256
Sarcopenia, 10, 19–20, 291, 331–32
Sauna, 54
Scuba diving, 56
Seaweed, 252, 258–59
Sedative drugs, 211–13
Sedentary lifestyle, 54, 56, 103, 158, 226, 246, 323
Seizures, 204, 220
Selenium, 7, 205, 257, 258, 260
Sepsis, 171–73
Serotonin, 295
Sertraline (Zoloft), 203
Sex
    erection problems, 49, 225–27
    following cancer, 48–49
    frequency and heart health, 54–55
    helpful resources, 49
    myths about men's sexuality, 221–23
    performance anxiety, 226–27
    practicing safer, 176
    toys, 49
    vaginal changes and, 48–49
SGLT2 inhibitors, 95, 97, 107–8
Shingles vaccine, 174
Shock, 80, 172, 323
Short-chain-fatty acids, 100, 115, 116, 189
SIBO (small intestinal bacterial overgrowth), 25, 121

Sick building syndrome, 6
Sildenafil (Viagra), 49
Simvastatin (Zocor), 218
Sinus infection, 213, 214, 294
Sinusitis, 4–6, 244
Sitting, 54
Skin cancers, 38–40
Skin conditions, 248–49
Sleep
    blood test for best bedtime,
        189–90
    bright-light exposure and, 41
    circadian rhythm and, 41, 196
    determining your chronotype,
        59
    diabetes control and, 97
    dinner time/bed time and
        cancer, 35
    disruptions and health
        problems, 59
    drooling during, 14
    essential oils for, 244
    foods disruptive to, 16
    immune system and, 7, 160–61,
        168
    lack of, weight gain and, 261
    lithium and, 195
    memory and, 16, 25
    pink noise for, 23
    position and pain, 314–15
    restorative, 219
    strategies for fatigue, 309
    testosterone levels and, 227
    triglyceride level and, 64
Sleep apnea, 13, 14, 64, 77, 78
Sleep diary, 213
Sleeping pills, 202
Smell, sense of, 286–88
Smiling, 271
Smoking, 44, 56, 107, 123, 233, 288
Smoothies, 255–56
Snacks, 127, 264
Snoring, 13, 14, 23
Social media, social isolation and,
    137–39
Sodium, salt, 126, 256, 301
Sore throat, 175, 213, 244–45
Soy foods, 229–30, 253
Spinal cord injury, 199–200
Spontaneous coronary artery
    dissection, 323
Sports drinks, 267
SSRIs (selective serotonin reup-
    take inhibitors), 203
Statin drugs, 55–56, 63, 64, 65,
    206, 218, 250
STDs (sexually transmitted
    diseases), 175–81, 329
    See also HPV; HTLV-1
Stem cell therapy, 187–89, 197

Steroids. See corticosteroids
Stevens-Johnson syndrome,
    216–17
Stomach cancer, 36, 191
Stomach ulcer, 127
Strep throat, 175
Stress
    beta-blocker drugs for, 130
    clutter and, 16–17
    daily stress relief, 319
    digestive disorders and, 125, 300
    facing a stressful task, 141–42
    holding hands for, 157
    immune system and, 319
    RA and, 309
    reducing, for heart health, 56
    relaxation techniques, 309
    relaxation techniques vs. pills,
        213
Stroke, 64
    AFib and, 68–69
    blood type and, 191
    diet drinks and, 70
    eczema and, 65
    heart attacks and risk, 70
    hydrogen therapy for, 277
    ischemic stroke, 324
    low-dose aspirin and, 215
    ministroke symptoms, 71–72
    prevention, 71–72, 324
    risk factors, 71
    risk for women, 324
    stem cell therapy for, 188
    TIAs, 296
    VNS for, 240
    "yo-yo" danger, 197
Sufentanil (Dsuvia), 210–11
Sugar, 63, 127
    cutting down on, 16, 249, 261–62
    daily limit for, 262
Suicide, 101–3, 133, 140, 195
    finding a psychiatrist, 132–33
    help after a suicide attempt,
        154–57
    resources, 156–57
Sulfonylureas, 95, 202, 204
Sumatriptan (Imitrex), 242, 295
Sun protection, 39–40, 83–84,
    89–90
Surgery
    ASCs and, 77–78
    circadian rhythm and, 196
    older surgeons and death rates, 78
    post-op problems, warnings,
        79–80
    "simple" turning deadly, 77–78
    3-D medical printing and, 193

T

Tamoxifen, 204, 219

Tea, 19, 309
Teeth, kids and toothpaste, 164
Telomeres, 277
Tennis, 271
Testicular cancer, 232–33
Testosterone
    abdominal fat and, 227
    boosting, 225, 228, 228n
    migraines and, 233–34
    prostate cancer caution, 229
    range of, normal levels, 228–29
    sex, frequency of, and, 228
    signs of low levels, 228
    sleep and, 227
    testicular cancer and, 232
Thiamine, 258
Thiazolidinediones, 95
Thoracic outlet syndrome (TOS),
    298–300
3-D medical printing, 193–94
Throat cancer, 51
Throat Coat tea, 161
Thyroid disorders, 196
TIAs (transient ischemic attacks,
    ministrokes), 296
Time-outs, 163
Tonsil and adenoid removal,
    risks, 162
Tonsillectomy, 77
Toxic epidermal necrolysis,
    216–17
Traditional Chinese medicine
    (TCM), 236, 247
Transvaginal ultrasound, 328
Travel, air quality and, 11–13
Trigger finger, 218
Triglycerides, 63–65, 261, 264
Trimethoprim/sulfamethoxazole
    (Septra, Bactrim), 173–74
Turmeric, 6, 16

U

Ulcerative colitis, 205
Ulcers, 191
Ulnar tunnel syndrome (Guyon's
    canal syndrome), 302
Upper-respiratory-tract infections,
    6, 162, 213
Urinary incontinence, 223–24,
    246–47
Urox, 247
Uterine cancer, 328

V

Vaginal dryness, 48–49, 331
Vaginal moisturizers, 48–49
Vagus nerve, 239–41
Vaping, e-cigarettes, 10–11
Varuna (Ayurvedic medicine), 247
Vascepa, 55, 63, 64–65

Vegetables
   amount of per day, 252
   antioxidants and, 326
   colorizing your plate, 318
   cruciferous vegetables, 326
   dietary fiber and, 100, 128
   fiber, potassium, and, 260
   finding more variety in, 252
   green smoothies, 255–56
   hydration and, 255–56
   nonstarchy, 265
   potassium-rich foods, 206
   rainbow colors, 252
   raw foods and, 126, 301
Vegetarian diet, 258–59, 318
Venlafaxine (Effexor), 203
Virta Health telemedicine, 109–10
Vision. *See* Eyes
Vitamin A, 219, 252
Vitamin B-6, 219, 257, 260
Vitamin B6, 302
Vitamin B-12, 7, 15, 164, 205, 206,
   219, 252, 258, 260, 302–3
Vitamin B-complex, 206, 236,
   260, 326
Vitamin C, 7, 219, 249, 252
Vitamin D, 9, 22–23, 164, 168,
   205, 219, 228, 260–61, 302
Vitamin E, 249, 257
Vitamin K, K-2, 206, 253, 254
VNS (vagus nerve stimulation),
   240
VOC's (volatile organic com-
   pounds), 85–87

W
Walking
   frequency, duration, and pace,
      103–4
   health benefits, 269
   to help depression, 141
   HIIT and, 270–71
   longevity and, 269–70
   to lower diabetes risk, 103–4,
      105

pace and, 269–70
   while in pain, 313
Walnuts, 115–16, 126, 257, 301
Warfarin (Coumadin), 144, 250
Water, hydration, 255
   for constipation, 118
   hydrogen-infused water, 278
   immunity and, 7
   mealtime caution, 118, 124,
      126, 301
   micromovements and, 256
   reducing cancer risks, 44
   urinary incontinence and, 246
   well water caution, 45, 85
   for wrist pain, 303
Weight gain
   food variety and, 262
   lack of sleep and, 261
   medications and, 203–5
   pregnancy and, 158
   See also obesity
Weight loss
   alternate-day fasting, 265
   caloric restriction and, 264
   cayenne, cayenne tea for,
      242, 243
   counselor for, 266
   diet mistakes of exercisers,
      267–68
   exercise and, 268–69
   intermittent fasting for, 264–65
   ketogenic diet and, 199
   nonstarchy vegetables and, 265
   periodic fasting and, 265
   "three-quarter" challenge, 263
   time-restricted eating and, 265
   when to eat and, 262–64
West Nile virus, 118
Whiplash, 298
Whole grains, 16, 19, 64, 84, 97,
   99, 100, 117, 128, 226, 264, 292
Wine, red, 318
Women's health, 317–32
   avoiding heart attack traps,
      322–24

calling an ambulance, 324–25
   cervical cancer surgery, 327–28
   DNA testing and breast cancer,
      320–21
   endometriosis-cancer link,
      326–27
   endometriosis pain relief,
      325–26
   fewer breast cancer treatment
      side effects, 320
   licorice root for hot flashes, 330
   mammograms, 3-D, 319–20
   meatless meals and, 319
   menopause and diet, 321
   muscle weakness and alcohol,
      331–32
   opioid addiction, 332
   opting out of chemo, 321–22
   perimenopause depression,
      330–31
   post-menopausal bleeding,
      326, 328–29
   reducing breast cancer risk,
      317–19
   stroke risk in women, 324
   uterine cancer rise warning, 328
Wrist pain, 301–3

Y
Yeast, yeast infection, 6, 248, 249
Yoga, 56, 123–24, 241, 271
Yogurt, 6, 26, 54, 116, 128, 258,
   264, 268, 292
"Yo-yo" cardio danger, 197

Z
Zaleplon (Sonata), 211
Zeranol (growth hormone), 318
Zika virus, 118
Zinc, 205, 228, 236, 249, 252,
   257, 258
Zolmitriptan (Zomig), 295
Zolpidem (Ambien), 211